30 Update in Intensive Care and Emergency Medicine

Edited by J.-L. Vincent

Springer-Verlag Berlin Heidelberg GmbH

J. J. Marini   T. W. Evans (Eds.)

Acute Lung Injury

With 97 Figures and 56 Tables

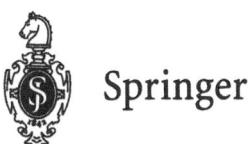 Springer

Series Editor

Prof. Dr. Jean-Louis Vincent
Clinical Director, Department of Intensive Care
Erasme University Hospital
Route de Lennik 808, B-1070 Brussels, Belgium

Volume Editors

Prof. Dr. John J. Marini
St. Paul Ramsey Medical Center, Pulmonary and Critical Care
640 Jackson Street, St. Paul MN 55101, USA

Prof. Dr. Timothy W. Evans
Royal Brompton Hospital, Anaesthesia and Critical Care
Sydney Street, London SW3 6NP, United Kingdom

ISSN 0933-6788

ISBN 978-3-642-64532-7   ISBN 978-3-642-60733-2 (eBook)
DOI 10.1007/978-3-642-60733-2
Library of Congress Cataloging-in-Publication Data
Acute lung injury / J. J. Marini, T. W. Evans (eds.). (Update in intensive care and emergency
medicine : 30)
Based on the proceedings of the Round Table Conference on Acute Lung Injury, Brussels,
Mar. 1997. Includes bibliographical references and index. ISBN 978-3-642-64532-7 (hardcover :
alk. paper) 1. Respiratory distress syndrome, Adult–Congresses. 2. Respiratory intensive
care–Congresses. I. Marini, John J. II. Evans, Timothy W. III. Round Table Conference on
Acute Lung Injury (1997 : Brussels, Belgium) IV. Series. [DNLM: 1. Respiratory Distress
Syndrome, Adult–physiopathology–congress. 2. Lung–injuries–congresses. 3. Lung–physiopathology–congresses.   W1 UP66H v.40 1997 / WF 140 A1827 1997]   RC776.R38A274 1997
616.2'4–dc21   DNLM/DLC

© Springer-Verlag Berlin Heidelberg 1998

Softcover reprint of the hardcover 1st edition 1998

The use of general descriptive names, registered names, trademarks, etc. in this publication
does not imply, even in the absence of a specific statement, that such names are exempt from
the relevant protective laws and regulations and therefore free for general use.

Product liability: The publisher cannot guarantee the accuracy of any information about dosage and application contained in this book. In every individual case the user must check such
information by consulting the relevant literature.

Typesetting: Zechnersche Buchdruckerei, Speyer

SPIN: 10568377   19/3133-5 4 3 2 1 0 – Printed on acid-free paper

Table of Contents

The Alveolar Epithelial Barrier

Mechanical Ventilation

Liquid Ventilation

Extra-Pulmonary Adjuncts to Ventilatory Support

Pharmacological Manipulation of V/Q in ALI and ARDS

Clinical Trials in ARDS

List of Contributors

Artigas A
Department of Intensive Care,
Sabadell Hospital,
Parc Tauli s/n,
Sabadell 08208, Spain

Abraham E
Department of Critical
Care Medicine,
University of Colorado Health
Sciences Center,
4200 East Ninth Avenue,
Denver, CO 80262, USA

Albert RK
Department of Medicine,
University of Washington
Medical Center,
Box 356522,
Seattle, WA 98195-6522, USA

Amato MB
Department of Pulmonary
and Critical Care,
University Hospital of Sao Paulo,
Av Dr. E. De Carvalho Aguiar,
2555 - Cerqueira Cesar,
Sao Paulo, Brasil

Bernard GR
Department of Allergy,
Pulmonary and Critical
Care Medicine,
The Center for Lung Research,
Vanderbilt University
School of Medicine,
Room T-1217 MCN
Nashville, TN 37232, USA

Bitterman PB
Department of Medicine,
UMHC, Box 276,
420 Delaware Street SE,
Minneapolis, MN 55455, USA

Brazzi L
Department of Anesthesiology
and Intensive Care,
Ospedale Maggiore di Milano,
Via Sforza 35,
Milan 20122, Italy

Brochard L
Department of Intensive Care,
Henri Mondor Hospital,
51 Avenue du Maréchal de Lattre
de Tassigny,
Créteil 94010, France

Brower R
Department of Pulmonary
and Critical Care Medicine,
Johns Hopkins University, Ross 858,
720 Rutland Avenue,
Baltimore, MD 21205, USA

Brunet F
Department of Intensive Care,
Cochin Hospital,
27 Rue du Faubourg St Jacques,
Paris 75679 Cedex 14, France

De Backer D
Department of Intensive Care,
Erasme University Hospital,
Route de Lennik 808,
Brussels 1070, Belgium

Dellinger RP
Department of Internal Medicine,
University of Missouri-Columbia,
Environmental Medicine,
Columbia, MO 65212, USA

Dhainaut JF
Department of Intensive Care,
Cochin Hospital,
27 Rue du Faubourg St Jacques,
Paris 75679 Cedex 14, France

Dinh-Xhuan AT
Department of Intensive Care,
Cochain Hospital,
27 Rue du Faubourg St Jacques,
Paris 75679 Cedex 14, France

Donnelly SC
Department of Respiratory Medicine,
University of Edinburgh,
Lauriston Place,
Edinburgh, EH3 9YW,
United Kingdom

Evans TW
Department of Intensive Care,
Royal Brompton Hospital,
Sydney Street,
London SW3 6NP,
United Kingdom

Falke K
Department of Anesthesiology
and Intensive Care,
University Hospital Charité-Virchow,
Augustenburger Platz 1,
Berlin 13353, Germany

Fuhrman BP
Department of Pediatric
Intensive Care,
Children's Hospital of Buffalo,
219 Bryant Street Buffalo,
New York, NY 14222, USA

Fumagalli R
Department of Anesthesiology
and Intensive Care,
Nuovo Ospedale San Gerardo,
Via G. Donizetti 106,
Monza MI 20052, Italy

Gattinoni L
Department of Anesthesiology
and Intensive Care,
Ospedale Maggiore di Milano,
Via Sforza 35,
Milan 20122, Italy

Gerlach H
Department of Anesthesiology
and Intensive Care,
University Hospital Charité-Virchow,
Augustenburger Platz 1,
Berlin 13353, Germany

Grasso S
Department of Anesthesiology,
University Hospital of Bari,
Piazza G. Cesare,
Bari 70124, Italy

Greene KE
Department of Pulmonary
and Critical Care Medicine,
University of Colorado School
of Medicine,
Denver Health and Hospitals,
Bannock Street 777,
Denver, CO 80204, USA

Günther A
Department of Internal Medicine,
Justus-Liebig University,
Klinikstrasse 36,
Giessen 35392, Germany

Haslett C
Department of Respiratory Medicine,
University of Edinburgh,
Lauriston Place,
Edinburgh, EH3 9YW,
United Kingdom

Hirschl RB
Department of Surgery,
The University of Michigan,
F3970 Mott Children's Hospital,
Ann Arbor, MI 48109-0245, USA

Hudson LD
Department of Pulmonary
and Critical Care Medicine,
Harborview Medical Center,
325 Ninth Avenue,
Seattle, WA 98104, USA

Jubran A
Department of Pulmonary
and Critical Care Medicine,
Loyola University Medical Center,
South First Avenue 2160,
Maywood, IL 60153, USA

Keh D
Department of Anesthesiology
and Intensive Care
University Hospital Charité-Virchow,
Augustenburger Platz 1,
Berlin 13353, Germany

Laghi F
Department of Pulmonary
and Critical Care Medicine,
Loyola University Medical Center,
South First Avenue 2160,
Maywood, IL 60153, USA

Levin B
Cardiovascular Research Institute,
University of California,
Box 0130,
San Francisco, CA 94143-0130, USA

Mangialardi RJ
Department of Allergy, Pulmonary
and Critical Care Medicine,
The Center for Lung Research,
Vanderbild University School
of Medicine,
Room T-1217 MCN,
Nashville, TN 37232, USA

Marini JJ
Department of Pulmonary Diseases,
University of Minessota,
St Paul-Ramsey Medical Center,
640 Jackson Hall,
St Paul, MN 55101-2595, USA

Matthay MA
Cardiovascular Research Institute,
University of California,
Box 0130,
San Francisco, CA 94143-0130, USA

Morris AH
Department of Pulmonary
and Critical Care,
LDS Hospital,
8th Avenue and C. Street,
Salt Lake City, UT 84143, USA

Parsons PE
Department of Pulmonary
and Critical Care Medicine,
University of Colorado School
of Medicine, Denver Health
and Hospitals,
Bannock Street 777,
Denver, CO 80204, USA

Payen D
Department of Anesthesiology,
Lariboisière University Hospital,
Rue Ambroise Paré 2,
Paris 75475, France

Pelosi P
Department of Anesthesiology
and Intensive Care,
Ospedale Maggiore di Milano,
Via Sforza 35,
Milan 20122, Italy

Pesenti A
Department of Anesthesiology
and Intensive Care Medicine,
Nuovo Ospedale San Gerardo,
Via G. Donizetti 106,
Monza MI 20052, Italy

Ranieri VM
Department of Anesthesiology,
University Hospital of Bari,
Piazza G. Cesare,
Bari 70124, Italy

Ribeiro SP
Samuel Lunefeld Research Institute,
Mount Sinai Hospital,
600 University Avenue, Suite 656 A,
Toronto, ON M5G 1X5, Canada

Ricou B
Department of Surgical Intensive Care,
Cantonal Hospital,
Rue Micheli-du-Crest 24,
1211 Geneva 14, Switzerland

Schuster DP
Department of Respiratory
and Critical Care Medicine,
Washington University School of
Medicine, Box 8052, 600 N Euclid,
St Louis, MO 63110, USA

Seeger W
Department of Internal Medicine,
Justus-Liebig University,
Klinikstrasse 36,
Giessen 35392, Germany

Sing S
Department of Intensive Care,
Royal Brompton Hospital,
Sydney Street,
London SW3 6NP, United Kingdom

Slutsky AS
Department of Respiratory Medicine,
Mount Sinai Hospital,
600 University Avenue, Suite 656 A,
Toronto, ON M5G 1X5, Canada

Steinberg KP
Department of Pulmonary
and Critical Care Medicine,
Harborview Medical Center, Room
10C-20, 325 Ninth Avenue,
Seattle, WA 97104, USA

Suter PM
Department of Surgical Intensive Care,
Cantonal Hospital,
Rue Micheli-du-Crest 24,
1211 Geneva 14, Switzerland

Tobin MJ
Department of Pulmonary
and Critical Care Medicine,
Loyola University Medical Center,
South First Avenue 2160,
Maywood, IL 60153, USA

Tortorella C
Department of Anesthesiology,
University of Bari, Piazza G. Cesare,
Bari 70124, Italy

Verghese G
Cardiovascular Research Institute,
University of California,
Box 0130,
San Francisco, CA 94143-0130, USA

Vincent JL
Department of Intensive Care,
Erasme University Hospital,
Route de Lennik 808,
Brussels 1070, Belgium

Walmrath HD
Department of Anesthesiology
and Intensive Care,
Ospedale Maggiore di Milano,
Via Sforza 35,
Milan 20122, Italy

Common Abbreviations

ALI	Acute lung injury
ARDS	Acute respiratory distress syndrome
BAL	Broncho-alveolar lavage
BPI	Bactericidal/permeability-increasing protein
CAM	Cell adhesion molecules
cAMP	Cyclic adenosine monophosphate
cGMP	Cyclic guanosine monophosphate
cNOS	Constitutive NOS
COPD	Chronic obstructive pulmonary disease
CPAP	Continuous positive airway pressure
DIC	Disseminated intravascular coagulation
DO_2	Oxygen delivery
EDRF	Endothelium-derived relaxant factor
ELAM	Endothelial leukocyte adhesion molecule
EN	Enteral nutrition
eNOS	Endothelial NOS
FRC	Functional residual capacity
GSH	Glutathione
HPV	Hypoxic pulmonary vasoconstriction
ICAM	Intercellular adhesion molecule
IFN-γ	Interferon gamma
IL	Interleukin
IL-1ra	IL-1 receptor antagonist
iNOS	Inducible NOS
ISS	Injury severity score
L-NAME	N^G-nitro-L-arginine methyl ester
L-NMMA	N^G-monomethyl-L-arginine
L-NNA	N^G-nitro-L-arginine
LPS	Lipopolysaccharide
LV	Left ventricular

MAP	Mitogen activated protein
MODS	Multiple organ dysfunction syndrome
MOF	Multiple organ failure
MOSF	Multiple organ system failure
MVEC	Microvascular endothelial cell
NAC	N-acetylcysteine
NADPH	Nicotinamide adenine dinucleotide phosphate
NF-κB	Nuclear factor kappa B
nNOS	Neuronal NOS
NO	Nitric oxide
NOS	NO synthase
P-V	Pressure-volume
PAC	Pulmonary artery catheter
PAF	Platelet activating factor
PAH	Pulmonary artery hypertension
PAP	Pulmonary artery pressure
PCWP	Pulmonary capillary wedge pressure
pHi	Intramucosal pH
PLV	Partial liquid ventilation
PMN	Polymorphonuclear
PVR	Pulmonary vascular resistance
RV	Right ventricular/ventricle
SIRS	Systemic inflammatory response syndrome
SOD	Superoxide dismutase
SVR	Systemic vascular resistance
TGF-β	Transforming growth factor-beta
TNF-α	Tumor necrosis factor-alpha
TPN	Total parenteral nutrition
VO_2	Oxygen consumption
VT	Tidal volume
EVLW	Extravascular lung water

Epidemiology of Acute Lung Injury

Epidemiology of ARDS. Incidence and Outcome: A Changing Picture

L. D. Hudson and K. P. Steinberg

Introduction

The incidence of ARDS remains unclear, but most studies suggest that it is an order of magnitude less than the initial estimates made by the National Institutes of Health (NIH) in the USA [1]. In 1972 NIH estimated that there were 150000 new cases per year in the USA, roughly an incidence of 60 per 100000 population per year [2]. It is difficult to study the incidence of ARDS due to changing definitions and unclear accuracy of diagnosis in large population areas, failure to capture complete data and a poor ability to know the true population base or denominator (some patients managed with ARDS within the population area may come from outside; others from the population base may develop the syndrome while outside the geographic area and would fail to be identified).

Several recent studies with a prospective cohort design have found incidence rates much lower than the NIH estimate. The incidence in these studies vary from $1.5/10^5$/year in a study in the Canary Islands [3] to a range of 4.8 to 8.3 cases/10^5/year identified in the state of Utah in the USA [4]. Other studies found incidences of $4.5/10^5$/year in the U.K. [5] and $3.0/10^5$/year in Berlin [6]. It is likely that these investigations underestimate the incidence of ARDS, and certainly that of acute lung injury (ALI) because they used definitions which generally captured only severe ARDS.

Villar and Slutsky [3] in 1989 in a prospective cohort study investigated the incidence of ARDS in the Canary Islands (a population of 700000). The advantage to this study was that the Islands have a socialized medical system with universal access and only one of the hospitals performs mechanical ventilation. Thus, all patients requiring mechanical ventilation are admitted to only one hospital and could be prospectively screened. The study was performed over a two year period. The definition of ARDS was quite strict, requiring a recognized predisposing illness and a PaO_2 < 55 mmHg while receiving an FiO_2 > 0.5 on 5 cmH$_2$O of PEEP without improvement in 24 h. The definition also required bilateral infiltrates on chest radiograph, no evidence of left ventricular failure, and no improvement in a 24-h period. The American-European Consensus Conference definition which was generated several years after this study uses a PaO_2/FiO_2 of < 200 and no time period is required. The authors did present data on an alternative oxygenation criterion using a PaO_2/FiO_2 ratio of less than 150 but the 24-h period without improvement remained. Patients < 15 years of age, were excluded, although the denominator was not adjusted to reflect this exclusion, as were patients with chronic obstructive pulmonary disease (COPD) who also developed ARDS. An incidence of ARDS of $1.5/10^5$/year was identified using the more severe definition and $3.5/10^5$/year using the more liberal oxygenation definition. In addition to the severe ARDS definition, this study raises a question in regard to patients at risk, including whether immunosuppression rates predisposing to sepsis and the incidence of trauma would be similar in other populations.

Thomsen and Morris [4] carried out a prospective cohort study over one year in the state of Utah (population 1 720 000). Their definition of ARDS included an oxygenation criteria of PaO_2/PAO_2 > 0.2 roughly equivalent to a PaO_2/FiO_2 > 110. They excluded patients < 12 years of age but did not adjust the denominator to reflect this exclusion but did report that 75% of the population was > 12 years of age so that the reader could make these adjustments. They screened ICU patients in 6 of the 40 general acute care hospitals in Utah. All 6 were referral hospitals of moderate to large size. They made the following corrections: 1) subtracting non-Utah residents who developed ARDS; 2) adding unidentified Utah residents with ARDS treated in non-screened hospitals; and 3) adding Utah residents leaving Utah for treatment of ARDS. They made the second and third corrections by using ICD-9 codes recorded with the Utah Hospital Association computerized hospital discharge database which included hospitals in Utah and adjacent states. ICD-9 codes had 85% sensitivity and 98% specificity for the diagnosis of ARDS in the 6 screened hospitals, and were assumed to behave similarly in the non-screened centers. However, experience with ICD-9 codes for the definition of ARDS challenges this assumption, in that a greater awareness of the diagnosis of ARDS in large referral hospitals night be expected. They calculated a lower limit of incidence, by using only the screened and identified Utah patients ($4.8/10^5$/year) and an upper limit by adjusting for estimates in non-screened hospitals and patients hospitalized in neighboring states ($8.3/10^5$/year). Potential problems of this study include the definition of very severe ARDS by oxygenation criteria, the fact that only 6 of 40 hospitals were screened directly, and the adjustments for other hospitals were made by ICD-9 codes based on the assumption that they would perform the same way as the screened hospitals.

Webster and colleagues [5] in 1988 studied the incidence of ARDS in one British health region with a population of 3 599 400. Their study involved a retrospective questionnaire to the consultants of all intensive therapy units in the region over a 1-year period. They received an 88% response to their questionnaire, representing 14 of the 17 intensive therapy units. They did not use a standard definition but accepted the diagnosis by the consultant in charge of the intensive therapy unit. Most consultants used an oxygenation criteria with a PaO_2 of > 8 kPa while receiving an $FiO_2 = 0.5$. No lower age limit was reported in their study, which recorded an incidence of $4.5/10^5$/year. Weaknesses in this study include the lack of a standard definition and relying on retrospective data gathering.

Lewandowski and co-authors [6] in 1995 reported a prospective cohort study of the incidence of ARDS in Berlin, Germany (population 3 440 000). They carried out the study over a 2-month period and were able to include 72 of the 74 intensive care units in Berlin. Data were captured by physicians in each of the units who were contacted twice a week. There was also a periodic check of logbooks in these units to ensure that patients were not missed. The diagnosis of ARDS was limited to patients aged 14 or greater but the denominator was not corrected for this. They based the definition on the Murray Lung Injury Score (LIS) (greater than 2.5) and also required that patients be on mechanical ventilation for >24 h. They found the incidence of ARDS was $3.0/10^5$/year. If they used a LIS >1.75, the incidence was $17.1/10^5$/year, and using a LIS >1.5, the incidence was $28.2/10^5$/year. The mortality for patients with a LIS >1.75 to 2.5 was identical to those with a LIS of 2.5 (62 and 59%, respectively). The mortality was also high for patients with a LIS >1.5 to 1.75 (47%). The authors pointed out that there were several reasons for possible underestimation: 1) they excluded patients <14 years but did not adjust the population denominator 2) they excluded patients receiving continuous or mask continuous positive airway pressure (CPAP); 3) they excluded patients who either died before 24 h of mechanical ventilation or were removed from mechanical ventilation before that time; 4) they missed patients dying at home or on the ward; 5) they missed patients that might have been excluded by the physician in charge of the data collection in each ICU; and 6) finally, they missed patients living in Berlin but treated elsewhere for ARDS.

In summary, these studies have reported an incidence of ARDS that was an order of magnitude lower than that estimated by the NIH in 1972. However, it is likely that they underrepresent the incidence of ARDS using current accepted definitions and they certainly underestimate the incidence of ALI because of problems of definition and study methodology. The definitions included only patients with severe ARDS by oxygenation criteria in all of the prospective studies; definitions of ARDS in two of the studies were restrictive in that they required a period of time with severe oxygenation without improvement. The problems with methodology included incomplete screening [4], retrospective questionnaires with no set criteria for the definition of ARDS [5], a short study period of two months [6], exclusion of patients under the age of 12 to 15 without correction of the denominator [3, 4, 6] or without stating any age limitation [5]. These studies may reflect the incidence of very severe ARDS. Experience indicates, however, that initial severity of oxygenation has little effect on outcome [6, 7] and that patients fulfilling the American–European Consensus Conference definitions of ALI (PaO_2/FiO_2 <300) and ARDS (PaO_2/FiO_2 <200) have similar outcomes. This suggests that identification of patients with the more liberal oxygenation criterion is important if mortality is to be reduced. The recent experience in the NIH. sponsored ARDS Clinical Centers Network in the USA suggests that the incidence of ALI is likely to be considerably greater than the above incidences of severe ARDS. In a 1-year period, the 10 participating centers (including a total of 26 hospitals) in the Network identified 2338 patients with ALI (this figure is based on 1-years experience at some centers and is extrapolated from 11 months experience in others). This presumably only represents a small fraction of the patients fulfilling this diagnosis in the USA (there are approximately 4500 hospitals in the USA of which 962 are teaching hospitals with residency programs) and does not include any hospitals in large metropolitan areas such as New York City, Los Angeles, Chicago, Houston, and Washington DC.

Patients At Risk for ARDS

A wide variety of conditions have been reported to be associated with ARDS. These can be divided into two broad groups according to the nature of the pulmonary insult (Table 1). Direct injuries are those in which a toxic substance directly damages lung epithelium. Examples include aspiration of gastric contents or inhalation of toxic gases. The risk of ARDS is dependent on the toxicity, concentration and dose of the substance. The more common pathophysiologic mechanism of ARDS is indirect, via a blood-born systemic inflammatory mechanism which has been referred to as "malignant systemic inflammation" [8] or "rogue inflammation" [9, 10], in which usually beneficial inflammatory mechanisms cause organ injury.

Most of the information regarding conditions which place a patient at risk come from retrospective analyses; series in which ARDS might be prospectively identified, but the risk conditions are retrospectively identified, or small series or case reports of a given condition occurring together with ARDS. These provide information on the conditions associated with ARDS, but do not allow calculation of a true incidence for developing ARDS since the denominator, the size of the population with the given condition of interest, is not known [1, 11]. However, two relatively large single center studies have prospectively examined carefully defined risk conditions for ARDS and identified the incidence of the syndrome with each of these conditions [12, 13]. These suggest that the conditions with the highest incidence of ARDS include severe sepsis or sepsis syndrome, severe trauma and aspiration of gastric contents. Table 2 shows the incidence of ARDS associated with all the precipitating conditions examined in these two studies. One series, but not the other, found pneumonia severe enough to warrant

Table 1. Clinical disorders associated with ARDS

Direct lung injury	Indirect lung injury*
Aspiration of gastric contents	Severe sepsis
Pulmonary contusion	Major trauma
Toxic gas (smoke) inhalation	Multiple long bone fractures
Near-drowning	Hypovolemic shock
Diffuse pulmonary infection	Hypertransfusion
Reperfusion injury	Acute pancreatitis
	Drug overdose
	Post-lung transplantation
	Post-cardiopulmonary bypass

* Due to activation of an acute, systemic inflammatory response with hematogenous delivery of inflammatory mediators to the lung

Table 2. Clinical disorders associated with ARDS (From [12, 13] with permission)

Disorder	Estimated Incidence (%)
Frequent causes	
– Sepsis	
– Bacteremia without sepsis syndrome	4
– Severe sepsis/sepsis syndrome	35–45
– Major trauma	25
– Multiple long-bone fracture	5–10
– Pulmonary contusion	17–22
– Hypertransfusion	5–36
– Aspiration of gastric content	22–36
Less frequent causes	
– Drug overdose	5–8
– Pancreatitis	
– Burn/smoke inhalation	
– Near-drowning	
– Viral pneumonia	
– Irritant gas inhalation	

admission to the ICU (so-called "ICU pneumonia") to be associated with ARDS. This discrepancy is possibly explained by the difficulty in distinguishing diffuse pulmonary infection from pneumonia associated with the criteria for sepsis.

Although these prospective investigations provide an incidence of ARDS occurring with specific risk factors found in the two institutions involved in the studies, others may differ considerably in their patient mix and thus risk conditions for ARDS. Thus these studies cannot provide information on how commonly a particular condition is the cause of ARDS. That would depend on the incidence and distribution of the risk conditions at a particular institution or throughout a population. In North America, sepsis appears to be the most common cause of ARDS as well as being the risk condition associated with the highest incidence of the established syndrome. This may differ considerably in other countries or regions. For example, in tropical countries, malaria and leptospirosis are common causes of ARDS.

Severe Sepsis

Infection was the most frequent cause of ARDS in both prospective series. However, the definitions used to identify infection varied between the two providing additional useful information. It appears that bacteremia alone does not place a patient at a significant risk for ARDS [12, 14, 15] but the clinical syndrome of severe sepsis does [13]. Patients with bacteremia (defined as 2 positive blood cultures growing pathogens) had only 4% incidence of ARDS in the Denver study

[12]. Identification of a syndrome of sepsis in that from Seattle yielded an incidence that was tenfold higher (42%) [13]. The sepsis syndrome definition used in this study re-presents the first attempt to define this condition for research purposes [16] and required:

1) either infection or inflammation, evidenced by two of the following
   a) evidence of local infection
   b) positive blood culture
   c) abnormal white blood cell count; or
   d) abnormal temperature

plus

2) some evidence of deleterious systemic effect, requiring one of the following findings
   a) hypotension for longer than 2 h
   b) systemic vascular resistance less than 800 dynes/sec/cm^5; or
   c) unexplained metabolic acidosis

This definition preceded the introduction of a widely used consensus conference definition of severe sepsis which was based on the same principles [17]. However, the Seattle definition required evidence which presumably reflected inadequate tissue perfusion, implying the presence of at least a mild degree of septic shock, and thus was more severe than the consensus conference criteria which accepted other organ failure (i.e. not necessarily cardiovascular insufficiency) as evidence of a deleterious systemic effect. Presumably, the sepsis syndrome definition reflecting inadequate tissue perfusion would be associated with a higher incidence of ARDS than less stringent criteria. The placebo arms of several intervention trials using varying definitions of severe sepsis based on or similar to the consensus conference definition show an incidence of ARDS of 25–38% [18–20].

Severe Trauma

Severe trauma is a common risk for ARDS. Although the mechanism is thought to be intravascular activation of inflammation, similar to sepsis, the exact mechanisms and the specific markers for injury that are associated with development of ARDS have not been clearly defined. Hemorrhagic shock is associated with both ARDS and multiple organ failure (MOF) in several series [21–25]. It is not clear, however, whether shock is necessary in order to develop trauma-associated ARDS. The trauma risks evaluated in the prospective Seattle study were:

1) multiple blood transfusions for the purposes of emergency resuscitation (>15 units in the 24-h period).
2) multiple fractures (requiring either multiple long bone fractures or an unstable pelvic fracture).

3) pulmonary contusion (defined by the appearance of a localized infiltrate on chest radiograph underlying an external manifestation of trauma such as ecchymosis of the chest wall, occurring within a 6-h period from the time of trauma) [13].

In this series, multiple transfusions were associated with the highest incidence of ARDS of these risk factors (25% as a single risk, 47% when transfusions occurred with another risk, for an overall total of a 37% incidence). Whether multiple transfusions reflect the presence of hemorrhagic shock, whether they are a marker of severe injury, or whether they play a mechanistic role in causing ARDS and MOF is not clear. Interestingly, the same multiple transfusion criteria for non-trauma patients also was associated with a high incidence of ARDS in this series: 44%. Transfusion practices have changed substantially in trauma since these data were collected, raising the possibility that the associated incidence of ARDS may now be different. In this study, pulmonary contusion was associated with a 22% incidence of ARDS whereas multiple fractures was associated with the lowest (11%). Less stringent criteria for fractures and transfusions in the prospective Denver series resulted in a lower associated incidence of ARDS [12]. Fractures, which could be a single long bone fracture by the definition used, were associated with only a 5% incidence of ARDS and multiple transfusions (defined as 10 units in 24 h) carried only a 5% incidence.

A subsequent smaller series using either combinations of the above risk factors as defined in the Seattle study, or a single risk factor plus an injury severity score (ISS, a commonly used scoring system evaluating the global severity of multiple trauma) of > 20 were evaluated [26]. Compared to the previous prospective study, the requirement of an ISS > 20 added to a single risk factor reduced the sensitivity from 87 to 67%, but increased the incidence of ARDS from 25 overall to 41%. Combinations of clinical trauma risks were more frequently associated with ARDS than were single risks with ISS > 20 (50 versus 35%), although this difference did not achieve statistical significance.

Sepsis occurring in trauma patients represents a significant risk for both ARDS and MOF [13, 21]. Trauma cohort studies examining predictors of MOF have found age, the transfusion requirement, presence of hypovolemic shock and ISS > 25 to be significant among others [21–25]. Obviously, several of these factors are interrelated. In a study using multiple logistic regression, age > 55, ISS > 25, and > 6 units of blood transfusion in 12 h were found to be independent predictors of development of MOF [25].

Aspiration of Gastric Contents

Aspiration of gastric contents either directly observed by medical personnel, or identified by the suctioning of gastric contents from the trachea were associated with a 36% and 26% incidence of ARDS development in the Denver and Seattle studies respectively. The combination of aspiration of gastric contents and drug overdose requiring intensive care was associated with a higher incidence of

ARDS than aspiration of gastric contents alone, raising the possibility that drug overdose may be associated with other mechanisms of ARDS development.

Other Conditions

A wide variety of other associated conditions for ARDS have been reported. Many of these reflect specific infections which could be associated with either a sepsis-like syndrome, or with diffuse direct pulmonary involvement [1, 11]. Others may represent varying mechanisms by which the lung could be diffusely injured as part of either a systemic or localized disease process. These are discussed in more detail in the section dealing with differential diagnosis below. A history of alcohol abuse appears to be associated with a higher incidence of ARDS when present in combination with some other underlying risk factors, particularly sepsis [27].

The epidemiology of a given condition is often continually changing and this is likely true for ARDS. Changes in the population admitted to ICU, the conditions placing the patient at risk and treatments for these conditions may all contribute. The prospective studies identifying risk factors were both based on data collected in the early 1980's. Newer studies are required to improve our understanding of the epidemiology of ARDS and to improve the reliability of our current information regarding patients at risk.

Duration of Mechanical Ventilation

Once a patient develops ARDS, the clincal course is extremely variable, lasting from a few days to several months. Even in patients who resolve their underlying illness or injury and respond readily to supportive therapy, the course usually lasts several days, in contrast to patients with cardiogenic pulmonary edema who, if they respond to therapy, improve in a few hours to a few days. The mean duration of mechanical ventilation is generally 10 to 14 days, but approximately 10 to 20% of patients remain ventilator-dependent for longer than 3 weeks [7, 28, 29]. Most of those who die with ARDS do so within the first 2 weeks of their illness [28–30]. Recovery for survivors can take several weeks or longer. In fact, duration of mechanical ventilation is inversely correlated with survival. Patients alive but mechanically ventilated after 3 weeks have a very high survival rate [30]. In one study, 95% of the non-survivors had expired by 5 weeks, and the survival of those remaining in the hospital after 5 weeks was independent of ventilator status [7].

Fatality Rate and Causes of Death

Until recently, the fatality rate of ARDS was widely considered to have remained high, generally in excess of 50% and usually about 60%, since its original description. Fatality rates are even higher in patients over 60 years of age and in those with sepsis-induced ARDS [7, 31]. Other factors associated with mortality are severity of underlying illness, such as ISS in trauma patients or advanced malignancy, and presence or development of MOF. While initial severity of lung injury, measured as an index of gas exchange such as PaO_2/FiO_2 ratio or a composite LIS, is not predictive of outcome, improvement in PaO_2/FiO_2 ratio over the first 3 days to 1 week, however, is associated with survival [7, 32].

Recently, an analysis of temporal trends in ARDS fatality rates at one institution (Harborview Medical Center, a major regional trauma and critical care center in Seattle, Washington, USA) indicates a decline that has occurred since 1989 to a low of 36% in 1993 [31]. Subsequent rates for 1994–1996 have fluctuated, but have remained within the range 28–42% (Fig. 1). The observation was made in all risk groups but was most notable in patients with sepsis-induced ARDS and in those under 60 years of age. Comparison of APACHE II scores in sepsis patients and ISS in trauma patients in years for which complete data were available (1983–85, 1990, and 1994) indicated that patient severity of illness at ARDS onset had not changed in more recent years. Further analysis comparing three cohorts (1983–85, 1990, and 1994) from this institution has demonstrated that fatality is similar in the 3 groups for the first 3 days following ARDS onset, but significantly improves after 3 days in the more recent cohorts (Fig. 2) [33]. The period of less than 3 days following ARDS onset corresponds to a period previously demonstrated to be associated with causes of death related to underlying illness or injury [28]. Deaths after 3 days were generally related to complications of ARDS, primarily development of sepsis syndrome and MOF. Causes of death in the study of the 3-time period cohorts were divided into those related to underlying illness or injury (defined as being present prior to ARDS onset) or related to complications (defined as having onset simultaneous with or subsequent to ARDS onset). This confirms that underlying illnesses continue to account for nearly all deaths in the first 3 days (Fig. 3). Although "complications" remain the leading cause of death after 3 days, both septic and non-septic complications as causes of death have significantly decreased in the later cohorts compared to the earliest time period studied (Fig. 4). Only a relatively small fraction of patients, 6 to 11%

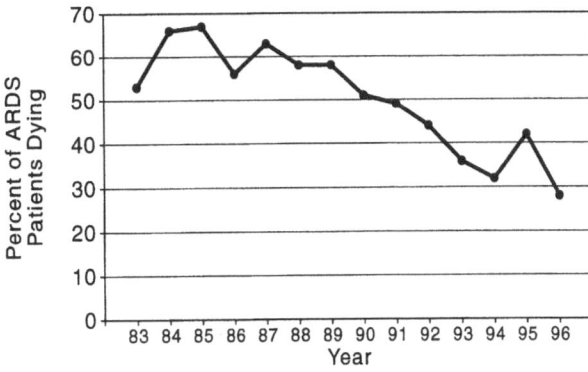

Fig. 1. Fatality rate in prospectively identified patients at Harborview Medical Center, Seattle, Washington, USA, using the same definition of ARDS from 1983 through 1996

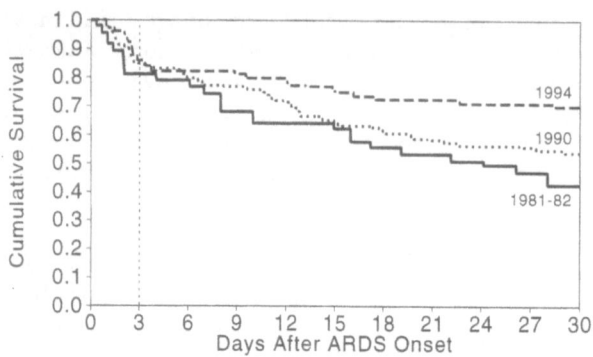

Fig. 2. Survival curves over the first 30 days following onset of ARDS in 3 cohorts of patients at Harborview Medical Center, Seattle, Washington, USA, using the same definition of ARDS. The 3-time cohorts are 1981–82, 1990, and 1994. The survival curves are approximately the same for the first 3 days following ARDS onset for the 3 cohorts. Following 3 days, the survival curves are significantly different (p = 0.002), with progressive improvement in the later 2 cohorts compared to the earlier one

of all ARDS patients in the two studies, die a respiratory death due to insupportable hypoxemia or refractory respiratory acidosis [28, 33]. These findings suggest that the reduction in mortality in this institution is related to fewer deaths related to complications, suggesting either a lower rate of complications or a lower mortality associated with those complications that do develop. Since there have been no randomized controlled trials of single interventions in ARDS showing benefit, improvements in mortality rate might be related to several changes in supportive therapy resulting in small but additive effects on mortality. Other investigators have reported similar reductions in mortality [34] in patients enrolled in control or placebo arms of clinical trials [35, 36].

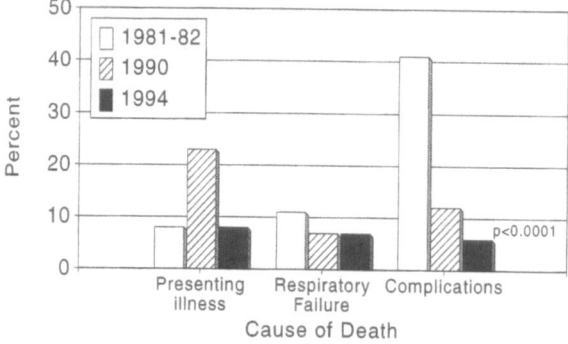

Fig. 3. Causes of death during the first 3 days following the onset of ARDS in 3 cohorts of patients (see Fig. 2) at Harborview Medical Center, Seattle, Washington, USA. The cause of death in the first 3 days following the onset of ARDS is primarily related to the presenting illness or injury

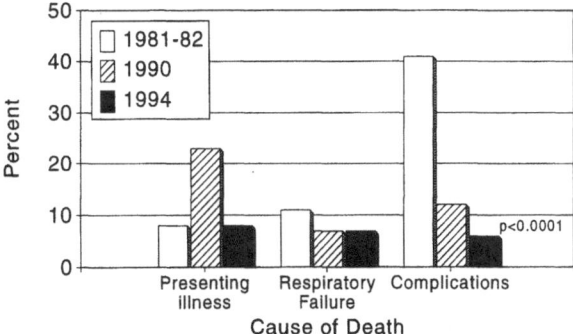

Fig. 4. Causes of death after 3 days from onset of ARDS in 3 cohorts of patients (see Fig. 2) at Harborview Medical Center, Seattle, Washington, USA. There has been little change in the number of deaths related to the presenting illness and to respiratory failure in these "late" deaths but the deaths from complications, i.e. conditions that have their onset simultaneously with or subsequent to the onset of ARDS, have significantly decreased

Sequelae

An early impression held by many investigators and clinicians was that pulmonary function in most survivors returned to normal or near normal levels. Studies in ARDS survivors are difficult to perform because they require a long period of follow-up and a high degree of patient cooperation. This is further complicated by the fact that many patients do not live in the city where they were hospitalized, but have been transported to institutions with the specialized ability to manage patients with ARDS. Several recent studies, though, have demonstrated that the picture is indeed generally optimistic [37–41]. Nearly all patients have reached their maximal recovery by 6 months following endotracheal extubation with few displaying further improvement after that time. Thus, 6 months following extubation could be used as a single time point for evaluation of pulmonary function recovery following ARDS. Although most patients markedly improve their pulmonary function during recovery approximately half continue to have some abnormality of pulmonary function at this time. This is either a mild restrictive impairment or, more often, a mild impairment in diffusing capacity, though more marked abnormalities can occur. Those patients who have continuing pulmonary dysfunction are more apt to have had more severe lung injury, identified either by failure to improve physiologic variables several days into the course of ARDS, or by the duration of mechanical ventilation [40, 41]. There are occasional patients, fortunately rare, who continue to have severe pulmonary functional abnormalities and who may require long-term home oxygen therapy. Finally, survivors of ARDS continue to have impairments in overall physical and psychosocial function but these are mild, are not perceived by the patients to be related to their pulmonary condition, and are often related to other aspects of their acute injury or illness [41].

References

1. Garber BG, Hébert PC, Yelle JD, Hodder RV, McGowan J (1996) Adult respiratory distress syndrome: A systematic overview of incidence and risk factors. Crit Care Med 24:687–695
2. National Heart and Lung Institute: Task Force on Problems, Research Approaches, Needs: The Lung Program. Washington, DC, Department of Health, Education, and Welfare (1972) Publication No. (NIH) 73–432, pp 165–180
3. Villar J, Slutsky AS (1989) The incidence of the adult respiratory distress syndrome. Am Rev Respir Dis 140:814–816
4. Thomsen GE, Morris AH (1995) Incidence of the adult respiratory distress syndrome in the state of Utah. Am J Respir Crit Care Med 152:965–971
5. Webster NR, Cohen AT, Nunn JF (1988) Adult respiratory distress syndrome – How many cases in the UK? Anaesthesia 43:923–926
6. Lewandowski K, Metz J, Deutschmann C, et al (1995) Incidence, severity and mortality of acute respiratory failure in Berlin, Germany. Am Rev Respir Dis 151:1121–1125
7. Sloane PJ, Gee MH, Gottlieb JE, et al (1992) A multicenter registry of patients with acute respiratory distress syndrome. Am Rev Respir Dis 2:419–426
8. Pinsky MR (1989) Multiple systems organ failure: Malignant intravascular inflammation. Crit Care Clin 5:195–198
9. Hudson LD (1989) Multiple systems organ failure (MSOF): Lessons learned from the adult respiratory distress syndrome (ARDS). Crit Care Clin 5:697–670
10. Goodman RB, Strieter RM, Martin DP, et al (1996) Inflammatory cytokines in patients with persistence of the acute respiratory distress syndrome. Am J Respir Crit Care Med 154:602–611
11. Hudson LD (1982) Causes of the adult respiratory distress syndrome: Clinical recognition. Clin Chest Med 3:195–212
12. Fowler AA, Hamman RF, Good JT, et al (1983) Adult respiratory distress syndrome: Risk with common predispositions. Ann Intern Med 98:593–597
13. Hudson LD, Milberg JA, Anardi D, Maunder RJ (1995) Clinical risks for development of the acute respiratory distress syndrome. Am J Respir Crit Care Med 151:293–301
14. Fein AM, Lippmann M, Holtzman H, et al (1983) The risk factors, incidence and prognosis of ARDS following septicemia. Chest 83:40–42
15. Kaplan RL, Sahn SA, Petty TL (1979) Incidence and outcome of the respiratory distress syndrome in Gram-negative sepsis. Arch Intern Med 139:867–869
16. Pepe PE, Potkin RT, Holtman Reus D, Hudson LD, Carrico CJ (1982) Clinical predictors of the adult respiratory distress syndrome. Am J Surg 144:124–130
17. Bone RC, Balk RA, Cerra FB, et al and the ACCP/SCCM Consensus Conference Committee (1992) Definitions for sepsis and organ failure and guidelines for the use of innovative therapies in sepsis. Chest 101:1644–1655
18. The Veterans Administration Systemic Sepsis Cooperative Study Group (1987) Effect of high-dose glucocorticoid therapy on mortality in patients with clinical signs of systemic sepsis. N Engl J Med 317:659–665
19. Bone RC, Fischer CJ Jr, Clemmer TP, Slotman GJ, Metz CA (1987) Early methylprednisolone treatment for septic syndrome and the adult respiratory distress syndrome (published erratum appears in Chest (1988) 94:448). Chest 92:1032–1036
20. Luce JM, Montgomery AB, Marks JD, Turner J, Metz CA, Murray JF (1988) Ineffectiveness of high-dose methylprednisolone in preventing parenchymal lung injury and improving mortality in patients with septic shock. Am Rev Respir Dis 138:62–68
21. Faist E, Baue AE, Dittmer H, et al (1983) MOF in polytrauma patients. J Trauma 23:775–787
22. Henao FJ, Daes JE, Dennis RJ (1991) Risk factors for multiorgan failure: A case-control study. J Trauma 31:74–80
23. Tran DD, Cuesta MA, van Leeuwen DAM, et al (1993) Risk factors for multiple organ system failure and death in critically injured patients. Surgery 114:21–30
24. Dunham CM, Damiano AM, Wiles CE, et al (1995) Post-traumatic multiple organ dysfunction syndrome: Infection is an uncommon antecedent risk factor. Injury 26:373–378

25. Sauaia A, Moore FA, Moore EE, et al (1994) Early predictors of postinjury MOF. Arch Surg 129:39–45
26. Steinberg KP, Davis DR, Milberg JA, Barton JA, Martin DP, Hudson LD (1995) Prediction of acute respiratory distress syndrome (ARDS) in trauma patients using combined clinical risk factors. Am J Respir Crit Care Med 151:A668 (Abst)
27. Moss M, Bucher B, Moore FA, Moore EE, Parsons PE (1996) The role of chronic alcohol abuse in the development of acute respiratory distress syndrome in adults. JAMA 275:50–54
28. Montgomery AB, Stager MA, Carrico CJ, Hudson LD (1985) Causes of mortality in patients with the adult respiratory distress syndrome. Am Rev Respir Dis 132:485–489
29. Kollef MH, Schuster DP (1995) Medical progress: The acute respiratory distress syndrome. N Engl J Med 332:27–37
30. Steinberg KP, Rubenfeld G, Milberg JA, Hudson LD (1996) ARDS fatality rate by duration of mechanical ventilation. Am J Respir Crit Care Med 153:A590 (Abst)
31. Milberg JA, Davis DA, Steinberg KP, Hudson LD (1995) Improved survival of patients with acute respiratory distress syndrome (ARDS): 1983–1993. JAMA 273:306–309
32. Moss M, Goodman PL, Heinig M, Barkin S, Ackerson L, Parsons PE (1995) Establishing the relative accuracy of three new definitions of the adult respiratory distress syndrome. Crit Care Med 23:1629–1637
33. Wang BM, Steinberg KP, Hudson LD (1996) Causes of mortality in patients with the acute respiratory distress syndrome (ARDS): 1981–1994. Am J Respir Crit Care Med 153:A593 (Abst)
34. Schuster DP (1995) What is ALI? What is ARDS? Chest 107:1721–1726
35. Gattinoni L, Pesenti A, Mascheroni D, et al (1986) Low frequency positive pressure ventilation with extracorporeal CO_2 removal in severe acute respiratory failure. JAMA 256:881–886
36. Morris AH, Wallace CJ, Menlove RL, et al (1994) Randomized clinical trial of pressure-controlled inverse ratio ventilation and extracorporeal CO_2 removal for adult respiratory distress syndrome. Am J Respir Crit Care Med 149:295–305
37. Elliott CG, Morris AH, Cengiz M (1981) Pulmonary function and exercise gas exchange in survivors of adult respiratory distress syndrome. Am Rev Respir Dis 123:492–495
38. Elliott CG, Rasmusson BY, Crapo RO, Morris AH, Jensen RL (1987) Prediction of pulmonary function abnormalities after adult respiratory distress syndrome (ARDS). Am Rev Respir Dis 135:634–638
39. Ghio AJ, Elliott CG, Crapo RO, Berlin SL, Jensen RL (1989) Impairment after adult respiratory distress syndrome: An evaluation based on American Thoracic Society recommendations. Am Rev Respir Dis 139:1158–1162
40. Peters JI, Bell RC, Prihoda TJ, Harris G, Andrews C, Johanson WG (1989) Clinical determinants of abnormalities in pulmonary functions in survivors of the adult respiratory distress syndrome. Am Rev Respir Dis 139:1163–1168
41. McHugh LG, Milberg JA, Whitcomb ME, Schoene RB, Maunder RJ, Hudson LD (1994) Recovery of function in survivors of the acute respiratory distress syndrome. Am J Respir Crit Care Med 150:90–94

Pronostic Factors and Outcome of ALI

A. Artigas

Introduction

The acute respiratory distress syndrome (ARDS) is an acute, severe alteration in lung structure and function characterized by hypoxemia, low-compliance lungs with a low funcional residual capacity, and diffuse radiographic infiltrates due to increased lung microvascular permeability [1]. Since first described in 1967 [2], the syndrome has been associated with a high mortality, and it is disappointing that despite many clinical and laboratory investigations the survival rates have remained virtually unchanged. Patients with the syndrome usually die either from the severity of lung impairment or from common complications. Whether the hypoxemia of acute respiratory failure is the usual cause of death in patients with ARDS is controversial. However, supportive measures such as mechanical ventilation with positive end-expiratory pressure (PEEP) [3] or extracorporeal membrane oxygenation [4, 5], although technically successful at increasing arterial oxygenation, have had no obvious effect on reducing mortality. This suggests a need to focus on the prevention or treatment of other aspects of this syndrome, in addition to respiratory support measures.

Definitions

The usual definition of ARDS includes only the most severe cases of permeability pulmonary edema. Since the clinical presentation of patients with ARDS has changed little from its original description in 1967, the development of physiologic indices for an accurate definition of the syndrome has been essential for the standardization of "entry criteria" into various clinical studies. These additional features of clinical diagnosis usually include the presence or absence of PEEP ventilation, specific values for the alveolar-arterial oxygen tension gradient (or the arterial-alveolar ratio) or calculated right-to-left pulmonary shunt fraction, and measurements of pulmonary compliance. These physiologic criteria are not universally accepted and vary widely among investigators (Table 1).

Following the introduction of bedside pulmonary artery catheterization with the measurement of pulmonary arterial occlusion pressure (PAOP) as a guide to pulmonary capillary and left atrial pressure, it has been possible to quantify the contribution of a raised capillary pressure to the formation of pulmonary edema. Indeed, it is believed essential to measure PAOP in ARDS, especially as these pa-

Table 1. ARDS definitions used in clinical studies investigating outcome of conventionally treated ARDS patients

Authors	Ref.	Definitions
Ashbaugh et al.	[2]	Severe dyspnea, tachypnea, cyanosis that is refractory to oxygen therapy, loss of lung compliance, and diffuse alveolar infiltration seen on CXR
NHLBI	[30]	Fast entry criteria: PaO_2 < 50 mmHg > 2 h at FiO_2 1.0, PEEP $\geq$ 5 H_2O; Slow entry criteria: PaO_2 < 50 mmHg > 12 h at FiO_2, 0.6, PEEP $\geq$ 5 cmH_2O and shunt > 30%; maximal medical therapy > 48 h
Bone	[26]	Mechanical ventilation for > 48 h, severe respiratory failure (PaO_2 < 60 mmHg at FiO_2 $\geq$ 0.5)
Bell et al.	[8]	Clinical respiratory distress, mechanical ventilation, infiltrates on CXR, hypoxemia (FiO_2 $\geq$ 0.5 to maintain a PaO_2 > 50 mmHg and a PCWM" < 15 mmHg
Zapol et al.	[49]	Infiltrates on CXR intubated (CMV + PEEP), PaO_2 < 50 mmHg with FiO_2 1.0 for $\geq$ 8 h or FiO_2 > 0.6 for $\geq$ 48 h
Fein et al.	[32]	PaO_2 < 50 mmHg with FiO_2 > 0.5, infiltrates on CXR no clinical evidence of heart failure, and/or a PCWP $\leq$ 15 mmHg and total pulmonary compliance < 50 ml/cmH_2O
Kaplan et al.	[33]	ARDS + gram negative sepsis (no further definitions given)
Fowler et al.	[22]	Acute respiratory failure, mechanical ventilation, infiltrates on CXR, appropriate predisposition, PCWP $\leq$ 12 mmHg, CT_{stat} $\leq$ 50 ml/cmH_2O, PaO_2/PAO_2 $\leq$ 2
Montgomery et al.	[7]	(1) PaO_2/FiO_2 < 150, (2) infiltrates on CXR, (3) PCWP < 18 mmHg and (4) no other cause to explain the above
Mancebo & Artigas	[24]	(1) Dyspnea, tachypnea, and cyanosis requiring mechanical ventilation, (2) infiltrates on CXR, (3) PaO_2 < 50 mmHg when FiO_2 > 0.5, (4) PCWP < 16 mmHg
Pepe et al.	[6]	(1) PaO_2 < 75 mmHg with FiO_2 $\geq$ 0.5, (2) infiltrates on CXR, (3) PCWP < 18 mmHg, (4) no other explanation for these findings
Artigas et al.	[16]	Patients with respiratory distress and infiltrates on CXR and severe hypoxemia defined by PaO_2 < 75 mmHg FiO_2 > 0.5 + PEEP 5 cmH_2O for $\geq$ 24 h
Rinaldo	[11]	(1) Predisposition to ARDS, (2) infiltrates on CXR, (3) mechanical ventilation with FiO_2 > 0.4, (4) absence of a clinical history of roentgenologic findings of congestive heart failure
Hickling et al.	[54]	(1) Appropriate clinical setting, (2) PaO_2/FiO_2 < 150, (3) infiltrates on CXR, (4) the condition was thought not to be due to heart failure, ateletasis or chronic disease processes
Morris et al.	[5]	Same criteria as in NHLBI study [30]
Anzueto et al.	[18]	(1) Sepsis, (2) Diffuse infiltrates on CXR, (3) PaO_2/FiO_2 < 250, (4) no evidence of left ventricular failure
Murray et al.	[57]	Severe lung injury with a LIS > 2.5
Bernard et al.	[12]	(1) Acute onset of ALI, (2) PaO_2/FiO_2 < 200, (3) bilateral infiltrates on CXR, (4) PCWP < 18 mmHg or no evidence of left ventricular failure
Knaus et al.	[67]	Acute respiratory distress, PaO_2/FiO_2 < 300
Kollef et al.	[14]	Bilateral infiltrates on CXR, increased lung vascular permeability, appropriate clinical setting
Milberg et al.	[10]	(1) PaO_2/FiO_2 $\leq$ 200 with PEEP $\geq$ 5 cmH_2O, (2) infiltrates in 3–4 lung quadrants, (3) PCWP < 18 mmHg or no evidence of congestive heart failure

CXR = chest roentgenogram; PCWP = pulmonary capillary wedge pressure; CT_{stat} = total static pulmonary compliance; COPD = chronic obstructive pulmonary disease

tients tend to develop acute pulmonary hypertension and right ventricular dysfunction, limiting the value of isolated measurements of central venous pressure. This invasive technology, although widely applied, has brought with it a number of problems: 1) Although usually reliable, PAOP is occasionally not an accurate measurement of either capillary pressure or left ventricular filling pressure in ARDS; 2) PAOP is rarely related to the prevailing plasma colloid oncotic pressure; and 3) since pulmonary artery catheterization is usually reserved for the most severely ill, a selection bias favoring the entry of severe cases of ARDS into clinical studies has occurred.

Unfortunately, we do not have the means to diagnose ARDS in its early stages. Mild hypocapnia is common in ARDS as well as hypoxemic respiratory failure due to other causes. Furthermore, many patients at high risk of developing ARDS develop severe transitory hypoxemia but never progress to the syndrome. Pepe et al. [6] found that 55% of patients considered at high risk for ARDS who developed "critical hypoxemia" did not progress to ARDS.

The intuitive impression of many clinicians is that most patients at high ARDS risk groups (e.g. post-trauma) who develop pulmonary infiltrates and require mechanical ventilation are now treated more successfully and with a higher survival rate than reported in the majority of published studies [6–10].

The discrepancy between the present perception of practitioners and the clinical literature suggests that the entry criteria for ARDS into published studies have increasingly selected an atypical population with a high incidence of severe underlying disease(s) or multiple extrapulmonary organ system failure [11].

Two criteria, severe hypoxemia (alveolar/arterial PO, ratio < 0.3) and a simultaneous indwelling pulmonary artery catheter (PAC), have introduced bias into published clinical studies, selecting out a small subset of ARDS patients with an unusually poor prognosis. In order to qualify as having ARDS in many recent published series, poor gas exchange refractory to PEEP, a high FiO_2 and a pulmonary artery catheter needed to be present. Because of increasing awareness of the uncertain risk/benefit ratio for the use of PAC, different groups treat ARDS patients with PEEP and reduce the FiO_2 to a non-toxic level without employing invasive monitoring of the cardiovascular system. If the supportive initial therapy is effective, these patients will not be diagnosed as having ARDS. To better assess the prognosis of acute lung injury (ALI), standard criteria for ARDS requiring a low alveolar/arterial PO_2 ratio and a PAC may need to be modified. Elimination of measurements obtained with a PAC will increase the risk of occasionally including in an ARDS study a patient with unsuspected cardiogenic edema. However, it may be necessary to accept this limitation in order to assess prognosis more accurately in a wider population and evaluate new treatments. The selection of an ARDS group with a high percentage of predictably moribund patients with severe underlying organ failure or irreversible underlying diseases will virtually guarantee that promising drugs undergoing clinical therapeutic trials in ARDS will not be shown to improve outcome. Rinaldo has emphasized this point in 27 patients using broad clinical criteria for ARDS [11]. Patients with "non-publishable" ARDS criteria (including young trauma patients without pre-

Table 2. Survival rates for patients with different ARDS criteria

	ARDS		Mortality	
	Number	%	Number	%
Non-publishable	20	74	6	30
Publishable	7	26	5	71
Total	27	100	11	40

existing disease) have a markedly increased ARDS survival rate approximating 70% (Table 2).

Recently the Committee of the American-European Consensus Conference on ARDS recommended that "ALI be defined as a syndrome of inflammation and increased permeability that is associated with a constellation of clinical, radiologic and physiologic abnormalities that cannot be explained by, but may coexist with, left atrial or pulmonary capillary hypertension." [12]. ARDS was defined as a more severe form of ALI according to the severity of gas exchange deteriotion and a cutoff of $PaO_2/FiO_2 < 200$ mmHg (Table 3).

Some authors proposed methods to identify the presence of pulmonary edema and increased vascular permeability. Different techniques have been proposed such as the measurement of extravascular lung water (EVLW) by indicator-dilution method, the chest X-ray and computed tomography, nuclear magnetic resonance imaging and positon emission tomography. EVLW measurements and the protein concentration of alveolar edema fluid are used in clinical practice but are associated with problems in accuracy, cost and complexity [13, 14].

Until an accurate, simple and clinical useful method is available to measure lung edema and vascular permeability, identification of ARDS will continue to be based on clinical criteria, which correspond to moderate and severe forms of the classification of acute respiratory failure.

Table 3. Recommended criteria for acute lung injury (ALI) and acute respiratory distress syndrome (ARDS)

Criteria	Timing	Oxygenation	Chest Radiograph	Pumonary Artery Wedge Pressure
ALI	Acute onset	$PaO_2/FIO_2 \leq 300$ mmHg (regardless of PEEP level)	Bilateral infiltrates seen on frontal chest radiograph	≤ 18 mmHg when measured or no clinical evidence of left atrial hypertension
ARDS	Acute onset	$PaO_2/FIO_2 \leq 200$ mmHg (regardless of PEEP level)	Bilateral infiltrates seen on frontal chest radiograph	≤ 18 mmHg when measured or no clinical evidence of left atrial hypertension

Mortality and Prognostic Factors

ARDS continues as a contributor to the morbidity and mortality of patients in intensive care units, imparting tremendous human and financial cost. The publised mortality rate of patients with ARDS varies from 10 to as high as 90%. The mortality rate in the European study was 59% and lower than the 1976 NHLBI sponsored Study (Table 4) [15, 16]. Recently it has been reported in one institution a decline in fatality rates to a lower mortality rate of 36% [10]. Krafft et al [17] analized 101 papers investigating 3264 patients between 1967 and 1994 who reported mortality and oxygenation index (PaO_2/FiO_2). The mean PaO_2/FiO_2 ratio remained unchanged throughout the observation period (118 ± 47 mmHg) and the mortality was $53 \pm 22\%$ with no apparent trend towards a higher survival [17]. Mortality rate in recent large multicenter ARDS studies was between 40% and 75% [18–20].

The prognosis for ARDS, as determined at the time of either hospital or ICU admission, is based on a variety of key factors such as the acute underlying diagnosis (e.g. head trauma, metastasic cancer, etc.), etiology, severity of illness as measured by pulmonary and non-pulmonary factors, the physiologic reserve as measured by chronologic age, and the morbidities and preexisting conditions such as AIDS, leukemia or other diseases that affect the patient's immune status [16].

Table 4. Etiologies: Comparison between American (NHLB, 1979) and European (1987) Studies

	United States (NHLB)			Europe		
	Number Patients	%	Mortality, %	Number Patients	%	Mortality, %
Aspiration	93	12.5	66.6	65	11.1	60
Extraabdominal infections	—	—	—	45	7.7	56
Intraabdominal infections	94	12.6	72.4	97	16.6	68
Trauma	55	7.4	47.2	109	18.9	38
Opportunistic pneumonia	—	—	—	50	8.5	86
Interstitial pneumonia	18	2.4	88.9	—	—	—
Other pneumonia	166	22.4	68.6	129	22.1	61
Cardiogenic shock	135	18.2	63.7	—	—	—
Hypovolemic shock	94	12.6	68.1	—	—	—
Miscellaneous	86	11.6	61.6	88	15.1	59
Total	741	100	65.9	583	100	59

Most deaths occurring in the first days of illness can be attributed to the underlying illness or injury. The majority of late deaths has been related to complications mainly septicemia (Fig. 1). The initial pathogenetic mechanisms are different, depending on the etiology (septicemia versus trauma). The highest mortality rates were due to ALI caused by diffuse infectious processes and pneumonias [16–21]. ARDS following chest trauma or associated with local abdominal or urinary sepsis carries an intermediate risk of death. Diffuse peritonitis and severe acute pancreatitis reached the highest mortality rates (> 70%) perhaps related to surgical problems. When an infectious ARDS developed in an immunocompromised host, the survival rate was very low [21].

Irreversible respiratory failure is responsible for only 10–16% of ARDS deaths, because of failure to maintain a degree of oxygenation and CO_2 elimination compatible with life. At autopsy, the lungs of these patients were severely injured and exhibit extensive pulmonary fibrosis.

Different authors have recently studied various factors and indicators of poor prognosis in ARDS patients [7, 15, 22]. The main factors correlating with survival are age and the extent of multisystem organ failure [23–25]. Eighty-two percent of patients over 70 years of age did not survive (Fig. 3). The mortality rate directly relates to the number of complications and increases to 83% when three or more complications are present (Fig. 4). Patiens without complications during their clinical management had lower mortality rate (38%). Shock and acute renal failure at ICU admission are associated with a high mortality rate.

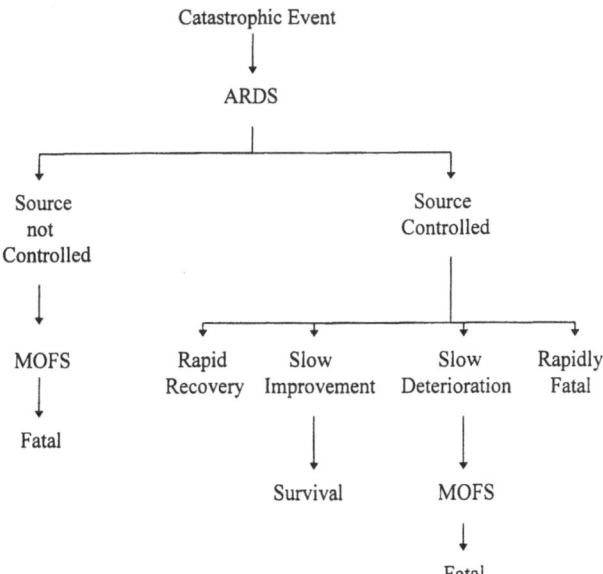

Fig. 1. When ARDS occurs as an isolated organ failure, patients follow one of several distinct clinical courses. When the source of the injury is not controlled, MOFS ensues, leading to death. Even when the source is controlled, however, clinical courses and outcomes span a wide spectrum. This diversity reflects differences in the alveolar repair process occurring after the onset ALI

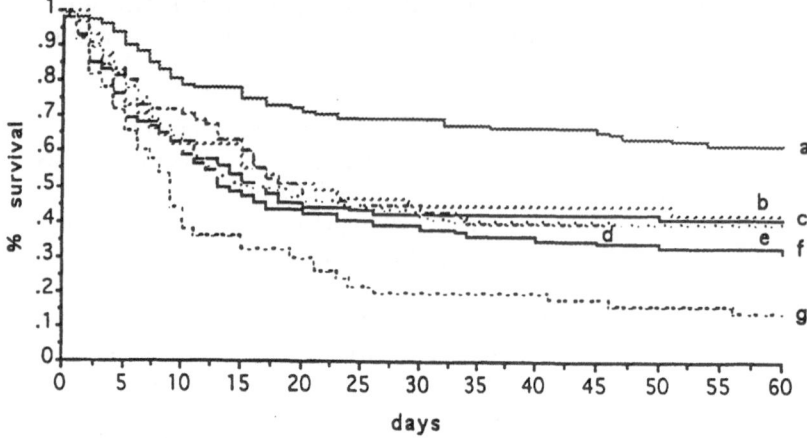

Fig. 2. Survival at 60 days in 583 patients with ARDS according to etiology. **a** Trauma; **b** Extra-abdominal sepsis; **c** Non-opportunistic pneumonia; **d** Aspiration; **e** Miscellaneous; **f** Intra-abdominal infections; **g** Opportunistic pneumonia. Traumatic patients have a higher survival rate, while patients with an ARDS due to an opportunistic pneumonia have a higher mortality $(p < 0.0001)$

Once treatment and patient support has begun, prognostic factors relate to serially obtained data that measure the patient's response to therapy. There are published data suggesting that although oxygenation (PaO_2/FiO_2) is an unreliable prognostic factor at the onset of ARDS, it does appear to be predictive of outcome when examined at 24 to 48 h after onset [16, 26, 27]. It is important to evaluate gas exchange parameters as prognostic factors, relating gas exchange with the response to PEEP and its evolution during the course of ARDS. In one study only [28], survivors decreased Qs/Qt after PEEP was applied. A higher mortality rate was reported by Lamy et al. [29] in ARDS patients having a "fixed shunt" with severe and irreversible alterations of pulmonary morphology. Oscillations of arterial PO_2 and $AaDO_2$ may indicate the evolution of the ARDS and allow us to prognosticate. The prognostic value of gas exchange variables improved at 24 h with significant differences between survivors and non-survivors in the ARDS European Study [16]. Consistent $AaDO_2$ values greater than 500 mmHg at FiO_2 1 predicted a fatal outcome and were associated with 100% mortality. A progressive increase of $PaCO_2$ despite increased ventilatory volume, an increase of the VD/VT ratio over 70%, an increase of arterial end-tidal CO_2 difference, and a persistently high pulmonary vascular resistance are associated with a poor prognosis and with morphologic destruction of the pulmonary circulation [28].

In the European Study, at admission, three hemodynamic variable provided independent prognostic information: diastolic SAP, systolic PAP and SvO_2. Regarding hemodynamic evolution during time, high systolic PAP, low diastolic SAP and low SaO_2 remained independent negative prognostic indicators [16].

Linear discriminant analysis has been performed for several physiologic cardiopulmonary variables during the first days of ARDS and correlated with

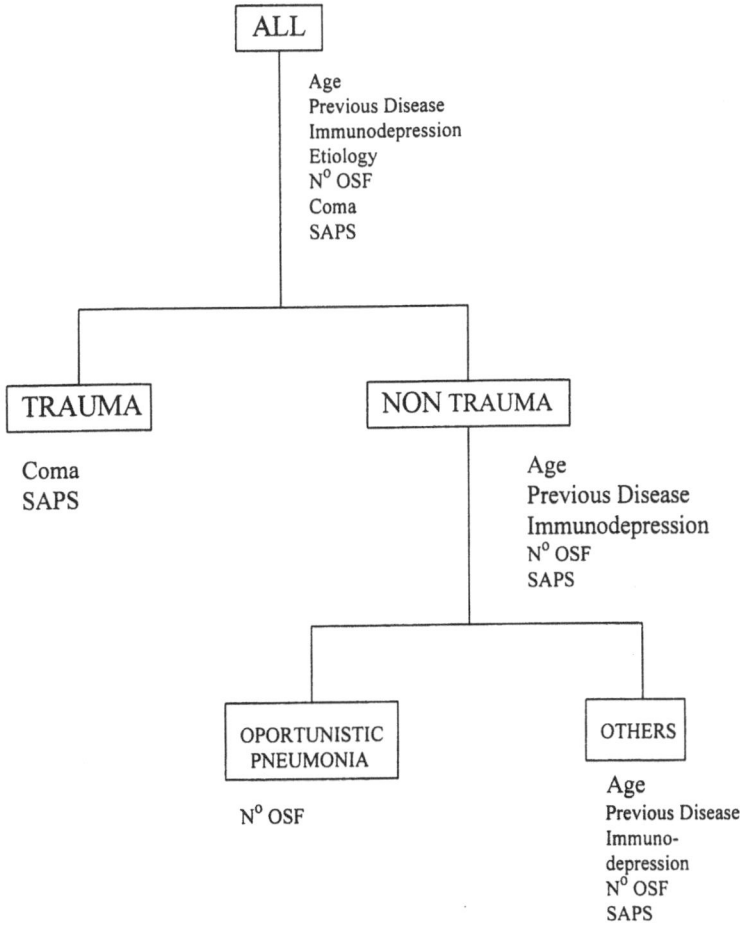

Fig. 3. A multivariate analysis of different prognostic factors and physiologic variables separated into two ARDS etiology groups (traumatic versus non-traumatic ARDS) and the presence of prior immunosuppression

mortality to define prognostic factors. In the NHLBI ARDS study, no variable or combination of variables were able to predict the survival or death reliably for all groups [30, 31]. However, in the subgroup of ARDS patients with the highest mortality rates, effective respiratory compliance, alveolar-arterial O_2 tension difference ($AaDO_2$), and buffer-base deviation were the best predictors. In another study, all patients with an effective compliance below 25 mL/cmH$_2$O on the first day of study died [31].

Fowler et al. [22] reported four variables were significantly associated with ARDS mortality: 1) presence of less than 10% band forms on the initial peripheral blood smear, 2) persistent acidemia with arterial pH less than 7.40, 3) calculated HCO_3^- less than 20 mg/dL, and 4) a blood urea nitrogen greater than

65 mg/dL. After eliminating those variables that did not contribute significantly to mortality in the presence of the others, only low ban forms, low pH and low HCO_3^- were significantly associated with increased mortality.

The development of secondary diagnoses and/or complications (e.g. acute myocardial infarction or single or multiple organ failure) have a profound impact on the ultimate outcome. The most frequent complications appearing during the course of ARDS are shock and acute renal failure, each associated with a mortality rate over 90%. The majority of late deaths are related to a sepsis syndrome, present in 73% of ARDS patients [7, 24], where the predominant site is the lung. Several investigators indicate that sepsis syndrome, rather than respiratory failure, is the leading cause of death in patients with ARDS [6–8, 24, 25, 32, 33]. These data indicate the importance of general supportive care and the use of accurate methods to determine the presence of a nosocomial pulmonary infections establishing an appropiate antibiotic treatment. Prevention and treatment of such complications during ARDS is probably the cause of the actual declining of death rate in ARDS.

Table 5. Classification of ARF (according to severity) used at the Massachusetts General Hospital, sponsored Center of Research in Adult Respiratory Failure

Category of ARF	Chest radiograph	Tracheal intubation and positive airway pressure	Oxygenation
At risk of developing ARF (abdominal sepsis, long bone or pelvic fractures, other nonthoracic trauma)	Normal or minimal changes, e.g., segmental atelectasis	None, except for short-term routine support, e.g., postoperative therapy	O_2 administeration only for short-term routine support, e.g. postoperative therapy
Mild	Minimal diffuse or lobar infiltrates or edema	May or may not be intubated and require positive airway pressure (CMV, IPS, CPAP)	$FiO_2 < 0.5$
Moderate (meets criteria for entry to NHLBL multicenter Additional Data Collection but not criteria for severe ARF)	Panlobar alveolar infiltrates of one or both lungs	Intubated > 24 h and need positive airway pressure (CMV, IMV, PEEP, CPAP)	$FiO_2 < 0.5$
Severe (meets rapid or slow criteria for entry into nHLBI multicenter study for ECMO)	Bilateral panlobar alveolar infiltrates	Intubated and need CMV with PEEP	$PaO_2 < 50$ mmHg with $FiO_2 = 1.0$ for 8 h or longer or $FiO_2 \geq 0.6$ for 48 h or longer

Abbreviations: CPAP: Continuous positive airway pressure; CMV: Continuous mandatory ventilation, also referred to as controlled mechanical ventilation; IMV: Intermittent mandatory ventilation; PEEP: Positive end-expiratory airway pressure; FiO_2: Fraction of oxygen inspired; IPS: Intermittent pressure support

Biochemical and Cellular Mediators

An intense inflammatory process in the lungs is a characteristic histologic feature of ARDS [34, 35]. In these patients, there is an accumulation of polymorphonuclear neutrophils (PMN) and macrophages in the air spaces and bronchoalveolar lavage (BAL) fluid [36–42]. There is evidence in humans and animal models that PMN can participate in the initiation and propagation of ALI [43, 44]. High PMN counts in BAL are associated with more severe lung dysfunction [39]. Steinberg reported that patients who still require mechanical ventilatory support 7 and 14 days after the onset of ARDS have increased PMN in BAL; moreover, the magnitude of this increase is associated with mortality, particularly in patients with sepsis syndrome [45]. By contrast, patients with sepsis-associated ARDS in whom BAL macrophages increase over time have lower lung injury scores and improved survival. These observations are consistent with the interpretation that persistence of the acute inflammatory response is associated with persistence of clinical manifestations of ARDS, whereas successful recruitment of monocytes and macrophages is important to the repair process. Cytokines are significantly increased regardless of the duration of ARDS and interleukin (IL)-8 and ENA-78, two potent PMN chemoattractants, significantly correlates with PMN concentration in BAL [46].

The mean cytokine values on each day were always higher in patients who died, although there was considerable overlap. Although neither IL-8 nor ENA-78 was associated with outcome, levels of IL-1β measured on day 7 were associated with an increased risk of death. It seems likely that persistent elevation of these inflammation prolongs their requirement for invasive ventilatory support and contributes to the high morbidity and mortality seen in patients with ARDS [46].

In a prospective study wherein different mediators were analyzed, antithrombin III, protein C, and α-2-macroglobulin demonstrated differences between survivors and non-survivors in an early phase of ARDS. Progressive normalization of these measurements occurred with improvement of ARDS [47, 48].

Severity Scoring Systems

The introduction of standard and accurate methods of scoring the severity of respiratory failure and the disturbances of overall physiology with or without specific and sensitive assays of some mediator(s) predicting the severity of lung injury may make possible the comparison of patient populations and examining the efficiency of therapeutic interventions. However, at present the determination of severity of illness or injury can be given by both specific and general indices.

Specific Pulmonary Scoring Indices

Interest in scoring systems for patients suffering from ALI has increased in recent years because there is a definite need for classifying severity stages and predicting the further course and outcome of ALI. ARDS is a manifestation of systemic disease produced by widespread increases in endothelial permealitity where lung dysfunction dominates the early clinical course. Lung is a very sensitive organ to any inflammatory insult producing an impairment in oxygenation and lung compliance. These physiological consequences of pulmonary edema in ARDS induced different authors to describe severity scores based on gas exchange, lung compliance and the needs for mechanical ventilation (tidal volume, PEEP, FiO_2) to maintain an adequate gas exchange.

MGH-ARF Classification

The Specialized Center of Research (SCOR) in adult respiratory failure at the Massachusetts General Hospital categorized the severity of ARF within 24 h ICU admission as at risk, mild acute respiratory failure, moderate ARDS, or severe ARDS according to the standarized radiographic, ventilatory, and arterial gas tension criteria outlined in Table 5. From 1978 to 1988, Zapol et al. [49] reported mortality rates according to severity of acute respiratory failure in 535 patients. The mortality rate paralleled the degree of severity of lung inflammation at ICU admission. The overall mortality rate was 39.3%, 352 patiens had mild respiratory failure with a mortality rate of 28.1%, 131 patients were classified as moderate respiratory failure with a mortality of 55% and 52 patients with a severe respiratory failure presented a highest mortality rate of 75%. The authors identified 227 at high risk to develop acute respiratory failure with a total mortality rate of 24.7%. Eighty-seven (38.4%) of the 227 high risk patients developped ALI with a mortality of 51.7%. The 140 at risk patients who remained at high risk of ALI but did not develop acute respiratory failure had a 7.9% mortality, whereas at high risk patients who developped mild respiratory failure had a four-fold increased (31.0%) mortality rate.

This categorization scheme for acute respiratory failure is a simple one designed for easy classification at the bedside and it introduces the concept of at risk of ALI patients that allows early identification of a subset of patients who are

Table 6. Evolution of Respiratory Severity index (RSI) and simplified acute physiological score (SAPS) in 35 ARDS patients in Spanish pilot study (Mancebo and Artigas, 1987)

		Day		
		1	3–5	5
SAPS	Survivors	12.6 ± 4.3	10 ± 3.46	8.78 ± 1.56
	Non-survivors	14.3 ± 4.1	15.06 ± 3.46[a]	16.25 ± 5.56[b]
RSI	Survivors	0.8 ± 0.09	0.5 ± 0.11	0.47 ± 0.01
	Non-survivors	0.8 ± 0.08	0.5 ± 0.11	0.47 ± 0.01

[a] $p < 0.025$;   [b] $p < 0.001$

very likely to develop acute respiratory failure and therefore candidate to different preventive therapeutical strategies.

Pulmonary Insufficiency Index

Batlett et al. [50] proposed a method for mortality prediction for use in patients with acute respiratory failure based on a graph of $AaDO_2$ (alveolar-arterial oxygen gradient) against time. The authors found a significant correlation between patient survival and the "pulmonary insufficiency index (PII)". The PII was calculated for each patients by integrating the $AaDO_2$/time curve for the period during which the $AaDO_2$ exceeded 300. In 45 acute respiratory failure patients the authors reported a mean PII of 0.84 in survivors and 11.3 in non-survivors. Retrospective analysis of acute respiratory failure patients from two major hospitals showed uniform mortality in all patients with PII over 6.0 [50]. By using the PII, Shimada et al. [51] found that in 10 ARDS patients who died a score value > 6.0 was measured. Two of 4 patients who survived, however, were also scored > 6.0. Barlett et al. proposed their system for use in a larger data base for possible prediction of mortality and evaluating management and new treatment options in ARDS patients. Up to now, this score has been seldom established in clinical practice or research. Limited positive experience in small patient populations and the influence of FiO_2 and PEEP on $AaDO_2$ calculation warrants further validation in larger controlled studies.

Severity Index

In 1982, Jardin et al. [52] proposed a simple score based on measurements of PaO_2, alveolar oxygen tension (PAO_2), FiO_2 and PEEP, performed twice daily in mechanically ventilated patients. The so-called "severity index (SI)" is defined as:

$$SI = OI + 0,014 \, PEEP \, (cmH_2O)$$

whereas oxygenation index (OI) is calculated by the formula:

$$OI = (PAO_2 - PaO_2)/[(\text{barometric pressure} + 47) \times FiO_2]$$

In a retrospective study in 50 ARDS patients, the authors tested the predictive value of this severity index and demonstrated that it reliably predicted the patient's survival or death from acute respiratory failure. If the SI exceeded 0.86 on the second day, the probability of death was 85%; if it exceeded this value on the third day, the patient's probability of death was 92%. The predictive value of this score was later confirmed by Artigas and Mancebo [23] in 35 ARDS patients (Table 6), and by the European ARDS study enrolling 583 patients were OI was evaluated after 24 h of ICU admission [16]. The influence of PEEP on SI is very small, and the score is based primarily on OI. The calculation of OI by the $AaDO_2/PAO_2$ avoids

Table 7. Pulmonary Failure Scoring System

Score	Chest roentgenogram	AaDO$_2$/FiO$_2$ (mmHg)[a]	Crs ml (cmH$_2$O)$^{-1}$	PAP (mmHg)
0	Normal	<300	>80	<20
	Moderately increased interstitial markings	300–375	70–80	20–25
2	Markedly increased interstitial markings	375–450	50–70	25–30
3	Patchy air-space consolidation	450–525	30–50	30–35
4	Extensive air-space consolidation	>525	<30	>35

[a] Continuous positive pressure ventilation with continuous positive airway pressure (CPAP) or positive end-expiratory pressure (PEEP) or more than 5 cmH$_2$O increases this particular score by +1.

AaDO$_2$/FiO$_2$: alveolar-arterial oxygen tension difference divided by inspired oxygen fraction; Crs: static compliance of the respiratory system; PAP: mean pulmonary arterial pressure

the influence of different FiO$_2$ settings on the AaDO$_2$ measurement. This simple and reliable predictive score is based in a large number of ARDS patients and allow the clinician to evaluate the clinical evolution of ALI. Patients without improvement of SI after 3 days of treatment have a poor prognosis.

Ventilator Score

In 1986, Smith and Gordon [53] suggested an index to predict outcome in ARDS. From the peak upper airway pressure (Paw), the oxygen gradient, and the age of the patient, the following ventilator score was obtained:

Ventilator score $= 0.5 \times$ age $+ 0.6 \times$ oxygen gradient $+ 1.2 \times \Delta$Paw

(difference between Paw in a given ARDS patient and a control value measured in healthy adults). In their series of 30 ARDS patients, this score reliably discriminated between the survivors and those who died from the pulmonary lesions of the syndrome. Later, Hickling et al. confirmed the ventilator score to be predictive for outcome in ARDS in a retrospective [54] and in a prospective [55] study. The ventilator score can be calculated at the bedside from data easily available on these patients. This score combines 3 parameters, age, oxygenation and airway resistance, evaluated by peak Paw which is not reflecting changes of lung compliance rather than total airways resistances including the resistance due to the artificial airways.

Pulmonary Failure Scoring System

To characterize the severity of lung damage in ARDS patients, Morel et al. [56] in 1982 proposed a "pulmonary failure scoring system (PFSS)", the "Genève" ARDS

Scoring System, using 4 independent variables, each of which is assigned a score between 0 and 4. A score of 0 corresponds to a normal state, 4 to the most diseased state. The authors added one point to the specific severity score for Aa-DO_2/FiO_2 if a patient received continuous possitive airway pressure (CPAP) or PEEP >5 cmH$_2$O. The final score value is calculated by dividing the sum of the score values of each variable by 4 (Table 7). The score discriminated between patients at risk of ARDS and those with established ARDS according to a cut off score of two. By dividing the total number of points scored by the value obtained for each patient, they found a significant correlation between the mean score and first-pass lung serotonin uptake. The value of the PFSS was confirmed in the European ARDS study when it was measured after 24 h of ICU admission [16]. This score needs the measurement of PAP and a PAC in place as well as the meas-

Table 8. Lung Injury Score

	Value	
1. Chest roentgenogram score		
No alveolar consolidation		0
Alveolar consolidation confined to 1 quadrant		1
Alveolar consolidation confined to 2 quadrants		2
Alveolar consolidation confined to 3 quadrants		3
Alveolar consolidation in all 4 quadrants		4
2. Hypoxemia score		
PaO$_2$/FiO$_2$	≥ 300	0
PaO$_2$/FiO$_2$	225–299	1
PaO$_2$/FiO$_2$	175–224	2
PaO$_2$/FiO$_2$	100–174	3
PaO$_2$/FiO$_2$	<100	4
3. PEEP score (when ventilated)	≥ 5 cmH$_2$O	0
PEEP	6–8 cmH$_2$O	1
PEEP	9–11 cmH$_2$O	2
PEEP	12–14 cmH$_2$O	3
PEEP	215 cmH$_2$O	4
4. Respiratory system compliance score (when available)		
Compliance	≥ 80 ml/cmH$_2$O	0
Compliance	60–79 ml/cmH$_2$O	1
Compliance	40–59 ml/cmH$_2$O	2
Compliance	20–39 ml/cmH$_2$O	3
Compliance	≤ 19 ml/cmH$_2$O	4

The final value is obtained by dividing the aggregate sum by the number of components that were used

	Score
No lung injury	0
Mild-to-moderate lung injury	0.1–2.5
Severe lung injury (ARDS)	>2.5

Abbreviations: PaO$_2$/FiO$_2$, arterial oxygen tension to inspired oxygen concentration ratio; PEEP: positive end-expiratory pressure

urement of static compliance of the respiratory system, both necessary only for patients with severe forms of ALI.

Lung Injury Score

In1988, Murray et al. [57] described the lung injury score (LIS), to assess and quantify the severity of ALI. LIS is calculated by the total points obtained and divided by the number of parameters assessed. Oxygenation is quantified by the ratio PaO_2/FiO_2, chest X-ray is scored according to the number of quadrants in which alveolar consolidation can be recognized, static respiratory system compliance is calculated using the formula VT/Pplateau-PEEP and additional points are assigned for the PEEP level applied (Table 8). Lung injury is classified as not present (0 points), mild-moderate (0.1–2.5 points), and severe ARDS (>2.5 points). This score, similar to the Genève Score, is widely used in clinical practice and research to assess severity of ALI because it is simple and non-invasive. Nevertheless, LIS has never been evaluated in a large number of patients. Recently, in a 12-month prospective study of 123 ALI patients, Matthay et al. [58] demonstrated that LIS on day 1 did not reliably predict mortality which was more closely related to non-pulmonary factors such as systemic hypotension, chronic liver disease and non-pulmonary organ dysfunction developed between hospital admission and admission to the ICU.

General Illness Scoring Indices

During the last years, considerable advances have been made in the refinement and application of severity-of-illness models to describe patients admitted to ICUs. These models can provide a method for risk stratification for important clinical research trials and for making quality of care comparisons among ICUs

Table 9. Multivariate prognosis analysis, using Cox's model in 583 ARDS patients

Model	RR[a]	p-value at the last step (LRT[b])
Age		0.004
Group (A, B)	1.8	0.003
Pre-existent disease	1.2	0.10
Trauma	0.7	0.05
SAPS		0.008
Immunodepression	1.8	<0.0001
PaO_2/FIO_2 (day 1)		0.01
Coma	1.3	0.09

[a] For binary variables, the relative risk is estimated by the exponential of the Cox's coefficient, at the last step. [b] Only significant variables at the 10% level are retained in the model of the last step

with a similar case mix [58]. The various severity scores for critical care patients have been substantially updated in the past few years. The new versions of these scores are based on much larger databases and have used better statistical methods for development, validation, and field testing. Appropiate methods for measuring discrimination and callibration are now widely used and logistic regression has become the dominant method for converting a score to a probability, for scaling physiologic variables, and for selecting and weighing clinical variables. Although some criticisms have raised concerns about the use of severity scores (even for important subgroups of patients), the use of severity scores has achieved a wide level of acceptance, particulary for auditing clinical practice and outcomes within the ICU of an individual hospital, and for risk stratification for large-scale clinical trials that include ICU patients.

In order to rigorously develop and assess a model, a large database must be available. A separate database using different patients must be employed for validation and field testing. Variables should be clearly defined and reliable. The model should reflect accurately the mortality experience of the patient sample as assessed by objective criteria. The criteria for assessing the reliability of a model are well established and include discrimination, using the area under the receiver/operator curve, and calibration, using formal goodness-of-fit testing [59]. Models should contain a minimum number of variables to reduce the burden of data collection and the potential for error. The common endpoint for the general ICU severity models is vital status at hospital discharge.

There has been a proliferation of general severity scoring systems but many of these models are based on intuitive selection of variables or are based on small samples on highly selected patients. The 3 most widely used gereral severity and prognostic scoring systems are the current versions of the Mortality Probability Model (MPM) [60], the Simplified Acute Physiologic Score (SAPS) [61], and the Acute Physiology and Chronic Health Evaluation (APACHE) Prognostic System [62].

The Mortality Probability Model (MPM II)

MPMII was developed from a large database of 19 124 patients from 137 hospitals [60]. The methodology used the statistical technique of multiple logistic regression to identify, as well as to weigh the clinical variables. This system is not primarily physiologic and no score is involved. The MPM system is a series of models availables at ICU admission, as well as at 24, 48, and 72 h [63]. The admission model (MPMo) is the only system available for estimating the probability of hospital mortality at the time of ICU admission and contains 15 easily obtainable variables without the requirement for a single primary precipitating diagnosis in order to calculate the probability. An ICU presentation model should provide an ideal tool for evaluating ICU quality performance and for stratifying patients prior to randomization in clinical trials before differential ICU treatment patterns have had an opportunity to alter physiology. The 24, 48, and 72 h models reflect patient status after treatment and predict hospital mortality based on 8 new variables collected at those times and used in conjunction with age, type of admission, cirrhosis, metastasic cancer and intracranial mass effect. The same variables, but with a different statistical constant value for each time period, comprise the models for calculation of probabilities at 24, 48 and 72 h.

The Simplified Acute Physiologic Score

SAPS was developed as an independent method for simplifying the original APACHE severity-of-illness scoring system [64]. An updated version, SAPSII, was validated using an international database similar to that used for MPM II [61]. The system includes 17 variables – 12 physiologic measurements, age, type of admission (scheduled surgical, unscheduled surgical, or medical), and 3 chronic disease variables (adquired immunodeficiency syndrome, metastasic cancer, and hematologic malignancy). The score ranges from 0 to 182 points and on algerithm converts the score to a probability of hospital mortality for bedside availability, this method eliminates the need for expensive computer equipment and specialized software and maintains the overall concept of a simple approach. The calibration and discrimination ability of SAPSII are comparable to the more complex APACHE physiology approach.

The APACHE System

Originally introduced in 1981 [65], APACHE provided a reliable and valid method for severity measurement and risk stratification but was complex and required multihospital validation. The APACHE III [62] was introduced in 1991 to expand and improve the prognostic estimates provided by APACHE II based on 1979–1982 data [66]. The APACHE III system consists of two parts – an APACHE III score, which contains points for 17 physiologic abnormalities, age, and chronic health status, and a series of predictive equations linked to ICU admission diagnosis, patient selection criteria, and the APACHE III database. The APACHE III score can be used to measure severity of disease and to risk-stratify patients within a single diagnostic category or independently defined patient group. APACHE III scores also can be used to compare group outcomes, but only for ICU admissions meeting diagnostic and selection criteria similar to those in the APACHE III study. A series of APACHE III equations predict outcomes by linking patient characteristics to a 1988 through 1990 nationally representative database of 17 440 ICU admissions at 42 ICUs in the United States. One such equation combines the first-day APACHE III score, diagnosis, and patient selection for intensive care to predict risk of hospital death for multidiagnostic patient groups.

Conversion of the score to a probability of hospital mortality is accomplished using a logistic regression equation requiring the specification of one of 79 specific diagnostic categories, as well as one of 9 patient locations [...]. The score will have a different associated probability of hospital mortality for patients in two different disease categories and for patients in the same disease category but admitted from two different locations. The APACHE III system is proprietary and the statistical weights to convert a score to a probability have not been made public. As a result, performance of the APACHE III system has not been tested independently. The same is true for the statistical equations that convert the score to an estimated length of ICU stay.

It has been suggested that daily physiology scores within diagnostic categories can provide useful information for dynamic modeling and for looking at the change in probability of mortality over time. Again, independent confirmation within specific diagnostic groups has not been performed.

The APACHE III system is more complex than APACHE II. A much larger database has been accumulated with APACHE III through a proprietary network, but it is unclear whether the additional data collection and resultitig costs represent a significant improvement over the APACHE II system.

All of the currently popular severity models are built on a broad base of heterogeneous medical and surgical patients from a large number of participating multipurpose ICUs. In reality, however, ICUs often are highly specialized. It is, therefore, not surprising that general models may not perform well within subgroups of patients concentrated in special ICUs, even though the models were originally intended for such patients.

What can be done about these special subgroups? The first is to test the general models using formal goodness-of-fit methods to determine whether the model over- or under-predicts across the spectrum of probability ranges. It may be possible to customize or recalibrate for these specialized groups of patients. As long as comparisons are made among similar types of patients, it may be possible that quality testing can be performed. Another approach may be to develop modified models that build on physiologic terms (APACHE/SAPS) and conditions (MPM) but add unique variables related specifically to aspects of the particular subgroups of patients in question.

Recently, Knaus et al. [67] demonstrated that the reliance on pulmonary deterioration alone was less accurate in its predictive value than was the use of overall physiologic derangement, as represented by risk of death calculated by the APACHE III method. Artigas et al. [27] evaluated the accuracy of general severity indexes (SAPS II and MPM II) and respiratory severity index (PaO_2/FiO_2) in predicting outcome of 8378 patients with ALI. After customization both general severity indexes were useful to predict mortality and PaO_2/FiO_2 correlated well with extrapulmonary organ system dysfunction and observed/predicted mortality ratio. The two studies indicate that successful estimation of risk of hospital mortality in patients with ALI can be obtained using a general severity score that accounts for both important pulmonary and extrapulmonary organ system dysfunction.

Relationship Between Prognostic Factors and Stratification of ALI

It is important to remember that the various factors influencing the outcome of ARDS are not independent. For instance, previous health status is statistically more vital as age increases [68]; severity of illness is more important when previous health status worsens; some diagnoses are more frequent in younger or older patients. Diagnosis markedly influences outcome: the SAPS score correlates with mortality in diagnosis-related groups of patients, but for the same SAPS score the outcome varies according to the primary diagnosis [64]. The multivariate analysis of the European ARDS Study demonstrated the value of many prognostic factors and physiologic variables in two etiology groups (post-traumatic versus non-traumatic ARDS), especially the presence or absence of prior immunosuppression (Fig. 2).

Age, previous disease, immunodepression, etiology of ALI, number and type of organ system failures at the ICU admission and during the clinical evolution of the disease, coma, gas exchange after 24 h of mechanical ventilation and SAPS were the independent variables related to mortality (Table 9, Fig. 3). Recently, the American-European Consensus Conference on ARDS proposed the GOCA stratification system which deals with the entire continuum of ALI, and incorporates additional important factors that have an important influence on prognosis (Table 10). In order to assess the magnitude of the public health problem posed by ARDS and to define the location of patients with ARDS, thereby facilitating future clinical and therapeutic studies, we believe that epidemiologic study of ARDS is the highest priority.

In collecting epidemiologic data, it will be useful to record, for consecutively observed patients: 1) information relating to etiology (at a minimum, direct or indi-

Table 10. Stratification system of acute lung injury (GOCA)

Letter	Meaning		Scale	Definition
G	Echange		0	$PaO_2/FiO_2 \geq 301$
			1	PaO_2/FiO_2 201–300
			2	PaO_2/FiO_2 101–200
			3	$PaO_2/FiO_2 \leq 100$
	Gas exchange		A	Spontaneousbreathing, no PEEP
	(to be combined		B	Assisted breathing, PEEP 0–5 cmH_2O
	with the numeric		C	Assisted breathing, PEEP 6–10 cmH_2O
	descriptor)		D	Assisted breathing, PEEP ≥ 10 cmH_2O
O	Organ failure	0	Lung only	
			1	Lung +1 organ
			2	Lung +2 organs
			3	Lung +3 organs
C	Cause	0	Unknown	
			1	Direct Lung Injury
			2	Indirect Lung Injury
A	Associated Diseases		0	No coexisting diseases that will cause death within 5 years
			1	Coexisting disease that will cause death withing 5 years but not within 6 months
			2	Coexisting disease that will cause death within 6 months

rect cause of lung injury); 2) mortality, including cause of death and wether death was associated with withdrawal of care; 3) presence of failure of other organs and other time-dependent covariates; and 4) follow-up information including fraction of patients for whom such data are available, recovery of lung function, and quality of life. The collection of epidemiologic data should be based on clear definition, as well as on a system that stratifies severity of ALI. The epidemiologic studies will require participation of investigators trained in sophisticated epidemiologic techniques. Concurrent with study of the epidemiology of ARDS, efforts to coordinate and/or facilitate study of various therapies for ARDS should go forward.

References

1. Loyd JE, Newman JH, Brigham KL (1984) Permeability pulmonary edema: Diagnosis and management. Arch Intern Med 144:143–147
2. Ashbaugh DG, Bigelow DB, Petty TL, Levine BE (1967) Acute respiratory distress in adults. Lancet 2:319–323
3. Pepe PE, Hudson LD, Carrico CJ (1984) Early application of positive end-expiratory pressure in patients at risk for the adult respiratory distress syndrome. N Engl J Med 311:281–286
4. Zapol WM, Snider MT, Hill JD, et al (1979) Extracorporeal membrane oxygenation in severe acute respiratory failure: A randomized prospective study. JAMA 242:2193–2196
5. Morris AH, Wallace CJ, Menlove RL, Clemmer TP, Orme JF, Weaver LK, Dean NC, Thomas F, East TD, Pace NL, Suchyta MR, Beck E, Bombino M, Sitting DF, Böhm S, Hoffmann B, Becks H, Butler S, Pearl J, Rasmusson B. Randomized Clinical Trial of Pressure-controlled Inverse Ratio Ventilation and Extracorporeal CO_2 Renoval for Adult Respiratory Distress Syndrome. Am J Respir Crit Care Med 1994, 149:295–305
6. Pepe PE, Potkin RT, Reus DH, Hudson LD, Carrico CJ (1982) Clinical predictors of the adult respiratory distress syndrome. Am J Surg 144:124–130
7. Montgomery B, Stager MA, Carrico CJ, Hudson LD (1985) Causes of mortality in patients with the adult respiratory distress syndrome Am Rev Respir Dis 132:485–489
8. Bell RC, Coalson JJ, Smith JD, Johanson WG (1983) Multiple organ system failure and infection in adult respiratory distress syndrome. Ann Intern Med 99:293–298
9. Fowler AA, Hamman RF, Good JT, et al (1983) Adult respiratory distress syndrome: Risk with common predisposition. Ann Intern Med 98:593–597
10. Milberg JA, Davis DR, Steinberg KP, Hudson LD (1995) Improved survival of patients with ARDS. 1983–1993. JAMA, 273:306–309
11. Rinaldo JE (1986) The prognosis of the adult respiratory distress syndrome. Inappropriate pessimism? Chest 90:470–471
12. Bernard GR, Artigas A, Brigham KL et al (1994). The American-European consensus conference on ARDS. Am J Respir Crit Care Med 149:818–824
13. Shuster DP (1995). What is acute lung injury? What is ARDS? Chest 107:1721–1726
14. Kollef MH, Shuster DP (1995). The acute respiratory distress syndrome. N Engl J Med 332:27–37
15. Artigas A, Carlet J, Chastang C, Le Gall JR, Blanch L, Fernández R. Adult respiratory distress syndrome: clinical presentation, prognostic factors and outcome. In: Artigas A, Lemaire F, Suter PM, Zapol WM (eds) Adult respiratory distress syndrome. Churchill Livingstone, Edinburgh 1992, pp 509–525
16. Artigas A, Carlet J, Le Gall JR, Chastant C, Blanch L, Fernández R. Clinical presentation, prognostic factors and outcome of ARDS in the European Collaborative Study (1985–1987). In: Zapol W, Lemaire F (eds) Adult respiratory distress syndrome. Marcel Dekker. New York 1991, pp 37–63

17. Krafft P, Fridrich T, Pernerstorfer RD, Fitzgerald D et al (1996) The acute respiratory distress syndrome: definitions, severity and clinical outcome. An analysis of 101 clinical investigations. Intensive Care Med 22:519-529
18. Anzueto A, Baughman R, Guntapalli K et al (1996) Aerosolized surfactant in adults with sepsis-induced acute respiratory distress syndrome. N Engl J Med 334:1417-1421
19. Brochard L, Roudot-Thoraval F, and the collaborative group on Vt reduction (1997) Tidal volume (Vt) reduction in acute respiratory distress syndrome (ARDS): a multicenter randomized study. Am J Respir Crit Care 155:A505
20. Stewart E, Meade M, Granton J et al (1997) Pressure and volume limited ventilation strategy (PLUS) in patients at high risk for ARDS: Results of a multicenter trial. Am J Respir Crit Care 155:A505.
21. Hudson LD, Milberg JA, Anardi D, Maunder RJ (1995) Clinical risks for development of the acute respiratory distress syndrome. Am J Respir Crit Care 151:293-301
22. Fowler AA, Hamman RF, Zerbe GO, Benson KN, Hyers TM (1985) Adult respiratory distress syndrome: Prognosis after onset. Am Rev Respir Dis 132:472-478
23. Artigas A, Mancebo J (1987) Etiology and multiple organ system failure as prognostic factors in ARDS. In: Vincent JL (ed) Update in Intensive Care and Emergency Medicine. Springer-Verlag, Berlin, pp 163-169
24. Mancebo J, Artigas A (1987) A clinical study of the adult respiratory distress syndrome Crit Care Med 15:243-246
25. Bone RC, Balk R, Slotman G, Maunder R, Silverman H, Hyers TM, Kerstein MD (1992) Adult Respiratory Distress Syndrome: Sequence and importance of development of multiple organ failure. Chest 101:320-326
26. Bone RC, Maunder R, Slotman G, Silverman H, Hyers TM, Kerstein MD, Ursprung JJ (1989) An early test of survival in patients with the adult respiratory distress syndrome. The PaO_2/FIO_2 ratio and its differential response to conventional therapy. Chest 96:849-851
27. Artigas A, Lemeshow S, Rue M, Avrunin J, Mestre J, Le Gall JR and ICU Scoring Group (1994) Risk stratification and outcome assessment of patients with acute lung injury. Am J Respir Crit Care Med 149:A1029
28. De Latorre FJ, Estopá R, Artigas A (1983) Intercambio gaseoso como factor pronóstico en el sín-drome de distress respiratorio del adulto. Med Intensiva 7:1-6
29. Lamy M, Fallat RJ, Koeniger E, et al (1976) Pathologic features and mechanisms of hypoxemia in adult respiratory distress syndrome. Am Rev Respir Dis 114:267-284
30. National Heart, Lung and Blood Institute, Division of Lung Discases (1979) Extracorporeal Support for Respiratory Insufficiency: A Collaborative Study. Bethesda, MD, NIH
31. Barlett RH, Morris AH, Fairley BF, Hirsh R, O'Connor N, Pontoppidan H (1986) A prospective study of acute hypoxic respiratory failure. Chest 89:684-689
32. Fein AM, Lippmann M, Holtzman H, Eliraz A, Goldberg SK (1983) The risk factors, incidence, and prognosis of ARDS following septicemia. Chest 83:40-42
33. Kaplan RL, Sahn SA, Petty TL (1979) Incidence and outcome of the respiratory distress syndrome in Gram-negative sepsis. Arch Intern Med 139:867-869
34. Idell S, Cohen AB (1983) Bronchoalveolar lavage in patients with the adult respiratory distress syndrome. Clin Chest Med 6:459-71
35. Bachofen M, Weibel ER (1982) Structural alterations of lung parenchyma in the adult respiratory distress syndrome. Clin Chest Med 3:35-56
36. Holter JF, Weiland JE, Patch ER, Gadek JE, Davis WB (1986) Protein permeability in the adult respiratory distress syndrome. Loss of size selectivity of alveolar epithelium. J Clin Invest 78:1513-22.
37. Sprung CL, Long WM, Marcial EH et al (1987) Distribution of proteins in pulmonary edema. The value of fractional concentrations. Am Rev Respir Dis 136:957-63
38. Fowler AA, Hyers TM, Fisher BJ, Bechard DE, Centor RM, Webster RO (1987) The adult respiratory distress syndrome cell populations and soluble mediators in the air spaces of patients at high risk. Am Rev Respir Dis 136:1225-31
39. Weiland JE, Davis WB, Holter JF, Mohammed JR, Dorinsky PM, Gadek JE (1986) Lung neutrophils in the adult respiratory distress syndrome: clinical and pathophysiologic significance. Am Rev Respir Dis 133:218-25

40. Martin TR, Pistorese BP, Hudson LD, Maunder RJ (1991) The function of lung and blood neutrophils in patients with the adult respiratory distress syndrome: implications for the pathogenesis of lung infections. Am Rev Respir Dis 144:254–62
41. Repine JE, Beehler CJ (1991) Neutrophils and adult respiratory distress syndrome: two interlocking perspectives in 1991. Am Rev Respir Dis 144:251–2
42. Suter PM, Suter S, Girardin E, Roux-Lombard P, Grau GE, Dayer JM. High bronchoalveolar levels of tumor necrosis factor and its inhibitors, interleukin^{-1}, interferon, and elastase, in patients with respiratory distress syndrome after trauma, shock, or sepsis. Am Rev Respir Dis 145:1016–22
43. Lee CT, Fein AM, Lippman M, Holtzman H, Kimbel P, Weinbaum G (1981) Elastalytic activity in pulmonary lavage fluid from patients with the adult respiratory distress syndrome. N Engl J Med 304:192–196
44. Shasby DM, Fox RB, Harada RN, Repine JE (1982) Reduction of the edema of acute hyperoxic lung injury by granulocyte deplation. J Appl Physiol 52:1237–1244.
45. Steinberg KP, Milberg JA, Martin TR, Maunder RJ, Cockrill BA, Hudson LD (1994) Evolution of bronchoalveolar cell populations in the respiratory distress syndrome. Am J Respir Crit Care Med 150:113–122
46. Goodman RB, Strieter RM, Martin DP, et al (1996) Inflammatory cytokines in patients with persistence of the acute respiratory distress syndrome. Am J Respir Crit Care Med 154:602–611
47. Artigas A, Fontcuberta J, Castella J, Rutllant M (1985) Coagulation disorders in the adult respiratory distress syndrome. In: Vincent JL (ed) Update in Intensive Care and Emergency Medicine. Springer-Verlag, Berlin, pp 84–89
48. Fontcuberta J, Artigas A, Sala N, et al (1986) Inhibitors of blood coagulation in adult respiratory distress syndrome. Intensive Care Med 12:224 (Abst)
49. Zapol WM, Frikker MJ, Pontoppidan H, Wilson RS, Lynch KE (1991) The adult respiratory distress syndrome at Massachusetts General Hospital: Etiology, progression and survival rates 1978–1988. In: Adult respiratory distress syndrome. De. WM Zapol, F Lemaire. Marcel Dekker, New York, pp 367–380
50. Bartlett RH, Gazzaniga AB, Wilson AF, Medley T, Wetmore N (1975) Mortality prediction in adult respiratory insufficiency. Chest 6:680–684
51. Shimada Y, Yoshiya I, Tanaka K, Sone S, Sakurai M (1979) Evaluation of the progress and prognosis of adult respiratory distress syndrome. Chest 76:180–186
52. Jardin F, Prost JF, Bazin M, Desfond P, Ozier Y, Margairez A (1982) Modalités évolutives du syndrome de détresse respiratoire aigüe de l'adulte: Valeur pronostique d'un indice de gravité tiré de l'oxygenation artérielle. Nouv Press Med 11:29–33
53. Smith PEM, Gordon IJ (1986) An index to predict outcome in adult respiratory distress syndrome. Intensive Care Med 12:86–89
54. Hickling KG, Henderson SJ, Jackson R (1990) Low mortality associated with low volume pressure limited ventilation with permissive hypercapnia in severe adult respiratory distress syndrome. Intensive Care Med 16:372–377
55. Hickling KG, Walsh J, Henderson S, Jackson R (1994) Low mortality rate in adult respiratory distress syndrome using low-volume, pressure-limited ventilation with permissive hypercapnia: a prospective study. Crit Care Med 22:1568–1578
56. Morel D, Dargent F, Bachmann M, Suter PM, Junot AF (1985) Pulmonary extraction of serotonin and propanolol in patients with ARDS. Am Rev Respir Dis 132:479–484
57. Murray JF, Matthay MA, Luce JM, Flick MR (1988) An expanded definition of the adult respiratory distress syndrome Am Rev Respir Dis 138:720–723
58. Schuster DP (1992) Prediction outcome after ICU admission: The art and science of assessing risk. Chest 102:1861
59. Lemeshow S, Le Gall JR (1994) Modeling the severity of illness of ICU patients: a system update. JAMA 272:1049–1055
60. Lemeshow S, Teres D, Klar J et al (1993) Mortality probability models (MPM II) based on an international cohort of intensive care unit patients. JAMA 270:2478–2486
61. Le Gall JR, Lemeshow S, Saulnier F et al (1993) A new simplified acute physiology score (SAPS II) based on an European/North American multicenter study. JAMA 270:2957–2963

62. Knauss WA, Wagner DP, Drapper ET et al (1991) The APACHE III prognostic system: Risk prediction of hospital mortality for critically ill hospitalized adults. Chest 100:1619–1636
63. Lemeshow S, Klar J, Teres D et al (1994) Mortality probability models for patients in the intensive care unit for 48 or 72 hours: A prospective, multicenter study. Crit Care Med 22: 1351–1358
64. Le Gall JR, Loirat P, Alperovitch A et al (1984) A simplified acute physiology score for ICU patients. Crit Care Med 12:975–977
65. Knaus WA, Zimmerman JE, Wagner DP et al (1981) APACHE – Acute physiology and chronic health evaluation: A physiologically based classification system. Crit Care Med 9: 591–597
66. Knaus WA, Draper EA, Wagner DP et al (1985) APACHE II: A severity of disease classification system. Crit Care Med 13:818–829
67. Knaus WA, Sun X, Hakim RB, Wagner DP (1994) Evaluation of definitions for adult respiratory distress syndrome. Am J Respir Crit Care 150:311–317
68. Le Gall JR, Brun-Buisson C, Trunet P, et al (1982) Influence of age, previous health status and severity of illness on outcome from intensive care. Crit Care Med 10:575–577

Basic Mechanisms of Injury and Response

Cytokines and Lung Injury

P. M. Suter and B. Ricou

Introduction

Among the many groups of mediators involved in the pathogenesis and clinical expression of acute lung injury (ALI) and acute respiratory distress syndrome (ARDS), cytokines occupy a central place. Since the discovery of the role of these substances in inflammatory processes of different types and locations of the human body, a number of experimental and clinical investigations suggest that they play an important role in ARDS.

Leukocyte activation and priming, as well as granulocyte recruitment within the lung, are among the earliest pathophysiological events in ALI, and are at least in part due to the effects of tumor necrosis factor-α (TNF-α), interleukin-1 (IL-1) and IL-8. As a consequence, bronchoalveolar lavage (BAL) fluid from patients with ARDS contains oxidant activity [1] and neutrophil enzymes such as elastase, myeloperoxidase and collagenase [2–5].

The local release of these enzymes which contributes to the marked lung tissue injury characteristic of the disease, appears to be the final step in a cascade of events, apparently triggered by TNF-α [6].

Polymorphonuclear Leukocytes (PMNL)

Indeed, among many other effects, TNF-α *in vivo* induces the production of IL-1α by vascular endothelium [7–9]; it has chemotactic activity from PMNL [10], stimulates PMNL degranulation and leads to increased pulmonary capillary permeability and interstitial edema [11–13]. The gross histopathological damage found in lungs, intestine, kidneys, pancreas and adrenals of TNF-α-treated mice resembles that induced by endotoxemia [14]. These properties in animal studies suggest a prominent role for TNF-α in the pathogenesis of inflammatory reactions, septic shock and ARDS.

The hypothesis that TNF-α could be involved in the pathogenesis of ARDS in man is supported by reports by Millar et al. [15] and Hyers et al. [16] who measured elevated levels of TNF-α in BAL fluid in patients with ARDS. Plasma levels of TNF-α in septic patients developing ARDS were elevated in only 27 out of 74 patients, the highest values being observed in the earliest phases [17, 18]. In patients with Gram-negative sepsis [19–21], bacterial lipopolysaccharide is thought to stimulate TNF-α secretion (Fig. 1). In non-septic ARDS, it is not clear what

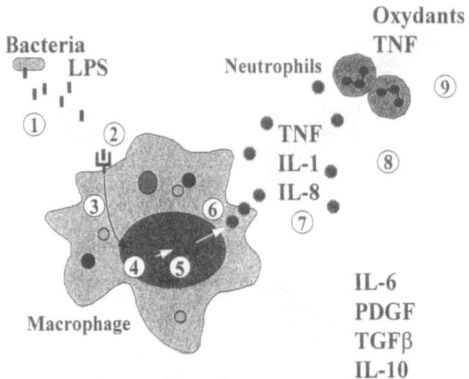

Fig. 1. Different steps of induction of inflammation.
① Microbial invasion, ② Receptor stimulation, ③ Biological cascade, ④ DNA stimulation, ⑤ RNA expression, ⑥ Protein synthesis, ⑦ Protein secretion, ⑧ Chemotaxis of neutrophils, ⑨ Induction of new synthesis by neutrophils.
Abbreviations: IL-1: Interleukin-1 – LPS: Lipopolysaccharide – PDGF: Platelet derived growth factor – TGFβ: Transforming growth factor – TNF: Tumor necrosis factor

triggers the release of this cytokine; a possible responsible mechanism is activation of macrophages by fibrin, leading to increased permeability of pulmonary vascular endothelial cells for albumin [22]. It is not established if systemic or local levels of these mediators are more important in the pathogenesis of this syndrome. In addition, the sequence and relation of mediator and cellular interactions in the development and clinical course of ALI/ARDS in man remains incompletely understood. The distribution of cytokines in ARDS may be very different from that observed in septicemia without ARDS.

TNF-α can be produced by activated pulmonary macrophages. These cells are located in lung interstitium, alveolar space and capillaries in man [23]. There is growing experimental evidence that cytokines bound to cell surfaces operate only at the local level and may be involved in cell-to-cell communication in the remodeling lung [24]. Lung macrophages obtained by BAL from healthy adult volunteers produce much larger quantities of TNF-α on stimulation than blood monocytes [25–27].

Jacobs et al. [28] reported that macrophages obtained by BAL from patients with ARDS release larger amounts of IL-1β than those obtained from patients with pneumonia or from controls. IL-1β can also be produced by epithelial cells [29], and it is possible that bronchial epithelial cells can secrete IL-1β. More recently, Van Nhieu et al. [30] and Donnelly et al. [31] confirmed that alveolar macrophages from patients were actively synthesizing TNF-α or IL-8 *in situ*. In animal models, systemic injection or intratracheal instillation of cytokines induce acute lung inflammation [32,33].

However, the precise role of each cytokine detected in human ARDS is not clear, nor is the sequence of events leading to ALI. Furthermore, through the concept of a cytokine network, more than one responsible molecule must be considered [34]. In addition, the role of natural cytokine inhibitors such as IL-1 receptor antagonist (IL-1ra), soluble IL-1, and TNF-α receptors as well as the anti-inflammatory cytokines such as IL-6, IL-10, or IL-13 in ARDS is still unknown. In animal models however, the possibility of influencing local inflammation by the use of anti-inflammatory cytokines has been reported [33, 35, 36].

At least 3 pro-inflammatory cytokines, namely TNF-α, IL-1 and IL-8, are instrumental in the PMN-microvascular endothelial cell (MVEC) interaction. IL-8, induced by TNF-α, IL-1 or lipopolysaccharide (LPS), is a potent neutrophil chemoattractant and can thus contribute to neutrophil influx during the initial stages of ALI [37], although a variety of other mediators, including leukotrienes, monokines and bacterial products are present in the inflamed lung.

Apart from inducing IL-8, TNF-α and IL-1 can dramatically modify the cell surface molecules of both leukocytes and MVEC. On the one hand, they increase the constitutive expression of intercellular adhesion molecule (ICAM)-1, and trigger the neo-expression of endothelial adhesion molecule (ELAM)-1 on MVEC. On the other, they enhance the expression of one of the recognition sites for ICAM-1, namely the β2 integrins (CD11/CD18 complex), on PMN. Several other modifications occur, which remain to be defined precisely. In addition, there is a high degree of complexity in these interactions, since, for instance, IL-8, in spite of its chemotactic activity on PMN, can cause inhibition of PMN-MVEC adhesion [38]. Finally, platelets and coagulation proteins expressed on MVEC may also modulate the leukocyte-MVEC interactions. The intricacy of these stimulating and inhibiting phenomena warrants further investigations.

Neutrophils are capable of synthesizing cytokines such as TNF-α [39] and produce free oxygen radicals which may enhance production of cytokines such as TNF-α or IL-1β [40]. Lung parenchymal cells are also involved in cytokine release: fibroblasts are able to produce IL-8 [41]; monocytes, macrophages as well as fibroblasts produce transforming growth factor-β (TGF-β) which could play a role in the remodeling process [42]. Moreover, extracellular matrix cell components such as endothelium and fibroblasts have been implicated in the inflammatory reaction observed in ALI/ARDS in rats [43].

Cytokine Network in Early ARDS

BAL fluid in early phases of human ARDS contains increased amounts of TNF-α, IL-1, and IL-8. Alveolar macrophages express the TNF-α gene, suggesting that those cells are synthesizing this cytokine at the site of the acute inflammation [30]. IL-1 has recently been shown to be the major pro-inflammatory agent during the acute phase of ARDS, rather than TNF-α [44]. IL-1 has been associated to higher risk of death in another work, but the ratio IL-1/IL-1ra was not predictive of outcome in this study [45]. The higher level of IL-8 in BAL of patients who subsequently develop ARDS compared to patients who do not, suggests that this chemokine might be a prognostic indicator of the development of ARDS [31]. Moreover, the level of IL-8 associated to the number of neutrophils in BAL samples correlates with the severity of lung injury and mortality [46]. Alveolar macrophage content in IL-8 was also increased in ARDS patients indicating that these cells are actively producing this chemotactic factor inside the alveolar space, and thus are responsible for the recruitment of the BAL neutrophils found in a great number in these subjects [31].

Natural Cytokine Inhibitors

The actions of many cytokines are regulated *in vivo* by their own natural inhibitor: TNF-α by soluble TNF-α receptors (TNF-α sR55 and sR75), IL-1 by IL-1 receptor antagonist (IL-1Ra), IL-1 soluble receptors (IL-1sRI and sRII), IL-6 by IL-6 soluble receptor (IL-6sR). The balance between cytokines and their inhibitors is probably more important than the effect of any single cytokine itself.

Chemoattractant Cytokines

As increased numbers of inflammatory cells are associated with the persistence of ARDS, chemoattractant cytokines were investigated [47]. Neutrophil attractants IL-8 and epithelial cell-derived neutrophil activator-78 (ENA-78) as well as 2 potent monocyte chemoattractants, monocyte chemotactic peptide-1 (MCP-1) and macrophage inflammatory peptide-1a (MIP-1a) were all increased in prolonged ARDS. Moreover, MCP-1 was associated with an increased lung injury score up to 21 days after onset, suggesting that it may be a contributor to the inflammatory process [45].

Pro- and Anti-inflammatory Cytokines

Cytokines can be divided into 2 major groups; the so-called pro-inflammatory cytokines including TNF-α, IL-1, and IL-8, and the anti-inflammatory cytokines including IL-4, IL-10, IL-13.

IL-10 is synthesized by T-cells, B-cells or monocytes and can inhibit the production of pro-inflammatory cytokines from monocytes *in vitro*. By contrast, it stimulates the production of IL-1ra. In an animal model of lung injury induced by instillation of IgG concomitant to an intravenous injection of an antigen, the co-instillation of IL-10 inhibits the development of ALI [35]. More recently, Donnelly and al. [48] demonstrated an association between mortality rates and decreased concentration of IL-10 and IL-1ra in BAL from patients with ARDS. They concluded that failure of localized intrapulmonary anti-inflammatory response early in the pathogenesis of ARDS might contribute to more severe lung injury and worse prognosis. IL-13 is synthesized by T or B cells and can inhibit the production of all the pro-inflammatory cytokines, but also of IL-10 [49].

Growth factors (Fig. 2)

The action of other molecules such as TGF-β and IL-6 are less clear. TGF-α has been shown to possess a dual role in the regulation of cytokine production *in vitro* [50]. In an animal model, TGF-β co-instilled intratracheally with LPS can decrease the amount of TNF-α produced, reduce the number of neutrophils and inhibit the development of lung injury [33]; in another work blocking TGF-β prevented lung injury in hemorrhaged mice, suggesting that this cytokine has potent pro-inflammatory and immunoregulatory properties [51].

Cytokines as Markers of Inflammatory Response

IL-6 is a good marker of inflammation in sepsis and multiple organ failure. However its exact role is not well understood. IL-6 seems to act more as a modulator than as a pro- or anti-inflammatory cytokine. It can inhibit TNF-α or IL-1, and induce synthesis of acute phase proteins. Recent investigations showed that C-reactive protein enhances or inhibits IL-1 and IL-1ra production depending on the cell considered [52].

Adhesion Molecules

Adhesion molecules complicate cellular interactions and influence the effects of cytokines as well as other mediators on inflammatory cells and lung parenchymal cells [53]. For example, ICAM-1 is expressed at various degrees in lung parenchymal cells of animals tracheally instilled with TNF-α or interferon-gamma (IFN-γ). Neutrophil infiltration depends on the density of adhesion molecules induced [54].

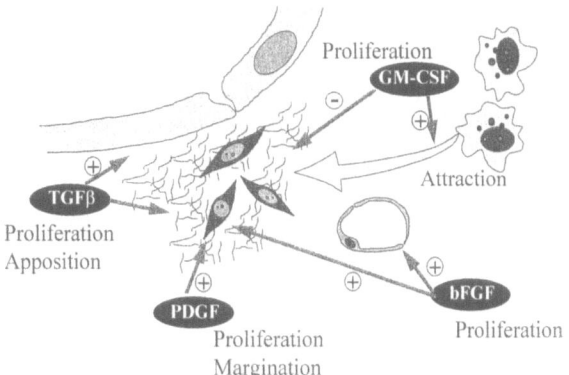

Fig. 2. Schematic representation of lung remodeling. Several factors such as platelet-derived growth factor (PDGF), basic fibroblast growth factor (bFGF), granulocyte-macrophage colony stimulating factor (GM-CSF) and transforming growth factor (TGFβ) modulate proliferation of matrix fibroblasts, endothelial or epithelial cells as well as apposition of extracellular matrix

Other Mediators Interacting with Cytokines

Oxidants

Oxygen free radicals such as $-OH, O_3^-, H_2O_2$ belong to the defense mechanisms of the cells [55]. Neutrophils are the major providers of oxygen metabolites and infiltrate the lung at a very early stage of ALI. However, in the uncontrolled inflammation encountered in ARDS, the original aim of the defense system seems to be surpassed and oxygen metabolites become deleterious to the lung parenchyma itself. Protein, DNA and lipid oxidation result in pulmonary cell injury enhancing the inflammatory process [1]. The usual antioxidant system composed of O_2 scavengers such as superoxide dismutase (SOD), glutathione (GSH) peroxidase or catalase which counterbalances this aggressive double edge sword system is lacking in ARDS [56], while oxidized GSH was shown to be increased in BAL fluid of such patients [57].

Neutrophils submitted to various stimuli, including cytokines, are able to release a huge amount of free radicals which in turn react with the environment. *In vitro*, endothelial cell susceptibility to superoxide and its permeability are increased by TNF-α which induces a decrease in glutathione content [58]. However, TNF-α can also increase the gene expression of manganese SOD, an enzymatic O_2 radical scavenger found in mitochondria, suggesting it has a role in cell protection against oxidant injury [59].

Many cytokines can induce inflammatory cells such as macrophages or parenchymal cells such as endothelial cells, to secrete nitric oxide (NO). The role of NO in modulating oxidative reactions is still unclear, but recent studies provide evidence that NO might play an antioxidant role *in vivo*. NO can reduce the production of superoxide anion by neutrophils via a direct action on NADPH oxidase [60]. Moreover, NO induces production of endothelial antioxidants such as heme-oxygenase, which adds to the evidence of its protective action [61]. In the mesenteric circulation of animals, NO decreases leukocyte adherence [62] and can prevent the increase of microvascular permeability [63]. P-selectin on the surface of endothelial cells is a possible molecular target of NO, since inhibition of NO synthesis by N^G-nitro-L-arginine-methyl ester (L-NAME) increases expression of P-selectin and promotes leukocyte rolling and adherence.

Another interaction of oxidants exists with lipid-derived mediators: Platelet activating factor (PAF) can prime neutrophils for enhanced superoxide production [64].

Lipid Mediators: Leukotrienes (LTB4), eicosanoids (TBX, PGE2, PGI2), and platelet activating factor (PAF).

Arachidonic acid metabolites are involved in the development of ALI/ARDS. Among them LTB4, a leukotriene, is a potent activator of neutrophils and plays a major role in lung injury [65]: inducing lung edema by increasing vascular permeability, enhancing chemotaxism and migration of PMN cells, and participating in the development of pulmonary arterial hypertension by its vasoconstrictive action. These effects are enhanced by PAF, a cell membrane-derived ether lipid produced, not only by inflammatory cells such as macrophages, but also by endothelial and epithelial cells, and fibroblasts [66]. Even small amounts of PAF can induce an ARDS-like lung injury in rats when given in combination with LPS, while it is insufficient to induce any inflammation by itself [67]. In humans, PAF has been shown to be increased in the BAL fluid from ARDS patients and TNF-α enhances PAF production by neutrophils [68].

TNF-α induces release of thromboxane A2 (TBX2), prostaglandin E2 and prostacyclin. Much of its known action takes place through other mediators: The increase of pulmonary capillary pressure has been shown to be mediated by TBX2 and PAF, while its effect on capillary permeability seems to be mediated by PAF only [69]. Inversely, PAF is able to increase the synthesis of TNF-α by B cells in humans [70]. Since inflammatory and tissue cells can all secrete either TNF-α or PAF, it is hard to distinguish which component is primarily responsible for acute inflammation.

As with many mediators, PAF seems to be wearing a 2 face mask: priming neutrophils for enhanced superoxide production and arachidonic acid release during their adhesion to endothelial cells [64], a common feature of lung injury where neutrophils play a major role. By contrast, PAF is present in natural surfactant and was recognized as a necessary molecule in the replacement therapy used in neonatal respiratory distress syndrome because of its physiological effects and is recommended to be added in future synthetic preparations [71].

High frequency oscillatory ventilation prevented the release of PAF and TBX2 and resulted in less lung injury than conventional mechanical ventilation suggesting that not only mediators present at inflammatory sites, but even mechanical factors can influence the course of events [72].

Extracellular Matrix and Cytokines

Extracellular matrix (ECM) is a dynamic lung parenchymal component crucial in maintaining pulmonary structure in order to preserve its primary function. Its components; collagen, fibronectin and proteoglycan, are injured during ALI/ARDS and participate actively to inflammation [73]. Matrix metalloproteinases (MMPs) and their selective inhibitor, the tissue inhibitor of metalloproteinases (TIMP) are significant in maintenance of ECM integrity and participate actively to the remodeling processes in lung injury [74]. Enzymes such as 92 kDa or 72 kDa gelatinases (MMP-9 and MMP-2) are produced by inflammatory cells such as monocytes, macrophages, neutrophils, and connective tissue cells like fibroblasts, and have been found to be increased in several chronic lung diseases such as sarcoidosis and idiopathic pulmonary fibrosis. The MMPs, 92 kDa gelatinase and its specific inhibitor TIMP-1 have recently been found to be increased in BAL from ARDS patients [75]. Their levels were higher than in controls, suggesting an important role in the development and course of lung injury. Moreover, the balance between the 92 kDa gelatinase and TIMP seemed more relevant than their absolute amount *per se*. More recently, we looked at the early phase of patients with ARDS and found that MMP-2 and MMP-9 were both increased in BAL fluid from ARDS patients, but to a lesser extent in patients who did not develop the syndrome, although they had the same risk factors [76].

Cytokines and Metalloproteinases

From studies on ECM, we learned that the effects of typical inflammatory factors such as cytokines are probably entertained by other mediators. Indeed, when looking at the time course of the pro-inflammatory cytokines such as TNF-α, IL-1, or IL-8 *in vitro*, their action decreases in a few hours, whilst in patients, inflammation is ongoing for days. Moreover, not only inflammatory cells but such as fibroblasts, epithelial cells or endothelial cell constituents of the lung parenchyma also play a role in the acute inflammatory reaction. The extracellular matrix can influence the production of cytokines. Indeed, macrophage capacity for production of IL-1 and IL-6 differs depending on the material upon which they are cultured. A fibroblast-induced extracellular matrix seems to enhance cytokine production in response to LPS, whilst inert materials such as plastic or collagen decrease the cell reactivity [77]. These results suggest that a complex regulation coordinates action of these MMPs which could result in degradation of ECM or fibroproliferation.

Activities of MMPs can be modulated by cytokines such as TNF-α, TGF-β or IL-6. IL-6 is known to induce the production of TIMP *in vitro*, which would favor the inhibition of lytic events; whether this inhibition equals fibrin apposition and fibroproliferation is not known [78]. IL-4 or IFN-γ can suppress the metalloproteinase biosynthesis in human alveolar macrophages [79, 80]; their effect *in vivo* has not been investigated so far.

MMPs, as key factors of ECM remodeling, might be of major interest in the late phase of ARDS. Interactions between these enzymes and cytokines in late ARDS has not been reported. The question of whether MMPs play a role in the resolution of lung inflammation at this stage or influence the occurrence of fibrosis should be addressed.

Metalloproteinase activities are not only modulated locally by the presence of their antagonist TIMP, but their action must be initiated by positive stimulation. Indeed, a number of factors such as elastase, cathepsin or enzymes of the coagulation cascade are able to cut the proforms of MMPs to render them active [74].

Recent reports suggest that levels of type-III procollagen peptide [81] are increased in BAL fluid of patients with ARDS and that their levels correlated with increased risk of death. This peptide results from the cleavage of procollagen to collagen and reflects the ongoing remodeling processes of lung parenchyma. These findings suggest that the components of extracellular matrix, such as fibroblasts and smooth muscular cells not only represent an inert scaffolding of the parenchyma but are implicated actively in lung inflammation occurring in ARDS.

In an animal study, PAF induced the gene expression of MMPs at corneal epithelium [82]. PAF can thus play a role not only in acute inflammation but may participate in the remodeling mechanisms.

Hyperoxic exposure of murine lungs increased expression of TIMP, which suggests that oxidative reactions may influence ECM remodeling [83].

Therapeutic Implications

Anti-cytokines

Since TNF-α and IL-1 seem to play an important role in the development of ALI, theoretical benefits might be expected from their antagonism. However, *post hoc* analysis of large multicentric trials with TNF-α antibodies did not report any beneficial effect of those antagonists in preventing the occurrence of ARDS, nor any reduction in mortality of the septic patients investigated. In an unconfirmed study using IL-1ra, the mortality of patients with septic shock and ARDS was decreased [84].

Small animal studies have shown a positive effect of antagonizing the effects of LPS by the anti-inflammatory cytokines IL-10, IL-13 or TGF-β [33, 35, 49]. However, more understanding of the complex interactions between all those mediators seems necessary before undertaking rigorous investigations in human ARDS.

Conclusion

Cytokines seem to play an important role in the complex inflammatory reaction that characterizes ALI/ARDS. However, the importance of initial lung damage, the clinical course and the resolution of injury depend on a network of pro- and anti-inflammatory cytokines and their inhibitors, as well as the interaction with a variety of other mediators. It is more and more recognized that not only leukocytes, but also vascular endothelial cells, alveolar epithelial and pulmonary interstitial cells participate actively in the production, release, inactivation and metabolism of cytokines. Finally, therapeutic interventions aiming at modulating the inflammatory reaction are not ready for clinical use and may be markedly less efficient than physiological autoregulatory mechanisms.

References

1. Cochrane CG, Spragg R, Revak SD (1983) Pathogenesis of the adult respiratory distress syndrome. Evidence of oxidant activity in bronchoalveolar lavage fluid. J Clin Invest 71: 754–761
2. Weiland JE, Davis WB, Holter JF, Mohammed JR, Dorinsky PM, Gadek JE (1986) Lung neutrophil in the adult respiratory distress syndrome. Clinical and pathophysiological significance. Am Rev Respir Dis 133:218–225

3. Lee CT, Fein AM, Lippman M, Holtzman H, Kimbel P, Weinbaum G (1981) Elastolytic activity in pulmonary lavage fluid from patients with adult respiratory distress syndrome. N Engl J Med 304:192–196.

4. Mc Guire WW, Spragg RC, Cohen AB, Cochrane GG (1982) Studies on the pathogenesis of the adult respiratory distress syndrome. J Clin Invest 69:543–553

5. Idell S, Kucich U, Fein A, (1985) Neutrophil elastase-releasing factors in bronchoalveolar lavage from patients with adult respiratory distress syndrome. Am Rev Respir Dis 132:1098–1105

6. Tracey KJ, Lowry SF, Cerami A (1988) Cachetin/TNF-α in septic shock and septic adult respiratory distress syndrome. Am Rev Respir Dis 138:1377–1379

7. Pober JS (1988) Cytokine-mediated activation of vascular endothelium. Physiology and pathology. Am J Pathol 133:426–433

8. Libby P, Ordovas JM, Auger KR, Robbins AH, Biriyi LK, Dinarello CA (1986) Endotoxin and tumor necrosis factor induce interleukin-1 gene expression in adult human vascular endothelial cells. J Pathol 124:179–185

9. Nawroth PP, Bank I, Handley D, Cassimeris J, Chess L, Stern D (1986) Tumor necrosis factor/cachectin interacts with endothelial cell receptors to induce release of interleukin 1. J Exp Med 163:1363–1375

10. Harmsen AG, Havell EA (1990) Roles of tumor necrosis factor and macrophages in lipopolysaccharide-induced accumulation of neutrophils in cutaneous air pouches. Infect Immun 58:297–302

11. Stephens KE, Ishizaka A; Larrick JW, Raffin TA (1988) Tumor necrosis factor causes increased pulmonary permeability and edema. Comparison to septic acute lung injury. Am Rev Respir Dis 137:1364–1370

12. Moser R, Schleiffenbaum B, Groscurth P, Fehr J (1989) Interleukin 1 and tumor necrosis factor stimulate human vascular endothelial cells to promote transendothelial neutrophil passage. J Clin Invest 83:444–455

13. Goldblum SE, Sun WL (1990) Tumor necrosis factor-α augments pulmonary arterial transendothelial albumin flux in vitro. Am J Physiol (Lung Cell Mol Physiol) 2:L57–L67

14. Tracey KJ, Beutler B, Lowry SF, et al (1986) Shock and tissue injury induced by recombinant human cachectin. Science 234:470–474

15. Millar AB, Foley NM, Singer M, Johnson McI, Meager A, Rook GAW (1989) Tumour necrosis factor in bronchopulmonary secretions of patients with adult respiratory distress syndrome. Lancet 2:712–724

16. Hyers TM, Tricomi SM, Dettenmeier PA, Fowler AA (1991) Tumor necrosis factor levels in serum and bronchoalveolar lavage fluid of patients with the adult respiratory distress syndrome. Am Rev Respir Dis 144:268–271

17. Marks JD, Berman Marks C, Luce JM et al (1990) Plasma tumor necrosis factor in patients with septic shock. Mortality rate, incidence of adult respiratory distress syndrome, and effects of methylprednisolone administration. Am Rev Respir Dis 141:94–97

18. Roten R, Markert M, Feihl F, Schaller MD, Tagan MC, Perret C (1991) Plasma levels of tumor necrosis factor in the adult respiratory distress syndrome. Am Rev Respir Dis 143:590–592

19. Calandra T, Baumgartner JD, Grau GE et al (1990) and the Swiss-Dutch J5 group. Kinetics and prognostic values of tumor necrosis factor, IL-1, IFN-α and IFN-γ in the serum of patients with septic shock. J Infect Dis 161:982–987

20. Girardin E, Grau GE, Dayer JM, Roux-Lombard P, The J5 study group, Lambert PH (1988) Tumor necrosis factor and interleukin-1 in the serum of children with severe infectious purpura. N Engl J Med 319:397–400

21. Waage A, Halstensen A, Espevik T (1987) Association between tumour necrosis factor in serum and fatal outcome in patients with meningococcal disease. Lancet 1:335–357

22. Ferro TJ, Lynch JJ, Malik AB (1989) Macrophages activated by fibrin increase albumin permeability across pulmonary artery endothelial monolayers. Am Rev Respir Dis 139:940–945

23. Dehring DJ, Wismar BL (1989) Intravascular macrophages in pulmonary capillaries of humans. Am Rev Respir Dis 139:1027–1029

24. Kelley J (1990) Cytokines of the lung (State of the art). Am Rev Respir Dis 141:765–788

25. Strieter RM, Remick DG, Lynch JP III, et al (1989) Differential regulation of tumor necrosis factor-α in human alveolar macrophages and peripheral blood monocytes: A cellular and molecular analysis. Am J Respir Cell Mol Biol 1:57–63

26. Rich EA, Panuska JR, Wallis RS, Wolf CB, Leonard ML, Ellner JJ (1989) Dyscoordinate expression of tumor necrosis factor-α by human blood monocytes and alveolar macrophages. Am Rev Respir Dis 139:1010–1016

27. Martinet Y, Yamauchi K, Crystal RG (1988) Differential expression of the tumor necrosis factor/cachectin gene by blood and lung mononuclear phagocytes. Am Rev Respir Dis 138:650–665

28. Jacobs RF, Tabor DR, Burks AW, Campbell GD (1989) Elevated interleukin-1 release by human alveolar macrophages during the adult respiratory distress syndrome. Am Rev Respir Dis 140:1686–1692

29. Tracey KJ, Lowry SF, Cerami A (1988) Cachectin: A hormone that triggers acute shock and chronic cachexia. J Infect Dis 157:413–420

30. Tran Van Nhieu J, Misset B, Lebargy F, Carlet J, Bernaudin JF (1993) Expression of tumor necrosis factor-alpha gene in alveolar macrophages from patients with the adult respiratory distress syndrome. Am Rev Respir Dis 147:1585–1589

31. Donnelly SC, Strieter RM, Kunkel SL, (1993) Interleukin-8 and development of adult distress syndrome in at risk patient groups. Lancet 341:643–647

32. Okusawa S; Gelfand JA, Ikejima T, Connolly RJ, Dinarello CA (1988) Interleukin 1 induces a shock-like state in rabbits. Synergism with tumor necrosis factor and the effects of cyclooxygenase inhibition. J Clin Invest 81:1162–1172

33. Ulich TR, Yin S, Guo K, Yi ES, Remick D, Del Castillo J (1991) Intratracheal injection of endotoxin and cytokines. II. Interleukin-6 and transforming growth factor-β inhibit acute inflammation. Am J Pathol 138:1097–1101

34. Xing Z, Jordana M, Kirpalani H, Driscoll KE, Schall TJ, Gauldie J (1994) Cytokine expression by neutrophils and macrophages in vivo: Endotoxin induces necrosis factor-α, macrophage inflammatory protein 2, IL-1β and IL-6 but not RANTES or TGF-β1 mRNA expression in acute lung inflammation. Am J Respir Cell Mol Biol 10:148–153

35. Mulligan MS, Jones ML, Vaporciyan AA, Howard MC, Ward PA (1993) Protective effects of IL-4 and IL-10 against immune complex-induced lung injury. J Immunol 151:5666–5674

36. De Waal Malefyt R, Abrams J, Bennett B, Figdor CG, De Vries JE (1991) Interleukin 10 (IL-10) inhibits cytokine synthesis by human monocytes: An autoregulatory role of IL-10 produced by monocytes. J Exp Med 174:1209–1220

37. Kunkel SL, Standiford T, Kasahara K, Strieter RM (1991) Interleukin-8 (Il-8) – The major neutrophil chemotactic factor in the lung. Exp Lung Res 17:17–23

38. Gimbrone MA, Obin MS, Brock AF, et al (1989) Endothelial interleukin-8. A novel inhibitor of leukocyte-endothelial interactions. Science 246:1601–1603

39. Xing Z, Kirpalani H, Torry D, Jordana M, Gauldie J (1993) Polymorphonuclear leucocytes as a significant source of tumor necrosis factor-α in endotoxin challenged lung tissue. Am J Pathol 143:1009–1015

40. Schwartz MD, Repine JE, Abraham E (1995) Hemorrhagic shock and ARDS: Blood loss rapidly induces pulmonary cytokine expression through an oxygen-radical dependent mechanism. Crit Care Med 23:A110 (Abst)

41. Standiford TJ, Kunkel SL, Phan SH, Rollins BJ, Strieter RM (1991) Alveolar macrophage-derived cytokines induce monocyte chemoattractant protein-1 expression from human pulmonary type II like epithelial cells. J Biol Chem 266:9912–9918

42. Roberts AB, Sporn MB (1989) Regulation of endothelial cell growth, architecture, and matrix synthesis by TGF-β. Am Rev Respir Dis 140:1126–1128

43. Xing Z, Jordana M, Gauldie J (1992) IL-1β and IL-6 gene expression in alveolar macrophages: Modulation by extracellular matrices. Am J Physiol 262:L600–L605

44. Pugin J, Ricou B, Steinberg KP, Suter PM, Martin TR (1996) Proinflammatory activity in bronchoalveolar lavage fluid from ARDS patients: A prominent role for interleukin-1. Am J Respir Crit Care Med 153:1850–1856

45. Goodman RB, Strieter RM, Martin DP, et al (1996) Inflammatory cytokines in patients with presistence of the acute respiratory distress syndrome. Am J Respir Crit Care Med 154:602–611

46. Miller EJ, Cohen AB, Nagao S, et al (1992) Elevated levels of NAP-1/Interleukin-8 are present in the airspaces of patients with the ARDS and are associated with increased mortality. Am Rev Respir Dis 146:427–432

47. Strieter RM, Zank K, Phan SH, Standiford TJ, Lukacs NW, Kunkel SL (1995) A role for C-C chemokines in fibrotic lung disease. L Leukoc Biol 57:782–787

48. Donnelly SC, Strieter RM, Reid PT, et al (1996) The association between mortality rates and decreased concentrations of interleukin-10 and interleukin-1 receptor antagonist in the lung fluids of patients with the adult respiratory distress syndrome. Ann Intern Med 125: 191–196

49. De Waal Malefyt R, Figdor CG, Huijbens R, et al (1993) Effects of IL-13 on phenotype, cytokine production, and cytotoxic function of human monocytes. J Immunol 151:6370–6381

50. Chantry D, Turner M, Abney E, Feldmann M (1989) Modulation of cytokine production by transforming growth factor-β. J Immunol 142:4295–4300

51. Shenkar R, Coulson WF, Abraham E (1994) Anti-transforming growth factor-β monoclonal antibodies prevent lung injury in hemorrhaged mice. Am J Respir Cell Mol Biol 11:351–357

52. Pue CA, Mortensen RF, Marsh CB, Pope HA, Wewers MD (1996) Acute phase levels of C-reactive protein enhance IL-1β and IL-1ra production by human blood monocytes but inhibit IL-1β and IL-1ra production by alveolar macrophages. J Immunol 156:1494–1600

53. Dayer JM, Isler P, Nicod LP (1993) Adhesion molecules and cytokine production. Am Rev Respir Dis 148 (Suppl S):S70–S74

54. Kang BH, Manderschied BD, Huang YCT, Crapo JD, Chang LY (1996) Contrasting response of lung parenchymal cells to instilled TNF-α and IFN-γ: The inducibility of specific cell ICAM-1 *in vivo*. Am J Respir Cell Mol Biol 15:540–550

55. Heffner JE, Repine JE (1989) Pulmonary strategies of antioxidant defense. Am Rev Respir Dis 140:531–554

56. Pacht ER, Timerman AP, Lykens MG, Merola AJ (1991) Deficiency of alveolar fluid glutathione in patients with sepsis and the adult respiratory distress syndrome. Chest 100: 1397–1403

57. Bunnell E, Pacht ER (1993) Oxidized glutathione is increased in the alveolar fluid of patients with the adult respiratory distress syndrome. Am Rev Respir Dis 148:1174–1178

58. Ishii Y, Partridge CA, Del Vecchio PJ, Malik AB (1992) Tumor necrosis factor-α mediated decrease in glutathione increases the sensitivity of pulmonary vascular endothelial cells to H_2O_2. J Clin Invest 89:794–802

59. Warner BB, Burhans MS, Clark JC, Wispé JR (1991) Tumor necrosis factor-α increases Mn-SOD expression: Protection against oxidant injury. Am J Physiol 260:L296–L301

60. Clancy RM, Leszczynska-Piziak J, Abramson SB (1992) Nitric oxide, an endothelial cell relaxation factor, inhibits neutrophil superoxide anion production via a direct anion on the NADPH oxidase. J Clin Invest 90:1116–1121

61. Motterlini R, Foresti R, Intaglietta M, Winslow RM (1996) NO-mediated activation of heme oxygenase: Endogenous cytoprotection against oxidative stress to endothelium. Am J Physiol 270 (Heart Circ Physiol 39):H107–H114

62. Kubes P, Suzuki M, Granger DN (1991) Nitric oxide: An endogenous modulator of leukocyte adhesion. Proc Natl Acad Sci USA 88:4651–4655

63. Kubes P, Granger DN (1992) Nitric oxide modulates microvascular permeability. Am J Physiol 262 (Heart Circ Physiol 31):H611–H615

64. Hill ME, Bird IN, Daniels RH, Elmore MA, Finnen MJ (1994) Endothelial cell-associated platelet-activating factor primes neutrophils for enhanced superoxide production and arachidonic acid release during adhesion to but no transmigration across IL-1β-treated endothelial monolyers. J Immunol 153:3673–3683

65. Gadaleta D, Davis JM (1994) Pulmonary failure and the production of leukotrienes. J Am Coll Surg 178:309–319

66. Henson PM, Barnes PJ, Banks-Schlegel SP (1992) Platelet-activation factor: Role in pulmonary injury and dysfunction and blood abnormalities. Am Rev Respir Dis 145:726–731

67. Rabinovici R, Bugelski PJ, Esser KM, Hillegass LM, Vernick J, Feuerstein G (1993) ARDS-like lung injury produced by endotoxin in platelet-activating factor-primat rats. J Appl Physiol 74:1791–1802

68. Matsumoto K, Taki F, Kondoh Y, Taniguchi H, Takagi K (1992) Platelet-activating factor in bronchoalveolar lavage fluid of patients with adult respiratory distress syndrome. Clin Exp Pharmacol Physiol 19:509–515
69. Hocking DC, Phillips PG, Ferro TJ, Johnson A (1990) Mechanisms of pulmonary edema induced by tumor necrosis factor-α. Circulation Research 67:68–77
70. Smith CS, Parker L, Shearer WT (1994) Cytokine regulation by platelet activating factor in a human B cell line. J Immunol 153:3997–4005
71. Moya FR, Hoffman DR, Zhao B, Johston JM (1993) Platelet activating factor in surfactant preparations. Lancet 341:858–860
72. Imai Y, Kawano T, Miyasaka K, Takata M, Imai T, Okuyama K (1994) Inflammatory chemical mediators during conventional ventilation and during high frequency oscillatory ventilation. Am J Respir Crit Car Med 150:1550–1554
73. Campbell EJ, Senior RM, Welgus HG (1987) Extracellular matrix injury during lung inflammation. Chest 92:161–167
74. Woessner JF Jr (1991) Matrix metalloproteinases and their inhibitors in connective tissue remodeling. FASEB J 5:2145–2154
75. Ricou B, Nicod L, Lacraz S, Welgus HG, Suter PM, Dayer JM (1996) Matrix metalloproteinases and TIMP in acute respiratory distress syndrome (ARDS). Am J Respir Crit Care Med 154:346–352
76. Kossodo S, Gasche Y, Ricou B, et al (1997) Do BAL fluid levels of metalloproteinases predict the development of ARDS? Am J Respir Crit Care Med (In press)
77. Perez RL, Roman J (1995) Fibrin enhances the expression of IL-1β by human peripheral blood mononuclear cells. Implications in pulmonary inflammation. J Immunol 154:1879–1887
78. Lotz M, Guerne PA (1991) Interleukin-6 induces the synthesis of tissue inhibitor of metalloproteinases-1/erythroid potentiating activity (TIMP-1/EPA). J Biol Chem 266:2017–2020
79. Lacraz S, Nicol L, Galve-de Rochemonteix B, Baumberger Ch, Dayer JM, Welgus HG (1992) Suppression of metalloproteinase biosynthesis in human alveolar macrophages by interleukin-4. J Clin Invest 90:383–388
80. Shapiro SD, Campbell EJ, Kobayashi DK, Welgus HG (1990) Immune modulation of metalloproteinase production in human macrophages. Selective pretranslational suppression of interstitial collagenase and stromelysin biosynthesis by interferon-γ. J Clin Invest 86:1204–1210
81. Clark JG, Milberg JA, Steinberg KP, Hudson LD (1995) Type III procollagen peptide in the adult respiratory distress syndrome. Association of increased peptide levels in bronchoalveolar lavage fluid with increased risk for death. Ann Intern Med 122:17–23
82. Tai Y, Bazan HE, Bazan NG (1995) Platelet activating factor induces the expression of metalloproteinases-1 and -9, but not -2 or -3, in the corneal epithelium. Invest Ophtalmol Vis Sci 36:345–354
83. Piedboeuf B, Johnston CJ, Watkins RH, et al (1994) Increased expressionof tissue inhibitor of metalloproteinases (TIMP-I) and metallothionine in murine lungs after hyperoxic exposure. Am J Respir Cell Mol Biol 10:123–132
84. Fisher CJ, Dhainaut JFA, Opal SM, et al (1994) for the phase III rhIL-1ra sepsis syndrome study group. Recombinant human interleukin 1 receptor antagonist in the treatment of patients with sepsis syndrome. Results from a randomised, double-blind, placebo-controlled trial. JAMA 271:1836–1843

Complement and Endotoxin in Lung Injury

K. E. Greene and P. E. Parsons

Introduction

The acute respiratory distress syndrome (ARDS) is characterized by progressive hypoxemia, decreased pulmonary compliance, and roentgenographic evidence of diffuse pulmonary infiltrates. The mechanisms that initiate, and then perpetuate the lung inflammation seen in ARDS remain poorly understood. Initially the syndrome was thought to involve only the lungs and to be the result of a single process; activation of the complement cascade. Subsequent investigations have shown that the injury is neither limited to the lungs nor is the pathogenesis simple. Neutrophil sequestration and migration within the lung remain histologic hallmarks of ARDS. It is likely that neutrophil recruitment and subsequent retention are the result of both chemotactic stimuli released within the lungs and activation of neutrophils by circulating mediators. Both complement components and lipopolysaccharide (LPS), a major component of the outer membrane of Gram-negative bacteria, have been implicated as important agents in the induction of ARDS.

Complement

The Complement Cascade

More than 25 proteins make up the complement system, and several of these have the potential to substantially contribute to ARDS. The first component of potential interest is C3. As shown in Fig. 1, cleavage of C3 occurs with activation of both the classical and alternative pathways. One of the resultant products, C3a, is effectively an anaphylatoxin which stimulates histamine release and thereby increases both vascular permeability and smooth muscle contraction. C3b, another product of the cleavage of C3, can bind to C3 convertase enzymes, generating C5 convertase which cleaves C5a and C5b from C5. C5a is a potent stimulus which could enhance neutrophil-mediated injury via chemotaxis, adherence, and the release of potentially injurious mediators including oxidants, proteases and arachidonate metabolites [1]. C5b sequentially binds to C6, C7, C8 and C9 to form the terminal membrane attach complex, C5b-9. This terminal complex creates pores in cell membranes which could contribute to lung permeability, and the complex may stimulate the release of oxidants from neutrophils further aggravat-

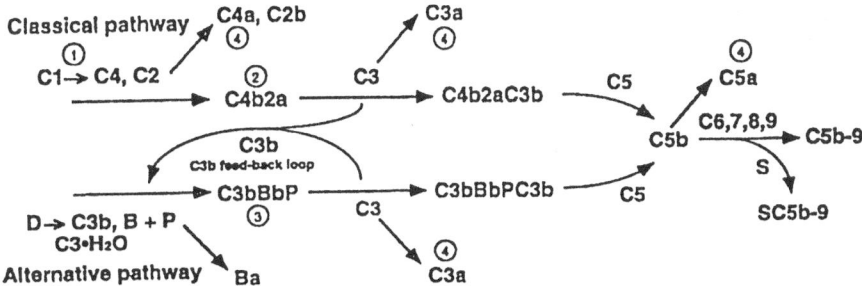

Fig. 1. This diagram illustrates the classical and alternative activation pathways of the human complement system, showing where some of the biologically active split products are produced. The numbered points indicated where the control proteins influence activation: 1, C1–INH binds to the active enzyme forms of C1r and C1s, removing them from the circulation and blocking further cleavage of C4 and C2; 2, C4bp binds to C4b, causing dissociation of the C4b2a enzyme complex, and I cleaves C4b to form iC4b, C4c, and C4d inactive fragments; 3, H binds to C3b causing dissociation of the C3bBb enzyme complex (P prevents H binding), and I cleaves C3b to form iC3b, C3c, and C3dg, 4, anaphylatoxin inactivator cleaves the C-terminal arginine from C3a, C4a, and C5a. (From [73] with permission)

ing injury [2]. Another component of the system which is important to consider in ARDS is complement receptor type 1 (CR1). CR1 can inhibit both the classical and alternative pathways by increasing the rate of decay or destruction of both C3 and C5 convertases and could, therefore, be a potentially important modulator of inflammation. Although many of the other complement components shown in Fig. 1 could contribute, their role has been less extensively studied in ARDS and they will not be discussed here.

Complement Components in ARDS

One of the first hypotheses generated to explain the pathogenesis of ARDS was that complement components activated neutrophils. This hypothesis was generated from observations made from patients undergoing hemodialysis. Early investigators noted that during the initiation of hemodialysis, patients developed transient pulmonary dysfunction in concert with complement-mediated neutropenia and increased neutrophil sequestration within the lung [3, 4]. A series of animal experiments provided further support for this hypothesis. Varying degrees of lung injury could be induced by the infusion of activated complement fragments in sheep [3], the intravascular activation of complement in rats [5], and the infusion of C5a into rabbits [6]. However, in the rabbit model, although neutrophils were retained within the lung microvasculature in response to the infusion of C5a, pulmonary vascular permeability did not increase unless the animal was exposed to a second insult. By contrast, in mice specifically deficient in C5, lung injury induced by pneumococcal sepsis, burns and hyperoxia was significantly attenuated [7–9]. Furthermore, the administration of antibodies to C5a decreased mortality in baboons with Gram-negative sepsis [10] and pretreatment with CR1 abrogated lung injury in rats with Gram-negative infections. [11]. These, and other studies, strongly suggested that complement activation was an important component of the inflammatory process which leads to the development of ARDS. However, they also suggested that other mediators of inflammation needed to be identified and considered.

Defining the role of complement activation in patients with ARDS has been complex. Early studies which relied on bioassays for the determination of complement activity found a strong association between complement activation and the development of ARDS in patients at risk for the syndrome [12]. However, when immunoassays for specific complement components became available, the association was less clear in that some studies again found an apparent relationship [13, 14], whereas others found that circulating levels of activated components of complement did not differentiate those patients at risk who did and did not develop ARDS [15, 16]. In fact, in one study in which multiple complement components were simultaneously measured in patients at risk, there was evidence that complement activation had occurred in 99% of those patients and in 100% of patients with ARDS [16]. Again, like the animal studies, these data suggested that complement activation should be considered in the pathogenesis of ARDS, but that further investigation into additional mediators of inflammation was necessary.

Endotoxin

Endotoxin was recognized as a potentially important mediator in the pathogenesis of ARDS in 1974 when the infusion of *Pseudomonas* into sheep was shown to produce increased pulmonary permeability [17]. Thereafter, it was found that infusion of *E. coli* endotoxin in sheep produced a similar picture of non-cardiogenic pulmonary dysfunction [18]. These observations led to the hypothesis that endotoxin, perhaps in addition to complement activation, was an important mediator in the development of lung injury.

Endotoxin is the LPS component of the cell walls of Gram-negative bacteria. It is comprised of three major components: an oligosaccharide chain (O antigen) which is species specific; a core polysaccharide; and the lipid A region which anchors the complex to the cell. The lipid A region accounts for the majority of the biologic activity of endotoxin. Unlike the O antigen, the core lipid A complex is virtually identical antigenically for all Gram-negative bacteria and therefore, not species-specific. LPS has numerous effects which could contribute to the pathogenesis of lung injury.

The Mechanism of LPS Effects

Recent studies have established that LPS triggers inflammatory responses by interacting with specific host proteins that initiate cytokine production. There is an "endotoxin paradox" when the *in vitro* effects of endotoxin are compared to the *in vivo* effects. In the absence of serum, relatively high concentrations of LPS are required to stimulate macrophages to secrete cytokines. By contrast, in the presence of serum, nannogram amounts of LPS activate macrophages.

LPS-binding Protein

Studies by Tobias and Ulevitch in the 1980's [19, 20] demonstrated that during acute-phase responses, endotoxin is bound by a plasma protein which they isolated and named LPS-binding protein (LBP). Experiments by Schumann and colleagues [21] demonstrated that when rabbit blood was immunodepleted of LBP prior to adding endotoxin, the endotoxin dose response for TNF-α production was shifted dramatically to the right. These data suggested that LBP might account for the differences between endotoxin dose responses in the presence and absence of serum. LBP enhances several LPS-stimulated responses which could contribute to ARDS, including up-regulation of CD18 [22], an adherence glycoprotein on neutrophils, the adherence of neutrophils [23], and the production of TNF-α from alveolar macrophages [20].

CD14 Receptor

LPS/LBP complexes interact with a specific cell surface receptor that has been identified as CD14. The model for LPS/LBP/CD14 interactions on monocytes and macrophages is shown in Fig. 2. CD14, originally found as a cell surface marker for differentiation of myelomonocytic cells, is expressed by monocytes, macrophages, granulocytes and non-myeloid cells as a 55 kDa membrane protein. The biological function of CD14 was not known until it was suggested that membrane bound CD14 (mCD14) was a "receptor" for LPS stimulation of leukocyte production of inflammatory cytokines such as TNF-α [24]. However, the status of mCD14 has now changed to an LPS acceptor since binding of LPS to mCD14 does not transduce the LPS signal in 70Z/3 cells [25], and mCD14 is not required for LPS to exert its activity [26, 27].

Soluble CD14

CD14 and other glycosyl-phosphatidylinosoitol-linked surface proteins are shed from cell membranes and circulate in plasma. Soluble CD14 (sCD14) can interact with circulating LPS/LBP complexes and confer LPS responsiveness to cells such as endothelial cells, that normally lack surface CD14 [28]. In order to understand the participation of sCD14 in endothelial cell activation by LPS, Zhang et al [29] examined sCD14 binding to human umbilical vein endothelial cells (HUVEC), which do not express mCD14. These authors demonstrated that sCD14 binding was inhibited by anti-human CD14 mAbs UCHM-1 and RM052, and that inhibiting sCD14-receptor binding also blocked the potentiation of LPS activity by

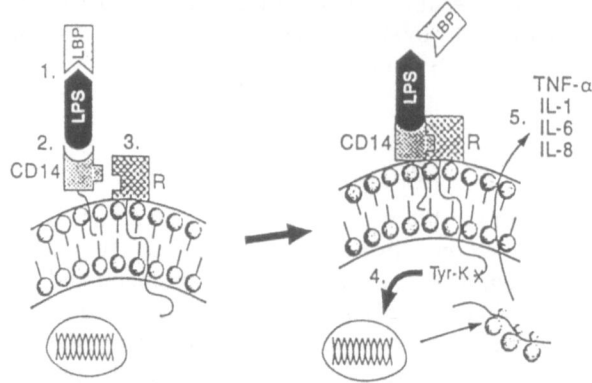

Fig. 2. Model for LPS/LBP/CD14 interactions on monocytes and macrophages. 1) LPS in solution interacts with circulating LBP. 2) The LPS-LBP complex interacts with CD14 on the cell surface. 3) This complex may associate with a second, yet unidentified protein on the cell surface, which results in the transmission of intracellular signals that involve tyrosine phosphorylation reactions 4) & 5). This results in the transcription of cytokine genes and the secretion of the mature cytokine proteins. (From [49] with permission)

sCD14 in these cells. The authors proposed that bridging or crosslinking between the putative LPS-receptor complex with the sCD14-acceptor complex via LPS-sCD14 interactions was the mechanisms of CD14-dependent activation of endothelial cells, and that this mechanism might also apply to leukocytes and lymphocytes. Clearly, the concepts outlined in Fig. 2 are in evolution. There is also evidence that suggests sCD14 can be protective [30], reducing cytokine secretion in whole blood.

Although the exact mechanism by which LPS/LBP complexes interact with CD14 to trigger intracellular responses to LPS is unknown, there is good evidence that this pathway is highly relevant to the lung. Martin and colleagues [31] have demonstrated that that the LPS-LBP-CD14 pathway is crucial to the interaction of LPS with cells in the lungs, and they have recently reported that CD14-dependent mechanisms may contribute to pulmonary inflammation in patients with ARDS [32]. These authors reported significantly increased levels of LBP and sCD14 in broncho-alveolar lavage (BAL) fluid of patient with ARDS. They went on to show that BAL sCD14 is strongly related to total protein; and polymorphonuclear (PMN) concentration, major indices of lung inflammation.

LPS and Neutrophils

There is evidence in humans and animal models that neutrophils can participate in the initiation and propagation of lung injury [33–36]. High neutrophil counts in BAL are associated with more severe lung dysfunction [37]; moreover, the magnitude of this increase is associated with mortality, particularly in patients with the sepsis syndrome [38]. The process that eventually leads to the accumulation of neutrophils within the alveolar airspace includes recruitment and retention of neutrophils within the lung, migration of neutrophils through the vascular endothelium and the alveolar epithelium, and the release of toxic mediators. There is evidence that endotoxin affects all of these processes.

Neutrophil Priming. In the systemic circulation, endotoxin activates complement, and both primes and stimulates neutrophils as well as monocytes. The priming of neutrophils is potentially an extremely important phenomenon in ARDS. Exposure to nannogram concentrations of endotoxin does not cause apparent neutrophil activation, but if they are then exposed to a second stimulus the responsiveness is significantly increased (Fig. 3). Cells can be primed for secretory, adherence, and synthetic responses. Numerous stimuli can serve as the secondary stimulus, but those frequently used *in vitro* include complement fragments, specifically C5a, and formyl-methionyl-leucyl-phenylalanine (FMLP) [39]. In both isolated perfused lungs and intact rabbit models [40, 41], LPS priming of neutrophils has been shown to contribute to lung injury. The data in patients is less conclusive. As discussed previously, C5a itself is present in many patients at risk

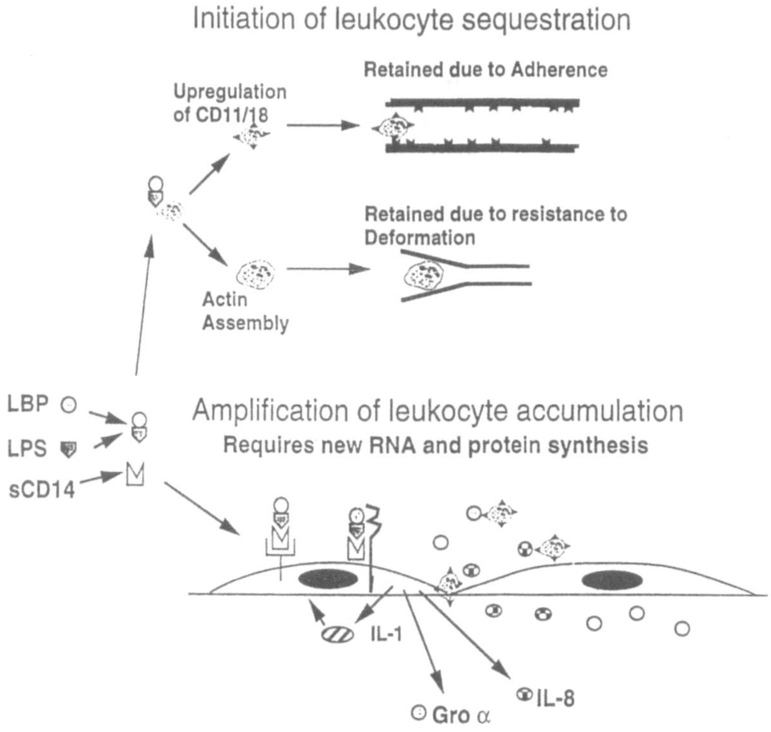

Fig. 3. This diagram outlines the effects of LPS on 1) the initiation of leukocyte sequestration by up-regulating adhesion glycoproteins CD11/18 and inducing actin assembly; and 2) the amplification of leukocyte accumulation by stimulating IL-1, IL-8 and Gro-a. (From Scott Worthen MD with permission)

for and with ARDS [15] and some evidence of complement activation is present in virtually all critically ill patients [16]. Endotoxin is also present in the circulation in patients at risk for ARDS [42], and there is an association between circulating endotoxin and the development of the syndrome [15]. Therefore, it is reasonable to hypothesize that LPS priming of neutrophils followed by stimulation with complement fragments could contribute to the development of ARDS. However, whether or not circulating neutrophils from patients at risk for and with ARDS are primed and/or activated is currently unclear. Neutrophils from patients with ARDS displayed increased chemotaxis, chemiluminescence, and superoxide release but decreased adherence compared to those from normal subjects in one study, and increased oxidant production and decreased chemotaxis compared to normals in another [43]. We recently found that unstimulated neutrophils isolated from patients at risk for and with ARDS did not spontaneously produce superoxide and were not primed for superoxide production, but produced the same amount of superoxide as cells from normal individuals when stimulated with phorbolmyristate acetate (PMA). When primed with LPS and stimulated with FMLP, however, patient neutrophils produced less superoxide than did cells from normal subjects (Fig. 4) [44]. To evaluate the mechanism for this decreased response to LPS, the expression of CD14 on neutrophils from patients with ARDS was examined. Compared with neutrophils from normal subjects, neutrophils from patients had both decreased baseline CD14 expression and less CD14 up-regulation after LPS stimulation. Two possible mechanisms to account for these results were examined. The first was that CD14 receptors could have been previously up-regulated and either internalized, or shed. *In vitro* experiments indicated that the receptors could be up-regulated and shed, and when sCD14 was measured in the patients' plasma, it was found to be increased, further

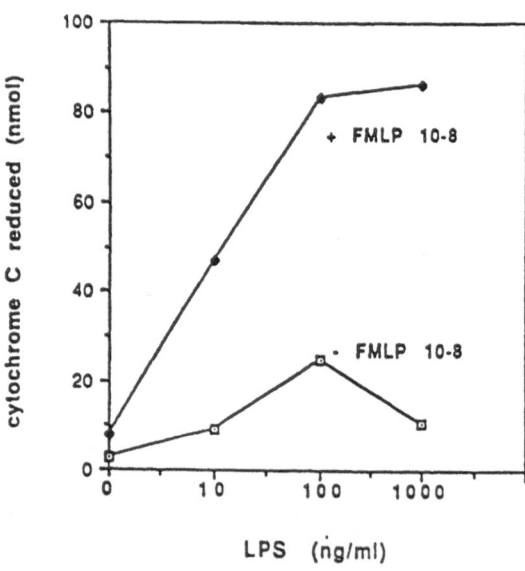

Fig. 4. In normal subjects, neither LPS at doses of 10, 100 or 1000 ng/mL nor 10^{-8} M FMLP alone stimulated significant superoxide production (open squares). However, if the cells were first primed with increasing doses of LPS and then stimulated with 10^{-8} FMLP, superoxide production was significantly increased (closed diamonds). (From [59] with permission)

supporting this mechanism. The alternative mechanism investigated was that neutrophil subpopulations existed that varied in CD14 expression, such that those most responsive to LPS were preferentially sequestered within the lung, and the cells available for study in the peripheral circulation represented a less responsive population. The data supported this mechanism as well. Neutrophil subpopulations which varied in responsivity to LPS were demonstrated *in vitro*, and there was evidence that those subpopulations existed in patients at risk for and with ARDS. These results suggested that neutrophil heterogeneity could be important in ARDS.

Neutrophil Retention. Neutrophils are recruited to and retained within the lung during the development of lung injury. LPS effects both these processes, as shown in Fig. 5. To traverse the lung even under normal conditions, neutrophils must alter their shape because their average diameter (8 μm) is larger than that of the average pulmonary capillary (5.5-6 μm) [45], and the perfusion pressure of the capillary bed is low. *In vitro*, LPS induces actin assembly in neutrophils which increases cell stiffness, thereby decreasing the ability of the neutrophil to deform and increasing neutrophil retention [46]. If neutrophils are pretreated with cytocholasin B, which prevents the assembly of actin, neutrophil retention is not increased. LPS also up-regulates adhesion glycoproteins such as CD11/18 on the neutrophil [20, 47] as well as glycoproteins such as E-selectin on the endothelium

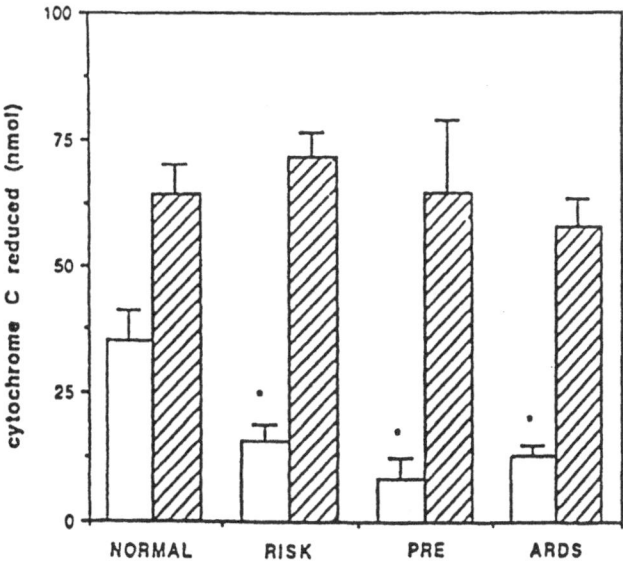

Fig. 5. When patient neutrophils were primed with LPS (100 ng/mL) and subsequently stimulated with 10^{-8} FMLP, superoxide production was increased above baseline but was less in all patient groups (p < 0.05) than in normal neutrophils (open bars). However, when neutrophils were stimulated with PMA (133 ng/mL) (striped bars), maximal superoxide was preserved in all patient groups. Data shown are mean ± SEM. (From [59] with permission)

[48], which could further increase neutrophil retention within the lung. LPS-induced actin assembly, alterations in cell stiffness, adherence to endothelial cells, and neutrophil retention within filters [46] are prevented if CD14 is blocked [23]. By contrast, if CD18 is blocked with mAb 60.3, neutrophil retention is not altered even though their adherence to surfaces is [49]. Both LPS-stimulated assembly of actin and adherence of neutrophils to endothelial cells occur within minutes, whereas the up-regulation of endothelial cell adherence glycoproteins takes hours. Thus, LPS-induced modulation of neutrophil deformability could initiate the process of neutrophil sequestration, and LPS up-regulation of endothelial cell adhesion molecules could prolong their retention within the lung.

Neutrophil Stimulation. LPS directly stimulates neutrophils to release toxic mediators including oxygen radicals, proteases, platelet activating factor (PAF), and eicosanoids, which can all contribute to lung injury through both direct and indirect mechanisms.

LPS and Surfactant Proteins

Pulmonary surfactant-associated proteins are emerging as important modulators of host defense and alveolar inflammation, in addition to their role in reducing alveolar surface tension. Both surfactant protein A (SP-A) and surfactant protein D (SP-D) bind LPS [50, 51]. Van Iwaarden et al [51] reported that the binding of SP-A to LPS-coated beads was saturable, both time and concentration-dependent, and required both calcium and sodium. The binding of SP-A to LPS was not affected by mannan and heparinizing or by deglycosylation of the SP-A, indicating that the carbohydrate-binding domain and the carbohydrate moiety of SP-A are not involved in its interaction with LPS. They also reported that SP-A bound to the lipid A moiety of LPS and to LPS from either *Salmonella minnesota* or the J5-mutant of E. coli. By contrast, it did not bind to 0111 LPS *E. coli*, suggesting that SP-A binds only to rough LPS. In further support of the role of SP-A in the alveolar defense system, Pikaar et al [52] reported that SP-A acted as an opsonin in the phagocytosis of rough LPS-containing bacteria by alveolar macrophages. Recent experiments demonstrate that SP-A is capable not only of binding LPS, but can also modulate its inflammatory effects on THP-1 cells, a macrophage cell line [53]. In these experiments, the effects of SP-A on LPS-induced stimulation of THP-1 cells was tested. THP-1 cells, induced to exhibit cell surface CD14 by incubating with vitamin D3, resembled tissue macrophages. The cells were then incubated with either LPS alone or LPS and LBP, in the presence or absence of increasing concentrations of SP-A. Cellular stimulation was measured as supernatant interleukin-8 (IL-8) concentration. The addition of SP-A resulted in a dose-dependent inhibition of IL-8 release from THP-1 cells incubated with LPS and LBP, but did not affect those cells incubated with LPS alone. These inhibitory effects were seen with Re595 LPS (rough) but not with 011:B4 (smooth). These data suggest that SP-A, one of the most abundant alveolar fluid proteins, may serve as a naturally occurring inhibitor of LPS-induced lung inflammation. We, and others, have found decreased concentrations of SP-A in BAL fluid of patients at risk and with documented ARDS [54, 55]. SP-A deficiency in the alveolar airspace may be important in determining the "balance" of inflammatory mediators, allowing lung inflammation to progress unchecked.

LPS as a Modulator of Inflammation

The effects of LPS discussed can all lead to the initiation and perpetuation of lung inflammation, but LPS can also induce tolerance. Tolerance occurs when exposure to a sublethal dose of LPS is associated with a relative hyporesponsiveness to subsequent exposure, the mechanisms of which have only partially been elucidated.

The tolerance of the immune response in endotoxemia is probably dependent on two different "mechanisms" that result in an early and late tolerant state. Late tolerance can be induced by repeated exposure to LPS and occurs within days or weeks after the first endotoxin exposure. This form of tolerance results from the generation of anti-endotoxin antibodies, and is, therefore, antigenically specific. By contrast, early tolerance develops within hours after a single dose of endotoxin and resolves within hours. This state of endotoxin tolerance is perhaps more relevant to the development of lung injury. *In vitro* and in animal models, an initial sublethal dose of endotoxin causes an increase in both TNF-α and IL-1 levels. Interestingly, cross tolerance has been found for endotoxin and these two cytokines [56, 57]. In the *in vitro* and animal models, a subsequent dose of endotoxin results in the decreased production and release of TNF-α, IL-1, and IL-6 from alveolar macrophages [58] compared to macrophages which have not been previously exposed to LPS.

The extent to which endotoxin tolerance could modulate the development of ARDS in humans remains unclear although a number of studies suggest it may occur. In patients with sepsis, both circulating monocytes [59] and neutrophils [56] exhibit decreased LPS-stimulated cytokine production. The mechanism commonly thought to contribute to this tolerance is the down-regulation of CD14 expression, which has been shown on circulating monocytes from septic patients. However, it was normal in one study of circulating neutrophils [56], and as discussed above, decreased on circulating neutrophils from septic patients in a third [44]. *In vitro* studies suggest that the mechanism may be more complex as there is evidence that the defect may be distal to CD14, i.e. post-transcriptional [56, 60] or post-translational [61]. Alternatively, LPS could indirectly confer tolerance by stimulating the release of mediators/modulators which themselves influence the cellular responses to LPS. Recently, Kimmings and colleagues studied this mechanism in humans [62]. The LPS-stimulated release of TNF-α from whole blood was significantly decreased 2 h following the intravenous administration of endotoxin to normal volunteers and returned to normal within 6 h. Serum obtained from these volunteers following endotoxin administration had increased levels of TNF-α, IL-10, soluble TNF-α receptors, bactericidal/permeability-increasing protein (BPI) and cortisol but did not significantly decrease LPS-stimulated TNF-α production from peripheral blood monocytes isolated from a healthy individual who had not received endotoxin. Thus, the mechanisms that confer tolerance continue to be investigated.

Sources of Endotoxin

LPS has been implicated as an important agent in the induction of lung injury, and is present in the plasma of many patients with sepsis and ARDS, even in the absence of positive blood cultures. The question remains: Where does the endotoxin come from? As previously discussed, LPS is a major component of the outer membrane of Gram-negative bacteria, and Gram-negative sepsis is a major risk factor for the development of ARDS. However, there are a number of patients with measurable circulating endotoxin who do not have Gram-negative infections [15]. In those patients, it was initially hypothesized that bacterial translocation could account for the presence of endotoxin in the circulation. This popular theory was originally put forth by Fine [63], who showed in the 1960's that gut-derived endotoxin gained access to the systemic circulation in shocked animals. Subsequent animal research has supported the concept that the gut is a likely source of endotoxin in the development of multiple organ failure (MOF) due to shock. The main problem with this theory is that it has never been demonstrated in humans, although in patients with severe burns, intestinal permeability is increased and correlates with septic complications [64], and in trauma patients the preservation of the integrity of the gastrointestinal mucosa results in fewer infectious complications [65]. In addition, multiple studies have been performed to analyze whether alteration of the gastrointestinal flora decreases the incidence of nosocomial infection, with conflicting results. These studies do not, however, distinguish between a decrease in infectious complications due to bacterial translocations, or decreased aspiration of bacteria, and do not directly address the question of endotoxemia. Two different studies have addressed the issue of whether endotoxin is present in the serum of patients with trauma, and whether endotoxin levels correlate with disease outcome. In both studies, there was no detectable serum endotoxin, despite the fact that there were patients who developed MOF [66] and that intestinal permeability was increased [67]. A recent study by Riddington [68] examined the relationship between intestinal permeability and endotoxemia in patients undergoing cardiopulmonary bypass. Endotoxin was detectable in the plasma of 42% of patients undergoing cardiopulmonary bypass, and there were increases in gut permeability, but there was no evident relationship between the degree of gut permeability and endotoxemia. Collectively, these studies suggest that the role of bacterial translocation as a source for endotoxin in patients without Gram-negative sepsis may not be as important as initially proposed, and that further studies are needed to better characterize the source of endotoxin in patients with ARDS.

Anti-endotoxin Therapy

There have been numerous studies, both in animal models and humans, using antibodies to endotoxin as a strategy for immunologic intervention in Gram-negative shock. These studies are based on the hypothesis that although antibiotics are required to clear bacteremia, they do not reverse evolving shock, because endotoxin free in the bloodstream or exposed on the surface of circulating bacteria continues to activate mediators of cell damage until natural clearance and detoxification mechanisms in the host are able to handle the load. As previously discussed, the lipid A moiety of endotoxin is the most toxic part of LPS and is presumed to be highly conserved among various species of Gram-negative bacilli. Therefore, monoclonal antibodies to the core have been developed to oppose the systemic manifestations of severe infections caused by these organisms and improve outcome. Despite the high expectations of scientists and industry, multiple clinical trials of anti-endotoxin therapies for sepsis have failed to demonstrate any benefit, and in some cases the agents used were actually harmful to patients [69, 70.] There are a variety of reasons why these therapies have not been successful. One problem may be that the binding properties of the antibodies may not be as specific for endotoxin as initially proposed [71]. In addition, the *in vitro* data and data from animals could not be reproduced [72]. Finally, strategies directed at modulating host defenses in sepsis may be a "two-edged" sword, and the indications for their use must be clearly defined. It may be that some aspect of the LPS response in humans is beneficial, such that its modulation or elimination may be similarly deleterious. Further work needs to be done in other models and with other anti-endotoxin strategies.

Conclusion

We have made tremendous advances in our understanding of the pathogenesis of ARDS. It is now clear that ARDS represents a spectrum of clinical disease which affects not only the lung but virtually every other organ. Although we appreciate lung inflammation is important, the factors that initiate and then perpetuate the inflammatory response remain unclear. We do not understand how the inflammatory process is different in those patients with (for example) severe sepsis who develop ARDS compared to those with apparently equally severe sepsis who are spared. It is likely that the mediators and cellular interactions that are involved in inflammation are extremely complex, and that the process is confounded by factors such as tolerance. In this chapter, we reviewed the role of both complement and endotoxin in the development of ARDS. Although complement activation alone does not itself cause lung injury, it is ubiquitous in critically ill patients, and thus it would be a mistake to dismiss its potential involvement. Similarly, it is likely that endotoxin is involved in the development of lung injury as it can stimulate inflammatory cells to release mediators which both cause and propagate injury. In addition, endotoxin stimulates the retention of inflammatory cells within the lung and may also cause injury directly. Finally, there is evidence that endotoxin interacts with specific host proteins that can either enhance the effects of LPS (LBP) or diminish the effects of LPS (SP-A). The balance of these host proteins in the alveolar air space may be more important than endotoxin itself in regulating the inflammatory response in ARDS.

References

1. Warren J, Johnson K, Ward P (1992) Immunoglobulin- and complement-mediated immune injury. In: R Crystal, JB West (eds). Lung injury. Raven Press, New York. pp 179–186
2. Muller-Eberhard H (1984) The membrane attach complex. Springier Seminars. Immunopathology 7:93–118
3. Craddock, PR, Fehr J, Dalmasso A, Brighham K, Jacob H (1977) Hemodialysis leukopenia: Pulmonary vascular leukostasis resulting from complement activation by dialyzer cellophane membrane. J Clin Invest 59:879–888
4. Craddock PR, Hammerschmidt DE, White JG, Dalmasso AP, Jacob AJ (1977) Complement (C5a)-induced granulocyte aggregation in vitro: A possible mechanisms of complement-mediated leukostasis and leukopenia. J Clin Invest 60:260–264
5. Till GO, Johnson KJ, Kunkel R (1982) Intravascular activation of complement and ALI: Dependency on neutrophils and toxic oxygen metabolites. J Clin Invest 69:1126–1135
6. Henson PM, Larsen GL, Webster RO, Mitchell BC, Goins AJ, Henson JE (1982) Pulmonary microvascular alterations and injury induced by complement fragments: Synergistic effect of complement activation, neutrophil sequestrations and prostaglandins. Ann NY Acad Sci 348:287–300
7. Hosea S, Brown E, Hammer C, Frank M (1980) Role of complement activation in a model of adult respiratory distress syndrome. J Clin Invest 66:375–382
8. Gelfand J, Donelan J, Hawiger A, Burke J (1982) Alternative complement pathway activation increases mortality in a model of burn injury in mice. J Clin Invest 70:1170–1176
9. Parrish D, Mitchell B, Henson PM, Larsen G (1984) Pulmonary response of fifth component of complement-sufficient and deficient mice to hyperoxia. J Clin Invest 74:956–965
10. Stevens, J, O'Hanley PT, Shapiro J, et al (1986) Effects of anti-C5a antibodies on the adult respiratory distress syndrome in septic primates. J Clin Invest 77:1812–1816
11. Rabinovic R, Yah C, Hillegass L, et al (1992) Role of complement in endotoxin/platelet activity factor-induced lung injury. J Immunol 149:1744–1750
12. Hammerschmidt D, Weaver L, Hudson L, Craddock PR, Jacob H (1980) Association of complement activation and elevated plasma C5a with adult respiratory distress syndrome: Pathophysiological relevance and possible prognostic value. Lancet 1:947–949
13. Duchteau J, Haas J, Schreyen H, et al (1984) Complement activation in patients at risk of developing the adult respiratory distress syndrome. Am Rev Respir Dis 130:1058–1064
14. Langlois PF, Gawryl MS (1988) Accentuated formation of the terminal Cfb-9 complement complex in patient plasma precedes development of the adult respiratory distress syndrome. Am Rev Respir Dis 138:368–375
15. Parsons PE, Worthen G, Moore E, Tate R, Henson PM (1989) The association of circulating endotoxin with the development of the adult respiratory distress syndrome. Am Rev Respir Dis 140:294–301
16. Parsons PE, Giclas PC (1990) The terminal complement complex (sC5b-9) is not specifically associated with the development of the adult respiratory distress syndrome. Am Rev Respir Dis 141:98–103
17. Brigham K, Woolverton W, Glake L, et al (1974) Increased sheep lung vascular permeability caused by Pseudomonas bacteremia. J Clin Invest 54:792–804
18. Brigham K, Bowers R, Haynes J (1979) Increased sheep lung vascular permeability caused by E. coli. Endotoxin. Circulation 45:292–297
19. Tobias PS, Ulevitch RJ (1983) Control of lipopolysaccharide-high density lipoprotein binding by acute phase proteins(s). J Immunol 131:1913–1916

20. Tobias PS, Soldau K, , Ulevitch RJ (1986) Isolation of a lipopolysaccharide-binding acute phase reactant from rabbit serum. J Exp Med 164:777–793
21. Schumann RR, Leong SR, Flaggs GW, et al (1990) Structure and function of lipopolysaccharide binding protein. Science 249:1429–1431
22. Wright S, Ramos R, Hermanowski-Vasatka A, Rockwell P, Detmers P (1991) Activation of the adhesive capacity of CR3 on neutrophils by endotoxin: Dependence on lipopolysaccharide-binding protein and CD14. J Exper Med 173:1281–1286
23. Worthen G, Avdi N, Vukajlovich S, Tobias P (1993) Neutrophil adherence induced by lipopolysaccharide. J Clin Invest 90:2526–2535
24. Wright S, Ramos R, Tobias P, Ulevitch RJ , Mathison JC (1990) CD14 a receptor for complexes of lipopolysaccharide (LPS) and LBP-binding protein. Science 249:1431–1433
25. Maliszewski CR, Ball ED, Grazino RF, Fanger MW (1985) Isolation and characterization of My23, a myeloid cell-derived antigen reactive with the monoclonal antibody AML-2-23. J Immunol 135:1929–1935
26. Lynn WA, Liu Y, Golenbock DT (1993) Neither CD14 nor serum is absolutely necessary for activation of mononuclear phagocytes by bacterial lipopolysaccharide. Infect Immun 61: 4452–4461
27. Golenbock DT, Bach RR, Lichenstein H, Juan TSC, Tadavarthy A, Moldow CF (1995) Soluble CD14 promotes LPS activation of CD14-deficient PNH monocytes and endothelial cells. J Lab Clin Med 125:662–671
28. Gray PW, Flaggs G, Leong SR (1989) Cloning of the cDNA of a human neutrophil bactericidal protein. Structural and functional correlations. J Biol Chem 264:9505–9509
29. Zhang JK, Morrison TK, Falk MC, Kang, YH, Lee CH (1996) Characterization of the binding of soluble CD14 to human endothelial cells and mechanisms for CD14-dependent cell activation by LPS. J Endotoxin 3:307–315
30. Ramadori G, Meyer zum Buschenfelde KH, Tobias PS, Mathison JC, Ulevitch RJ (1990) Biosynthesis of lipopolysaccharide-binding protein in rabbit hepatocytes. Pathobiology 58: 89–94
31. Martin TR, Mathison JS, Tobias PS, et al (1992) Lipopolysaccharide binding protein enhances the responsiveness of alveolar macrophages to bacterial lipopolysaccharide. Implications for cytokine production in normal and injured lungs. J Clin Invest 90:2209–2219
32. Martin TR, Rubenfeld GD, Ruzinski JT et al (1997) Relationship between soluble CD14, lipopolysaccharide binding protein and the alveolar inflammatory response in patients with acute respiratory distress syndrome. Am J Respir Crit Care Med (In press)
33. Shasby DM, Fox RB, Harada RN, Repine JE (1982) Reduction of the edema of acute hyperoxic lung injury by granulocyte depletion J Appl Physiol 52:1237–1244
34. Rinaldo JE, Borovetz H (1985) Deterioration of oxygenation and abnormal lung microvascular permeability during resolution of leukopenia in patients with diffuse lung injury. Am Rev Respir Dis 131:579–583
35. Lo SK, Everitt J, Gu J, Malik AV (1992) Tumor necrosis factor mediates experimental pulmonary edema by ICAM-1 and CD18-dependent mechanisms. J Clin Invest 89:981–988
36. Windsor AC, Walsh CJ, Mullen PG, et al (1993) Tumor necrosis factor-alpha blockade prevents neutrophil CD18 receptor up-regulation and attenuates ALI in porcine sepsis without inhibition of neutrophil oxygen radical generation. J Clin Invest 91:1459–1468
37. Goodman RD, Strieter RM, Martin DP, et al (1996) Inflammatory cytokines in patients with persistence of the acute respiratory distress syndrome. Am J Respir Crit Care Med 154: 602–611
38. Steinberg KP, Milberg JA, Martin TR, et al (1994) Evolution of bronchoalveolar cell populations in the adult respiratory distress syndrome. Am J Respir Crit Care Med 150:113–122
39. Haslett CL, Guthrie LA, Kopaniak MM, Johnston RB, Henson PM (1985) Modulation of multiple neutrophil functions by preparative methods or trace concentrations of bacterial lipopolysaccharide. Am J Pathol 119:101–110
40. Worthen G, Hasslet C, Rees A, Gumbay R, Henson J, Henson PM (1987) Neutrophil-mediated pulmonary vascular injury. Synergistic effect of trace amounts of lipopolysaccharide and neutrophil stimuli on vascular permeability and neutrophil sequestration within the lung. Am Rev Respir Dis 136:19–28

41. Hasslet C, Worthen G, Giclas P, Morrison D, Henson J, Henson PM (1987) The pulmonary vascular sequestration of neutrophils in endotoxemia is initiated by an effect of endotoxin on the neutrophil in the rabbits. Am Rev Respir Dis 136:9–18

42. Donner RL, Elin RJ, Hossein SM, Wesley RA, Reilly JM, Parillo JE (1991) Endotoxin in human septic shock. Chest 99:169–175

43. Fowler AA, fisher B, Center R, Carchman R (1983) Development of ARDS, progressive alteration of neutrophil chemotactic and secretory processes. Am J Path 166:427–435

44. Parsons PE, Gillespie MK, Moore EE, Moore FA, Worthen GS (1995) Neutrophil response to endotoxin in the adult respiratory distress syndrome: Role of CD14. Am J Respir Cell Mol Biol 13:152–160

45. Guntheroth W, Lachter D, Kawaburi I (1982) Pulmonary microcirculation: Tubules rather than sheet and post. J Appl Physiol 53:510–515

46. Erzurum S, Downey G, Schwab B, Elson D, Worthen GS (1992) Mechanisms of lipopolysaccharide-induced neutrophil retention. Relative contributions of adhesive and cellular mechanical properties. J Immun 149:154–162

47. Tonnesum JG, Anderson DC, Springer TA, Knedler A, Avdi N, Henson PM (1989) Adherence of neutrophils to cultured human microvascular endothelial cells. Stimulation by chemotactic peptides and lipid mediators and dependence upon the Mac-1, LFA-1, p-150.95 glycoprotein family. J Clin Invest 83:637–646

48. Bevilacqua M, Nelson R (1993) Selectins. J Clin Invest 91:379–387

49. Henson PM, Doherty DE, Riches DWH, Parsons PE, Worthen GS (1994) LPS, cytokines. In: Brigham KL (ed) Endotoxin and the lungs. Marcel Dekker, New York, NY pp 267–304

50. Kuan Df, Rust K, Crouch E (1992) Interactions of surfactant protein D with bacterial lipopolysaccharides. J Clin Invest 90:97–106

51. Van Iwaarden JF, Pikaar JC, Storm J, et al (1994) Binding of surfactant protein A to the lipid A moiety of lipopolysaccharides. Biochem J 303:407–411

52. Pikaar JC, Voorhout WF, van Golde LMG, Verhoef J, Van Strijp JAG, van Iwaarden JF (1995) Opsonic activities of surfactant protein A and D in phagocytosis of Gram-negative bacteria by alveolar macrophages. J Infect Dis 172:481–489

53. Greene KE, Wong VA, Mongovin SM, Goodman RB, Martin TR (1996) SP-A inhibits the bioactivity and release of IL-8. Am J Respir Crit Care Med 153:A662 (Abst)

54. Gregory TJ, Longmore WJ, Moxley MA, et al (1991) Surfactant chemical composition and biophysical activity in acute respiratory distress syndrome. J Clin Invest 88:1976–1981

55. Greene KE, Wright JR, Wong WB, et al (1995) Serial SP-A levels in BAL and serum of patients with ARDS. Am J Respir Crit Care 153:A587 (Abst)

56. McCall C, Grosso-Wilmouth L, LaRue K, Guzman R, Cousart S (1993) Tolerance to endotoxin-induced expression of the interleukin-1 beta gene in blood neutrophils of humans with the sepsis syndrome. J Clin Invest 91:853–861

57. Alexander H, Sheppard B, Jensen J, et al (1991) Treatment with recombinant human tumor necrosis factor-alpha protects rats against the lethality, hypotension, and hypothermia of gram negative sepsis. J Clin Invest 88:34–39

58. Mathison J, Walfson E, Ulevitch R (1988) Participation of tumor necrosis factor in the mediation of Gram-negative bacterial lipopolysaccharide-induced injury in rabbits. J Clin Invest 81:1925–1937

59. Munoz C, Carlet J, Fitting C, Misset B, Bierot J, Cavaillon J (1991) Dysregulation of in vitro cytokine production by monocytes in sepsis. J Clin Invest 88:1747–1754

60. Mathison J, Virca G, Wolfson E, Tobias P, Glaser K, Ulevithch R (1990) Adaptation of bacterial lipopolysaccharide controls lipopolysaccharide-induced tumor necrosis factor production in rabbit macrophages. J Clin Invest 85:1108–1118

61. Zuckerman S, Evans G, Snyder Y, Roeder W (1989) Endotoxin-macrophage interaction: Post-translational regulation of tumor necrosis factor expression. J Immunol 143:1223–1227

62. Kimmings AN, Pajkrt D, Zaaijer K, et al (1996) Factors involved in early in vitro endotoxin hyporesponsiveness in human endotoxemia. J Endotoxin Research 3:283–289

63. Fine J (1967) The intestinal circulation in shock. Gastroenterology 52:454–460

64. Ziegler T, Smith R, O'Dwyer S, Demling, Wilmore D (1988) Increased intestinal permeability associated with infection in burn patients. Arch Surg. 123:1313–1319

65. Moore F, Moore E, Jones T, et al (1989) TEN versus TPN following major abdominal trauma-reduced septic mortality. J Trauma 29:916–23

66. Moore F, Moore E, Poggetti R, et al (1991) Gut bacterial translocation via the portal vein: A clinical perspective with major torso trauma. J Trauma. 31:629–638

67. Roumen R, Hendriks T, Wevers R , Goris J (1993) Intestinal permeability after severe trauma and hemorrhagic shock is increased without relation to septic complications. Arch Surg 128:453–457

68. Riddington, DW, Venkatesh B, Boivin CM, et al (1996) Intestinal permeability, gastric intra-mucosal pH, and systemic endotoxemia in patients undergoing cardiopulmonary bypass. JAMA 275:1007–1012

69. McCloskey RV, Straube RC, Sanders C, Smith SM, Smith CR (1994) Treatment of septic shock with human monoclonal antibody Ha-1A. Ann Inter Med 121:1–5

70. Ziegler EJ, Fisher CJ, Sprung, et al (1991) Treatment of Gram-negative bacteremia and septic shock with Ha-1A human monoclonal antibody against endotoxin. N Engl J Med 324: 429–436

71. Baumgartner JD (1991) Immunotherapy with antibodies to core lipopolysaccharide: A critical appraisal. Infec Dis Clin North Am 5:915–927

72. Baumgartner JD, Heumann D, Gerain J, Weinbreck P, Grau GE, Glauser MP (1990) Association between protective efficacy of anti-lipopolysaccharide (LPS) antibodies and suppression of LPS-induced tumor necrosis factor alfa and interleukin 6. J Exp Med 171:889–896

73. Manual of clinical laboratory immunology (1997) Rose NR et al. (eds) 5th ed. Washington, DC, ASM Press

Protective Effects of the Stress Response in Sepsis and ALI

S. P. Ribeiro and A. S. Slutsky

Introduction

Sepsis and its clinical consequences, such as the acute respiratory distress syndrome (ARDS) and multiple organ dysfunction syndrome (MODS), are major contributors to morbidity and mortality in most intensive care units despite the use of specific therapies [1–4]. In recent years, there have been novel approaches to the management of some of these conditions with agents other than antimicrobials. For example, sepsis prophylaxis has been shown to be promising when antibodies to tumor necrosis factor (TNF) were injected in animal models of sepsis [5–7]. Similarly, the administration of interleukin-1 receptor antagonist (IL-1ra) into rabbits prevented death in a septic model [8]. Unfortunately, results of studies using these agents in patients have been relatively disappointing [9–12].

In this chapter, we review studies demonstrating that a natural defense mechanism, called the stress response or the heat shock response, is protective against experimental sepsis and lung injury. Although the exact mechanisms are unknown, we provide further evidence that the heat shock proteins might be key components of the protective machinery.

Sepsis and ARDS: The Problem

Infection and injury are often accompanied by significant metabolic, immune and vascular derangements that in the worst cases present as a devastating syndrome of hemodynamic collapse, shock, and death. The cascade of events during the systemic inflammatory response syndrome (SIRS) is very complex and our knowledge of all its details is rudimentary. However, from the use of experimental animal models of sepsis, we now know that the immune system is activated in an uncontrolled manner. It is believed that there is overproduction of various proinflammatory mediators which is perpetuated in the septic shock state. There is a great deal of evidence implicating endotoxin, a bacterial outer membrane segment, as the principal factor initiating the "sepsis cascade" [13, 14]. Lipid A, the lipopolysaccharide (LPS) toxic substance, is probably responsible for various systemic host responses seen in Gram-negative endotoxemia. Upon exposure to plasma, LPS binds to either lipoproteins or LPS-binding protein (LBP) [15, 16]. LBP is a 60 kDa glycoprotein with a high affinity binding site for the lipid A moiety of LPS. The LPS-LBP complex stimulates monocytes and macrophages by binding to a cell-surface glycoprotein, CD14 [17]. Although multiple pathways appear to regulate macrophage responsiveness to LPS, it has been shown that anti-CD14 antibodies reduce the responsiveness of monocytes to LPS by a factor of 10 [18]. Similarly, cellular responsiveness to LPS is diminished 100-fold by depletion of plasma and tissue culture media of LBP [19].

Endotoxin promotes the release of inflammatory mediators from mononuclear phagocytes and other cells, with a direct effect on the vascular endothelium. While endotoxin may be the initiating factor in sepsis, many endogenous inflammatory mediators contribute to maintain this state of injury. For many years, it has been recognized that one of the initiating events in the development of SIRS is the triggering of the body's defense mechanism by the invading microorganisms and their products [20]. These defense mechanisms include the release of cytokines (TNF, IL-1, IL-6, IL-8), activation of neutrophils and monocytes (chemotactic hormones, IL-8), and activation of plasma protein cascade systems such as the complement system (C5a, C3), the intrinsic (factor XII) and extrinsic (tissue factor, TF) pathways of coagulation, and the fibrinolytic system. The clinical consequences of this cascade are various, including disseminated intravascular coagulation (DIC), renal insufficiency, MODS, and ARDS [13, 21, 22]. The complex network of inflammatory mediators seen in SIRS causes, in some cases, the perpetuation of synthesis of most of these mediators, leading to septic shock.

The management of patients with sepsis and/or ARDS generally involves correction of tissue hypoxia, control of underlying infection, and supportive treatment. These goals are achieved by the use of the well known armamentarium, such as mechanical ventilation to provide adequate oxygenation, vasoactive drugs to maintain arterial pressure, and the use of specific antibiotics to combat infection. Although these strategies have been intensively studied for several years, it has been difficult to document improved mortality rates. With the advent of studies clarifying pathophysiologic mechanisms involving inflammatory mediators in sepsis, a new strategy termed immmunotherapy has gained some enthusiasm. Immunomodulation for sepsis, however, faces a major impediment: a central mediator of sepsis does not seem to exist, although TNF-α has been commonly proposed for this role. Thus, for many of the inflammatory mediators known to participate in the sepsis cascade, there appears to be an article showing that the blockade of its function – by means of the use of specific antibodies and other forms of antagonism – is protective against sepsis [5, 23–27]. Some of these novel immunotherapies have left the laboratory bench but results to date have been disappointing [12, 28].

The Heat Shock Response: The Potential Solution

One potential strategy that our laboratory has been studying for a number of years is a natural defense mechanism present in virtually all cells: the heat shock response or the stress response. The stress response, when triggered prior to an otherwise lethal injury, has been shown to be protective in a number of experimental systems. Among others, it has been shown that the induction of the stress response by brief hyperthermia (heat stress) or by non-thermal means (sodium arsenite injection) protects rats against the lethal effects of experimental sepsis [29, 30], intratracheal phospholipase A2 (PLA2) [31], and prolonged exposure to 100% O_2 [32]. The mechanisms of protection may be related directly to a set of proteins produced during the stress response – the heat shock or stress proteins (HSP).

The heat shock response was described in a series of studies by the geneticist Ritossa in 1962 [33]. Ritossa reported that when the larvae of *Drosophila busckii* and *Drosophila melanogaster*, which were normally raised at 25°C, were exposed to higher temperatures (30–32°C) for 30 min, several new "puffs" appeared on the giant salivary gland chromosomes. Experiments with radioactive precursors showed that the heat-induced puffs were the sites of intense RNA transcription of active, induced genes. When purified, heat shock mRNA fractions were added to *in vitro* systems for protein synthesis, they were translated into specific heat shock proteins [34]. These observations clearly indicated that the heat shock mRNA's, made at heat shock puff sites, were translated into heat shock proteins.

The potential importance of the heat stress response can be appreciated by the ubiquitous nature of this reaction; the response is remarkably well conserved throughout evolution, occurring in virtually all organisms, including prokaryotes, yeast, plants and all higher eukaryotes [35]. In addition, there is tremendous HSP homology across widely diverse lifeforms. The time course and relative magnitude of the heat shock response after a stress condition varies widely among different cell types in the same organism [36] and can even vary between individual HSP within a single cell type. In mammals, it is thought that the optimum temperature to turn on HSP gene expression is approximately 40°–45°C. Although thermal stress has been the most extensively characterized stimulus, other agents are also capable of inducing HSP protein production [37–39]. These include glucose deprivation, anoxia and prolonged ischemia, sodium azide (a poison of cellular respiration), hydrogen peroxide, transition series metals, different chemicals (sodium arsenite, ethanol), drugs, such as d-lysergic acid diethylamine (LSD), amino acid analogs, salicylates, and the normal cell cycle [40]. Also, there have been reports showing that viral [41] and bacterial infection [42] induce the stress response. It is important to note that the heat shock or stress response has been observed in all organisms examined from archaebacteria to eubacteria, yeasts, plants, invertebrates, and vertebrates, including humans.

Although there are differences among the various organisms, molecular weight and number of HSP, it is remarkable how similar the response has remained even in very distant species throughout evolution. Comparison of the sequences of the respective heat shock genes from *E. coli*, plants, yeasts, *Drosophila*, and man, have indicated that HSP are among the most highly conserved proteins in nature [43]. However, the threshold for initiating the response varies greatly with the type of organism and the duration of the stimulus. Similarly, the recovery time, or the time necessary for the cell to recover its normal function, is in accord with the type and duration of the stimulus [36, 44]. Taken together, these studies indicate that the major biological finding in cells experiencing stress is that the protein machinery is transiently affected with an interruption in protein processing and formation. It is important to note, however, that as the cell recovers from the stress event, and providing that the stress insult is not too severe, cellular function returns to normal.

Studies from Mitchel and Tissieres in 1974 [45] led to the recognition of the other major consequence of the stress response: The preferential transcription and translation of a set of proteins called HSP. This new set of polypeptides was named the heat shock proteins or stress proteins because they were thought to be induced mostly by heat stress. The heat shock proteins are classified according to their molecular weights (Table 1). Each class is composed of a number of proteins and the designation of the class refers to the "round number" approximating the molecular weights of its typical members (i.e. [20, 70, 90, 100]).

Table 1. The heat shock proteins (Adapted from [46])

Family	Name	Size kDa*	Localization	Functions
Low molecular weight	Ubiquitin	8	Cytosol/Nucleus	Involved in nonlysosomal protein degradation pathway
	HSP 10	10	Mitochondria/chloroplast	Cofactor for HSP60
	Low molecular weight HSP	20–30	Cytosol/nucleus	Proposed regulator of actin cytoskeleton; proposed molecular chaperone
HSP60	HSP47	47	Endoplasmic reticulum	Collagen chaperone
	HSP56	56	Cytosol	Part of steroid hormone receptor complex; binds FK506
	HSP60	60	Mitochondria/chloroplast	Molecular chaperone
	TCP-1	60	Cytosol/nucleus	Molecular chaperone related to HSP60
HSP70	HSP72	70	Cytosol/nucleus	Highly stress induced Molecular chaperone
	HSP73	70	Cytosol/nucleus	Constitutively expressed Molecular chaperone
	Grp75	70	Mitochondria/chloroplast	Constitutively expressed Molecular chaperone
	Grp78 (Bip)	70	Endoplasmic reticulum	Constitutively expressed Molecular chaperone
HSP100	HSP90	90	Cytosol/nucleus	Part of steroid hormone receptor complex; chaperone (?) for retrovirus-encoded tyrosine protein kinase
	HSP104/110	104/110	Cytosol/nucleus	Required for survive severe stress; molecular chaperone

* Approximate size by SDS-PAGE

Until relatively recently, much of the research pertaining to the stress response has focused on issues related to the regulation and mechanisms of gene transcription. It is only in recent years that the biologic changes coincident with the stress response, the properties of the individual stress proteins, and the protective effect of these proteins have been examined in greater detail. HSP are now thought to play a major role in many biological processes. In particular, there is a large body of data which suggests that HSP protect cells from the toxic effects of many stresses, including hyperthermia [47–50]. The evidence for this assertion comes from a number of sources. The induction of HSP is extremely rapid and intense and is associated with decreased production of all other proteins, a pattern highly suggestive that this is an "emergency response" [48]. More direct evidence that HSP subserve a protective function are data implicating these proteins in the development of thermotolerance, i.e. pretreatment with a sublethal exposure to heat protects against a subsequent heating schedule that is lethal in controls. Several lines of evidence suggest a role for HSP in the development of thermotolerance including correlation of tolerance with HSP levels, protection by non-thermal stimuli that induce HSP, and studies in mutant yeast containing a deletion in one specific HSP [51]. Interestingly, heating induces tolerance to a number of other stresses, including ethanol and anoxia; conversely, these later forms of stress can induce tolerance to heat as well.

Most data correlate the phenomenon of thermotolerance with the induction of the heat shock proteins, particularly with proteins from the 70 kDa family [52]. The collapse of intermediate filaments around the nucleus [53] and the redistribution of HSP70 family members from the nucleus into the nucleolus [54] have been associated with cytoprotection. However, these changes do not occur in the thermotolerant cell, i.e. in cells receiving a second heat stress challenge. Mizzen and Welch [54, 55] characterized thermotolerance using different mammalian cell lines. Their findings suggest that the major hallmarks of the thermotolerant cell are faster kinetics of both the synthesis and repression of HSP and their accelerated intracellular redistribution after a second and more severe heat-shock treatment. The specific involvement of HSP in thermotolerance was provided by the demonstration of a lack of thermotolerance in fibroblasts [56] and mouse oocytes microinjected with anti-HSP70 monoclonal antibodies [57]. The protective role of HSP appears to be related physically to association with proteins experiencing difficulties in proper folding, and also to newly synthesized proteins. Because of this specific function, the heat shock proteins are called "molecular chaperones".

Experimental Evidence

There is experimental evidence demonstrating that the stress response, if applied prior to an otherwise lethal stimulus, is protective *in vivo*. In most studies, the stress response was produced by exposing animals to a brief period of non-lethal heat stress. In our studies, rats were anesthetized and placed into a pre-warmed

(41°C) infant incubator until their rectal temperature reached 42.5°C. This protocol was well tolerated by the animals: there was no related mortality and it was sufficient to induce HSP in a number of organ systems in a time-related fashion [31, 32]. Using immunoblotting, we demonstrated that HSP 72 kDa, the most inducible of the stress proteins and used in most studies as a marker to determine the up-regulation of HSP, is present in whole lung homogenates as soon as 2 h after exposure to heat, peaking between 12 and 24 h, and remaining at high levels up to about 72 h [31, 32].

Using similar heating protocols, Ryan et al [58] used the intravenous injection of bacterial endotoxin as a model of experimental sepsis to determine whether this would be protective. The administration of lethal doses of bacterial endotoxin (20 mg/kg of *E. coli*) to rats that were exposed to heat stress 24 h before LPS stimulation resulted in a mortality rate of zero, in comparison with the group of animals exposed to LPS alone that demonstrated 72% mortality. In a similar study, mice were protected against the high mortality observed after bacterial endotoxin injection (*E. coli*, 20 mg/kg, ip), if a prior heat shock treatment had been applied [59]. We showed that heat stress was protective against a number of experimental models of lung injury. Winston et al. [32] exposed rats to a brief period of warming and, 18 h later, to 100% O_2 for 60 h, an experimental model of hyperoxic lung injury. The rats that were exposed to heat stress demonstrated less evidence of lung injury and also decreased mortality rates. Villar et al [31] preheated rats and instilled PLA2 into the trachea 18–24 h later. Under control conditions, 27% of the unheated animals died by 48 h after PLA2 instillation, compared with zero mortality in the group of animals that received heat treatment.

Using a more clinically relevant experimental model of sepsis, cecal ligation and perforation (CLP) [60, 61], Villar et al [29] demonstrated that preheating rats was also protective against CLP. In this study, 18 h after CLP, 25% of unheated animals had died compared with no mortality seen in the heated group. Seven days after CLP, the protection was still evident, with 69% mortality compared with 20%, respectively. The lungs of the septic animals were found to have evidence of acute inflammatory infiltrates, early hyaline membrane formation, and atelectasis. By contrast, lungs from heated and septic animals revealed a relatively normal architecture and less evidence of pulmonary edema.

After determining that a non-lethal and brief period of warming (heat stress) was sufficient to make rats tolerant to sepsis [29], we examined the hypothesis that these effects could be achieved by non-thermal means. Since heating could be associated with a number of non-specific mechanisms, unrelated to induction of the stress response, we used sodium arsenite, an arsenic compound used in pesticides. The injection of sodium arsenite was shown to be effective in inducing HSP 72 kDa in the lungs in a dose- and time-dependent fashion. The goal of our studies was to examine the protective effects of the stress response in lung injury, and thus we did not directly examine the presence of HSP (induced by sodium arsenite) in other target organs. However, this was well explored by Brown and Rush [37] who showed HSP expression in the kidney, heart and liver following sodium arsenite stimulation.

Using CLP as an experimental model of systemic and lethal injury, we demonstrated that rats could be protected from CLP with the injection of sodium arsenite [30]. In this study, rats were injected with 6 mg/kg of sodium arsenite, a treatment which did not induce a febrile response. Thereafter, they were exposed to CLP 18 h after injection. Eighteen hours after CLP, 42% of control animals had died, compared with 6% of sodium arsenite, septic rats. This protection could be extended up to 24 h, with 45% mortality rate versus 16%, respectively. Of interest, the protection in the sodium arsenite-treated animals appeared to follow the time course of HSP 72 kDa protein levels in the lung, such that mortality between the control and sodium arsenite-treated groups were essentially the same after 48 h, at a time when HSP levels returned to baseline (Fig. 1).

In studies in which heat stress was applied [29], survival rates were extended as long as one week, in contrast to sodium arsenite in which protection was achieved only up to 24 h after sepsis. This difference could be explained by HSP 72 kDa levels in the organs tested, i.e. although both heating and sodium arsenite induced the expression of HSP 72 kDa in the lungs, the pattern of expression was different between these two treatments. In sodium arsenite-injected animals, the protein concentrations had returned to baseline by 60 h after injection, whereas in heat-stressed animals there was persistence of protein accumulation for at

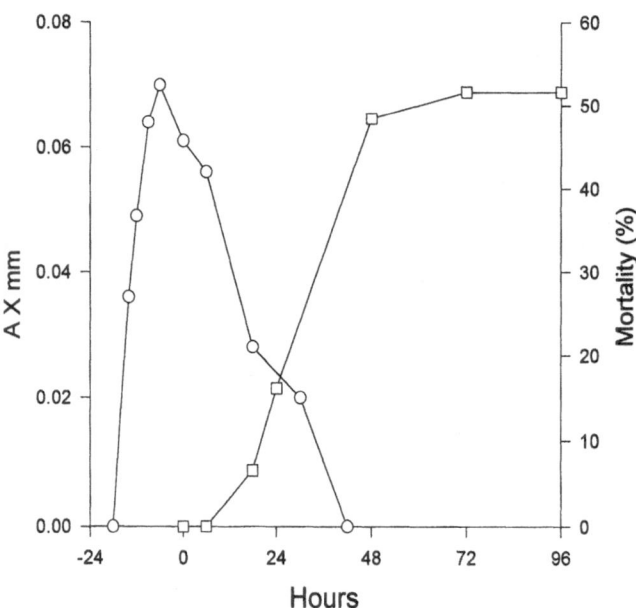

Fig. 1. Time course curve of HSP 72 kDa protein expression (open circles) in the lungs of sodium arsenite-injected animals was plotted with a mortality curve (open squares) from animals injected with sodium arsenite and exposed to cecal ligation and perforation. Note that as HSP expression starts to decrease, mortality rate increases, reaching a peak when HSP returned to baseline values. A X mm, absorbance units by mm wide. (From [30] with permission)

least 72 h. Although the dose of sodium arsenite used was the lowest that reliably induced HSP in the lungs with no signs of acute poisoning, we cannot discard the possibility of overlapping of stresses. In this case, the use of sodium arsenite in association with sepsis could be deleterious in the long term. Similarly, if a more sensitive method of detecting the synthesis of HSP 72 kDa had being used, a lower dose of sodium arsenite could have been selected. These studies, however, open up the possibility of eventually using such a therapeutic strategy in the clinical setting, although not with sodium arsenite which has substantial toxicity, or heating per se, which can be very stressful to the cardiovascular system.

Given the importance of TNF as a central mediator in sepsis and ARDS, we hypothesized that one mechanism by which the stress response could provide protection was by attenuation in plasma TNF levels, making the animals more resistant to sepsis [62]. To examine this hypothesis, we studied rats who were anesthetized and randomly allocated into 3 groups: controls, which initially received a saline injection; animals submitted to heat stress (H); and sodium arsenite injected rats (SA). Following the initial treatment, animals were returned to their cages for 18 h to recover and to provide time for the induction of HSP. At the end of this period, animals were injected with bacterial endotoxin (20 mg/kg, iv, *Salmonella typhosa*). We found significantly higher concentrations of plasma TNF-α at 1 and 2 h after LPS injection in the control group, compared to rats exposed to heat stress or to sodium arsenite injection 18 h prior to LPS challenge which demonstrated a significant decrease in plasma TNF-α levels (Fig. 2).

Using mechanical ventilation as an example of direct injury to the lungs, we have set up a system to determine the role of inflammatory mediators in ventilator-induced lung injury [63, 64]. From reports by Dreyfuss et al [65, 66], it has become clear that some strategies of mechanical ventilation (high pressures, high volumes) produce lung injury, with the presence of lung edema, hyaline membrane formation, and detachment of endothelial cells from their basement membrane (denudation). Also there is a concept that such forms of ventilation would worsen an already established lesion. In this regard, Hernandez et al [67] have studied the effects of oleic acid alone (an experimental model of ARDS), mechanical ventilation alone, and the combination of both on the capillary filtration coefficient and indices of edema (wet-dry weight ratio) in *ex vivo* rabbit lungs. When oleic acid administration was followed by mild overinflation during mechanical ventilation, a significant increase of filtration and in the wet-dry weight ratio was observed, suggesting that mechanical ventilation can worsen pre existing lung injury.

To determine whether inflammatory mediators were involved in this form of injury, we exposed rats to either bacterial endotoxin or saline and applied large-volume, high-pressure ventilation in an *ex vivo* rat lung model. Injurious ventilation strategies produced a rise in TNF lung lavage levels in LPS-injected animals, compared with animals treated with LPS and submitted to "standard" ventilation [63, 64]. Lung lavage IL-1β levels, however, were increased in both LPS and saline-treated animals which had been exposed to injurious forms of mechanical ventilation. Histopathologic specimens from lungs of LPS-stimulated rats demonstrated a marked presence of neutrophils in the lungs that had been ventilated us-

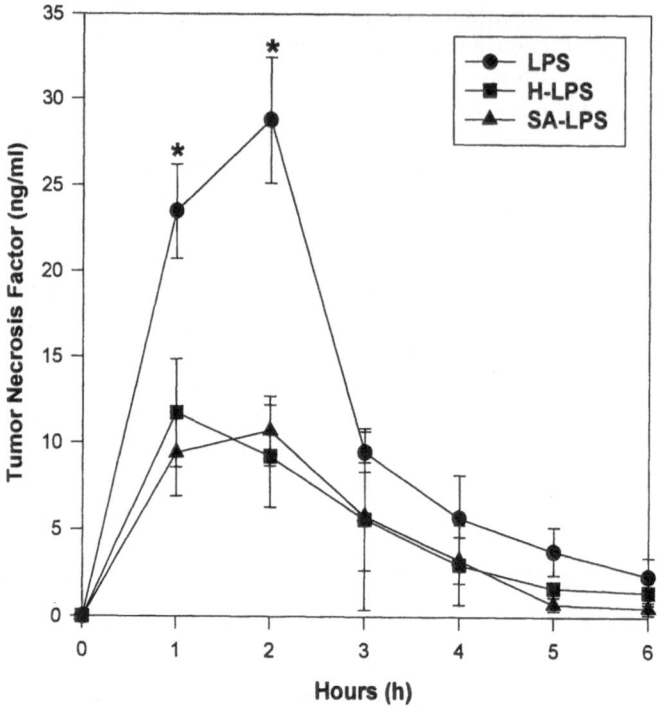

Fig. 2. Effects of the stress response on rat TNF-α protein levels. The animals treated with LPS alone had significant higher plasma TNF concentration compared to animals exposed to heat stress (H) or sodium arsenite (SA) injection 18 h prior to *S. typhosa* endotoxin (* different from the other two groups, p < 0.0001). (From [62] with permission)

ing injurious ventilatory parameters, suggesting recruitment of polymorphonuclear (PMN) cells to the lungs. In determining the mechanisms related to cytokine up-regulation by mechanical ventilation, one could postulate that overstretching lung cells would be the signal to produce inflammatory mediators. In support of this concept is the report from Liu et al [68, 69] in which stretching fetal rat lung cells (alveolar type II) caused the release of soluble growth factors which stimulated epithelial cell proliferation. Another possible mechanism is a direct form of injury by direct tissue damage and subsequent release of cytokines. Evidence for this hypothesis in association whith the use of high pressure ventilation [65] is the finding of denuded pulmonary epithelium, together with the presence of endproducts of cell damage which have been shown to activate alveolar macrophages to synthesize cytokines [70, 71]. Independent of the precise mechanism, these studies suggest that injurious ventilatory strategies promote and also worsen already established (sepsis) inflammatory responses.

Using the same *ex vivo* experimental model of ventilator-induced lung injury, we tested the hypothesis that the stress response would also be protective against mechanically induced lung injury. In this study [72], we randomly allocated rats to receive either sham treatment or to be exposed to heat stress. Eighteen hours later, the lungs were harvested and placed into a warmed (37°C) and humidified chamber. In a blinded fashion, a pressure-volume curve (PV) was constructed and an injurious mode of mechanical ventilation initiated: VT 40 cc/kg, for 2 h. At the end of this period, another PV curve was obtained and the lungs were subjected to a saline lavage for cytokines. In control lungs, we observed a 47% decrease in lung compliance, and high levels of TNF-α, IL-1β and MIP-2. By contrast, lungs from animals that were exposed to heat stress demonstrated a significant attenuation in lung injury, expressed by a smaller decrease in post-ventilation lung compliance (20% decrease, as compared to pre-ventilation values), and lower levels of cytokines in lung lavage. To our knowledge, this is the first demonstration that the stress response is also protective against a mechanically induced injury, and may be an important tool to attenuate ventilator-induced lung injury.

In all the studies cited above, the stress response was triggered before the onset of injury. Although these systems have been developed to study the mechanisms by which the stress response is protective, they were not designed to study the most common clinical situation: patients are identified after the disease has been initiated. Examples include septic shock and ARDS. If induction of the stress response is to be used clinically, it will be necessary to examine experimental protocols in which the stress response is initiated *after* the induction of injury. As discussed previously, most novel therapies for sepsis and ARDS which have been developed in the laboratory have failed to improve outcome in controlled studies in humans. There are probably many reasons for this failure including the complexity of the inflammatory cascade, our lack of detailed information about the interaction between mediators, and our inability to stop an ongoing inflammatory reaction of this complexity. In addition, the inflammatory cascade is generally a protective phenomenon and it is difficult to know how aggressively this cascade should be blocked to achieve an anti-inflammatory response.

The advantage of using the stress response is related to its universal presence. In contrast to TNF antibodies which block only TNF expression, the stress response has the potential to act on many cytokine pathways and other proteins, slowing down the inflammatory reaction. In support of this concept is the finding that the stress response also down-regulates IL-1 production in LPS-stimulated cells [73, 74]. However, against this approach are the findings of Buchman et al [75] who observed that when endothelial cells were treated with LPS for 18 h and *then* exposed to heat stress or sodium arsenite, a dose-dependent cytotoxicity was observed. This study suggests that triggering the stress response during the course of an ongoing inflammatory response can lead to apoptosis.

Based on the importance of Buchman's studies showing the induction of apoptosis in LPS-stimulated cells that were exposed to heat stress, we have explored the hypothesis that heat stress could also be protective if induced after the initiation of sepsis [76]. In contrast to Buchman's study, in which endothelial cells were stimulated with bacterial endotoxin for 18 h and were then exposed to a period of heat stress (43°C for 90 min), we decreased both stresses, by reducing the dose of endotoxin and the period of exposure to heat stress. In this prospective and randomized study, rats were anesthetized and injected with an LD50 iv dose of *E. coli* endotoxin (15 mg/kg – in our previous studies we administered 20 mg/kg of endotoxin). Immediately thereafter, animals were randomly assigned to 1 of 2 treatment groups: septic (control), or septic, and heated to 41°C (in our previous protocol, rats achieved Tr 42.5°C). The animals were then observed for the development of fever and survival rates monitored for 72 h. In another set of rats the same experimental protocol was used to determine plasma cytokine levels in heated and non-heated groups. Blood samples were obtained after LPS injection for TNF-α and IL-1β detection. LPS injection in the control group did not produce fever and animals exposed to heat stress increased the abundance of HSP 72 kDa in the lungs. Twelve hours after the initiation of experimental sepsis, the survival rates of the control group injected with LPS alone and the group heated to 41°C were 48 and 80%, respectively ($p = 0.039$). The increase in survival in septic animals that were exposed to artificial fever (heat stress) was associated with a significant attenuation in plasma TNF-α levels and plasma IL-1β levels. From this study, we concluded that heat stress after the initiation of sepsis can provide protection against an otherwise lethal stimulus and that the mechanism of protection may be related to the attenuation of plasma TNF-α and IL-1β levels.

Potential Cytoprotective Mechanisms

The major function of the heat shock proteins is to physically associate with other proteins [46], acting as molecular chaperones. This transient interaction is believed to be responsible for the cytoprotective effects of the stress response [77]. Also, the specific role of HSP 72 kDa in protection has been shown in *in vivo* studies in which transgenic mice overexpressing this particular protein were resistant to ischemic injury to the heart [78] and had improved post-ischemic myocardial recovery [79].

To determine the specific role of HSP 72 kDa in our studies, we conducted *in vitro* experiments in which a more controlled environment could be obtained. In this study [62], we exposed alveolar macrophages, obtained from normal rats, to heat stress or sodium arsenite stimulation. Eighteen hours later, the cells were challenged with bacterial endotoxin and TNF-α levels were obtained. A major advantage of the use of LPS as an experimental model for sepsis is its reproducibility either in *in vivo* or *in vitro* systems. LPS has been widely used in various cell lineages, and has been shown to be a potent stimulatory factor to induce the production of TNF and other cytokines from macrophages. The exposure of alveolar macrophages to heat stress or to sodium arsenite induced the synthesis of HSP 72 kDa in a time-related fashion. The stress response also attenuated the amount of TNF released from the cell under LPS stimulation (Fig. 3). Mechanistically, our findings that both animals and cells produced decreased amounts of TNF provides a plausible explanation as to how animals might be protected against the lethality of sepsis. By decreasing TNF levels in the circulation, the stress response abolishes the pivotal inflammatory mediator in the sepsis cascade (TNF).

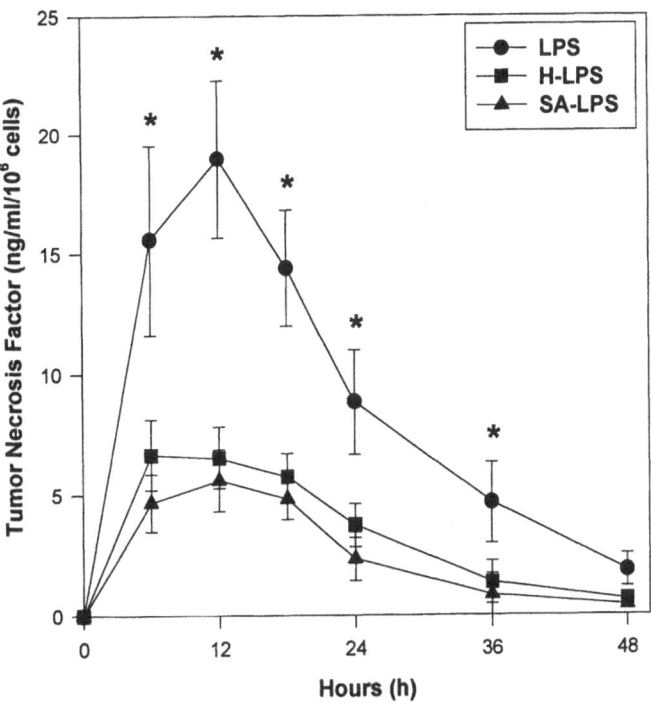

Fig. 3. Effects of the stress response on TNF-α production by LPS-stimulated alveolar macrophages (AM). Macrophages stimulated with LPS alone produced significantly higher levels of TNF (* different from the other two groups, p < 0.0001) compared to cells exposed to heat stress (H) or to SA 18 h prior to LPS stimulation. (From [62] with permission)

Interestingly, decreasd TNF release from the cell was not associated with a similar attenuation in TNF mRNA levels or in cell-associated TNF protein. These results are important in determining the mechanisms by which the stress response is protective. The demonstration that heat stress or sodium arsenite treatments did not alter TNF mRNA levels in LPS-stimulated cells suggests normal TNF transcription. In this regard, our results support the evidence that cell-membrane receptors, the signal transduction pathway, and mechanisms of TNF gene activation have regained their functions 18 h after the initial stress. Also, our findings that cell-associated TNF is present in both groups and follows similar dynamics levels, suggest a post-translational control for TNF under stress conditions. Finally, we observed that HSP 72 kDa and TNF-α form a protein/protein complex intracellularly, under stress conditions and LPS stimulation, but this complex was not observed under LPS challenge only. Given the chaperone function of HSP, we speculate that HSP are directly responsible for decreased TNF release, by binding TNF intracellularly and preventing its release from macrophages.

Possible involvement of HSP in protection against sepsis and septic lung injury can be summarized as in Fig. 4. Our studies suggest that when animals or cells are stimulated with bacterial endotoxin (LPS), there is production of high levels of TNF (Fig. 4). However, if the stress response is activated 18 h prior to LPS stimulation, there is a significant decrease in TNF released from the cell (Fig. 4). In determining the mechanism of TNF regulation by the stress response, we showed that the signals responsible for TNF synthesis were not affected by the stress response, since TNF messenger RNA levels were similar among experimental groups (Fig. 4), and cell-associated TNF was also similar in the groups studied. These data suggest that TNF regulation occurred at the post-translational level. The finding that TNF and HSP 72 kDa were physically associated in stressed and LPS-stimulated cells is compatible with the notion that HSP may bind to TNF and hence exert post-translational control over TNF release (Fig. 4). We speculate that HSP "determine" whether TNF is released from the cell or is sent the lysosomal machinery for degradation (Fig. 4).

These results, however, must be interpreted with caution. The demonstration that HSP 72 kDa and TNF-α form a complex of proteins in stressed and LPS-stimulated cells does not prove that HSP 72 kDa is responsible for TNF down-regulation. Also, although there are advantages of studies in *in vitro* systems, repro-

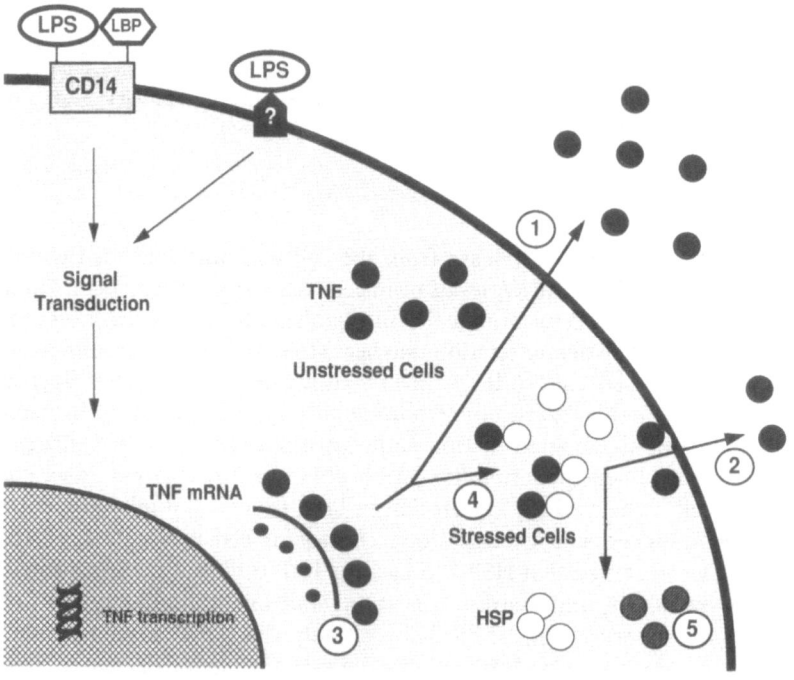

Fig. 4. Potential mechanisms involving HSP 72 kDa in cytoprotection against sepsis and ALI. See text for details

ducing the same data *in vivo* would certainly strengthen the findings. In future studies, the functional role of HSP in TNF regulation has to be determined. Since HSP are intracellular proteins, the use of a technique that antagonizes HSP function intracellularly is necessary. Antisense oligonucleotides and microinjection of antibodies to HSP are such examples. To be effective, however, these agents must successfully enter the cell, without being degraded by specific intracellular DNAases [80, 81]. Microinjection of antibodies to HSP directly into cells has been successfully used to block HSP70 protein expression [56]. Whichever approach is taken to abolish HSP expression, one has to be cognizant of the fact that HSP70 is not the only member of the heat shock protein family associated with cell protection [46]. Antagonizing the functions of one HSP might not be sufficient.

Conclusion and Potential Clinical Implications

There are a number of potential clinical uses related to our knowledge of the stress response and the heat shock proteins in disease processes other than sepsis and ARDS. The demonstration that physiologically relevant insults such as seizures [82], ischemia [83], hypoxia [84], ischemia/reperfusion [38], and fever [85] can induce the stress response *in vivo* opens up the possibility for using HSP as markers of disease activity. Also, using the induction of HSP as markers of toxic effects of different compounds in cells grown *in vitro* could reduce the use of animals for this purpose. More promising, however, is the use of the stress response in non-emergent situations. In particular, applying heat stress to donors has been shown to improve kidney function after transplantation [86], and reconstructive surgeons have found that skin flap survival improves if the flap is first made thermotolerant [87]. Pizarro et al [88] demonstrated that there is overexpression of TNF in rat cardiac transplants during allograft rejection. Their findings, in combination with our data demonstrating that the stress response prevents overexpression of TNF, suggest the possibility for the direct use of this natural defense mechanism (the stress response) to prevent organ rejection, although our studies demonstrated no improvement in lung function following pulmonary preservation in rabbits [89]. In addition, it is possible that patients at risk for developing sepsis and ARDS could benefit from the use of some strategy to trigger the stress response. Finally, in contrast to making use of overexpression of HSP as a cytoprotective tool, finding a way by which to down-regulate HSP might also have clinical utility. For example, tumor cells expressing HSP72 are more resistant to chemotherapeutic agents [90]. Thus, down-regulation of HSP in malignant cells could enhance the efficacy of many chemotherapeutic agents, allowing the use of lower doses of these agents, and minimizing the toxic side effects.

Acknowledgement. Dr. Ribeiro is a recipient of a Fellowship from The Will Rogers Foundation (USA). This work was supported in part by the Medical Research Council of Canada.

References

1. Bone RC (1991) Gram-negative sepsis. Background, clinical features, and interventions. Chest 100:802–808
2. Kollef MH, Schuster DP (1995) The acute respiratory distress syndrome. N Engl J Med 332: 27–37
3. Fowler AA, Hamman RF, Zerbe GO, Benson KN, Hyers TM (1985) Adult respiratory distress syndrome: Prognosis after onset. Am Rev Respir Dis 132:472–478
4. Montgomery AB, Stager MA, Carrico CJ, Hudson LD (1985) Causes of mortality in patients with the adult respiratory distress syndrome. Am Rev Respir Dis 132:485–489
5. Beutler B, Milsark IW, Cerami A (1985) Passive immunization against cachectin/tumor necrosis factor protects mice from lethal effect of endotoxin. Science 229:869–871
6. Mathinson JC, Wolfson E, Ulevitch RJ (1988) Participation of tumor necrosis factor in the mediation of Gram-negative bacteria lipopolysaccharide-induced injury in rabbits. J Clin Invest 81:1925–1937
7. Tracey KJ, Fong Y, Hesse HG (1987) Anti-cachectin/TNF antibodies prevent the fatal sequelae of experimental bacteremia in primates. Nature 330:662–664
8. Ohlsson K, Bjork P, Bergenfeldt M, Hageman R, Thompson RC (1990) Interleukin-1 receptor antagonist reduces mortality from endotoxin shock. Nature 348:550–552
9. Bone RC (1991) A critical evaluation of new agents for treatment of sepsis. JAMA 266: 1686–1691
10. Greenman RL, Schein RMH, Martin MA, et al (1991) A controlled clinical trial of E5 murine monoclonal IgM antibody to endotoxin in the treatment of Gram-negative sepsis. JAMA 266:1097–1102
11. Haupt MT, Jastremski MS, Clemmer TP, Metz CA, Goris GB (1991) Effect of ibuprofen in patients with severe sepsis: A randomized, double-blind, multicenter study. Crit Care Med 19:1339–1347
12. Cohen J, Carlet J (1996) INTERSEPT: An international, multicenter, placebo-controlled trial of monoclonal antibody to human tumor necrosis factor-α in patients with sepsis. Crit Care Med 24:1431–1440
13. Bone RC (1991) The pathogenesis of sepsis. Ann Intern Med 115:457–469
14. Fong Y, Lowry SF (1991) Modulation of the cytokine response in sepsis. In: Vincent JL (ed) Update in intensive care and emergency medicine. Springer-Verlag, Berlin, pp 223–231
15. Tobias PS, Mathinson J, Mintz D, et al. (1992) Participation of lipopolysaccharide-binding protein in lipopolysaccharide-dependent macrophage activation. Am J Respir Cell Mol Biol 7:239–245
16. Roine R, Luurila OJ, Soukas A, et al (1992) Alcohol and sauna bathing: Effects on cardiac rhythm, blood pressure, and serum electrolyte and cortisol concentrations. J Inter Med 231:333–338
17. Ziegler-Heitbrok HWL, Ulevitch RJ (1993) CD14: Cell surface receptor and differentiation marker. Immunol Today 14:121–125
18. Dentener MA, Bazil V, von-Asmuth EJU, Ceska M, Buurman WA (1993) Involvement of CD14 in lipopolysaccharide-induced tumor necrosis factor-α, IL-6 and IL-8 release by human monocytes and alveolar macrophages. J Immunol 150:2885–2891
19. Schumann RR, Leong SR, Flaggs GW, et al (1990) Structure and function of lipopolysaccharide binding protein. Science 249:1429–1431
20. Morrison DC, Ulevitch RJ (1978) The effects of bacterial endotoxins on host mediation systems. Am J Pathol 93:527–617
21. Said SI, Foda HD (1989) Pharmacologic modulation of lung injury. Am Rev Respir Dis 139: 1553–1564
22. Tracey KJ, Beutler B, Lowry SF (1986) Shock and tissue injury induced by recombinant human cachectin. Science 234:470–474
23. Silva AT, Bayston KF, Cohen J (1990) Prophylactic and therapeutic effects of a monoclonal antibody to tumor necrosis factor-alpha in experimental Gram-negative shock. J Infect Dis 162:421–427
24. Ashkenazi A, Marsters SA, Capon DJ, et al (1991) Protection against endotoxic shock by tumor necrosis factor receptor immunoadhesin. Proc Natl Acad Sci USA 88:10535–10539

25. Ziegler EJ, McCutchan JA, Fierer J, et al (1987) Treatment of Gram-negative bacteremia and shock with human antiserum to mutant *Escherichia coli*. N Engl J Med 307:1225–1230
26. Walsh CJ, Carey PD, Cook DJ, Bechard DE, Fowler AA, Sugerman HJ (1991) Anti-CD18 antibody attenuates neutropenia and alveolar capillary-membrane injury during Gram-negative sepsis. Surgery 110:205–212
27. Bone RC, Fisher CJ, Clemment TP, Slotman GJ, Metz CA, Balk RA (1987) A controlled clinical trial of high dose methylprednisolone in the treatment of severe sepsis and septic shock. N Engl J Med 317:653–658
28. Herdegen JJ, Bone RC (1995) Inflammatory mediators and the role of immunomodulation in sepsis. In: Bone RC (ed) Pulmonary and critical care medicine. 1st ed. Mosby, Toronto, pp 1–20
29. Villar J, Ribeiro SP, Mullen JBM, Post M, Slutsky AS (1994) Induction of heat shock response reduces mortality rate and organ damage in a sepsis-induced acute lung injury model. Crit Care Med 22:914–921
30. Ribeiro SP, Villar J, Downey GP, Edelson JD, Slutsky AS (1994) Sodium arsenite induces heat shock protein – 72 kilodalton expression in the lung and protects rats against sepsis. Crit Care Med 22:922–929
31. Villar J, Edelson J, Post M, Mullen JBM, Slutsky AS (1993) Induction of heat stress proteins is associated with decreased mortality in an animal model of acute lung injury. Am Rev Respir Dis 147:177–181
32. Winston BW, Villar J, Edelson JD, Piovesan J, Mullen JBM, Slutsky AS (1991) Induction of heat stress proteins (hsp) is associated with decreased mortality in an animal model of hyperoxic lung injury. Am Rev Respir Dis 143:A728 (Abst)
33. Ritossa F (1962) A new puffing pattern induced by temperature shock and DNP in drosophila. Experientia 18:571–573
34. Lindquist-McKenzie SL, Meselson M (1977) Translation *in vitro* of Drosophila heat shock messages. J Mol Biol 117:279–283
35. Welch WJ (1992) Mammalian stress response: Cell physiology, structure/function of stress proteins, and implications for medicine and disease. Physiol Rev 72:1063–1081
36. Blake MJ, Gershon D, Fargnoli J, Holbrook NJ (1990) Discordant expression of heat shock protein mRNA in tissues of heat stressed rats. J Biol Chem 265:15275–15279
37. Brown IR, Rush SJ (1984) Induction of a "stress" proteins in intact mammalian organs after the intravenous administration of sodium arsenite. Biochem Biophys Res Commun 120:150–155
38. Nowak TS Jr (1990) Synthesis of a stress protein following transient ischemia in the gerbil. J Neurochem 45:1635–1641
39. Clark BD, Brown IR (1982) Protein synthesis in the mammalian retina following intravenous administration of LSD. Brain Res 247:97–104
40. Nover L (1991) Heat shock response. CRC Press, Boston pp 1–509
41. Ashburner M (1970) Pattern of puffing activity in the salivary gland chromosomes of *Drosophila*: Response to environmental treatments. Chromossoma 31:356–376
42. Tomasovic SP, Klostergaard J (1991) Bacterial endotoxin lipopolysaccharide modulates synthesis of the 70 kDa heat stress protein family. Int J Hyperthermia 7:643–651
43. Morimoto RI, Tissieres A, Georgopoulos C (1990) Stress proteins in biology and medicine. Cold Spring Harbor Laboratory Press, pp 1–450
44. Henle KJ, Leeper DB (1976) Interaction of hyperthermia and radiation in CHO cells: Recovery kinetics. Radiat Res 66:505–518
45. Tissieres A, Mitchell HK, Tracy VM (1974) Protein synthesis in salivary glands of Drosophila melanogaster: Relation to chromossome puffs. J Mol Biol 84:389–398
46. Minowada G, Welch WJ (1995) Clinical implications of the stress response. J Clin Invest 95:3–12
47. Welch WJ (1987) The mammalian heat shock (or stress) response; A cellular defense mechanism. Adv Exp Med Biol 225:287–304
48. Lindquist S (1988) The heat-shock proteins. Ann Rev Genet 22:631–677
49. Lindquist S (1986) The heat-shock response. Ann Rev Biochem 55:1151–1191
50. Burdon RH (1986) Heat shock and the heat shock proteins. Biochem J 240:313–324

51. Sanchez Y, Lindquist S (1990) HSP104 is required for induced thermotolerance. Science 248:1112–1115
52. Li GC, Laszlo A (1985) Amino acid analogs while inducing heat shock proteins sensitize CHO cells to thermal damage. J Cell Physiol 122:91–97
53. Collier NC, Schlesinger MJ (1986) The dynamic state of heat shock proteins in chicken embryo fibroblasts. J Cell Biol 103:1495–1507
54. Welch WJ, Mizzen LA (1988) Characterization of the thermotolerant cell II. Effects on the intracellular distribution of heat-shock protein 70, intermediate filaments, and small nuclear ribonucleoprotein complexes. J Cell Biol 106:1117–1130
55. Mizzen LA, Welch WJ (1988) Characterization of the thermotolerant cell I. Effects on protein synthesis activity and the regulation of heat-shock protein 70 expression. J Cell Biol 106:1105–1116
56. Riabowol KT, Mizzen LA, Welch WJ (1988) Heat shock is lethal to fibroblast microinjected with antibodies against HSP 70. Science 242:433–436
57. Hendrey J, Kola I (1991) Thermolability of mouse oocytes is due to the lack of expression and/or inducibility of HSP70. Mol Reprod Dev 28:1–8
58. Ryan AJ, Flanagan SW, Moseley PL, Gisolfi CV (1992) Acute heat stress protects rats against endotoxin shock. J Appl Physiol 73:1517–1522
59. Hotchkiss R, Nunnally I, Lindquist S, Taulien J, Perdrizet G, Karl I (1993) Hyperthermia protects mice against the lethal effects of endotoxin. Am J Physiol 265:R1447–R1457
60. Wichterman KA, Baue AE, Chaudry IH (1980) Sepsis and septic shock: A review of laboratory models and a proposal. J Surg Res 29:189–201
61. Chaudry IH, Wichterman KA, Baue AE (1979) Effect of sepsis on tissue adenine nucleotide levels. Surgery 85:205–211
62. Ribeiro SP, Villar J, Downey GP, Edelson JD, Slutsky AS (1996) Effects of the stress response in septic rats and LPS-stimulated alveolar macrophages: Evidence for TNF-α post-translational regulation. Am J Respir Crit Care Med
63. Valenza F, Ribeiro SP, Slutsky AS (1995) Large-volume, high-pressure mechanical ventilation up-regulates the production of tumor necrosis-α in an *ex vivo* rat septic lung model. Crit Care Med 23:A159 (Abst)
64. Valenza F, Ribeiro SP, Mullen JBM, Slutsky AS (1995) Large-volume, high-pressure mechanical ventilation up-regulates the production of proinflammatory mediators in an *ex vivo* rat septic lung model. Am J Respir Crit Care Med A452 (Abst)
65. Dreyfuss D, Basset G, Soler P, Saumon G (1985) Intermittent positive-pressure hyperventilation with high inflation pressures produces pulmonary microvascular injury in rats. Am Rev Respir Dis 132:880–884
66. Dreyfuss D, Saumon G. (1994) Ventilator-induced injury. In: Tobin MJ (ed) Principles and practice of mechanical ventilation. McGraw-Hill, Toronto pp 793–811
67. Hernandez LA, Coker PJ, May S, Thompson AL, Parker JC (1990) Mechanical ventilation increases microvascular permeability in oleic acid-injured lungs. J Appl Physiol 69:2057–2061
68. Liu M, Skinner SJM, Xu J, Han RNN, Tanswell AK, Post M (1992) Stimulation of fetal rat lung cell proliferation *in vitro* by mechanical stretch. Am J Physiol 263:L376–L383
69. Liu M, Xu J, Tanswell AK, Post M (1993) Stretch-induced growth promoting activities stimulate fetal rat lung epithelial cell proliferation. Exp Lung Res 19:505–517
70. Laskin DL, Soltys RA, Berg RA, Riley D (1994) Activation of alveolar macrophages by native and synthetic collagen-like polypeptides. Am J Respir Cell Mol Biol 10:58–64
71. Murphy JK, Livinstong FR, Gozal E, Torres M, Forman HJ (1993) Stimulation of the rat alveolar macrophages respiratory burst by extracellular adenine nucleotides. Am J Respir Cell Mol Biol 9:505–510
72. Ribeiro SP, Rhee K, Tremblay L, Slutsky AS (1997) Heat stress prevents ventilator-induced lung injury. Am J Respir Crit Care Med (Abst) (In press)
73. Schmidt JA, Abdulla E (1988) Down-regulation of IL-1β biosynthesis by inducers of the heat shock response. J Immunol 141:2027–2034
74. Nahori MA, Morange M, Vargaftig BB (1992) Heat shock response of guinea-pig tracheal epithelium: Modulation by LPS. Am Rev Respir Dis 145:A364 (Abst)

75. Buchman TG, Abello PA, Smith EH, Bulkley GB (1993) Induction of heat shock response leads to apoptosis in endothelial cells previously exposed to endotoxin. Am J Physiol 265: H165–H170

76. Ribeiro SP, Chu E, Slutsky AS (1996) Heat stress after injection of LPS in rats decreases mortality. Am J Respir Crit Care Med 153:A252 (Abst)

77. Beckmann RP, Lovett M, Welch WJ (1992) Examining the function and regulation of HSP70 in cells subjected to metabolic stress. J Cell Biol 117:1137–1150

78. Marber MS, Mestril R, Chi S, Sayen R, Yellon DM, Dilman WH (1995) Overexpression of the rat inducible 70 kDa heat stress protein in transgenic mouse increases the resistance of the heart to ischemic injury. J Clin Invest 95:1446–1456

79. Plumier JCL, Ross BM, Currie RW, et al. (1995) Transgenic mice expressing the human heat shock protein 70 have improved post-ischemic myocardial recovery. J Clin Invest 95: 1854–1860

80. Toulme JJ, Helene C (1988) Antimessenger oligodeoxyribonucleotides: An alternative to antisense RNA for artificial regulation of gene expression – A review. Gene 72:51–58

81. Wickstrom EL, Bacon TA, Gonzalez A, Freeman DL, Lyman GH, Wickstrom E (1988) Human promyelocytic leukemia HL-60 cell proliferation and c-myc protein expression are inhibited by an antisense pentadecadoxynucleotide target against c-myc mRNA. Proc Natl Acad Sci USA 85:1028–1032

82. Vass K, Berger ML, Nowak TSJ, Welch WJ, Lassmann H (1989) Induction of stress protein HSP 70 in nerve cells after status epileticus in the rat. Neurosci Lett 100:259–264

83. Dilmann WH, Metha HB, Barrieux A, Guth BD, Neeley WE, Ross J Jr (1986) Ischemia of the dog heart induces the appearance of cardiac mRNA coding for a protein with migration characteristics similar to heat-shock/stress proteins. Circ Res 59:110–114

84. Howard G, Geoghegan TE (1985) Induction of stress proteins mRNA in mouse cardiac tissue by hypoxic hypoxia. Fed Proc 44:664–

85. Polla BS, Kantengwa S (1991) Heat shock proteins and inflammation. Curr Top Microbiol Immunol 167:93–105

86. Perdrizet GA, Hefferon TG, Buckingan FC (1989) Stress condition: A novel approach to organ preservation. Curr Surg 42:23–25

87. Koenig WJ, Lohner RA, Perdrizet GA, Lohner ME, Schweitzer RT, Lewis VL Jr (1992) Improving acute skin-flap survival through stress conditioning using heat shock and recovery. Plast Recontr Surg 90:659–664

88. Pizarro TT, Malinowska K, Kovacs EJ, Clancy J Jr, Robinson JA, Piccinini LA (1993) Induction of TNF-α and TNF-β gene expression in a rat cardiac transplants during allograft rejection. Transplant 56:399–404

89. Waddell TK, Hirai T, Piovesan J, et al. (1994) The effect of heat shock on immediate post-preservation lung function. Clin Invest Med 17:405–413

90. Hahn GM, Li GC. (1990) Thermotolerance, thermoresistance, and thermosen-sitization. In: Morimoto RI, Tissieres A, Georgopoulos C (eds) Stress proteins in biology and medicine. Cold Spring Harbor, New York pp 79–100

Alveolar Surfactant and ARDS

W. Seeger, A. Günther, and H. D. Walmrath

Introduction

The acute respiratory distress syndrome (ARDS) characterizes different states of acute impairment of pulmonary gas exchange. Underlying noxious events may directly affect lung parenchyma from the alveolar side (e.g. gastric acid aspiration), or – more classically – the lung vasculature may be the primary target site of circulating humoral or cellular mediators activated under conditions of systemic inflammatory events such as sepsis or severe polytrauma [1]. Key pathophysiological features of the initial "exudative" phase of ARDS include:

1) increased capillary endothelial and alveolar epithelial permeability.
2) leakage of protein rich edema fluid into interstitial and alveolar spaces.
3) increased pulmonary vascular resistance with maldistribution of pulmonary perfusion.
4) alveolar instability with formation of atelectases and ventilatory inhomogenities.
5) severe disturbances of gas exchange characterized by ventilation-perfusion mismatch and extensive shunt flow.

This exudative phase may persist for days to weeks, and full recovery without persistent loss of lung function is possible during this period. New inflammatory events, such as recurrent sepsis or acquisition of secondary (nosocomial) pneumonia, may repetitively worsen the state of lung function and then progressively trigger proliferative processes with mesenchymal cell activation and rapidly ongoing lung fibrosis. Thus, within a few weeks, the lung architecture may become dominated by thickened fibrotic alveolar septae and large interposed airspaces ("honeycombing"). Prognosis is very poor during this phase of ARDS, and only partial recovery of lung function may be achieved in the few survivors from this late phase of disease.

The alveolar space of all mammalian lungs is covered by a complex surfactant system, which is essential to make alveolar ventilation and gas exchange feasible at physiological transpulmonary pressures. It is mainly composed of lipids (90%) and proteins (10%) [2–5]. Apart from a minor amount of neutral lipids (10–20%), phospholipids (PL, 80–90%) represent the predominant class of lipids in this surface lining material. Among those, phosphatidylcholine (PC, 70–80% of PL, 50–60% substituted with the saturated palmitic acid) and phosphatidylglycerol (PG, 10% of PL, bearing a large percentage of unsaturated fatty acids) represent the predominant classes; phosphatidylethanolamine (PE), phosphatidylserine (PS), phosphatidylinositol (PI) and sphingomyelin (Sph) are regularly found in low percentages [2]. About half the protein mass of the alveolar lining layer represents the surfactant specific apoproteins (SP)-A (28 kDa), SP-B (8 kDa), SP-C (5 kDa), and SP-D (43 kDa) (all molecular weights given for reducing conditions [3–5]). The predominant, and with respect to some compounds, exclusive source of the different lipid and protein components of the alveolar surfactant system is the type II alveolar epithelial cell. A complex and yet not fully understood interaction between phospholipids and surfactant apoproteins results in far-reaching reduction in the alveolar surface tension, approximating to near zero (mN/m) values at end expiration, with a limited increase in surface tension upon alveolar surface enlargement during inspiration [6]. Such extreme low surface tension may only be achieved by dense "packing" of some rigid lipid material such as dipalmitoyl-PC in the surface film. However, characteristics of fluidity are similarly essential for removal of surface film compounds into the bulk phase during surface (over)-compression and rapid re-entry and re-spreading of these compounds upon re-expansion of the surface area. Studies focusing on the biophysical properties of individual surfactant compounds (for review see [2–6]) underlined the importance of dipalmitoyl-PC and unsaturated PG, and elaborate a key role for the highly hydrophobic low molecular weight apoproteins SP-B and SP-C in adsorption facilities and dynamic surface tension lowering properties [7–10].

More recent studies demonstrate a metabolic cycle of the secreted surfactant material within the alveolar space. Surfactant material retrieved by bronchoalveolar lavage (BAL) fluid may be separated by density or high speed centrifugation into different subfractions defined as small and large surfactant aggregates. The highly surface active large surfactant aggregates comprise lamellar bodies, tubular myelin and multilamellar vesicles, and are thought to represent the precursor fraction of the alveolar lining layer, whileas small surfactant aggregates consist mainly of small, unilamellar vesicles, which largely represent the degradation products of the lining layer and possess poor surface activity [11]. A conversion of the large to the small aggregates may be encountered upon periodic surface area changes and in presence of an enzymatic activity, which can be blocked in vitro and in vivo by serin protease inhibitors [12]. However, this enzyme, recently entitled surfactant convertase, has not been identified.

Although several authors reported on a cooperative effect of SP-A with the hydrophobic apoproteins on adsorption kinetics [7,13,14], the predominant function of this protein may be the regulation of the surfactant pool size in the alveolar space. SP-A binds to dipalmitoyl-PC, promotes the uptake of phospholipids into type II cells via receptor-operated events, and inhibits secretion of surfactant compounds by this cell type [15–17]. In addition, SP-D and SP-A might be involved in host defense mechanisms of the lower airways in vivo, as they function as opsonins for alveolar macrophage phagocytosis of bacteria and viruses in vitro [18–21].

Surfactant deficiency has been established as the primary cause of the respiratory distress syndrome in preterm infants (IRDS), and transbronchial application of natural surfactant preparations has been proven to be beneficial in this disease

[22, 23]. Surfactant abnormalities may also be involved in the sequelae of pathogenetic events in ARDS; however, due to the diversity of underlying triggering mechanisms and the complexity of pathophysiological events, any evaluation of the role of surfactant in this disease is much less certain. This review focuses on three questions:

1) What is the present evidence for surfactant abnormalities in patients with ARDS?
2) Which pathophysiological events encountered in the course of ARDS may be ascribed to surfactant abnormalities?
3) What are the acute effects of a transbronchial surfactant administration in ARDS in view of gas exchange and compliance?

These aspects aim to provide a rational basis for the question, whether transbronchial surfactant application might become a safe and general therapeutic approach in patients with ARDS as it is in IRDS.

Alteration of Surfactant in ARDS

Early post-mortem investigations in lungs from patients who had died with ARDS, provided the first evidence of severe impairment of surfactant function [24]. More direct proof was provided by biophysical analysis of BAL fluids obtained by flexible bronchoscopy during the active state of the disease [25–28]. Compared to normal volunteers, BAL samples of these patients showed increased minimal surface tension and decreased hysteresis of the surface tension/surface area relationship, two critical variables of surfactant function

Table 1. Impairment of surface activity in ARDS

Authors	Ref.	material	method	variable	change[a]
– Hallman et al.	[26]	protein-complexes[b]	BAL, lipid Balance	Wilhelmy	γ_{min} ↑_
– Pison et al.	[27]	BAL[c]	Wilhelmy Balance	Hysteresis γ_{min}	↓ ↑
– Gregory et al.	[25]	surfactant pellet[d]	BAL, crude Surfactometer	Bubble γ_{max}	γ_{min} ↑ ↑
– Günther et al.	[28]	surfactant pellet[d]	BAL, crude Surfactometer	Bubble γ_{max}	γ_{min} ↑ ↑

[a] Change as compared to normal volunteers
[b] BAL was centrifuged twice (140 × g, supernatant; 10 000 × g pellet) and was subjected to a discontinuous sucrose density gradient (100 000 × g). Material between 0.2 and 1.3 M sucrose ("lipid-protein complex") was used
[c] BAL was separated from cells by centrifugation at 300 × g, no further preparation
[d] BAL was separated from cells by centrifugation at 450 × g, supernatant was centrifuged at 48 000 × g, the resulting "crude surfactant pellet" was resuspended in saline and used for bubble measurements – γ_{min} – minimum surface tension, γ_{max} – maximum surface tension

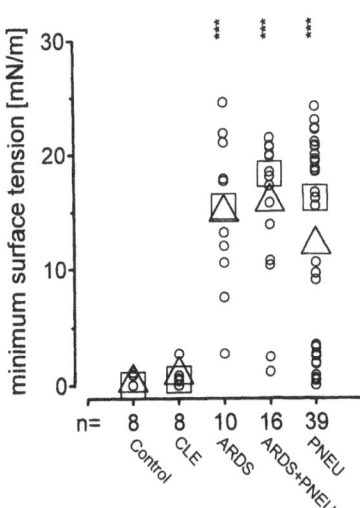

Fig. 1. Biophysical surfactant properties of isolated large surfactant aggregates. For controls and the different groups of patients, all single events (O), means (△) and median (□) values are indicated. Surface tension [mN/m] at minimum bubble size after 5min of film oscillation (γ_{min}) is given. Phospholipid concentration was 2 mg/mL; n-numbers are given in the x-axis. All groups were compared to controls; p is indicated by * (p < 0.05), ** (p < 0.01) or *** (p < 0.001). CLE: cardiogenic lung edema, ARDS : Acute respiratory distress syndrome, PNEU: Severe pneumonia necessitating mechanical ventilation, ARDS + PNEU: ARDS and lung infection. (From [28] with permission)

in vivo (Table 1, Fig. 1). Recently, elevated minimal surface tension values were also determined for surfactant samples obtained from patients being at risk for ARDS [25]. Several factors may underlay such a loss of surface activity in ARDS.

Lack of Surface-Active Compounds and Change in Phospholipid, Fatty Acid and Apoprotein Profiles

Clinical studies addressing the phospholipid composition of surfactant samples obtained from patients with ARDS revealed three important features. First, the overall content of phospholipids was found to be decreased in 2 of the 4 studies performed to date. In addition, this decrease appeared to be dependent on the severity of ARDS [25]. Second, the relative amounts of the 2 functionally most important phospholipids, PC and PG, were markedly depressed in all 3 studies (Table 2). Most strikingly, the PG levels decreased by > 80% in 3 of the studies; the decrease in the percentage of PC was more moderate in all investigations. However, the degree of palmitoylation, especially the relative amount of dipalmitoylated PC (DPPC), was found to be severely reduced in patients with ARDS (not given in detail). Third, all studies demonstrated an increase in the relative amounts of PI, PE and Sph.

Due to the late detection and – in case of SP-B and SP-C – the extreme hydrophobic nature of the surfactant apoproteins, appropriate analytical techniques for the measurement of these essential surfactant compounds have only recently become available; SP-C quantification in BAL samples is still an unresolved problem. Two recent studies measuring SP-A and SP-B in BAL samples from patients with ARDS demonstrated an impressive decline of SP-A (Table 3). SP-B loss was

Table 2. BAL phospholipid-profile[a]

%	PC	PG	PI	PE	PS	SPH	LPC
Control (n = 17)	83.1 ± 0.9	8.6 ± 0.6	3.2 ± 0.2	1.7 ± 0.2	1.2 ± 0.3	0.8 ± 0.2	0.1 ± 0.1
CLE (n = 10)	83.3 ± 0.8	7.3 ± 1.0	4.3 ± 0.7	1.5 ± 0.1	1.3 ± 0.2	1.2 ± 0.2	0.1 ± 0.1
ARDS (n = 15)	81.9 ± 1.1	3.5 ± 0.7[d]	6.5 ± 1.0[b]	1.9 ± 0.3	1.8 ± 0.5	3.5 ± 0.9[c]	0.3 ± 0.1
ARDS + PNEU (n = 28)	76.8 ± 2.6	2.4 ± 0.3[d]	8.0 ± 0.8[d]	2.6 ± 0.3	1.7 ± 0.3	5.2 ± 0.9[d]	0.2 ± 0.1
PNEU (n = 64)	79.2 ± 1.0	5.2 ± 0.4[d]	5.5 ± 0.4[b]	2.4 ± 0.3	2.4 ± 0.4	4.3 ± 0.6[d]	0.2 ± 0.1

[a] For controls and the various patient groups, the different phospholipid classes are given in percent of total phospholipids; mean values ± SE are depicted. All groups were compared to controls, and p is indicated by [b] (p < 0.05), [c] (p < 0.01) or [d] (p < 0.001).

PC: phosphatidylcholine, PG: phosphatidylglycerol, PI: phosphatidylinositol, PE: phosphatidylethanolamine, PS: phosphatidylserin, SPH: sphingomyelin, LPS: lysophosphatidylcholine, CLE :cardiogenic lung edema, ARDS: Acute respiratory distress syndrome, PNEU: Severe pneumonia necessitating mechanical ventilation, ARDS + PNEU: ARDS and lung infection. (From [28] with permission)

Table 3. BAL apoprotein contents[a]

	SP-B				SP-A			
	ng/ml	μg/ml[u]	% PL	% Prot	ng/ml	μg/ml	% PL	% Prot
Control (n = 20)	740 ± 85	94 ± 15	3.0 ± 0.3	1.4 ± 0.3	1533 ± 175	148 ± 31	6.2 ± 0.7	2.8 ± 0.4
CLE (n = 13)	628 ± 42	119 ± 13	2.5 ± 0.3	0.5 ± 0.1[c]	1013 ± 111	182 ± 21	4.5 ± 0.8	1.0 ± 0.3[c]
ARDS (n = 15)	867 ± 131	62 ± 16	3.3 ± 0.4	0.6 ± 0.2[c]	849 ± 96[b]	54 ± 14[b]	3.5 ± 0.5	0.7 ± 0.3[d]
ARDS + PNEU (n = 35)	818 ± 78	63 ± 22[b]	6.3 ± 0.8[c]	0.3 ± 0.0[d]	747 ± 79[c]	71 ± 35[c]	7.8 ± 1.5	0.3 ± 0.0[d]
PNEU (n = 86)	737 ± 43	58 ± 9[b]	5.5 ± 0.5[b]	0.4 ± 0.0[d]	876 ± 75[c]	66 ± 10[c]	6.2 ± 0.6	0.5 ± 0.1[d]

[a] BAL SP-B and SP-A levels are displayed for controls and the different groups of patients. Values are given for concentrations in the original lavage fluid (ng/ml), concentrations corrected for the urea quotient (μg/ml[u]), apoprotein-phospholipid ratios (%; wt/wt) and apoprotein-total protein ratios (%, wt/wt). All groups were compared to controls; p is indicated by [b] (p < 0.05), [c] (p < 0.01) or [d] (p < 0.001).

CLE: cardiogenic lung edema, ARDS: Acute respiratory distress syndrome, PNEU: Severe pneumonia necessitating mechanical ventilation, ARDS + PNEU: ARDS and lung infection. (From [28] with permission)

particularly prominent in the large surfactant aggregate fraction (see below). Again, some decrease of these functionally important compounds was also observed in patients at risk for ARDS [25].

The reported changes in lavage phospholipid and apoprotein content in patients suffering from ARDS are very much reminiscent of biochemical profiles characterized in neonates with immature lungs and IRDS [2]. They are thus likely to reflect injury of type II pneumocytes, with altered lipid and apoprotein metabolism and/or secretion by this cell type. In addition, the increase in PI, PE and Sph may be due to some surfactant "contamination" with membrane phospholipids from different injured cell types, and there may be leakage of plasma phospholipids under conditions of increased endothelial and epithelial permeability. Finally, as will be discussed below, incorporation of phospholipids into hyaline membranes might also contribute to the alterations in phospholipid and apoprotein profiles.

Alteration of Surfactant Subtype Distribution

Under physiological conditions, nearly 80–90% of the extracellular surfactant material is retrieved among the fraction of large surfactant aggregates (Fig. 2). This subfraction possesses a high SP-B content and excellent surface activity. Under conditions of ARDS, however, increase of the small surfactant aggregates at the expense of the large surfactant aggregates is encountered and is paralleled by a loss of SP-B and surface activity within the large surfactant aggregates (Fig. 2).

Inhibition of Surfactant Function by Plasma Protein Leakage

Leakage of plasma proteins into the alveolar space may contribute substantially to surfactant alterations in ARDS. Measurements of the protein content in BAL samples from these patients persistently show markedly increased levels when compared to normal controls. Protein leakage is an early event in the sequence of pathogenetic events in ARDS, and is related to the severity of the disease [28]. Experimental studies *in vitro* and *in vivo* have demonstrated that admixture of blood, serum, plasma or alveolar washings obtained during states of plasma leak-

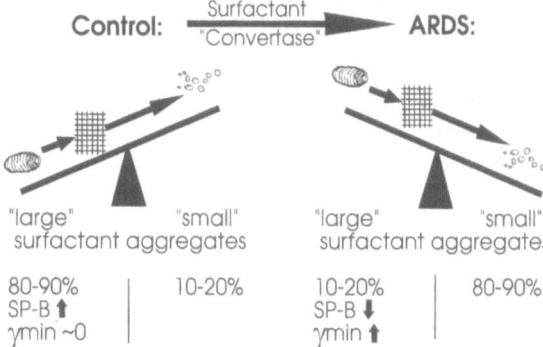

Fig. 2. Changes in the surfactant subtype distribution and the biophysical activity and SP-B content of large surfactant aggregates in the development of ARDS. (For details see text)

Table 4. Protein inhibition of pulmonary surfactant[a]

Varying degree of "protein-resistance" among different surfactants:
  relevant compounds SP-B > SP-C > SP-A
Inhibitory Capacity: Fibrinoligomers/-polymers ≫ Fb(g)lysisproducts > Fbmonomers,
  Fbg > Hemoglobin > Albumin
Polymerising Fibrin = "Surfactant-trap"
  (phospholipids and hydrophobic apoproteins)
"Specialized" alveolar Fibrinpolymer characterized by
  – incorporation of pulmonary surfactant with
  – promotion of alveolar collapse
  – lower susceptibility towards fibrinolytic enzymes
  – altered mechanical properties (e.g. rigidity ↓)
Restoration of regular surface tension properties by fibrinolytic approaches possible (release of
  surface active material)

[a] The table summarizes the current knowledge concerning the inhibition of surfactant function
  by plasma protein, especially the influence of fibrinogen (Fbg), fibrin monomers (Fb
  monomers) and fibrin oligo/polymers (Fb oligo/polymers). For details see text

age may severely compromise biophysical surfactant function (Table 4) [29–32]. Among different proteins involved, albumin [13, 29, 33, 34], hemoglobin [35], and in particular fibrinogen or fibrinmonomer [9, 13, 29, 34, 36, 37] possess strong surfactant inhibitory properties (Table 4). Concerning fibrinogen, it has been demonstrated that its potency to inhibit surfactant function depends on the surfactant apoprotein profile. Surfactant preparations lacking hydrophobic apoproteins are extremely sensitive to fibrinogen inhibition, and less sensitivity is noted in the presence of both SP-C and SP-B in near physiological quantities [9, 38]. In addition, a further reduction of surfactant sensitivity to fibrinogen is achieved by supplementation of phospholipid and hydrophobic apoprotein-based surfactants with SP-A [13].

"Incorporation" of Surfactant in Fibrin/Hyaline Membranes

Intra-alveolar accumulation of clot material, characterized as "hyaline membranes", is commonly found in ARDS and other acute or chronic inflammatory diseases of the lung [39–42]. In the alveolar milieu, the extrinsic coagulation pathway represents the predominant clotting sequence. Alveolar macrophages express and shed procoagulant activity, which is mainly attributable to tissue factor in compound with factor VII [43–46]. This alveolar procoagulant activity was found to be markedly increased in ARDS patients (possibly because of local macrophage activation [45–49]), and in several experimental models of lung injury (Fig. 3) [50–53]. By contrast, concentrations of urokinase-type plasminogen activator, representing the predominant fibrinolysis pathway within the alveolar spaces [45, 53–55], were noted to be decreased in lavage fluids from patients with ARDS. Concomitantly, increased levels of plasminogen-activator-inhibitor-1 and 2-antiplasmin were detected [45, 48, 53, 56]. Moreover, surfactant phospholipid mixtures

Alveolar Hemostatic Balance

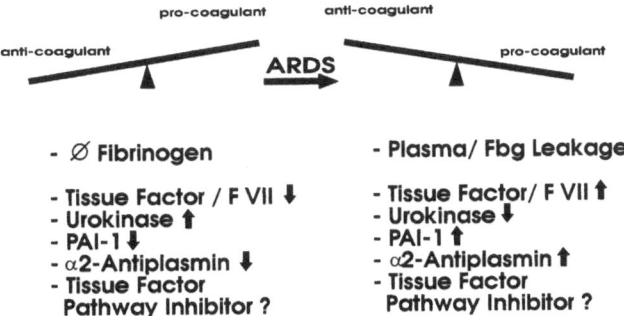

- ∅ Fibrinogen

- **Tissue Factor / F VII ↓**
- **Urokinase ↑**
- **PAI-1 ↓**
- **α2-Antiplasmin ↓**
- **Tissue Factor
  Pathway Inhibitor ?**

- **Plasma/ Fbg Leakage**

- **Tissue Factor/ F VII ↑**
- **Urokinase ↓**
- **PAI-1 ↑**
- **α2-Antiplasmin ↑**
- **Tissue Factor
  Pathway Inhibitor ?**

Fig. 3. Increase in procoagulant and decrease in fibrinolytic activity in the alveolar space under conditions of ARDS. (For details see text)

were found to inhibit plasmin-, trypsin- or elastase-induced fibrino(geno)lysis, in particular when combined with the surfactant apoproteins SP-B and SP-C [57,58]. Thus, the hemostatic balance within the alveolar milieu appears to be shifted towards predominance of procoagulant and antifibrinolytic activity in acutely or chronically inflamed lung regions, in particular in ARDS. Recent investigations performed by this group [59] demonstrated loss of surfactant phospholipids from the soluble phase due to binding to/within fibrin strands, when the process of fibrin polymerization occurred in the presence of surfactant material. In parallel, virtually complete loss of surface activity was noted, with fibrin dose-effect curves ranging two orders of magnitude below the corresponding efficacy range of soluble fibrinogen. ^{31}P-NMR-spectrum analysis suggested membrane-like, highly ordered arrangement of the fibrin-associated phospholipids. Overall, these findings obviously suggest "incorporation" of phospholipids (and possibly hydrophobic apoproteins) into nascent fibrin strands. This phenomenon may cause severe loss of functionally important surfactant compounds in areas with alveolar fibrin and hyaline membrane formation. Interestingly, surface activity may be largely restored by application of fibrinolytic agents *in vitro* [58] and *in vivo* (unpublished data), with release of formerly incorporated surfactant material into the soluble phase.

Damage of Surfactant Compounds by Inflammatory Mediators

A variety of inflammatory processes are assumed to underlie the microcirculatory disturbances of ARDS, and mediator generation has also been demonstrated in the alveolar compartment. Free elastase and collagenase activities were repeatedly detected in BAL fluids of patients with ARDS [60, 61]; oxidative inhibition of the alveolar α1–proteinase inhibitor indicated oxygen radical generation in this compartment, and increased levels of lysophospholipids (predominantly lyso-

Table 5. Impact of inflammatory mediators on surfactant function : *In vitro* studies

Mediator	Effects
phospholipases (A₂,C)	– generation of lysophospholipids (especially lysoPC) – loss of surface activity – higher sensitivity towards inhibition by plasma proteins – generation of free fatty acids (including arachidonic acid)
cytokines	
– TNF	– pretranslational inhibitory effect on the expression of SP-A and SP-B
proteases	
– elastase	– degradation of SP-A, indirect evidence for degradation of SP-B and SP-C; loss of surface activity
– mixed	– increased conversion of large to small surfactant aggregates?
– oxygen radicals	– decrease in surface activity – induction of lipid peroxidation
lipid mediators	
– arachidonic acid	– decrease in surface activity
– PMN	– decrease in surface activity – degradation of SP-A

PC) [26] suggested increased phospholipolytic activity in the alveolar space. A variety of *in vitro* studies have addressed putative direct inhibitory effects of inflammatory mediators on biophysical surfactant functions. Inhibitory potencies were demonstrated for phospholipases, proteases, oxygen radicals, free fatty acids and activated granulocytes (via release of oxygen radicals), as summarized in Table 5. Presently, however, no data are available to quantify the contribution of such surfactant-inhibitory effects of inflammatory mediators to the impairment of surfactant function in patients with ARDS.

Pathophysiological Consequences of Surfactant Alterations in ARDS

As outlined above, there is strong evidence of severe impairment of the alveolar surfactant system in ARDS, and several mechanisms may underlay this finding. Thus the question arises, whether and to what extent such surfactant alterations contribute to the sequence of pathogenetic events and the loss of lung functional integrity encountered in this disease.

Alteration of Lung Mechanics

Loss of alveolar surface activity increases surface tension thereby causing alveolar instability with formation of atelectases. These features must be expected to result in a marked decrease of lung compliance. This basic finding was, indeed, already described in the very early reports on altered mechanics of post-mortem analyzed lungs from patients dying with ARDS [24]. In addition, in a variety of experimental approaches using animal models of ARDS, induction of lung injury resulted in a significant decrease in compliance [62–67]. Accordingly, transbronchial application of surfactant was shown to completely or partially restore physiological lung compliance in some of these models [62–67]. In patients with severe ARDS, however, reliable measurements of lung compliance are still difficult to perform, mostly because of uncertainties concerning lung volumes (at which part of the pressure-volume curve does the lung actually range?) and transpulmonary pressures. Moreover, there is presently no reliable *in vivo* technique to differentiate the contribution of increased alveolar surface tension from that of interstitial congestion and on-going fibrosis to the reduction in lung compliance of ARDS patients. It is well conceivable that surfactant alterations predominate in the early phase of ARDS, whereas fibrotic events gain increasing importance in later states of the disease.

Impairment of Gas Exchange – V/Q Mismatch and Shunt Flow

Lack of surface active material has been established as a primary cause of severe gas exchange disturbances in IRDS, and dramatic improvements in arterial oxygenation are achieved by transbronchial surfactant application under these conditions [22, 23]. Similarly, experimental approaches in adult animals with removal of alveolar surfactant (lung lavage models [68]) and subsequent transbronchial reapplication of surface active material have underscored the fundamental significance of the alveolar surfactant system for ventilation-perfusion (V/Q) matching in adult lungs [68, 69, 70]. In more realistic models of ARDS, starting with induction of microvascular or alveolar injury, matters are more complex. Shunt (perfusion of atelectatic regions) and blood flow through lung areas with low V/Q ratios (partial closure of alveolar units or small airways) may well be related to an acute impairment of the alveolar surfactant system in such experiments, and transbronchial surfactant application was found to improve gas exchange in models with protein-rich edema formation due to cervical vagotomy [62], acid aspiration [63, 66, 71], induction of pneumonia [72], hyperoxic lung injury [73] and application of N-nitroso-N-methylurethane (NNNMU) [64, 65] or oleic acid [67]. The efficacy of surfactant replacement in these models with induction of lung inflammation is, however, lower than in those with primary surfactant depletion (lavage, preterm newborns), which is most probably attributable to the inhibitory capacities of leaked plasma proteins and inflammatory mediators, as discussed above. Larger amounts of surfactant material are apparently needed under these conditions, in order to surpass, at least partially, such inhibitory capacities.

Lung Edema Formation

Interstitial and alveolar edema is a key finding in ARDS, primarily ascribed to increased endothelial and epithelial permeability in the diseased lungs. Surfactant alterations may, however, contribute to the disturbances in fluid balance in ARDS. Any increase in alveolar surface tension must be expected to result in a decrease in interstitial and thus perivascular pressures and, according to Starling's law, increase transendothelial fluid fluxes into septal and interstitial spaces. Similarly, increased alveolar surface tension favors transepithelial fluid movement into the alveolar spaces. Several experimental studies have indeed demonstrated extensive lung edema formation due to inhibition of surfactant function *in vivo* by transbronchial detergent application [74, 75], intratracheal injection of bile acid [76], cooling and ventilating at low functional residual capacity (FRC) [77], or plasma lavage [78]. Moreover, the permeability characteristics of the epithelial membrane may be influenced by surfactant deficiencies. Increased transepithelial passage of ^{99m}Tc-DPTA (from alveolar to intravascular space) and labeled albumin (from intravascular to alveolar space) was observed under experimental conditions of surfactant impairment, and the increased fluxes could be reduced by transbronchial surfactant replacement [76, 79, 80]. Similarly, increased epithelial permeability for ^{99m}Tc-DPTA is noted in neonates with IRDS [81]. Concerning patients with ARDS, there is presently no conclusive study evaluating the impact of surfactant abnormalities on lung fluid balance and alveolar epithelial permeability characteristics.

Reduction of Host Defense Competence?

Next to the reduction of surface tension within the alveolar compartment, the pulmonary surfactant system is involved in many host defense properties of the lung. Although not fully understood at the present time, there is evidence that the hydrophilic apoproteins SP-A and SP-D might act as highly effective opsonins, thereby enhancing the phagocytosis of several strains of bacteria and viruses. By contrast, the lipid fraction of pulmonary surfactant is capable of suppressing the activation and proliferative response of lymphocytes, granulocytes and alveolar macrophages. Thus, these aspects are at best mosaics of a complex alveolar host defense system, which largely remains to be defined. The marked decrease in SP-A levels in lungs of ARDS patients (see above) may suggest a loss of opsonizing capacity and increased susceptibility to nosocomial infections.

"Collapse Induration", Mesenchymal Cell Proliferation and Fibrosis

The proliferative phase of ARDS is characterized by progressive mesenchymal cell activation and proliferation, predominantly in atelectatic regions, and may result in widespread lung fibrosis and honeycombing within weeks. Underlying mechanisms may include major roles for the alveolar surfactant system and alveolar fibrin deposition, as schematically depicted in Fig. 4. A corresponding sequence of events was suggested for the pathogenesis of lung fibrosis in general by Burkhardt [40] and termed "collapse induration". Basically, this concept starts with persistent atelectasis at sites of extensive loss of alveolar surfactant function,

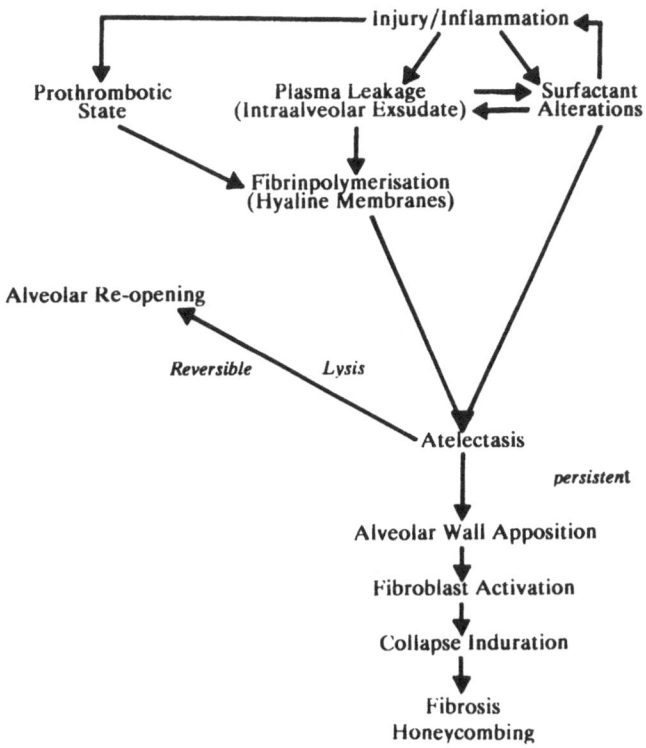

Fig. 4. Possible envolement of surfactant inhibition and alveolar fibrin deposition in the pathogenesis of fibrosis and honeycombing in protracted ARDS. (For details see text)

in particular regions with fibrin deposition. Alveolar wall apposition and the fibrin matrix represent a nidus for fibroblast activation, and the alveolar space is definitely lost through deposition of fibrous tissue (collapse induration). Thus, thick indurated septae (or conglomerates of several septae) may exist adjacent to widened (remaining) alveoli to provide the typical morphological image of fibrosis and honeycombing [39, 82]. This concept does not deny an important role of inflammatory mediators, such as TNF, and growth factors for the induction of mesenchymal cell activation in late ARDS. But it provides an explanation for the predominance of fibrosis at sites of persistent atelectasis and fibrin deposition.

Surfactant Replacement in ARDS: Current Status

Against the above background, improvement of alveolar surfactant function appears to be a reasonable approach to augment gas exchange in ARDS patients. Such attempts may include pharmacological approaches to stimulate the secretion of intact surfactant material from type II pneumocytes, but clear evidence that this approach may be effectively used under conditions of acute respiratory failure is lacking. In addition, transbronchial administration of exogenous (natural) surfactant preparations, commonly used in IRDS, may also be employed in ARDS, but will clearly demand larger quantities of material to overcome the surfactant inhibitory capacities in the alveolar space under these conditions. Two pilot studies in this field have been completed. Performing repetitive intratracheal application of Survanta, with cumulative doses between 300 and 800 mg/kg body weight, Gregory and colleagues [83] noted some improvement of gas exchange and even obtained some preliminary evidence for an increase in survival in adults with acute respiratory failure. Our group investigated the safety and efficacy of a bronchoscopic application of a natural surfactant extract (Alveofact) in patients with severe ARDS. All patients fulfilled extracorporeal membrane oxygenation (ECMO) criteria (mean Murray lung injury score ≈ 3.3) and were treated within the first 5 days of disease, i.e. before the onset of major fibrotic processes. Underlying diseases were mostly sepsis and severe pneumonia. At the present time, the study includes 26 patients. 300 mg/kg Alveofact was delivered bronchoscopically in divided doses to each segment of both lungs (total dose 22.5 ± 1.4 g in 375 mL saline), followed by a second application of 200 mg/kg (total dose 15.5 ± 1.05 g in 260 mL saline) 18–24 h later in selected patients. Measurements of gas exchange including ventilation-perfusion characteristics, hemodynamic measurements and BAL was performed before and after surfactant application. As given in Fig. 5, an acute and impressive improvement of the gas exchange was encountered, even during the application procedure. When analyzing the course of gas exchange among all patients, the first surfactant application resulted in an immediate increase of mean PaO_2/FiO_2 from <90 to ≈ 200 mmHg (Fig. 6), mainly due to a decrease in shunt flow (from ≈ 40 to ≈ 20 %). More than 2/3 of the patients "responded" with a PaO_2/FiO_2 increase of at least 25%. The effect was partially lost within the following hours in some of

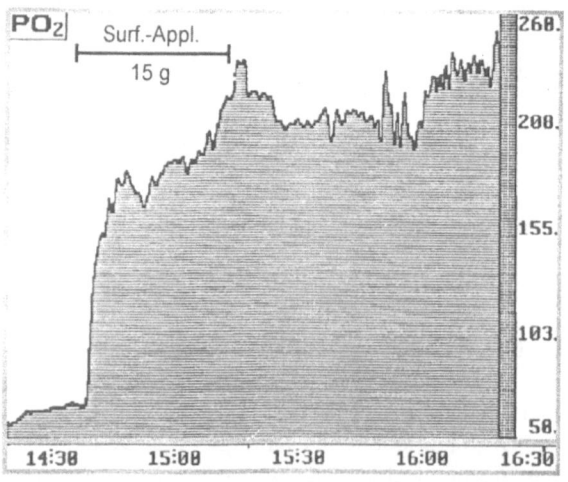

Fig. 5. On-line monitoring of PaO_2 during surfactant application in a 18–year old female with ARDS due to sepsis. As evident from the figure, a far-reaching improvement of oxygention was encountered already within the process of bronchoscopic surfactant application (300 mg/kg body weight Alveofact). The time period of the bronchoscopic procedure is indicated; FiO_2 was set 1.0 throughout. (From [84] with permission)

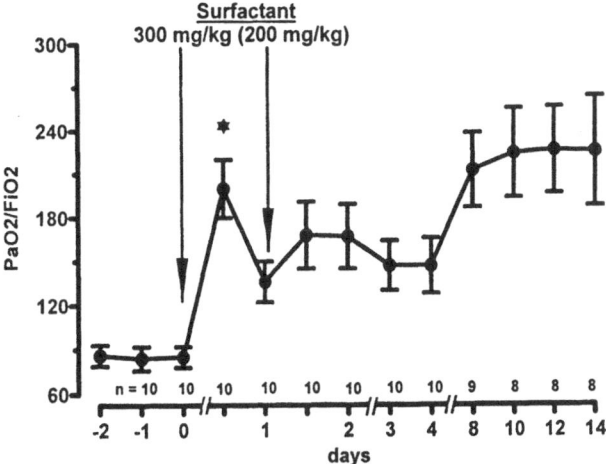

Fig. 6. Time course of oxygenation index (PaO_2/FiO_2) in response to surfactant application. Mean ± SEM of 10 patients are given. 300 mg/kg natural surfactant was delivered bronchoscopically in separate doses to each segment of both lungs in all patients (time zero). In 5 patients, in whom the surfactant-related increase in arterial oxygenation was partially lost within the next hours, a second dose of 200 mg/kg surfactant was applied 18–24 h later. The highest PaO_2/FiO_2 value is given for each day, and for every 12 h within the first 2 days. The number of surviving patients is indicated. (* $p < 0.001$ for comparison of the PaO_2/FiO_2 values before and after the first surfactant application). (From [84] with permission)

the responders, but restored with prolonged improvement of arterial oxygenation by the second application. Initial BAL showed severe alteration of surfactant composition and impaired biophysical surfactant function (Table 6). Surfactant application resulted in a marked, but still incomplete restoration of surfactant properties, with a profound improvement of the phospholipid (PL)-protein ratio, relative content of large surfactant aggregates, relative content of phosphatidylcholine, minimum surface tension in absence as well as in presence of the inhibitory BAL fluid proteins. Analysis of the ventilation-perfusion characteristics revealed that in response to the bronchoscopic surfactant application, formerly collapsed alveoli were re-aerated, yielding a reduction of the intrapulmonary shunt flow and an increase in regions with low and normal ventilation-perfusion ratios.

Conclusion

Profound alterations of the alveolar surfactant system are encountered in ARDS. There is now good evidence that these abnormalities contribute to the severe impairment of gas exchange under these conditions. Transbronchial surfactant application, performed by bronchoscopy by our group, may offer a feasible and safe approach to improve biochemical and biophysical properties of the endogenous

Table 6. BAL variables pre- and post-surfactant application : Comparison to controls and surfactant replacement material

Variables	Patients		Controls	AlveoFact®
	pre	post		
PPR	0.02 ± 0.01	$0.23^c \pm 0.1$	0.58 ± 0.1	—
LSA (%)	27.7 ± 5.3	$68.6^a \pm 8.8$	67.0 ± 7.1	> 90
PC (%)	72.6 ± 2.1	$85.3^c \pm 1.0$	83.1 ± 0.9	87.8 ± 0.4
PG (%)	3.1 ± 0.6	$7.2^c \pm 0.9$	8.6 ± 0.6	7.6 ± 0.1
SM (%)	7.7 ± 1.3	$2.4^c \pm 0.5$	0.8 ± 0.2	0.8 ± 0.1
SP-B (% of PL)	3.73 ± 1.15	4.9 ± 1.26	3.0 ± 0.3	3.8 ± 0.7
SP-A (% of PL)	1.0 ± 0.5	0.4 ± 0.1	6.2 ± 0.7	—
γ_{ads} (mN/m)	45.0 ± 1.6	$25.6^c \pm 2.8$	22.5 ± 0.7	22.2 ± 0.3
γ_{min} (mN/m)	21.6 ± 1.4	$9.2^b \pm 2.8$	0.25 ± 0.2	0.28 ± 0.3
$\gamma_{ads} + P$ (mN/m)	43.5 ± 1.5	37.6 ± 2.4	22.7 ± 0.7	—
$\gamma_{min} + P$ (mN/m)	34.4 ± 2.2	24.2 ± 3.6	0.5 ± 0.3	—

Variables are given for the BAL fluids obtained 3 h prior to (pre) and 15–21 h after (post) the first surfactant administration (mean ± SEM). For comparison, data from 10 healthy controls and the surfactant material used for replacement therapy (measured in triplicate) are displayed. (PPR: ratio of PL to protein in the BAL fluid, LSA: large surfactant aggregates (% of total PL), PC: phosphatidylcholine, PG: phosphatidylglycerol, SM: sphingomyelin, SP-B/A: surfactant protein-B/A (all % of total PL), γ_{ads} and γ_{min}: adsorption and minimum surface tension in the absence or presence (+P) of supernatant protein). Significance level (comparison of pre- and post-surfactant data) is indicated by [a] ($p < 0.05$) and [b] ($p < 0.01$). (From [84] with permission)

surfactant pool and, by this, the gas exchange conditions in most severe early-stage ARDS. However, a high and/or repetitive dosage regimen appears to be necessary to overcome inhibitory capacities in the alveolar space of these patients and to achieve sustained alveolar recruitment. Forthcoming studies will have to rule out the optimum timing and dosage regimen of such intervention and will have to address the question whether this therapy is capable of reducing the still high mortality of patients with most severe ARDS, and critically consider its impact on inflammation, host-defense and mesenchymal proliferation in the alveolar compartment.

References

1. Seeger W, Lasch HG (1987) Septic lung. Rev Infect Dis 9:570–579
2. Akino T (1992) Lipid components of the surfactant system. In: Robertson B, van Golde LMG, Batenburg JJ (eds) Pulmonary Surfactant, Elsevier Science, Amsterdam, pp 19–32
3. Whitsett JA, Baatz JE (1992) Hydrophobic surfactant proteins SP-B and SP-C: Molecular biology, structure and function. In: Robertson B, van Golde LMG, Batenburg JJ (eds) Pulmonary Surfactant, Elsevier Science, Amsterdam, pp 33–54
4. Possmayer F (1988) A proposed nomenclature for pulmonary surfactant-associated proteins. Am Rev Respir Dis 138:990–996

5. Hawgood S (1989) Pulmonary surfactant apoproteins: A review of protein and genomic structure. Am J Physiol 257 (Lung Cell Mol Physiol 1):L13–L22
6. Goerke J, Clements JA (1986) Alveolar surface tension and lung surfactant. In: Macklem PT, Mead J (eds) Handbook of physiology. American Physiological Society, Bethesda, pp 247–261
7. Hawgood S, Benson BJ, Schilling J, Damm D, Clements JA, White RT (1987) Nucleotide and amino acid sequences of pulmonary surfactant protein SP18 and evidence for cooperation between SP18 and SP28–36 in surfactant lipid adsorption. Proc Natl Sci USA 84:66–70
8. Revak SD, Merritt TA, Degryse E, et al (1988) Use of human surfactant low molecular apoproteins in the reconstitution of surfactant biologic activity. J Clin Invest 81:826–833
9. Seeger W, Günther A, Thede C (1992) Differential sensitivity to fibrinogen-inhibition of SP-C versus SP-B based surfactants. Am J Physiol (Lung Cell Mol Physiol 5):L286–L291
10. Yu SH, Possmayer F (1988) Comparative studies on the biophysical activities of the low molecular weight hydrophobic proteins purified from bovine pulmonary surfactant. Biochim Biophys Acta 961:337–350
11. Gross NJ, Schultz RM (1992) Requirements for extracellular metabolism of pulmonary surfactant: Tentative identification of serine protease. Am J Physiol 262:L446–L453
12. Gross NJ, Bublys V, D'Anza J, Brown C (1995) The role of (1–antitrypsin in the control of extracellular surfactant metabolism. Am J Physiol 268:L438–L445
13. Cockshutt AM, Weitz J, Possmayer F (1990) Pulmonary surfactant-associated protein A enhances the surface activity of lipid extract surfactant and reverses inhibition by blood proteins in vitro. Biochemistry 29:8424–8429
14. Ross GF, Notter RH, Meuth J, Whitsett JA (1986) Phospholipid binding and biophysical activity of pulmonary surfactant-associated protein (SAP)-35 and its non-collagenous COOH-terminal domains. J Biol Chem 261(30):14283–14291
15. Kuroki Y, Mason R, Voelker D (1988) Pulmonary surfactant apoprotein A structure and modulation of surfactant secretion by rat alveolar type II cells. J Biol Chem 263:3388–3394
16. Rice WR, Ross GF, Singleton FM, Dingle S, Whitsett JA (1987) Surfactant-associated protein inhibits phospholipid secretion from type II cells. J Appl Physiol 63:692–698
17. Wissel H, Looman AC, Fritzsche I, Rüstow B, Stevens PA. (1996) SP-A-binding protein BP55 is involved in surfactant endocytosis by type II pneumocytes. Am J Appl Physiol 271:L432–L440
18. Iwaarden JF van, Welmers B, Verhoef J, Haagsman HP, Golde van LMG (1990) Pulmonary surfactant protein A enhances the host defense mechanism of rat alveolar macrophages. Am J Respir Cell Mol Biol 2:91–98
19. Iwaarden JF van, Strijp van JAG, Erbskamp MJM, Welmers AC, Verhoef J, Golde van LMG (1991) Surfactant protein A is opsonin in phagocytosis of herpes simplex virus type 1 by rat alveolar macrophages. Am J Physiol (Lung Cell Mol Physiol) 5:L204–L209
20. Iwaarden JF van, Shimizu H, van Golde PHM, Voelker DR, van Golde LMG (1992) Rat surfactant protein D enhances the production of oxygen radicals by rat alveolar macrophages. Biochem J 286:5–8
21. Tenner AJ, Robinson SL, Borchelt J, Wright JR (1989) Human pulmonary surfactant protein (SP-A), a protein structurally homologous to C1q, can enhance FcR- and CR1-mediated phagocytosis. J Biol Chem 264:13923–13928
22. Collaborative European Multicenter Study Group (1988) Surfactant replacement therapy for severe neonatal respiratory distress syndrome: An international randomized clinical trial. Pediatrics 82:683–691
23. Hennes HM, Lee MB, Rimm AA, Shapiro DL (1991) Surfactant replacement therapy in respiratory distress syndrome. Am J Dis Chest 145:102–104
24. Petty TL, Silvers GW, Paul GW, Stanford RE (1979) Abnormalities in lung elastic properties and surfactant function in adult respiratory distress syndrome. Chest 75:571–575
25. Gregory TJ, Longmore WJ, Moxley MA, et al (1991) Surfactant chemical composition and biophysical activity in acute respiratory distress syndrome. J Clin Invest 88:1976–1981
26. Hallman M, Spragg R, Harrell JH, Moser KM, Gluck, L (1982) Evidence of lung surfactant abnormality in respiratory failure. J Clin Invest 70:673–683
27. Pison U, Seeger W, Buchhorn R, et al (1989) Surfactant abnormalities in patients with respiratory failure after multiple trauma. Am Rev Respir Dis 140:1033–1039

28. Günther AG, Siebert C, Schmidt R, et al (1996) Surfactant alterations in severe pneumonia, acute respiratory distress syndrome, and cardiogenic lung edema. Am J Respir Crit Care Med 153:176–184
29. Fuchimukai T, Fuchiwara T, Takahashi A, Enhorning G (1987) Artificial pulmonary surfactant inhibited by proteins. J Appl Physiol 62:429–437
30. Kobayashi T, Nitta K, Ganzuka M, Inui S, Grossmann G, Robertson B (1991) Inactivation of exogenous surfactant by pulmonary edema fluid. Pediatric Research 29:353–356
31. Seeger W, Walmrath D, Menger M, Neuhof H (1986) Increased lung vascular permeability after arachidonic acid and hydrostatic challenge. J Appl Physiol 61:1781–1789
32. Tierney DF, Johnson RP (1965) Altered surface tension of lung extracts and lung mechanics. J Appl Physiol 20:1253–1260
33. Holm BA, Notter RH, Finkelstein JN (1985) Surface property changes from interactions of albumin with natural lung surfactant and extracted lung lipids. Chem Phys Lipids 38:287–298
34. Seeger W, Stöhr G, Wolf HRD, Neuhof H (1985) Alteration of surfactant function due to protein leakage: Special interaction with fibrin monomer. J Appl Physiol 58:326–338
35. Holm BA, Notter RH (1987) Effects of hemoglobin and cell membrane lipids on pulmonary surfactant activity. J Appl Physiol 63:1434–1442
36. O'Brodovich HM, Weitz JI, Possmayer F (1990) Effect of fibrinogen degradation products and lung ground substance on surface function. Biol Neonate 57:325–333
37. Seeger W, Thede C, Günther A, Grube C (1991) Surface properties and sensitivity to protein-inhibition of a recombinant apoprotein C-based phospholipid mixture in vitro – Comparison to natural surfactant. Biochim Biophys Acta 1081:45–52
38. Venkitaraman AR, Baatz JE, Whitsett JA, Hall SB, Notter RH (1991) Biophysical inhibition of synthetic phospholipid-lung surfactant apoprotein admixtures by plasma proteins. Chem Phys Lipids 57:49–57
39. Bachofen M, Weibel EF (1982) Structural alterations of lung parenchyma in the adult respiratory distress syndrome. Clin Chest Med 3:35–56
40. Burkhardt A (1989) Alveolitis and collapse in the pathogenesis of pulmonary fibrosis. Am Rev Respir Dis 140:513–524
41. Jackson LK (1982) Idiopathic pulmonary fibrosis. Clin Chest Med 3:579–592
42. Spencer H (1977) Pathology of the lung. WB Saunders, Philadelphia, pp 235–240
43. Chapman HA, Reilly JJ, Kobzik L (1988) Role of plasminogen activator in degradation of extracellular matrix protein by live human alveolar macrophages. Am Rev Respir Dis 137:412–419
44. Gross TJ, Simon RH, Sitrin RG (1992) Tissue factor procoagulant expression by rat alveolar epithelial cells. Am J Respir Cell Mol Biol 6:397–403
45. Idell S, James KK, Levin EG, et al (1989) Local abnormalities in coagulation and fibrinolytic pathways predispose to alveolar fibrin deposition in the adult respiratory distress syndrome. J Clin Invest 84:695–705
46. Nakstadt B, Boye NP, Lyberg T (1987) Procoagulant activities in human alveolar macrophages. Eur J Respir Dis 71:459–471
47. Idell S, Gonzalez KK, Bradford H, et al (1987) Procoagulant activity in bronchoalveolar lavage in the adult respiratory distress syndrome. Am Rev Respir Dis 136:1466–1474
48. Idell S, Koenig KB, Fair DS, Martin TR, McLarty J, Maunder RJ (1991) Serial abnormalities of fibrin turnover in evolving adult respiratory distress syndrome. Am J Physiol (Lung Cell Mol Physiol) 5:L240–L248
49. Seeger W, Hübel J, Klapettek K, et al (1991) Procoagulant activity in bronchoalveolar lavage of severly traumatized patients – Relation to the development of acute respiratory distress. Thromb Res 61:53–64
50. Idell S, Gonzalez KK, MacArthur CK, et al (1987) Bronchoalveolar lavage procoagulant activity in bleomycin induced lung injury in marmosets. Am Rev Respir Dis 136:124–133
51. Idell S, James KK, Gillies C, Fair DS, Thrall RS (1989) Abnormalities of pathways of fibrin turnover in lung lavage of rats with oleic acid and bleomycin-induced lung injury support alveolar fibrin deposition. Am J Pathol 135:387–399

52. Idell S, Peterson BT, Gonzalez KK, et al (1988) Local abnormalities of coagulation and fibrinolysis and alveolar fibrin deposition in sheep with oleic acid-induced lung injury. Am Rev Respir Dis 138:1282–1294
53. Bertozzi P, Astedt B, Zenzius L, et al (1990) Depressed bronchoalveolar urokinase activity in patients with adult respiratory distress syndrome. N Engl J Med 322:890–897
54. Chapman HA, Bertozzi P, Sailor LZ, Nusrat AR (1990) Alveolar macrophage urokinase receptors localize enzyme activity to the cell surface. Am J Physiol 259 (Lung Cell Mol Physiol 3): L432–L438
55. Hasday JD, Bachwich PR, Lynch JP, Sitrin RG (1988) Procoagulant and plasminogen activator activities of bronchoalveolar fluid in patients with pulmonary sarcoidosis. Exp Lung Res 14:261–278
56. Nakstad B, Lydberg T, Skjonsberg OH, Boye NP (1990) Local activation of the coagulation and fibrinolysis systems in lung disease. Thromb Res 57:827–838
57. Günther A, Bleyl H, Seeger W (1993) Apoprotein-based synthetic surfactants inhibit plasmic cleavage of fibrinogen *in vitro*. Am J Physiol 265:L186–L192
58. Günther A, Kalinowski M, Elssner A, Seeger W (1994) Clot-embedded natural surfactant: Kinetics of fibrinolysis and surface activity. Am J Physiol 267:L618–L624
59. Seeger W, Elssner A, Günther A, Kraemer HJ, Kalinowski HO (1993) Lung surfactant phospholipids associate with polymerizing fibrin: Loss of surface activity. Am J Respir Cell Mol Biol 9:213–220
60. Christner P, Fein A, Goldberg S, Lippmann M, Abrams W, Weinbaum G (1985) Collagenase in the lower respiratory tract of patients with adult respiratory distress syndrome. Am Rev Respir Dis 131:690–695
61. Lee CT, Fein AM, Lippmann M, Holtzman H, Kimbel, Weinbaum G (1981) Elastolytic activity in pulmonary lavage fluid from patients with adult respiratory distress syndrome. N Engl J Med 304:192–196
62. Berry D, Ikegami M, Jobe A (1986) Respiratory distress and surfactant inhibition following vagotomy in rabbits. J Appl Physiol 61:1741–1748
63. Lamm WJE, Albert RK (1990) Surfactant replacement improves lung recoil in rabbit lungs after acid aspiration. Am Rev Respir Dis 142:1279–1283
64. Lewis JF, Ikegami M, Higuchi R, Jobe A, Absolom D (1991) Nebulized versus instilled exogenous surfactant in an adult injury model. J Appl Physiol 71:1270–1276
65. Lewis JF, Ikegami M, Jobe AH (1992) Metabolism of exogenously administered surfactant in the acutely injured lungs of adult rabbits. Am Rev Respir Dis 145:19–23
66. Strohmaier W, Redl H, Schlag G (1990) Studies of the potential role of a semisynthetic surfactant preparation in an experimental aspiration trauma in rabbits. Exp Lung Res 16:101–110
67. Zelter M, Escudies BJ, Hoeffel JM, Murray JF (1990) Effects of aerosolized artificial surfactant on repeated oleic acid injury in sheep. Am Rev Respir Dis 141:1014–1019
68. Robertson B, Lachmann B (1988) Experimental evaluation of surfactants for replacement therapy. Exp Lung Res 14:279–310
69. Berggren P, Lachmann B, Curstedt T, Grossmann G, Robertson B (1986) Gas exchange and lung morphology after surfactant replacement in experimental adult respiratory distress syndrome induced by repeated lung lavage. Acta Anaesthesiol Scand 30:321–328
70. Hall SB, Venkitaraman AR, Whitsett JA, Holm BA, Notter RH (1992) Importance of hydrophobic apoproteins as constituents of clinical exogenous surfactants. Am Rev Respir Dis 145:24–30
71. Kobayashi T, Ganzuka M, Taniguchi J, Nitta K, Murakami S (1990) Lung lavage and surfactant replacement for hydrochloric acid aspiration in rabbits. Acta Anaesthesiol Scand 34:216–221
72. van Daal GJ, So KL, Gommers D, et al (1991) Intratracheal surfactant administration restores gas exchange in experimental adult respiratory distress syndrome associated with viral pneumonia. Anesth Analg 72:589–595
73. Huang YC, Fawcett TA, Moon RE, et al (1992) Exogenous surfactant treatment improves V_A/Q abnormalities in hyperoxic lung injury. Am Rev Respir Dis 145:A609 (Abst)

74. Bredenberg CE, Paskanik AM, Nieman GF (1983) High surface tension pulmonary edema. J Surg Res 34:515–523
75. Nieman GF, Bredenberg CE (1985) High surface tension pulmonary edema induced by detergent aerosol. J Appl Physiol 58:129–136
76. Kaneko T, Sato T, Katsuya H, Miyauchi Y (1990) Surfactant therapy for pulmonary edema due to intratracheally injected bile acid. Crit Care Med 18:77–83
77. Albert RK, Lakshminarayan S, Hildebrandt J, Kirk W (1979) Increased surface tension favours pulmonary edema formation in anaesthetized dogs' lungs. J Clin Invest 63:1015–1018
78. Nieman GF, Goyette D, Paskanik A, Brendenberg C (1990) Surfactant displacement by plasma lavage results in pulmonary edema. Surgery 107:677–683
79. Evander E, Wollmer P, Jonson B, Lachmann B (1987) Pulmonary clearance of inhaled ^{99m}Tc-DTPA: Effects of surfactant depletion by lung lavage. J Appl Physiol 62:1611–1614
80. Ikegami M, Jobe AH, Tabor BL, Rider ED, Lewis JF (1992) Lung albumin recovery in surfactant-treated preterm ventilated lambs. Am Rev Respir Dis 145:1005–1008
81. Jefferies AL, Coates G, O'Brodovich H (1984) Pulmonary epithelial permeability in hyaline-membrane disease. N Engl J Med 311:1075–1080
82. Hasleton PS (1983) Adult respiratory distress syndrome: A review. Histopathology 7:327–332
83. Gregory TJ, Gadek JE, Weilnad JE, et al (1994) Survanta supplementation in patients with acute respiratory distress syndrome (ARDS). Am J Respir Crit Care Med 149:A567 (Abst)
84. Walmrath D, Günther A, Ghofrani AG, et al (1996) Bronchoscopic surfactant administration in patients with severe adult respiratory distress syndrome and sepsis. Am J Respir Crit Care Med 154:57–62

BAL Inflammatory Markers of Initiation and Resolution of ALI

C. Haslett and S. C. Donnelly

Introduction

Acute respiratory distress syndrome in adults (ARDS) is a catastrophic form of acute inflammatory lung injury which was first fully described clinically 30 years ago [1]. It is important as a disease in its own right; it has a significant mortality (up to 70% in some patient groups) and is a major burden on intensive care unit resources. ARDS also represents a remarkable "model" of human inflammatory disease that provides special opportunities for defining disease pathogenesis and for intervening with novel mechanism-based therapies.

There are a large number of potential predisposing conditions (Table 1), but in many of the most common, such as sepsis, multiple trauma and pancreatitis, the original insult is distant from the lungs. Despite the diversity of the predisposing conditions, the resultant pathological features appear to be common to all [2–4]. This suggests that in most cases the initiating insult sets in train a common series of humorally-mediated processes which ultimately impinge on the lung. It is now established that ARDS is merely part of a systemic disease involving inflammatory microvascular injury in several organs which sometimes leads to multiple organ failure syndrome (MOFS).

One remarkable aspect of ARDS is that in most cases there is a delay or "latent period" of several hours, or even days, between the development of a precipitating condition and the onset of clinically detectable lung injury, although at present it is difficult to predict which patients in the at risk groups will develop this catastrophic condition. The latent period provides an almost unique "win-

Table 1. ARDS disease etiology: Direct and indirect initiating events

Direct	Indirect
Pneumonia	Trauma
Contusion	Sepsis
Aspiration	Pancreatitis
Oxygen toxicity	Massive transfusion
Near-drowning	Burns
Smoke inhalation	Drug overdose
	Cardiopulmonary bypass

dow of opportunity" to investigate the earliest mechanisms of human inflammatory disease. In the studies described below, we capitalize on this opportunity to identify which of a variety of potentially important inflammatory mechanisms are central in the development of full-blown ARDS.

It has been recognized for some time that ARDS is a disease in which an inappropriate or excessive inflammatory response targets the lung microvascular endothelial and epithelial cells resulting in extensive injury; interstitial edema and hemorrhage; widespread epithelial denudation and attempts at repair; and extravasation of protein-rich fluid into the alveolar airspaces. Pathological and experimental animal studies suggest that the neutrophil and other acute inflammatory cells, influenced by mediators activated as a result of the precipitating event, become abnormally sequestered in the pulmonary microvessels as a result of an increased adhesive interaction with endothelial cells and reduced deformability [5–8]. Therein, they become primed and activated to secrete excessive amounts of injurious agents, including proteinases and reactive oxygen species (ROS), which damage the alveolar-capillary lining cells and begin the vicious cycle of events: injury →leak → more inflammation → more injury → more leak, etc. that is probably responsible for the classical pathological features of ARDS. Although there is considerable evidence of the importance of neutrophils in ARDS pathogenesis [9–15], a condition which is clinically indistinguishable from other forms of ARDS has been described in neutropenic patients [16]. Another difficulty is presented by the vast redundancy of the inflammatory response – most previous studies have been either in established ARDS or at variable times in the late risk period by which time it is clear that all the important inflammatory cascades (leukotrienes, prostaglandins, chemokines and their constituents) are implicated. This makes it extremely difficult to identify critically important mediators or to develop rational therapeutic strategies. For example, in established disease, to prevent neutrophil attraction to the lung it may be necessary to block the effects of complement (C) C5a, leukotriene (LT)B$_4$ and a large number of neutrophil chemokines. Similarly, a large number of neutrophils and endothelial surface molecules have been identified in what is now recognized to be the multi-staged event of neutrophil-endothelial adhesion [17–19]. Finally, the neutrophil can release more than 30 agents with known capacity to injure tissues, many of which have been implicated in the pathogenesis of ARDS, perhaps the most important being elastase (and other proteases) and the reactive oxygen intermediates (Table 2). Again this

Table 2. Potentially histotoxic neutrophil products

Oxidants and radicals	Proteolytic enzymes
Superoxide anion	Elastase
Hydrogen peroxide	Collagenase
Hypochlorous acid	Cathepsin
Chloramines	Lysozyme
Nitric acid	Heparanase

example of redundancy presents great difficulties for therapeutic targeting when we do not know which are the most important agents in human disease. Consequently, one of the key aims of our studies was to quantify the earliest inflammatory events in the ARDS-risk period of well-defined sub-groups of patients suffering from multiple trauma, pancreatitis, perforated bowel, and to relate them to whether or not the patient developed ARDS. By this approach, it might have been possible to identify key mechanisms which might be therapeutically targeted with the ultimate aim of ameliorating disease or even "stopping it in its tracks" before it is fully established. Furthermore, key early events might provide an index for identifying those patients at the very highest risk of developing full-blown ARDS. A strength of these studies is that we were permitted at the outset not only to study inflammatory events in the blood but also to obtain bronchoalveolar lavage fluid (BAL) to study pulmonary events at the very earliest stages (1–2 h) of the risk period in ARDS-risk patients.

The second element of our studies relates to the outcome of established ARDS. On clinical grounds, it is very difficult to predict which patients with ARDS are likely to continue to deteriorate or to join the 50% who survive, in whom the inflammatory lung disease presumably resolves and injury is repaired, since many of those who survive enjoy a return to excellent lung function [20, 21]. Because there were varying reports of whether levels of interleukin(IL)-8 and other pro-inflammatory mediators in blood or BAL were related to prognosis [22, 23] and our preliminary data did not support a definite relationship, we tested an alternative hypothesis, that, by contrast with the initiation of disease, in which IL-8 appears to be important, the outcome of established disease would relate more strongly to whether or not effective levels of anti-inflammatory cytokines such as IL-10 and IL-1ra were generated in the lungs, rather than whether there was persistent generation of pro-inflammatory chemokines.

Methods

ARDS was defined using Murray's expanded definition [24]. Over one hundred patients "at risk" for ARDS have been enrolled on presentation to the Royal Infirmary or Western General Hospitals, Edinburgh. Enrolled patients come from well defined "at risk" patient groups, namely, multiple trauma, acute pancreatitis, patients undergoing laparotomy for a perforated viscus, and patients undergoing coronary artery bypass surgery. In addition, over 40 patients with established ARDS have been studied. Informed consent was obtained from patients' relatives or guardians. Our studies were approved by the Lothian Health Board Ethics Committee. All patients had blood and BAL sampling performed when they were enrolled into the study. Patients "at risk" for ARDS following trauma were studied on initial hospital presentation (mean 97 min post-insult). Patients with perforated bowel were studied while under a general anesthetic prior to laparotomy. Patients with pancreatitis were studied within 12 h of hospital presentation. For patients with established ARDS, sampling was performed within 24 h of diagnosis.

On study enrolment, a 10 ml venous blood sample was taken prior to bronchoscopy. The venous samples were centrifuged at 400 g × 10 min at 4°C. The serum was aspirated and stored at − 70°C and assays were performed at a later time. A fiber optic bronchoscope was introduced through either the nasal passages or via an indwelling endotracheal tube for intubated patients. The distal end of the bronchoscope was wedged into the right middle lobe. Three 60 mL aliquots of 0.9% NaCl solution were instilled and immediately gently aspirated. On average 61% of instilled fluid was recovered (range 40–87%). All bronchoscopy procedures were performed by the same bronchoscopist. Recovered fluid and cells were stored at 4°C until processed. All venous and BAL samples were processed within 1 h of collection. For BAL, processing initially entailed straining the lavage fluid through sterile gauze to remove mucus. The strained fluid was then centrifuged at 400 × g at 4°C for 10 min to recover cells. Total cell counts were performed using a hemacytometer. Aliquots of cells were pelleted onto glass slides using a Cytospin-2 (Shandon Scientific, Cheshire, England) and then stained with Diff-Quick (Merz-Dade AG, Dudingen, Switzerland), a modified Wright-Giemsa stain. Differential counts were determined by counting 500 cells under oil immersion (× 100). The lavage fluid supernatant was respun at 400 g × 10 min at 4°C to remove cellular debris and stored at − 70°C until assayed at a later date for specific inflammatory mediators.

In collected samples, both pro- (IL-1β, TNF-α and IL-8) and anti- (IL-10 and IL-1ra) inflammatory cytokines were assayed via standard sandwich ELISA techniques [25, 26]. Circulating neutrophil surface adhesion expression was quantified by floss cytometric analysis after cell surface binding with appropriate fluorescent stained MoAbs directed against specific neutrophil selectin and integrin molecules. Soluble circulating receptors were assayed via ELISA technique [27, 28]. Circulating elastase levels were measured by radio-immunoassay [29].

Statistical Analysis: Patient group data and assay results are presented as medians with ranges in parentheses. Intergroup comparisons were made using nonparametric methods including the Mann-Whitney test or Spearman Rank Correlation Coefficient where appropriate. Significance was defined as $p < 0.05$.

Results

Early "at risk" Period – Studies on Peripheral Blood

We assayed circulating elastase as a marker of recent neutrophil degranulation and while we found significantly elevated elastase in trauma patients who progressed to ARDS compared to those who did not ($p = 0.009$) (Fig. 1), there was overlap between the groups and it seemed unlikely that peripheral blood elastase levels would be of value as a single predictive index of ARDS risk [29].

We found no significant correlation between circulating levels of the neutrophil chemokines IL-8 (Fig. 2) and ENA-78 in early blood samples and progression to ARDS [25]. Nor did we find any relationship between a wide range of other mediators (IL-1β, TNF-α, IL-6, MCP-1, MIP-1α, MIP-1β, ENA-78) in peripher-

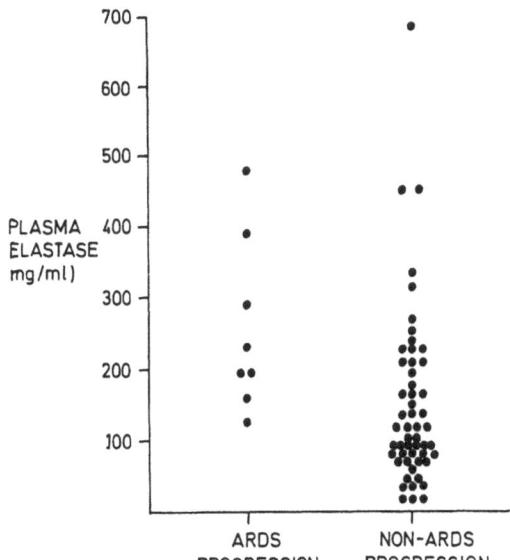

Fig. 1. Circulating elastase levels in blood samples obtained from trauma patients on initial hospital presentation. Comparing patients who subsequently progressed to ARDS with those who did not (p = 0.009)

al blood and ARDS progression. This is perhaps not suprising when it is considered that the risk patients had devastating systemic disease and we were seeking evidence of agents that related to injury of a specific organ – the lung – and it lent impetus to our studies using BAL.

With regard to surface adhesion molecules on circulating neutrophils (CD11a/18, CD11/CD18 and L-selectin) no significant difference was found in the level of surface expression on peripheral blood neutrophils between those who progressed to ARDS and those who did not. Again, this finding is not suprising given that activated "sticky" neutrophils in this early period of ARDS disease pathogenesis might be expected to become marginated within the lungs and thus not accessible to assay in peripheral blood neutrophils. This led us to propose that plasma levels of soluble receptors, in particular L-selectin, which is implicated in initial neutrophil margination and cleared to a soluble form during neutrophil transition from loose adhesion to tight adhesion, would reflect neutrophil/endothelial events within pulmonary capillaries and might correlate with ARDS progression. A highly significant correlation between low soluble L-selectin levels (sL-selectin) and ARDS development was found (p = 0.0001) (Fig. 3) [27]. These findings may reflect the sequestration of sL-selectin by widespread binding to activated endothelium in microvascular beds. Endothelial cells activated *in vitro* express a nascent ligand for L-selectin, which could be induced *in vivo* [30]. This is supported by preliminary immunohistochemical findings which show sL-selectin specifically bound to luminal surfaces of high endothelial venules at sites of inflammation [28]. Thus, reduced sL-selectin could represent a peripheral blood marker of widespread pan-endothelial activation – an important event in the pathogenesis of ARDS and MOFS [31]. This hypothesis was

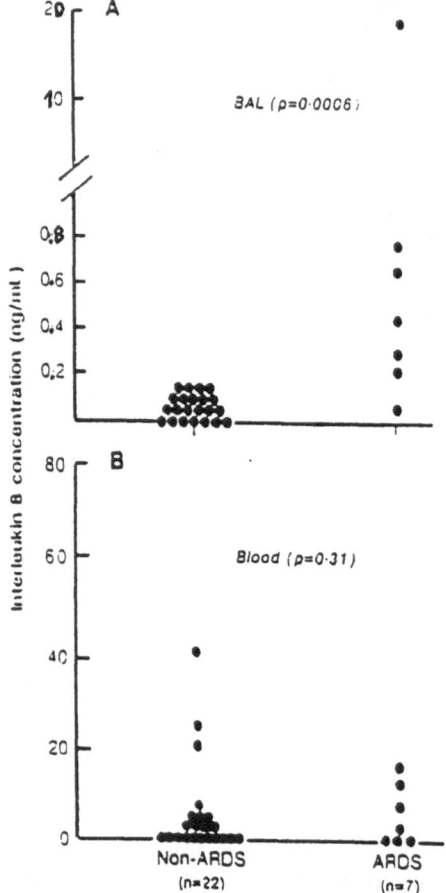

Fig. 2. Interleukin-8 in initial samples of BAL and blood

supported by our findings of a highly significant correlation (p = 0.0001) between a low initial circulating sL-selectin and the subsequent development of a more extensive and more severe form of organ failure (Fig. 4).

Early "at risk" Period – Studies on BAL

There is considerable evidence implicating the neutrophil in the pathogenesis of ARDS [32]. In ARDS, the normal preponderance of alveolar macrophages is replaced by an excess number of neutrophils, suggesting that at some time-point prior to the clinical presentation of ARDS, migration of neutrophils from the circulation into the pulmonary interstitium and ultimately into the alveolar airspaces has occurred. We therefore hypothesized that specific neutrophil chemokines would be evident in the alveolar airspaces in the early ARDS risk period. We

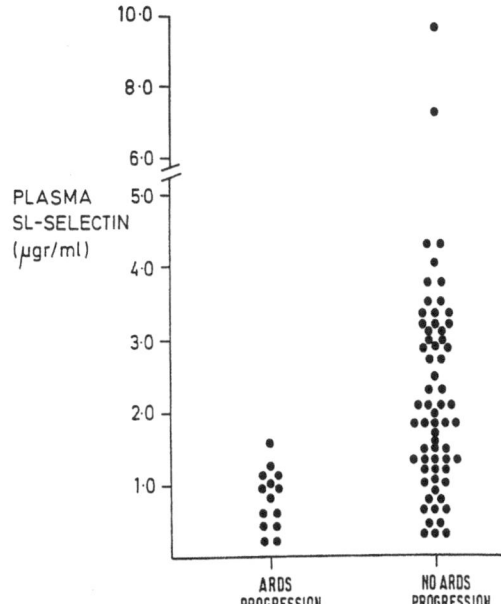

Fig. 3. Initial plasma sL-selectin in patients who subsequently progressed to ARDS compared to those who did not (p = 0.0001)

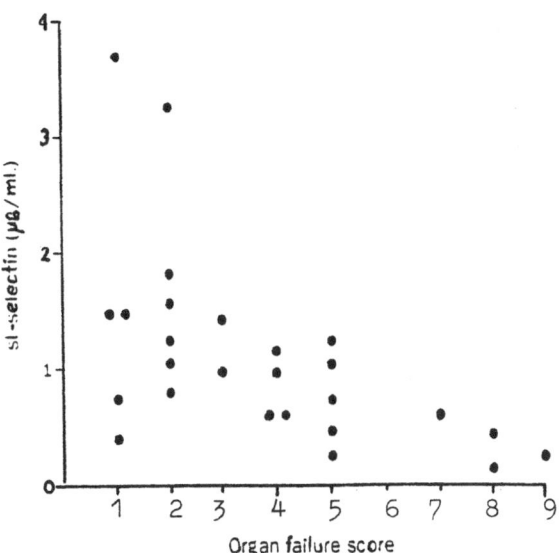

Fig. 4. Initial plasma sL-selectin levels and subsequent organ failure score (p = 0.0001)

found in BAL samples obtained from our ARDS "at risk" population, that levels of IL-8 (but not the neutrophil chemokine ENA-78) correlated with those patients who subsequently progressed to ARDS compared to those who did not (p = 0.0006) (Fig. 2) [25]. Analysis via our harvested BAL cell pellet showed the alveolar macrophage to be an important source of the raised IL-8 found. In our original publication, 29 patients were investigated. We have since enlarged our "at risk" patient population to over 90 patients and can report that the highly significant association is maintained (p = 0.0001). Indeed multivariate statistical analysis suggests that the measurement of this single inflammatory mediator within the alveolar airspace at this early time-point is associated with a positive predictive value for subsequent ARDS of 80% [33].

Our trauma patient "at risk" group were enrolled on average 95 min after the initiating trauma event. We found elevated levels of IL-8 in the alveolar airspaces at this early timepoint. These IL-8 levels did not correlate with BAL levels of IL-1β or TNF-α. This raises the possibility of a novel IL-1β or TNF-α independent pathway, perhaps involving neuropeptide/neuroendocrine mechanisms, in this rapid IL-8 release.

Established ARDS – Studies on BAL Mediators

We assayed selected pro-inflammatory mediators in established ARDS (IL-1β, TNF-α, IL-8, MCP-1, ENA-78, MIP-1a, MIP-1b) and found that the alveolar levels of these cytokines were of no prognostic significance. This led us to hypothesize that an inability by individual patients to mount an appropriate intra-alveolar anti-inflammatory cytokine response would be associated with an adverse prognosis. We assayed IL-10 and IL-1ra in BAL samples from patients with ARDS and

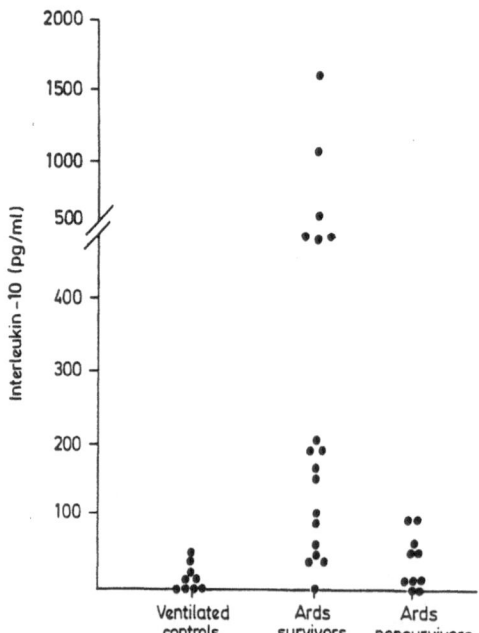

Fig. 5. IL-10 in BAL samples obtained from ventilated controls and survivors and non-survivors of ARDS

found that low levels of both anti-inflammatory cytokines were associated with subsequent patient mortality (p = 0.003 and p = 0.008, respectively) [26] (Fig. 5, Fig. 6).

Discussion

Our findings of a significant association between both levels of circulating neutrophil elastase (a specific marker of neutrophil degranulation) and sL-selectin and alveolar IL-8 (a specific neutrophil chemokine) and progression to ARDS, add considerable additional evidence implicating the neutrophil in the pathogenesis of early ARDS. Although the measurement of this individual product of recent neutrophil degranulation is of great value in identifying individuals at high risk of progression to ARDS, our study [29] implicates elastase in ARDS pathogenesis and an anti-elastase therapeutic approach may be valid, particularly in trauma patients, where the opportunity of therapeutic intervention exists within minutes of the initiating event.

Interleukin-8 in the alveolar airspaces is the only mediator measured which at this early stage correlates with impending disease. Indeed multivariate retrospective analysis of our data suggests that a high BAL IL-8 has a positive predictive value for ARDS of 80%. The importance of IL-8 has been highlighted in other examples of acute lung injury (ALI), in particular neonatal respiratory distress syndrome [34] and cystic fibrosis [35]. This suggests that despite the redundancy that exists in later stages of disease pathogenesis, IL-8 may be a genuine single target at the earliest stages of ARDS disease pathogenesis.

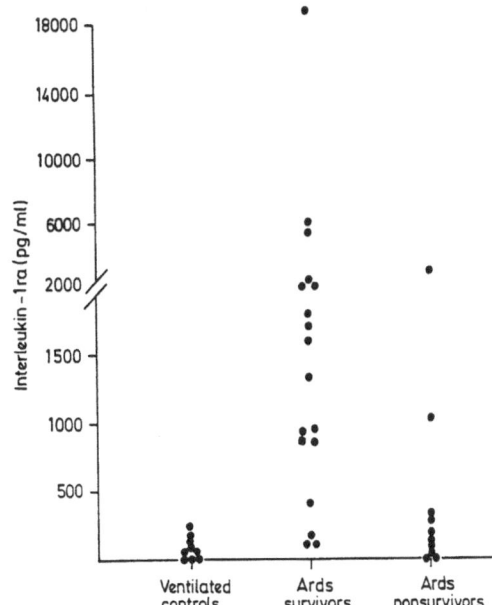

Fig. 6. IL-1ra in BAL samples obtained from ventilated controls and survivors and non-survivors of ARDS

One of the earliest events in neutrophil/endothelial transmigration is a transient adhesion phase mediated by L-selectin. Our findings of an association between circulating levels of this shed receptor and ARDS disease progression adds weight to the suggestion that levels of this receptor within the circulation may be an indirect marker of widespread endothelial activation, but further studies will be needed to prove this assertion.

Other investigators studying patients with established ARDS have found levels of alveolar pro-inflammatory cytokines to be of prognostic significance [22, 23]. We have investigated a wide variety of important pro-inflammatory mediators in the alveolar airspaces (IL-1β, TNF-α, IL-6, IL-8, MCP-1, and MIP-1α) and have found the levels to be elevated [36] but not related to mortality [26]. This led us to investigate the hypothesis that an insufficient anti-inflammatory response may predispose individual patients to a worse prognosis. IL-10 and IL-1ra are recently described cytokines [37, 38] with predominantly anti-inflammatory properties [39–43]. These properties play an important immuno-modulatory role in the function of inflammatory cells. Recent studies [44] have shown that the inhibition or endogenous IL-10 results in substantially enhanced lung injury. We measured IL-10 and IL-1ra in BAL samples in established ARDS, and found that low alveolar levels of these cytokines were associated with mortality (Fig. 5, Fig. 6) [26]. These important findings highlight a complementary therapeutic strategy, namely the augmentation of anti-inflammatory cytokine defenses. This has potential relevance not only in ARDS but in sepsis and other inflammatory diseases.

Conclusion

To date, our studies of inflammatory mechanisms of ARDS have been greatly illuminated by BAL. In particular, in the early risk period, this has enabled us to monitor pathogenetic events in the target organ of interest which revealed a key and highly predictive event – the local production of IL-8 – which was not reflected in peripheral blood levels of IL-8. Similarly, our BAL studies have shown that failure of the lung to produce high levels of the anti-inflammatory cytokines IL-10 and IL-1ra seems more important than continued generation of pro-inflammatory mechanisms in relating to patient mortality. Nevertheless, BAL is not a trivial procedure, particularly in the early risk period in critically ill patients with, for example, multiple trauma. In a recent retrospective analysis of multiple factors, we find that a combined index of "blood" levels of sL-selectin, elastase, and IL-8 give a positive predictive value for subsequent ARDS of 70% [45]. Clearly, the value of such indices needs to be established in major multicenter prospective studies.

References

1. Ashbaugh DG, Bigelow DB, Petty TL, Levine BE (1967) Acute respiratory distress syndrome. Lancet 2:319–323.
2. Lamy M, Fallat RJ, Koeniger E, et al (1976) Pathologic features and mechanisms of hypoxemia in adult respiratory distress syndrome. Am Rev Respir Dis 114:267–284
3. Fukudu Y, Ishizaki M, Masuda Y, Kimura G, Kawanami O, Masugi Y (1987) The role of intra-alveolar fibrosis in the process of pulmonary structural remodelling in patients with diffuse alveolar damage. Am J Path 126:171–182
4. Bachofen M, Weibel ER (1974) Basic pattern of tissue repair in human lungs following unspecific injury. Chest 65:14S–19S
5. Weiss SJ (1989) Tissue destruction by neutrophils. N Engl J Med 320:365–376
6. Henson PM, Johnston RB (1987) Tissue injury in inflammation. Oxidants, proteinases and cationic proteins. J Clin Invest 79:669–674
7. Haslett C, Savil JS, Meather L (1989) The neutrophil. Curr Opin Immunol 2:10–18
8. Selby C, Drost E, Wraith PK, MacNee W (1991) *In vivo* neutrophil sequestration within the lungs of man is determined by *in vitro* "filterability". J Appl Physiol 71:1996–2003
9. Rinaldo JE, Rogers RM (1982) Adult respiratory distress syndrome: Changing concepts of lung injury and repair. N Eng J Med 306:900–910
10. Warshawski FJ, Sibbald WJ, Driedger AA, Cheung H (1986) Abnormal neutrophil-pulmonary interaction in the adult respiratory distress syndrome. Am Rev Respir Dis 133:797–804
11. Weiland JE, Davis WB, Holter JF, Mohammed JR, Dorinsky PM, Gadek JE (1986) Lung neutrophils in the adult respiratory distress syndrome. Clinical and pathophysiological significance. Am Rev Respir Dis 133:218–225
12. Rocker GM, Wiseman MS, Pearson D, Shale DJ (1989) Diagnostic criteria for adult respiratory distress syndrome: Time for reappraisal. Lancet 1:120–123
13. Christner P, Fein A, Goldberg S, Zippman M, Abrams W, Weinbaum G (1985) Collagenase in the lower respiratory tract of patients with the adult respiratory distress syndrome. Am Rev Respir Dis 131:690–695
14. Parsons PE, Fowler AA, Hyers TM, Henson PM (1985) Chemotactic activity in bronchoalveolar lavage fluid from patients with the adult respiratory distress syndrome. Am Rev Respir Dis 132:490–493
15. Miller EJ, Naguo S, Cohen AB, et al (1992) Elevated levels of NAP-1/interleukin-8 are present in the airspaces of patients with the adult respiratory distress syndrome and are associated with increased mortality. Am Rev Respir Dis 146:427–432
16. McWhinney PHM, Gillespie SH, Kibbler CC, Hoffbrand AV, Prentice HG (1991) Streptococcus nutis and ARDS in neutropenic patients. Lancet 337:429
17. Tedder TF, Steeber DA, Chen A, Engel P (1995) The selectins: Vascular adhesion molecules. FASEB J 9:866–873
18. Mizgerd JP, Meek BB, Kutoski GJ, Bullard DC, Beaudet AL, Doerschuk CM (1996) Selectins and neutrophil traffic: Margination and streptococcus-induced emigration in murine lungs. J Exp Med 184:639–645
19. Wahl SM, Feldman GM, McCarthy JB (1996) Regulation of leukocyte adhesion and signaling in inflammation and disease. J Leuk Biol 59:789–796
20. Elliot CG, Morris AH, Cengiz M (1981) Pulmonary function and exercise gas exchange in survivors of adult respiratory distress syndrome. Am Rev Respir Dis 123:492–495
21. Elliot CG, Rasmusson BY, Crapo RO, Morris AH, Jensen RL (1987) Prediction of pulmonary function abnormalities after adult respiratory distress syndrome. Am Rev Respir Dis 135:634–638
22. Meduri GU, Kohler G, Headley S, Tolley E, Stenz F, Postlethwaite A (1995) Inflammatory cytokines in the BAL of patients with ARDS. Persistent elevation over time predicts poor outcome. Chest 108:1303–1314
23. Chollet-Martin S, Montravers P, Gilbert C, et al (1993) High levels of interleukin-8 in the blood and alveolar spaces of patients with pneumonia and adult respiratory distress syndrome. Infect Immunol 61:4553–4559

24. Murray JF, Matthay MA, Luce JM, Flick MR (1988) An expanded definition of the acute respiratory distress syndrome. Am Rev Respir Dis 138:720–723
25. Donnelly SC, Strieter RM, Kunkel SL, et al (1993) Interleukin-8 and development of adult respiratory distress syndrome in at risk patient groups. Lancet 341:643–647
26. Donnelly SC, Strieter RM, Reid PT, Kunkel SL, Burdick MD, Armstrong I, Mackenzie A, Haslett C (1996) The association between mortality rates and decreased concentrations of interleukin-10 and interleukin-1 receptor antagonist in the lung fluids of patients with the adult respiratory distress syndrome. Ann Int Med 125:191-196
27. Donnelly SC, Haslett C, Dransfield I, Robertson CE, Carter DC, Ross JA, Grant IS, Tedder TF (1994) Altered levels of soluble L-selectin adhesion receptor in plasma and the development of the adult respiratory distress syndrome (ARDS) in at-risk patient groups. Lancet 344:215–219
28. Spertini O, Schleiffenbaum B, White-Owen C, Ruitz P Jr, Tedder TF (1992) ELISA for quantitation of L-selectin shed from leukocytes in vivo. J Immun Methods 156:115–123
29. Donnelly SC, MacGregor I, Zamani A, Gordon MW, Robertson CE, Steedman DJ, et al (1995) Plasma elastase in multiple trauma and the adult respiratory distress syndrome (ARDS). Am J Respir Crit Care Med 151:1428–1433
30. Spertini O, Luscinkas FW, Munro JM et al (1991) Leukocyte Adhesion Molecule-1 (LAM-1, L-selectin) interacts with an inducible endothelial cell ligand to support leukocyte adhesion and transmigration. J Immunol 147:2565–2573
31. MacNaughton PD, Evans TW (1992) Management of adult respiratory distress syndrome. Lancet 339:469–472
32. Donnelly SC, Haslett C (1992) Cellular mechanisms of acute lung injury: implications for future treatment in the adult respiratory distress syndrome. Thorax 47:260–263
33. Reid PT, Donnelly SC, Haslett C (1995) Inflammatory predictors for the development of the adult respiratory distress syndrome (ARDS). Thorax 50:1023–1026
34. McColm JR, McIntosh N (1994) Interleukin-8 in bronchoalveolar lavage samples as predictor of chronic lung disease in premature infants. Lancet 343:729
35. McElvaney NG, Nakamura H, Birrer P, Hebert CA, Wong WL, Alphonso M, Baker JB, Catalano MA, Crystal RG (1992) Modulation of airway inflammation in cystic fibrosis. In vivo suppression of interleukin-8 levels on the respiratory epithelial surface by aerosolization of recombinant secretory leukoprotease inhibitor. J Clin Invest 90:1296–1230
36. Donnelly SC, Strieter RM, Kunkel SL, Walz A, Steedman D, Grant IS, Pollok AJ, Carter DC, Haslett C (1994) Chemotactic cytokines in the established adult respiratory distress syndrome and at-risk patients. Chest 105:98S–99S
37. Arend WP, Joslin FG, Thompson RC, Hannum CH (1989) An IL-1 inhibitor from human monocytes: Production and characterization of biological properties. J Immunol 143:1851–1858
38. Fiorentino DF, Bond MW, Mosmann TR (1989) Two types of mouse helper T-cell. IV. Th2 clones secrete a factor that inhibits cytokine production by Th1 clones. J Exp Med 170:2081–2095
39. Hannum CH, Wilcox CJ, Arend WP, Joslin FG, Dripps DJ, Heimdal PL, et al (1990) Interleukin-1 receptor antagonist activity of a human interleukin-1 inhibitor. Nature 343:336–340
40. Fiorentino DF, Zlotnik A, Mossmann TR, Howard M, O'Garra A (1991) IL-10 inhibits cytokine production by activated macrophages. J Immunol 147:3815–3822
41. de Waal Malefyt R, Yssel H, Roncarolo MG, Spits H, de Vries JE (1992) Interleukin-10. Curr Opin Immunol 4:314–320
42. Bogdan C, Vodovotz Y, Nathan C (1991) Macrophage deactivation by Interleukin-10. J Exp Med 174:1549–1555
43. te Velde AA, de Waal-Malefyt R, Huijbens PJF, de Vries JE, Figdor C (1992) IL-10 stimulates monocyte Fc gamma R surface expression and cytotoxic activity: distinct regulation of antibody-dependant cellular cytotoxicity by IFNg, IL-4 and IL-10. J Immunol 149:4048–4052
44. Shanley TP, Schmal H, Friedl HP, Jones ML, Ward PA (1995) Regulatory effects of intrinsic IL-10 in IgG immune complex-induced lung injury. J Immunol 154:3454–3460
45. Donnelly SC, Reid PT, Strieter RM, Burdick M, MacGregor I, Steedman D, Grant IS, Carter DC, Fernandez M, Tedder TF, Haslett C (1994) Early circulating predictors of progression to the adult respiratory distress syndrome. Eur Resp J 7:5S

Lung Repair

P. B. Bitterman

Introduction

Survival of patients with the acute respiratory distress syndrome (ARDS) depends on timely and effective alveolar repair. The biology of healing, whether integumentary or visceral, has traditionally attracted the attention of physician scientists since it lies at the interface of basic inquiry and clinical practice. Lung repair is no exception, having engaged cell biologists, molecular biologists, physiologists, and immunobiologists. One tangible outcome of this interdisciplinary focus is the recognition that biomechanical forces can profoundly influence the cell and molecular processes involved in organ repair. This information is currently shaping new therapeutic strategies focused on minimizing perturbing forces imposed by positive pressure mechanical ventilatory support. Additional therapeutic interventions based on a more complete understanding of the basic biology of lung repair are rapidly emerging.

In this report, the biological processes involved in lung repair will be highlighted, drawing heavily on two recently completed chapters [1, 2] to which the reader is referred for a more complete discussion and bibliography. This report will begin by summarizing the anatomy and pathophysiology of ARDS. A consideration of the key anatomic events involved in lung repair will follow. The discussion will continue with a brief overview of selected key cellular functions involved in repair including migration, proliferation and apoptosis. I will conclude with a consideration of the clinical implications of this information.

Anatomy and Pathophysiology of Injury

Whether from direct assault by pneumonia or indirectly by sepsis or trauma, ARDS is manifest in the context of transmural lung injury [3,4]. There is death of type I epithelial cells which cover 95% of the air lung interface and provide the primary barrier to the influx of solute and water into the normal alveolus. As a result, in many alveolar units, the air space is flooded leading to profound shunt physiology. Dysfunction of type II epithelial cells, which cover the remaining 5% of the air lung interface, has profound physiological impact. In some alveolar units, insufficient or chemically altered surfactant [5] results in alveolar collapse which contributes further to the venous admixture observed in the first several hours after lung injury. Production of new surfactant by the injured type II cell is insufficient to restore normal surface tension properties to the air lung interface. Also charged with the responsibility for active sodium transport from the airspace into the intersitium [6], type II cells display a diminished capacity to pump salt and water out of the flooded airspace. The lung interstitium expands with edema fluid distorting the mechanical properties of the lung and hence the distribution of gas to remaining functional alveolar units. Endothelial dysfunction and death in the microcirculation result in an augmented transfer of plasma and circulating cells from the vascular compartment into the lung. Basement membrane collagens are exposed to platelets leading to intravascular coagulation. This interrupts the flow of blood to many alveolar units resulting in increased wasted ventilation. The combination of flooded and collapsed air spaces along with an impaired microcirculation leads to gas exchange abnormalities so profound that they are unsurvivable outside of a contemporary critical care unit.

Lung Repair

The host response to this transmural tissue injury can be observed immediately. The elements of the response in the lung mirror closely those observed in nearly all integumentary and visceral wound healing. Contact of platelets and plasma from disrupted blood vessels with the alveolar basement membrane leads to intraalveolar coagulation followed by an acute explosive inflammatory response. Awakened by a defined set of inflammatory cytokines, interstitial myofibroblasts migrate into the alveolar clot, thus initiating the fibroproliferative response. These cell attach and proliferate in the airspace thereby effacing the gas exchange surface [3, 7]. Fibroproliferation is also seen in the microcirculation [8]. Fibroproliferation results in the durable physiological derangements characteristic of the interval of mechanical ventilatory support. In the airspace, fibroproliferation leads to shunt and in the microcirculation it causes rarefaction of the pulmonary circulatory cross sectional area and pulmonary hypertension. If patients are to survive, the fibroproliferative response abates with the orderly induction of programmed cell death among the mesenchymal cell population, with restoration of the alveolar epithelial and endothelial surface.

Locomotion

Fibroblasts and epithelial cells are normally sessile. After injury, significant changes are observed. Under the influence of peptide differentiation factors such as transforming growth factor-β (TGF-β), interstitial fibroblasts differentiate into myofibroblasts containing abundant smooth muscle cell actin and vinculin. There is an associated increase in cytoskeletal organization and display of new matrix receptors as a motile phenotype is acquired [9]. These receptors are especially suited to migration on the provisional matrix proteins associated with the injured air space. Important receptors include the fibronectin receptor $\alpha5$ $\beta1$ integrin, CD44, and the receptor for hyaluronic acid mediated motility (RHAMM) [10]. Similarly, epithelial cells change their degree of cytoskeletal organization and express α5 β1 integrin at their basal and lateral surface in preparation for re-populating the provisional matrix coating the air lung interface [11].

Endowed with an appropriate array of cell surface receptors, myofibroblasts egress from the edematous interstition into the provisional matrix within the air-space. Signaling molecules driving this migration include platelet-derived growth factor (PDGF) family ligands released from degranulated platelets and activated macrophages [12], as well as solid phase signals provided by matrix molecules recognizing both CD44 [13] and RHAMM [14]. Epithelial cells prob-ably utilize a repertoire of fibronectin binding integrins [15] including αV β6, α5 β1, and αV β3 to migrate on fibronectin in response to signals such as TGF-β [16]. Also important in the process of migration are basement membrane active proteinases such as MMP-9 which are rapidly expressed after injury. Such protei-nases have the potential to facilitate detachment of otherwise stably attached epi-thelial cells facilitating their migration. However, the precise molecular mecha-nism involved in coordinating matrix receptor expression, the ligands they uti-lize, the specific proteinases involved, and the cytoskeletal organization are not well defined.

Proliferation

Polypeptide growth factors regulate the transition from quiescence to a prolifera-tive state [17]. These peptide signals are also important in the early events of G1 cell cycle transit up to the latter portion of G1 designated the R point or restric-tion point. This tightly controlled transition which includes such important reg-ulatory molecules as the D cyclins, their partner kinases, their targets (e.g. the re-tinoblastoma protein) and their respective inhibitors demarcate the growth fac-tor-dependent portion of the cell cycle from that which is autonomously programmed and independent of exogenous input. For growth factors to influ-ence target cell function, appropriate cell surface receptors must be displayed. In addition, the target cell must have the appropriate matrix receptors displayed on its surface and be residing on an appropriate substratum. Sources of growth fac-tors in the injured microenvironment include those derived from the processes of coagulation, inflammation and autocrine or paracrine parenchymal cell produc-tion. Having arrived in the injured alveolar airspace, lung myofibroblasts are ex-posed to a set of positive proliferative signals. Two important signals, fibronectin and PDGF, are capable of signaling both directed migration and the emergence from quiescence [18, 19]. In response to these signals, the myofibroblast popula-tion expands. This leads to a spectrum of anatomic abnormalities within the air-space ranging from complete effacement and absolute shunt physiology, to par-tial effacement with varying degrees of impairment of the gas exchange process.

In this chapter, I will focus on PDGF, basic fibroblast growth factor (FGF), and TGF-β, three signals which have been closely linked with the *in vivo* process of fi-broproliferation.

PDGF family ligands are a dimeric group of peptides tightly connected with pathological fibroproliferation in the lung and vasculature as well in physiological wound healing [12, 20]. There are 2tPDGF genes designated A and B. Homodimeric or heterodimeric ligands bind to cognate receptors on the surface of target cells stimulating both migration and emergence from quiescence. The myofibroblast response to PDGF is determined by the cell surface receptor population. Ligand binding leads to receptor dimerization, auto-phosphorylation, and a cascade of events associated with signal transduction eventually leading to the phosphorylation and activation of mitogen activated protein (MAP) kinase. There are 2 types of PDGF receptor proteins designated α and β. Target cell responsiveness to a particular ligand varies with the receptor repertoire expressed. The α chain exhibits affinity for both PDGF A and B, whereas, the β subunit binds predominantly B chain. Myofibroblasts typically display mainly β type receptors explaining its more robust biological response to PDGF B. Following lung injury, PDGF probably derives from platelet α granules which are released when denuded epithelial and endothelial basement membranes are exposed to the circulation. As the process evolves, macrophages and parenchymal cells may produce and release PDGF family ligands. The specific signals that induce and regulate PDGF release are currently not completely defined, however, interleukin-1β (IL-1β) has the capacity to induce autocrine release of PDGF B by lung myofibroblasts.

Among the fibroblast growth factor family, basic FGF is found at the air lung interface following lung injury, and functional ligand has been recovered from the lungs of patients with ALI [21]. In general, receptor dimerization is required for a cellular response to basic FGF. Lacking a classical leader sequence, basic FGF is constitutively secreted through alternative secretory pathways binding to nearby glycosaminoglycans in the lung interstitium. FGF probably derives from both inflammatory and parenchymal cells although detailed metabolic labeling studies following ALI have not been carried out. In addition to its role as a growth factor, basic FGF has also been implicated in morphogenesis providing positional information to cells as they migrate from one region to another. This function may be equally important as its role as a proliferative signal as the remodeling process proceeds following ALI.

The TGF family of peptides includes at least 20 members [22]. TGF-β1 is a potent modulator of mesenchymal cell differentiated state and has been closed associated with a number of fibroproliferative processes including ALI. There are three TGF-β1 receptors which dimerize to form heteromeric protein kinase complexes which initiate the signal transduction process following ligand binding. Shortly following injury, TGF-β1, likely derived from platelet β granules, signals interstitial fibroblasts to differentiate into myofibroblasts. After the airspace fills with myofibroblasts, TGF-β1 derived from both inflammatory and parenchymal cells is capable of signaling the transition from a motile proliferative phenotype into a collagen synthetic phenotype. This process has the capacity to lead to intraalveolar deposition of collagens I and III, contraction of the airspace, and permanent alveolar collapse. TGF-β1 provides both positive and negative proliferative signals to myofibroblasts. During active alveolar fibroproliferation, TGF-β1 can indirectly promote the process by stimulating autocrine production of PDGF B. It may also signal cell cycle arrest as the airspace fills, by down-regulation of cyclin-dependent kinases 4 and 6 which are essential for the R point transition. After promoting fibroblast quiescence, TGF-β1 may function to stimulate fibroblast collagen synthesis.

While peptide growth factors have an essential role in the genesis of fibroproliferation after lung injury, the importance of these molecules in the maintenance of fibroproliferation is uncertain. A variety of investigations in a number of different systems have indicated that fibroblasts from fibroproliferative lesions, whether in the lung or elsewhere, are capable of displaying an enhanced proliferative or synthetic phenotype independent of continuous exogenous stimulation [23]. Following ALI, myofibroblasts assume and maintain an enhanced proliferative phenotype enabling them to proliferate with minimal exogenous stimulation [24]. Therapeutic strategies designed at ligand interdiction will clearly need to take into account the possibility that ligand may be only necessary to initiate the fibroproliferative response within the air space and vessel wall, and not necessarily to maintain it.

The process of re-epithelialization which is recognized as critical to re-establishing normal barrier function is less well understood than the process of fibroproliferation. It is assumed that similar biological mechanisms involving peptide growth factors, matrix receptors, and matrix ligands play a critical role in the migratory and proliferative response of the epithelial cell population. Type II epithelial cells are regarded as the alveolar epithelial progenitor cell and responsible for the re-epithelialization process. Type II cells also are important regulators of the provisional matrix serving as an important source of plasminogen activators capable of initiating the degradation of polymerized fibrin within the airspace [25, 26]. Among the peptide growth factors that may be involved in the re-epithelialization process, keratinocyte growth factor (KGF) has received the most attention [27]. Released by fibroblasts, KGF is active *in vitro* and *in vivo* to stimulate alveolar type II cell proliferation. In addition, experimental evidence points to an important role for KGF as a cytoprotective molecule, regulating the viability of target epithelial cells. Data have not yet been developed which tightly link the integrity of the KGF-epithelial cell axis with the effectiveness of lung repair.

Apoptosis

Apoptosis is one type of genetically regulated death [28]. It is recognized by a distinct sequence of morphological events. The nucleus and cytoplasm condense, followed by fragmentation and formation of membrane bound vesicles termed apoptotic bodies. Following severe lung injury, lung neutrophils undergo apoptosis. As part of this process there are alterations of the plasma membrane which provide recognition signals for macrophages as well as neighboring cells permitting orderly and prompt elimination of the products of apoptosis [29]. Apoptosis typically does not trigger an inflammatory response and thereby provides a biological mechanism for inflammatory cell elimination and tissue remodeling without the adverse consequences of additional inflammation during the later phases of lung repair. Apoptosis can be triggered by an intrinsic genetic program, lack of survival signals, or by specific death signals interacting with cell surface receptors.

While known to be important in the removal of acute inflammatory cells, apoptosis also appears to be one important mechanism for ridding the airspace of intraalveolar granulation tissue during repair after injury. Apoptosis of granulation tissue must be closely coordinated with re-epithelialization of the gas exchange surface. Available data suggests that similar to events in integementary wounds, myofibroblast apoptosis is one mechanism for elimination of granulation tissue from the airspace and the re-establishment of gas exchange [30]. A similar process is thought to occur in the muscularized microvessels where normal anatomic structure also seems to be restored by elimination of excess mesenchymal cells.

Fibroblasts have specific requirements to remain viable. These include signals provided by the extracellular matrix through integrins and proteoglycans as well as by peptide growth factors such as PDGF and insulin-like growth factors (IGF 1). This requirement however, seems to depend on a variety of physiological context variables including the type of matrix the cell resides on and whether the cell is in cycle or quiescent. Fibroblasts display receptors for death signals including TNF-α [31] and Fas [32]. The functional role of these receptors in intraalveolar tissue regression, however, has not been established. While the molecular details remain to be worked out, the interplay between matrix, polypeptide growth factors, and death signals has the potential to form an important foundation for new therapeutic directions.

A nearly universal observation in diffuse alveolar damage following injury is the presence of type II cell hyperplasia. Many alveolar units in both postmortem and biopsy specimens are lined with type II cells. This observation has two important implications: 1) following even the most severe ALI, the progenitor function of type II cells remains intact; and 2) if the alveolar structures are to be restored to their normal configuration, a large number of type II cells must be eliminated as they differentiate into type I cells. Using available morphometric data and simple geometric assumptions, alveoli lined by a hyperplastic epithelium contain somewhere between an 8- and 10-fold excess of type II cells. Type II cell loss and their differentiation into type I cells must occur in a manner that preserves barrier function. Thus, type II cell elimination must be coordinated with differentiation into type I cells. The molecular regulation of type II cell apoptosis and subsequent differentiation into type I cells remains to be defined.

Conclusion

The integration of molecular biology with physiology has led to important new insights regarding potential therapeutic directions in lung repair. While prevention and early therapy remain important goals, most patients enter our critical care units with much of the injury already inflicted. For that reason, a focus on aspects of the reparative process is very attractive to the physician scientist. Early on, molecular manipulation of the rate of sodium and water transport out of the alveolus as well as alteration of the microenvironment to promote fibrinolysis may represent important therapeutic directions. For those alveolar units in which intraalveolar coagulation and granulation tissue develop, understanding the regulatory signals involved in the induction of myofibroblast apoptosis and the impact of positive pressure ventilation on these biological processes hold significant promise. Similarly, identifying the regulatory signals which coordinate type II cell apoptosis with differentiation to a normal type I cell dominated alveolar surface is a logical direction to pursue. The convergence of molecular and cell biology with physiology and applied bioengineering has the potential to make significant inroads into the currently unacceptable mortality rate of our patients with ALI, and to improve the quality of life of those who survive.

References

1. Polunovsky V, Bitterman P (1997) Regulation of cell population size. The Lung 1:133–153
2. Wendt C, Bitterman P (1997) The pathogenesis of pulmonary fibrosis. In: Fishman (ed) Pulmonary Diseases and Disorders (In Press)
3. Fukuda Y, Ishizaki M, Masuda Y, Kimura G, Kawanami O, Masugi Y (1987) The role of intraalveolar fibrosis in the process of pulmonary structural remodeling in patients with diffuse alveolar damage. Am J Pathol 126:171–182
4. Bachofen M, Weibel ER (1982) Structural alterations of lung parenchyma in the adult respiratory distress syndrome. Clin Chest Med 3:35–36
5. Gunther A, Siebert C, Schmidt R, et al (1996) Surfactant alterations in severe pneumonia, acute respiratory distress syndrome, and cardiogenic lung edema. Am J Respir Crit Care Med 153:176–184
6. Bland RD, Nielson DW (1992) Developmental changes in lung epithelial ion transport and liquid movement. Ann Rev Physiol 54:373–394
7. Anderson RW, Thielen K (1992) Correlative study of adult respiratory distress syndrome by light, scanning and transmission electron microscopy. Ultrastructural Pathol 16:615–628
8. Meyrick B (1991) Structure function correlates in the pulmonary vasculature during ALI and chronic pulmonary hypertension. Toxicol Pathol 19:447–457
9. Kapanci Y, Desmouliere A, Pache JC, et al (1995) Cytoskeletal protein modulation in pulmonary alveolar myofibroblasts during idiopathic pulmonary fibrosis: Possible role of transforming growth factor beta and tumor necrosis factor alpha. Am J Respir Crit Care Med 152:2163–2169
10. Hall CL, Turley EA (1995) Hyaluronan: RHAMM mediated cells locomotion and signaling in tumor genesis. J Neuro Oncol 26:221–229
11. Fukuda Y, Basset F, Ferrans VJ, Yamanaka N (1995) Significance of early intraalveolar fibrotic lesions and intergrin expression in lung biopsy specimens from patients with idiopathic pulmonary fibrosis. Hum Pathol 26:53–61
12. Snyder LS, Hertz MI, Peterson MS, et al (1991) ALI: Pathogenesis of intraalveolar fibrosis. J Clin Invest 88:663–673
13. Svee K, While J, Valliant P, Jessurun J, et al (1996) ALI fibroblast migration and invasion into a fibrin matrix is mediated by CD44. J Lab Invest 98:1713–1727
14. McKee CM, Penno MB, Cowman M, et al (1996) Hyaluronon (HA) fragments induce chemokine gene expression in alveolar macrophages. The role of HA size and CD44. J Clin Invest 98:2403–2413
15. Shepperd D, Yokosaki Y (1996) Roles of airway epithelial integrins in health and disease. The Parker B. Francis Lectureship. Chest 109 (3 Suppl.):295–335

16. Spurzem JR, Sacco O, Richard KA, et al. (1993) Transforming growth factor-β increases adhesion but not migration of bovine bronchial epithelial cells to matrix proteins. J Lab Clin Med 122:92–102
17. Sherr CJ (199-) Mammalian G1 cyclins. Cell 73:1059–1065
18. Bitterman PB, Rennard SI, Adelberg S, Crystal RG (1983) Role of fibronectin as a growth factor for fibroblasts. J Cell Biol 97:1925–1932
19. Ross R, Raines EW, Bowen-Pope DF (1986) The biology of platelet derived growth factor. Cell 46:155–169
20. Ferns GAA, Raines EW, Spruge KH, et al (1991) Inhibition of neointimal smooth muscle accumulation after angioplasty by an antibody to PDGF. Science 253:1129–1132
21. Henke C, Marinelli W, Jessurun J, et al (1993) Macrophage production of basic fibroblast growth factor in the fibroproliferative disorder of alveolar fibrosis after lung injury. Am J Pathol 143:1190–1199
22. Brand T, Schneider MD (1996) Transforming growth factor-β signal transduction. Circulation Res 78:173–179
23. LeRoy EC (1974) Increased collagen synthesis by scleroderma skin fibroblasts *in vitro*: A possible defect in the regulation or activation of the scleroderma fibroblast. J Clin Invest 54:880–889
24. Chen B, Polunovsky V, White J, et al (1992) Mesenchymal cells isolated after ALI manifest an enhanced proliferative phenotype. J Clin Invest 90:1778–1785
25. Idell S, James KK, Levin EG, et al (1989) Local abnormalities in coagulation and fibrinolytic pathways predispose to alveolar fibrin deposition in the adult respiratory distress syndrome. J Clin Invest 84:695–705
26. Simon RH, Gross TJH, Edwards JA, Sitrin RG (1991) Fibrin degradation by pulmonary alveolar epithelial cells. Am J Physiol 262:L482–L488
27. Panos RJ, Bak PM, Simonet WS, et al (1995) Intratracheal instillation of keratinocyte growth factor decreases hyperoxia-induced mortality in rats. J Clin Invest 96:2026–2033
28. Wyllie AH (1993) Apoptosis (The 1992 Frank Rose Memorial Lecture). Br J Cancer 67:205–208
29. Haslett C, Savill JS, Whyte MK, Stein M, Dransfield I, Mengler LC (1994) Granulocyte apoptosis and the control of inflammation. Philosophical transactions of the Royal Society of London Series B. Biological Sciences 345:327–333
30. Polunovsky V, Chen B, Henke C, et al (1993) Role of mesenchymal cell death in lung remodeling following injury. J Clin Invest 92:388–397
31. Mackey F, Rotte J, Bluethmann H, Loetscher H, Lesslaver W (1994) Differential responses of fibroblasts from wild type and TNF-R55 deficient mice to mouse and human TNF-alpha activation. J Immunol 153:5274–5284
32. Aggarwal BB, Singh S, LaPushin R, Totpal K (1995) Fas antigen signals proliferation of normal huma diploid fibroblasts and its mechanism is different from tumor necrosis factor receptor. FEBS Letters 364:5–8

The Pulmonary and Systemic Circulation in ARDS

The Pulmonary Circulation in Acute Lung Injury

S. Singh and T. W. Evans

Introduction

In adults, lung injury may complicate a wide range of serious medical and surgical conditions, only some of which involve a direct pulmonary insult (Table 1). Although the extreme form, acute respiratory distress syndrome (ARDS) was first

Table 1. Clinical conditions associated with the development of ARDS

Respiratory	Non-respiratory
– Pneumonia (bacterial/viral/fungal)	Sepsis syndrome
– Aspiration of gastric contents	Major trauma/shock
– Pulmonary contusion	Massive burns
– Post-pneumonectomy	DIC
– Inhalation of smoke or toxins	Transfusion reactions
– Near-drowning	Fat embolism
– Thoracic irradiation	Pregnancy-associated (e.g. amniotic fluid embolism)
– Oxygen toxicity	Pancreatitis
– Ischemia/reperfusion	Drug/toxin reactions (e.g.paraquat, heroin)
– Vasculitis (eg. Goodpasture's)	Post-CP bypass
– Head injury/ raised ICP	Tumour lysis syndrome

DIC – disseminated intravascular coagulopathy; CP – cardiopulmonary; ICP – intracranial pressure

Table 2. Definitions: ALI and ARDS. (Adapted from [6])

	Timing	Oxygenation	Chest radiograph	Pulmonary artery occlusion pressure
– ALI criteria	Acute onset	PaO_2/FiO_2 < 300 mmHg (regardless of PEEP level)	Bilateral infiltrates seen on frontal CXR	< 18 mmHg when measured, or no clinical evidence of left atrial hypertension
– ARDS criteria	Acute onset	PaO_2/FiO_2 < 200 mmHg (regardless of PEEP level)	Bilateral infiltrates seen on frontal CXR	< 18 mmHg when measured, or no clinical evidence of left atrial hypertension

described formally some 30 years ago, a uniformally accepted clinical definition was not published until 1994 [1]. Simultaneously, acute lung injury (ALI) was also defined as a distinct clinical entity in recognition of the spectrum of severity of lung injury that may occur as a result of these precipitating conditions (Table 2). ALI and ARDS are distinguished only by the severity of the refractory hypoxemia that characterizes both conditions, and this distinction may prove to have little clinical relevance. Nevertheless, in terms of recognizing the incidence, epidemiology, and histopathological evolution of lung injuries; and in carrying out trials of new therapeutic interventions, the distinction is important.

Epidemiology

Lung injury is common. Some 35% of patients with sepsis have mild to moderate lung injury, whilst 25% have fully-developed ARDS, with an associated mortality of between 50 and 75%. Lung injury rarely occurs in isolation, and is increasingly recognized as the pulmonary manifestation of a panendothelial insult or inflammatory vascular dysfunction (Fig. 1) [1, 2]. ALI has been defined only in the relatively recent past and data regarding incidence and outcome are sparse. Nevertheless, from published data regarding the incidence of ARDS (about 6 cases per 100 000 population) it is likely that more cases of ALI occur. There are reasons to suppose that different precipitating factors lead to ALI as opposed to full-blown ARDS, in that the incidence of the latter is undoubtedly dictated by the underlying condition in a given patient population. Further, it is the associated clinical conditions and coexisting organ failures that appear to be the major determinants of survival in patients with lung injury [3, 4]. In one study, for example, respiratory failure accounted for only 16% of deaths, the majority being attributable to associated multiple organ system failure (MOSF). Although ALI and ARDS are characterized by impaired pulmonary gas exchange, there is also frequently a failure of oxygen utilization in the periphery, leading ultimately to MOSF. Whether this occurs through a failure of microvascular control leading to

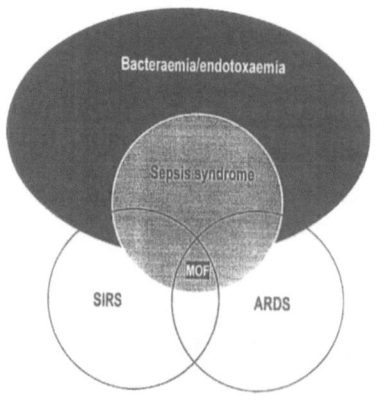

Fig. 1. The overlapping clinical syndromes associated with sepsis. Only a proportion of these syndromes are associated with the identification of an infective agent. More frequently there is detectable endotoxemia, but in some neither of these are present. SIRS: systemic inflammatory response syndrome, MOF: multiple organ failure, ARDS: acute respiratory distress syndrome. (From [14] with permission)

Fig. 2. ALI: The spectrum of disease. Lung injury can occur in response to a wide variety of insults. The response of an individual is unpredictable and the subsequent injury may present with characteristic clinical sequelae, the most severe form of which is full-blown ARDS, or it may be sub-clinical. Other organs may also be affected to a variable extent, and the most severe clinical end of this spectrum would be multiple organ failure. Currently the ability to predict those patients who are at high risk of developing significant lung injury (and other organ damage), as well as those with established ARDS who will survive, is seen as a research priority. MOF: multiple organ failure, ARDS: acute respiratory distress syndrome

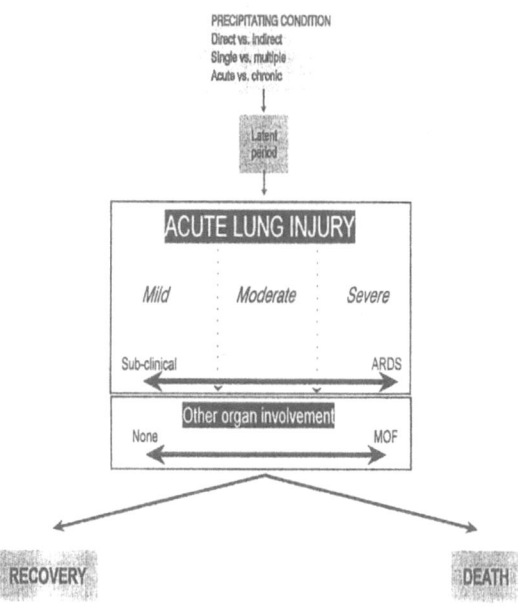

tissue hypoxia, or mitochondrial dysfunction preventing utilization of available oxygen, remains unclear. It is therefore not surprising that sepsis occurs up to 6 times more commonly in patients with ARDS compared to other critically ill patients, or that up to 25% of cases of established sepsis or systemic inflammatory response syndrome (SIRS) are complicated by ARDS. ALI and ARDS are thus clinically recognizable sequelae of a complex inflammatory reaction to diverse insults, so that very frequently other organs are involved in the clinical pathology (Fig. 2). It is the vascular endothelium that represents the interface between the inflammatory insult and its clinical manifestation.

Pathogenesis

ALI and ARDS represent the common endpoint of a wide variety of inflammatory pathways. Of these, the best characterized is initiated by endotoxin, a lipopolysaccharide (LPS) component of the cell wall of Gram-negative bacteria, which through endothelial cell activation leads to the generation and release of a cascade of inflammatory mediators such as tumor necrosis factor-α (TNF-α), interleukins (IL)-1, IL-8, and IL-16, and platelet activating factor (PAF); from neutrophils, macrophages, platelets, and endothelium. Infusion of LPS or TNF-α in animals reproduces some of the clinical features of sepsis, including lung injury. Critically ill patients with sepsis have high levels of serum LPS, and those with ARDS frequently have detectable endotoxemia. Further, raised levels of TNF-α and IL-1 have been demonstrated in both serum and bronchoalveolar lavage

(BAL) fluid from patients with ARDS [5]. Subsequent activation of neutrophils by endotoxin or other agents is one of the earliest events in the pathogenesis of lung injury, and BAL taken from patients with ARDS contains increased numbers of neutrophils, as well as excessive amounts of neutrophil-generated proteinase enzymes such as elastase and collagenase.

Injury to, and activation of the endothelium is central to the inflammatory response to endotoxin, and to the resultant functional and structural changes that occur in the pulmonary vasculature. Endotoxin, TNF-α and other cytokines are all capable of inducing endothelial cell injury [6], thereby stimulating ultrastructural changes within the cells leading to increased permeability. Endothelial cell activation also facilitates the adherence and subsequent migration of activated neutrophils from blood to tissue, mediated by adhesion molecules. This occurs principally in post-capillary venules, within which white cells marginate, as a result of loose tethering to the underlying endothelium. Subsequently, the neutrophils become more adherent, changing from spherical to a flatter shape. This facilitates their slow migration between endothelial cells through the basement membrane into the interstitium. This process is now known to be mediated by interaction of specific cell adhesion molecules (CAM) on the surface of both the

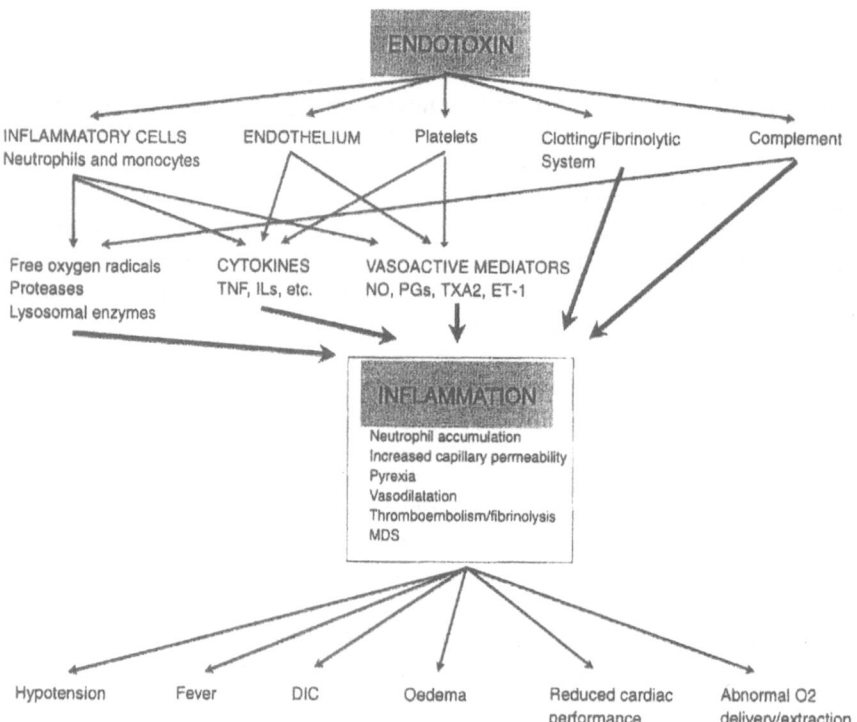

Fig. 3. The inflammatory vascular response to sepsis. DIC: disseminated intravascular coagulopathy

neutrophil and endothelial cell in a sequence known as the adhesion cascade. The endothelium has other facets of its inflammatory functions, most important of which are a group of endotoxin/cytokine-inducible genes which result in the expression of mRNA coding for a range of proteins, including cyclooxygenase, the constitutive (cNOS) and inducible (iNOS) forms of nitric oxide(NO) synthase (NOS) and endothelins (Fig. 3). It is the release of these potent vasoactive and inflammatory mediators that allows the endothelium to modulate the vascular response to sepsis. When the inflammatory response is widespread and severe, intense activation of the endothelium in some areas and damage to it in others contribute to the clinical syndromes described above.

Pathophysiology

Alveolar-Capillary Membrane Permeability

ALI and ARDS are clinical diagnoses designed to reflect the clinical spectrum of lung injury [7]. Pulmonary endothelial damage can lead to mild respiratory impairment or overwhelming alveolar edema, although the extent of the increase in alveolar capillary permeability does not predict outcome [8, 9]. Clinical studies have identified elevated pulmonary vascular resistance (PVR) as a universal finding in patients with acute respiratory failure [10]. In ARDS, PVR is increased via a combination of increased vascular tone and structural influences such as extrinsic compression by edema fluid, the application of positive pressure ventilation, thromboembolic phenomenon and vascular remodelling. In ARDS, pulmonary hypertension contributes to pulmonary edema formation and impaired right ventricular performance and has been identified with an increased mortality [11]. Further, impaired gas transfer coefficient has been identified as being of adverse prognostic significance in ARDS and is positively correlated with PVR [12].

Hypoxic Pulmonary Vasoconstriction

Hypoxic pulmonary vasoconstriction (HPV) is the physiological response by which blood is diverted away from underventilated alveoli, thereby improving the matching of perfusion (Q) and ventilation (V). This homeostatic control mechanism is disrupted in ALI/ARDS [13]. Using the multiple inert gas technique, investigators have demonstrated that the resultant intra-pulmonary shunting is large enough to account for the observed alveolar/arterial PO_2 gradient, even without invoking a reduction in diffusion capacity [14]. It has long been recognized that the endothelium has an inhibitory role on HPV. In some species HPV is dependent upon an intact pulmonary vascular endothelium, and hypoxia-induced contractions of pulmonary arteries in vitro are reduced by endothelial removal. Nevertheless, endothelial injury can also enhance HPV, and in the longer term, structural alterations in pulmonary endothelial cells may also con-

tribute to the development of hypoxic pulmonary hypertension [15]. The endothelium removes circulating vasoconstrictor substances [16], and more importantly releases a range of vasoactive agents locally. Any change in the dynamic
balance of these factors could modulate the vascular tonic response.

Endothelium-derived Factors Capable of Modifying PVR

Nitric Oxide

The vascular relaxation induced by acetylcholine was first shown to be dependent on the presence of intact endothelium and to be mediated via the release of
an endothelium-derived relaxant factor (EDRF) in 1980 [17]. The chemical and
pharmacological properties of EDRF are virtually identical to those of NO, which
is synthesized from the amino acid, L-arginine, by a group of flavin-containing
oxygenase enzymes commonly termed nitric oxide synthase (NOS) [18]. Endothelial cells were the first mammalian cells shown to release NO, a potent vasodilator. NO relaxes blood vessels by activating soluble guanylate cyclase, the resultant increase in cyclic guanosine monophosphate (cGMP) causing a quenching of
intracellular calcium (Fig. 4a) [19]. It is now accepted that various cell types can
release NO and that at least three distinct isoforms of NOS exist (Table 3). Endothelial NOS (eNOS) and neuronal NOS (nNOS) are constitutive and calcium-dependent enzymes, but a third isoform is induced (iNOS) by LPS and inflammatory cytokines. The cDNA for all three types of NOS has now been purified, cloned,
sequenced and expressed. Although differences exist in the biochemistry of the
three NOS isoforms, the basic pathway of metabolism of L-arginine to NO and L-
citrulline is well conserved and all are inhibited by the L-arginine analogs N^G-

Table 3. Vascular isoforms of NOS

	eNOS	iNOS
– Response in sepsis	Constitutive Immediate NO synthesis	Induced by LPS & cytokines Massive NO production after 2–6 h
– Location	Endothelial cell Membrane-bound	Mainly smooth muscle Cytosolic
– Regulation	Oestrogens, shear stress & exercise increase activity	Induction prevented by corticosteroids & inhibitors of protein synthesis
– Activation	Calcium-dependent	Calcium-independent
– Non-selective inhibitors	L-arginine analogs (e.g. N^G-monomethyl- L-arginine)	L-arginine analogs (e.g. N^G-monomethyl-L-arginine)
– Selective inhibitors	None known	Aminoguanidine L-canavanine

NO: nitric oxide, NOS: nitric oxide synthase: "e" - endothelial; "i" - inducible, LPS: lipopolysaccharide

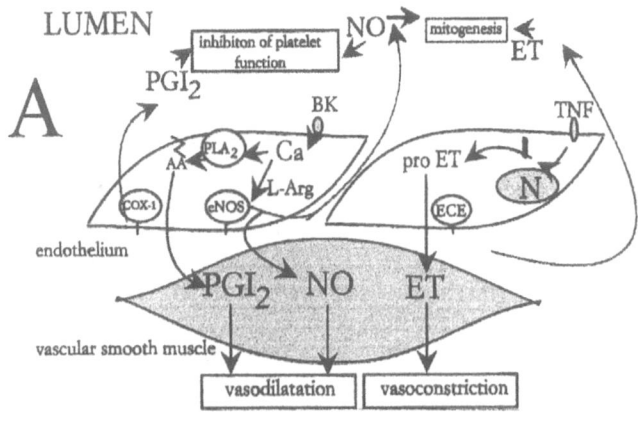

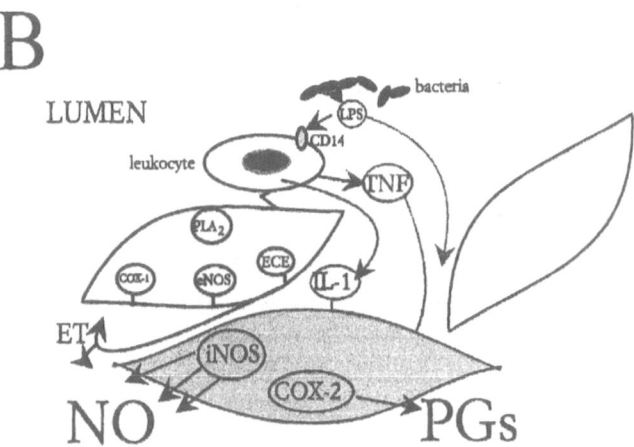

Fig. 4. The vasoactive factors released by the endothelium. **A.** The endothelial cell contributes to vascular tone and local anti-coagulation by the tonic release of several mediators including NO via eNOS, prostacyclin (PGI$_2$) via COX-1 and endothelin-1 (ET-1). These are released both basally and into the vessel lumen. **B.** In "sepsis", the presence of endotoxin and a variety of early inflammatory cytokines result in endothelial cell activation and disruption. The activated cells produce larger quantities of NO (via iNOS), PGI$_2$ (via COX-2) and ET-1. At the same time, however, the underlying smooth muscle undergoes iNOS induction resulting in the production of massive quantities of NO. It seems likely that the degree of local damage to the endothelium may determine the vascular response to the initial inflammatory insult, and that on a larger scale this may contribute to the clinical outcome

monomethyl-L-arginine (L-NMMA) , N^G-nitro-L-arginine (L-NNA) and/or N^G-nitro-L-arginine methyl ester (L-NAME) [19, 20]. Such inhibitors cause a rapid increase in blood pressure in animals and in man, suggesting that in health NO is required in order to maintain vascular tone.

NO in Sepsis: Suprabasal release of NO is known to occur in response to a diverse range of stimuli including endotoxin, cytokines, hypoxia, histamine, thrombin, bradykinin, calcium ionophore, endothelin and substance P (Fig. 4b). As a result, an increase of NO release during the inflammatory response to sepsis is inevitable. Patients and animals with septic shock lose peripheral vascular tone, and the responsiveness of systemic vessels to constrictor agents such as catecholamines is diminished, both *in vitro* and *in vivo*. The incubation of bovine aortic endothelial cells with LPS causes rapid release of an NO-like factor. Further, levels of NO metabolites are significantly elevated in patients with septic shock [21], and the administration of NOS inhibitors in these circumstances [22] , or in animal models of sepsis [23], can produce reproducible elevations in systemic vascular resistance (SVR) where other vasoconstrictors are ineffective. In fact, excess quantities of NO are produced in sepsis. Endotoxin leads to the induction of the calcium-independent NOS (iNOS) in both the endothelium and the vascular smooth muscle [24], as well as in the myocardium where the increase in NO production has been shown to reduce contractility [25] . Other cytokines (TNF, IL-1 and IL-2) also stimulate iNOS activity in vessel walls.

The time course of the increase in NO release in sepsis is the subject of considerable speculation. In isolated endotoxin-treated rat main pulmonary arteries, NOS inhibitors reverse the vascular hyporesponsiveness to phenylephrine [26], and there is little doubt that in established sepsis, NO is largely reponsible for this reduced reactivity. The NO-mediated hyporeactivity to norepinephrine starts within 60 min in a rat model of sepsis *in vivo* [27], and may therefore be too rapid to be explained by the induction of iNOS. Although it seems likely that this early increase in NO release is explained by an elevation in NO production by endothelial cNOS, this remains controversial and the early hyporesponsiveness may be caused not by NO, but by some other factor(s). It is clear, however, that from about 3 h after the endotoxic insult, there is massive NO production as a result of iNOS activity in the endothelium, and to an even greater extent in the vascular smooth muscle. The endothelium appears to be required for maximal NO response, such that its removal causes a significant delay in the onset of vascular responsiveness (6 compared with 4 h) and reduces the sensitivity of rat aorta to LPS *in vitro*. The application of the technique of reverse transcription polymerase chain reaction (rt-PCR) has allowed the demonstration of the widespread tissue expression of iNOS mRNA in a rat model at 4 h post-LPS injection compared with undetectable expression in control animals. In rat pulmonary artery, this rise can be attenuated by pretreatment with dexamethasone 30 min before the LPS challenge [28] . Further, preliminary evidence suggests that there is differential regulation of the cNOS and iNOS mRNAs in rats treated with LPS *in vivo*, such that whilst there is greatly increased expression of iNOS mRNA in rat heart, lung and aorta 4 h post-LPS, the expression of eNOS mRNA is simultaneously down-regulated when compared with levels from control animals [29].

NOS Inhibitors in Sepsis: The intravenous administration of L-NMMA has been shown to (temporarily) correct systemic hypotension in 2 patients with septic shock. Other L-arginine analogs such as L-NNA, that non-specifically block NOS, given to critically ill patients with sepsis can cause increases in systemic and pulmonary vascular resistance as well as in mean arterial pressure, with reduction in cardiac index. Theoretically, these non-specific inhibitors of NOS may augment a pre-existing overall reduction in regional blood flow in sepsis in some beds (notably renal, mesenteric and pulmonary) which could be amplified by NOS inhibition.

A gradual improvement in the understanding of the role of iNOS in sepsis has fueled investigation into the possibility of the selective blockade of the enzyme in sepsis [30] .The theoretical attraction of this as a therapeutic tool are obvious. In comparative studies between L-NMMA and aminoguanidine, the latter was found to be at least seven times more potent at inhibiting iNOS [31]. However L-NMMA was 15 times more potent at inhibition of the constitutive enzyme than aminoguanidine. Aminoguanidine produced a dose-dependent increase in phenylephrine-induced tension in intact and endothelium-denuded pulmonary artery rings from endotoxin-treated rats, but it had no effect on sham-treated controls [30]. Aminoguanidine-precipitated contraction in the endothelium-denuded vessels was abolished by L-arginine or L-NMMA pretreatment, suggesting that its mechanism of action involves the L-arginine/NO axis.

NO in HPV: A reduction in NO production or a decrease in its target receptor sensitivity could theoretically result in pulmonary vasoconstriction during hypoxia. Certainly, endothelium-dependent relaxation is impaired by hypoxia in rabbit and rat pulmonary artery rings [32]. However, there is no consistency between such in vitro results and those obtained in human tissue or in isolated lung experiments. In fact, the contraction induced by hypoxia in isolated human lobar arteries is potentiated by endothelial removal, while in isolated perfused lung preparations, inhibition of NO release under hypoxic conditions with methylene blue or L-NMMA potentiates the pressor response, suggesting that NO release may actually increase during HPV [33]. It is therefore possible that alterations in this shift of NO production in the most hypoxic areas of lung could disrupt appropriate blood diversion.

In sepsis, the induction of iNOS would be expected to reduce the degree of local HPV. However, recent evidence on pulmonary artery and aortic rings in vitro from LPS-treated rats suggests that not only does hypoxia inhibit cNOS, thus producing rapid vasoconstriction, but that it also inhibits LPS-induced iNOS [34] .

Endothelins

In 1988, an endothelially-derived vasoconstrictor was cloned and sequenced following its isolation from the culture medium of porcine aortic endothelial cells [35]. This substance, termed endothelin (ET), was found to elicit a slow, sustained contraction of isolated arteries from many different species. Three ET-related genomic loci have been identified that encode for three similar but distinct 21 amino acid ET peptides (ET-1, ET-2, ET-3) [36], produced following cleavage of a pre-propeptide via a propeptide. This conversion is mediated by the activity of one of a family of endothelin converting enzymes (ECE), of which there are several types: Preliminary evidence suggest that there is at least one form available on the cell membrane to handle circulating "Big ET", and two intracellular forms involved in mature ET-1 production and release.

ET-1 immunoreactivity cannot be demonstrated in homogenates of capillary endothelial cells, and release of ET from cultured endothelium can be prevented by a protein synthesis inhibitor, suggesting that ETs are not stored but rather synthesized de novo. Factors that have been found to be capable of stimulating ET release are diverse and include vessel wall shear stress, hypoxia, endotoxin, TNF-α, interferon, epinephrine, angiotensin, thrombin, activated platelets and some prostanoids (Fig. 5). Local ET release would therefore be expected during any inflammatory response. ET-induces smooth muscle contraction via several second messenger pathways whose final common pathway is to increase free intracellular calcium. Synthesis of inositol triphosphate and diaglycerol is thought to be the principal effector system, although protein kinase C is also involved [37].

Two ET receptor subtypes have so far been cloned and expressed. ET_A has a higher affinity for ET-1 than ET-2 or -3, and has widespread expression particularly on vascular smooth muscle, but has not been found on endothelial cells. ET_B is non-selective, binding all three endothelin isoforms equally avidly such that they are equipotent in their displacement of ^{125}ET-1. ET_B is found on vascular en-

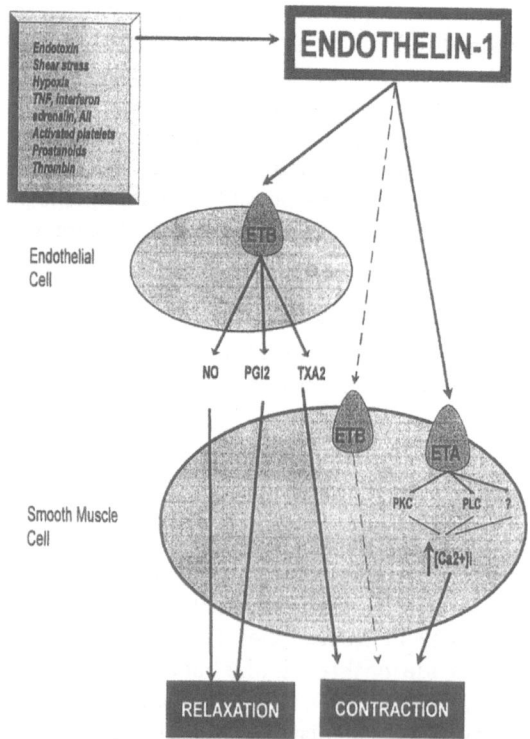

Fig. 5. Endothelin-1: Release and receptors.
TNF: tumor necrosis factor-α,
AII: angiotensin II,
PKC: phosphokinase C,
PLC: phospholipase C,
[Ca^{2+}]: intracellular free calcium

dothelium and also on smooth muscle in some vascular beds. At first it was thought that ET_A receptor stimulation was responsible for the direct constrictor effects of ET and that ET_B receptor stimulation resulted in the release of other vasoactive factors from those cells. ET-1 is certainly a potent vasoconstrictor in humans and animals by direct stimulation of ET_A receptors, a response which the endothelium can modulate via ET_B receptor stimulation. However, it has become apparent recently that ET_B receptors exist on some vascular smooth muscle and mediate contraction directly, and that some ET_A receptors are capable of stimulating prostanoid release. There is now also clear evidence from both *in vitro* and *in vivo* studies that ETs release NO from the endothelium by ET_B receptor stimulation. This gives rise to the characteristic hemodynamic responses of rats (and other species) to intravenous ET-1, in which there is an initial transient fall in systemic blood pressure followed by a sustained pressor response [35]. Only the former can be attenuated by L-NMMA pretreatment, and only the latter can be attenuated by ET_A receptor antagonists such as BQ123 [37]. There is also evidence that ET-1 can stimulate the release of prostacyclin and thromboxane from endothelial cells via ET_B receptors.

Low dose ET-1 infusion in man causes a rise in systemic and pulmonary arterial vascular resistances and a small fall in cardiac output [38]. ET-1 is largely metabolised in the pulmonary circulation, whilst some is eliminated by the kidneys. The plasma half-life of a bolus of radiolabelled ET-1 in anesthetised rats was 40 sec in one study, with 82% uptake in the lungs and 10% in the kidneys.

Endothelins in Sepsis: Plasma ET-1 levels are elevated in many animal models of sepsis, as well as in critically ill patients, possibly correlating with indicators of illness severity [39]. It is probable that ET-1 effects vascular tone as a result of autocrine and paracrine activity rather than as a circulating hormone, especially since release of ET-1 from endothelial cells appears to be polarised predominantly to the basal (abluminal) direction (Fig. 4b). The expression of ET-1 mRNA in several tissues from endotoxin-treated rats (heart, lung, aorta, pulmonary artery) is significantly increased when compared with controls, although the time course for this increase varies from tissue to tissue, and none was seen in skeletal muscle or kidney from the same [40]. Interestingly, the marked early increases in circulating [ET-1] in patients with acute lung injury seen in one study appeared to be due, at least in part, to reduced pulmonary metabolism of the peptide [41].

Despite potent effects on vascular tone, both direct and indirect, and unequivocal increases in ET-1 production and release in sepsis, the role of these peptides in sepsis remains unclear. Isolated pulmonary arteries from endotoxemic rats demonstrate hyporesponsiveness to exogenous ET-1, and complete contraction to ET-1 in these vessels is dependent upon the presence of the endothelium [42]. By contrast, the intact pulmonary circulation of septic rats is hypersensitive to ET-1, an effect exacerbated by pretreatment with L-NMMA [43]. Further, administration of non-selective ET antagonists has been shown to attenuate sepsis-associated pulmonary hypertension in pigs but not in rats. As potent vasoconstrictors, it is tempting to speculate that ETs contribute to the reduction of regional blood flow seen in certain organ beds such as the gut, kidney and lung during established sepsis, but further data are required. Administration of ET_A/ET_B antagonists to rats being infused with endotoxin exacerbates the systemic hypotensive response [44], implying that ET-1 may afford some protection against the loss of systemic vascular tone seen in sepsis.

Arachidonic Acid Metabolites

Arachidonic acid is the precursor of a variety of vasoactive and inflammatory mediators implicated in the pathogenesis of sepsis. The first step in arachidonic acid metabolism is its liberation from membrane-bound phospholipids, usually by the actions of phospholipase A2. Once free in the cell, arachidonic acid is metabolised by various oxygenase enzymes, such as cyclooxygenase to form prostaglandins (PG), thromboxanes (TX) and prostacyclin (PGI_2) or lipoxygenase (LO) to form leukotrienes (LT). Cyclooxygenase is now known to exist in constitutive and inducible isoforms [45]. It is thought that inducible cyclooxygenase predominates at the site of inflammation, including in the lung of rats 6 h after LPS challenge. Thus, inducible cyclooxygenase may represent the main source of prostanoids released in the lung during septic shock. The identification of inducible cyclooxygenase as a major inflammatory enzyme has promoted attempts to develop non-steroidal anti-inflammatory drugs (NSAIDs) which specifically inhibit this isoform.

Arachidonic Acid Metabolites in Sepsis: Cytokines stimulate prostanoid release both *in vivo* and *in vitro*. During the inflammatory response, generation of prostanoids and thromboxane A2 (TXA_2) occurs in inflammatory cells such as macrophages as well as in the endothelium. The release of PGI_2 and TXA_2 is controlled by individual cell types. Thus, endothelial cells form mainly PGI_2 whereas platelets and to a lesser extent, eiosinophils and neutrophils, are the main sources of TXB_2. Inducible cyclooxygenase-derived increases in PGI_2 have been demonstrated in intact human vessels treated with IL-1 and bovine endothelial cells treated with LPS, as well as in lung homogenates and aortic smooth muscle from rats treated with LPS [45, 46]. This increase of PGI_2 may therefore attenuate pulmonary hypertension associated with sepsis. Thus, the balance between the local production of vasodilator (PGI_2) and vasoconstrictor (TXA_2 and endoperoxides) agents in this way undoubtedly contributes to the vascular tone in that area [47]. The induction of cyclooxygenase occurs from about 6 h, and PGI_2 is released from cultured endothelial cells in response to endotoxin at about this time. More specifically, IL-1, known to be one of the principal mediators that amplifies the early inflammatory response in sepsis, induces PGI_2 production from human endothelial cells [46]. Both IL-1 and TNF induce cyclooxygenase mRNA expression in human endothelial cells. TXA_2 is a vasoconstrictor, and its inhibition has been shown to diminish the early pulmonary hypertension, but not the increased vascular permeability, in an experimental model of endotoxin-induced sepsis. Clinical studies of patients with ARDS have demonstrated increased serum levels of TXA_2

and leukotrienes in BAL [48]. The generation of cyclooxygenase products by the lung is suggested by the finding in endotoxemic sheep that lung lymph concentrations exceed plasma levels. Several animal studies of sepsis have successfully attenuated the early changes in pulmonary hemodynamics using cyclooxygenase inhibitors or thromboxane receptor antagonists with a corresponding improvement in survival [49].

Therapeutic Considerations

Despite recent advances in understanding the role of the endothelium in modulating the pathophysiology of lung injury, successful therapeutic intervention, as judged by a reduction in mortality, remains elusive. However, this enhanced understanding has led to the development of new strategies whose potential has not yet been fully realized.

Nitric Oxide Synthase (NOS) Inhibitors

The theoretical attraction of inhibiting NOS in sepsis is clear: The restoration of systemic vascular tone with elevation in the systemic vascular resistance and systemic blood pressure, hence resulting in improved organ perfusion. Non-specific inhibitors of NOS have been shown in small numbers of cases to improve systemic blood pressure in patients with refractory septic shock [22]. However, L-NNA has been shown to increase not only SVR, but also PVR. This highlights the theoretical disadvantage of non-selective NOS inhibition: Complete NOS inhibition, even in a patient with septic shock, may have deleterious cardiovascular side effects. In particular, the pulmonary hypertension that is characteristically seen in ALI/ARDS may be exacerbated. In addition, there is preliminary evidence that the balance between cNOS and iNOS isoforms is an important determinant of local vascular tone in the septic circulation [29], and that a sweeping disruption of this balance may be disadvantageous. Laboratory-derived data suggest that certain vascular beds may require NO to maintain perfusion, even in sepsis. For example, pretreatment with L-NMMA, but not phenylephrine, increased microvascular damage in the intestine of LPS-treated rats [50]. In the isolated, perfused pulmonary circulation, rats treated with LPS exhibit hypersensitivity to constrictors including ET-1, a response exacerbated by pretreatment with L-NMMA [43].

   The theoretical disadvantages of non-selective NOS inhibition could, to a great extent, be avoided if the inhibition was restricted to the inducible enzyme only. The use of aminoguanidine has theoretical advantages, having been shown to selectively inhibit iNOS in LPS-treated rats [28, 30, 31], although potential toxicity has hindered its clinical use. Clinical studies are now underway to investigate the therapeutic potential of NOS inhibitors in critically ill septic patients. Nevertheless, the universal application of any such agent may prove beneficial in only certain areas of the circulation whilst proving harmful in others.

Inhaled NO

The use of conventional, intravenous vasodilator therapy to reduce PVR and improve hypoxemia and right ventricular dysfunction in ALI/ARDS is limited by two problems. Firstly, the global pulmonary vasodilator effect of intravenous agents may abolish any residual (protective) HPV in underventilated alveoli, causing a further deterioration in V/Q mismatch and worsening hypoxemia. Secondly, the doses required to produce a beneficial effect in the pulmonary vascular bed frequently cause systemic vasodilatation and cardiovascular instability. The concept of using inhaled NO as a selective pulmonary vasodilator in patients with ALI/ARDS has therefore emerged. Any lack of pharmacological specificity for the pulmonary circulation becomes less relevant, in that NO is avidly bound by hemoglobin and thereby inactivated prior to it reaching and affecting the systemic circulation. The dilator action of inhaled NO is thus theoretically confined to the area of deposition, thereby recruiting blood to functional lung units to which the inspired gas has access, without deleterious systemic effects. This should lead to a simultaneous improvement in V/Q matching, a reduction in shunt fraction and a fall in PVR [51]. Indeed, early animal studies using inhaled NO (at concentrations of 5–80 parts per million) in acute hypoxic and pharmacologically-induced pulmonary hypertension demonstrated rapidly reversible pulmonary vasodilatation with no systemic effects [52, 53]. The effect of inhaled NO in human volunteers during hypoxia was similar except that much lower concentrations (10 ppm) of NO were required for maximum effect [54] . In a trial of inhaled NO in ARDS, concentrations of 18 ppm for 40 min produced significant reductions in mean pulmonary artery pressure, and an increase in arterial oxygen (PaO_2) to inspired oxygen (FiO_2) ratio, enabling FiO_2 to be reduced by 15% [55]. Similar results have been reported at lower concentrations (100 parts per billion – 18 ppm) [56]. Although no study has yet demonstrated a clear reduction in mortality or morbidity, a trend towards reduced mortality in a subgroup of inotrope/vasopressor resuscitated septic ARDS patients who responded to inhaled NO (> 20% rise in arterial oxygen tension and/or > 15% fall in mean pulmonary artery pressure) has been identified [57]. A response to NO was associated with increased right ventricular function, cardiac index and improved oxygen delivery while lack of response to NO and higher mortality were characteristic of a group with depressed cardiac reserves .

Although its potential utility for some patients is evident, the benefits of inhaled NO are not invariable and indeed it may impair gas exchange. Furthermore, issues of toxicity in the inflamed lung are not yet resolved. Ongoing trials have been designed to address outcome, although death is an insensitive endpoint for ARDS due to the influence of its diverse etiologies on mortality [58].

Cyclooxygenase Inhibitors

Experimental data derived from animal models suggest that mortality can be reduced by the application of cyclooxygenase (COX) inhibitors in sepsis [59]. A recent multicentre randomised control trial of the NSAID ibuprofen in sepsis demonstrated safety and physiologic reductions in fever, tachycardia , oxygen consumption and lactic acidosis but no improvement in overall survival [60]. This continues to be an area of dynamic research.

Endothelin Antagonists/Antibodies

As yet, there are no data to support the use of ET antagonists in sepsis or lung injury. Further evidence is required to dissect out the precise role of ET-1 in different vascular beds before such interventions could be justified clinically. Indeed, some animal experiments suggest that non-selective antagonism of ET receptors in endotoxemia may exacerbate systemic hypotension. By contrast, blood urea and creatinine levels, as well as urine output, were improved in a rat model of endotoxemia by the administration of an anti-ET-1 antibody. It is conceivable that tailored delivery of selective ET antagonists or antibodies may attenuate the pulmonary hypertension of ALI, as well as improving function of other organs, without simultaneously having deleterious effects on others.

Conclusion

ALI and ARDS occur in association with a variety of pulmonary and extra-pulmonary pathologies. Damage to the pulmonary vascular endothelium is a fundamental step in the initiation and mediation of the inflammatory process that produces tissue injury. Clearly, the endothelium and its release of NO, ET and eicosanoids represents a dynamic fulcrum during sepsis, and the balance of these factors determines both the local pulmonary vascular tone and the extent of the inflammatory reaction. However, it is increasingly evident that other cell types, including vascular smooth muscle, can release these substances after exposure to LPS or cytokines. Thus, during inflammatory events, the vascular smooth muscle may serve to compensate for a failing and damaged endothelium. Research is currently concerned with identifying therapeutic ways of altering the balance of these vasoactive and inflammatory mediators in a favorable way, to dampen the inflammatory response and restore the usually beneficial effects of HPV, which is disrupted in lung injury.

Acknowledgements. Supported in part by the British Heart Foundation.

References

1. Bernard GR, Artigas A, Brigham KL, et al (1994) The American-European consensus conference on ARDS: Definitions, mechanisms, relevant outcomes and clinical trial co-ordination. Am J Respir Crit Care Med 149:818–824
2. Bone RC, Balk R, Slotman G, et al (1992) Adult respiratory distress syndrome. Sequence and importance of development of multiple organ failure. The Prostaglandin E1 Study Group. Chest 101:320–326

3. Seidenfeld JJ, Pohl DF, Bell RC, et al (1986) Incidence, site, and outcome of infections in patients with the adult respiratory distress syndrome. Am Rev Respir Dis 134:12-16
4. Bone RC, Fisher CJ Jr., Clemmer TP, Slotman GJ, Metz CA, Balk RA (1989) Sepsis syndrome: A valid clinical entity. Methylprednisolone Severe Sepsis Study Group. Crit Care Med 17: 389-393
5. Hyers TM, Tricomi SM, Dettenmeier PA, Fowler AA (1991) Tumor necrosis factor levels in serum and bronchoalveolar lavage fluid of patients with the adult respiratory distress syndrome. Am Rev Respir Dis 144:268-271
6. Curzen NP, Griffiths MJD, Evans TW (1994) The role of the endothelium in modulating the vascular response to sepsis. Clin Sci 86:359-374
7. Macnaughton PD, Evans TW (1992) Management of adult respiratory distress syndrome. Lancet 339:469-472
8. Murray JF, Matthay MA, Luce JM, Flick MR (1988) An expanded definition of the adult respiratory distress syndrome. Am Rev Respir Dis 138:720-723
9. Sloane PJ, Gee MH, Gottlieb JE et al (1992) A multicenter registry of patients with acute respiratory distress syndrome. Physiology and outcome. Am Rev Respir Dis146:419-426
10. Zapol WM, Snider MT (1977) Pulmonary hypertension in severe acute respiratory failure. N Engl J Med 296:476-480
11. Bernard GR, Rinaldo J, Harris T et al (1985) Early predictors of ARDS reversal in patients with established ARDS. Am Rev Respir Dis 131:A143 (Abst)
12. Pallares LCM, Evans TW (1992) Oxygen transport in the critically ill. Respir Med 86: 289-295
13. Schoemaker WC, Appel PL, Kram HB (1988) Prospective trial of supranormal values of survivors as therapeutic goals in high risk surgical patients. Chest 94:1176-1186
14. Dantzker DR, Brook CJ, Dehart P, Lynch JP, Weg JG (1979) Ventilation-perfusion distributions in the adult respiratory distress syndrome. Am Rev Respir Dis 120:1039-1052
15. Rodman DM, Yamaguchi T, Hasunuma K, O'Brien RF, McMurtry IF (1990) Effects of hypoxia on endothelium-dependent relaxation of rat pulmonary artery. Am J Physiol 258: L207-L214
16. Liu SF, Dewar A, Crawley DE, Barnes PJ, Evans TW (1992) Effect of tumor necrosis factor on hypoxic pulmonary vasoconstriction. J Appl Physiol 72:1044-1049
17. Furchgott RF, Zawadzki JV (1980) The obligatory role of endothelial cells in the relaxation of arterial smooth muscle by acetylcholine. Nature 288:373-376
18. Palmer RM, Ferrige AG, Moncada S (1987) Nitric oxide release accounts for the biological activity of endothelium-derived relaxing factor. Nature 327:524-526
19. Moncada S, Higgs A (1993) The L-arginine-nitric oxide pathway. N Engl J Med 329:2002-2012
20. Salter M, Knowles RG, Moncada S (1991) Widespread tissue distribution, species distribution and changes in activity of Ca^{2+}-dependent and Ca^{2+}-independent nitric oxide synthases. FEBS Letters 291:145-149
21. Evans T, Carpenter A, Kinderman H, Cohen J (1993) Evidence of increased nitric oxide production in patients with the sepsis syndrome. Circ Shock 41:77-81
22. Petros A, Bennett D, Vallance P (1991) Effect of nitric oxide synthase inhibitors on hypotension in patients with septic shock. Lancet 338:1557-1558
23. Rees DD, Palmer RM, Moncada S (1989) Role of endothelium-derived nitric oxide in the regulation of blood pressure. Proc Natl Acad Sci USA 86:3375-3378
24. Fleming I, Gray GA, Schott C, Stoclet JC (1991) Inducible but not constitutive production of nitric oxide by vascular smooth muscle cells. Eur J Pharmacol 200:375-376
25. Brady AJB, Warren JB, Poole-Wilson PA, Williams TJ, Harding SE (1993) Nitric oxide attenuates cardiac myocyte contraction. Am J Physiol 265:H176-H182
26. Fox GA, Paterson NAM, McCormack DG (1994) Effect of inhibition of NO synthase on vascular reactivity in a rat model of hyperdynamic sepsis. Am J Physiol 267:H1377-H1382
27. Szabo C, Mitchell JA, Thiemermann C, Vane JR (1993) Nitric oxide-mediated hyporeactivity to noradrenaline precedes the induction of nitric oxide synthase in endotoxin shock. Br J Pharmacol 108:786-792
28. Griffiths MJD, Liu S, Curzen N, Messent M, Evans TW (1995) *In vivo* treatment with endotoxin induces nitric oxide synthase in rat main pulmonary artery. Am J Physiol 268:L509-L518

29. Liu S, Adcock IM, Barnes PJ, Evans TW (1995) Differential regulation of the constitutive and inducible NO synthase mRNA by endotoxin *in vivo* in the rat. Am J Respir Crit Care Med 151: A15 (Abst)
30. Griffiths MJD, Messent M, MacAllister RJ, Evans TW (1993) Aminoguanidine selectively inhibits inducible nitric oxide synthase. Br J Pharmacol 110: 963–968
31. Misko TP, Moore WM, Kasten TP, et al (1993) Selective inhibition of the inducible nitric oxide synthase by aminoguanidine. Eur J Pharmacol 233: 119–125
32. Johns RA, Linden JM, Peach MJ (1989) Endothelium-dependent relaxation and cGMP accumulation in rabbit pulmonary artery are selectively impaired by moderate hypoxia. Circ Res 65: 1508–1525
33. Liu SF, Crawley DE, Barnes PJ, Evans TW (1991) Endothelium-derived relaxing factor inhibits hypoxic pulmonary vasoconstriction in rats. Am Rev Respir Dis 143: 32–37
34. Zelenkov P, McLoughlin T, Johns RA (1993) Endotoxin enhances hypoxic constriction of rat aorta and pulmonary artery through induction of EDRF/NO synthase. Am J Physiol 9: 346–354
35. Yanagisawa M, Kurihara H, Kimura S, et al (1988) A novel potent vasoconstrictor peptide produced by vascular endothelial cells. Nature 332: 411–415
36. Haynes WG, Webb DJ (1993) The endothelin family of peptides: Local hormones with diverse roles in health and disease? Clin Sci 84: 485–500
37. Rubanyi GM, Polokoff MA (1994) Endothelins: Molecular biology, biochemistry, pharmacology, physiology, and pathophysiology. Pharmacol Rev 46: 325–415
38. Weitzberg E (1993) Circulatory responses to endothelin-1 and nitric oxide. Acta Physiol Scand 148: S61–S72
39. Pittet JF, Morel DR, Hemsen A, et al (1991) Elevated plasma endothelin-1 concentrations are associated with the severity of illness in patients with sepsis. Ann Surg 213: 261–264
40. Curzen NP, Kaddoura S, Sugden PH, Poole-Wilson PA, Evans TW (1995) Vascular expression of endothelin-1 mRNA increases in sepsis. Br Heart J 73: P46 (Abst)
41. Langleben D, DeMarchie M, Laporta D, Spanier AH, Schlesinger RD, Stewart DJ (1993) Endothelin-1 in acute lung injury and the adult respiratory distress syndrome. Am Rev Respir Dis 148: 1646–1650
42. Curzen NP, Griffiths MJD, Evans TW (1995) Contraction to endothelin-1 in pulmonary arteries from endotoxin-treated rats is modulated by endothelium. Am J Physiol 37: H2260–H2266
43. Curzen NP, Griffiths MJD, Evans TW (1996) Is the pulmonary circulation hypersensitive to endothelin-1 in sepsis? Heart 75: P9 (Abst)
44. Gardiner SM, Kemp PA, March JE, Bennett T (1996) Effects of the non-peptide, non-selective endothelin antagonist, bosentan, on regional haemodynamic responses to N^G-mono-methyl-L-arginine in conscious rats. Br J Pharmacol 118: 352–354
45. Mitchell JA, Larkin S, Williams TJ (1995) Cyclooxygenase-2; regulation and relevance in inflammation. Biochem Pharmacol 50: 1535–1542
46. Hla T, Neilson K (1992) Human cyclooxygenase-2 cDNA. Proc Natl Acad Sci USA 89: 7384–7388
47. Petrak RA, Balk RA, Bone RC (1989) Prostaglandins, cyclo-oxygenase inhibitors, and thromboxane synthetase inhibitors in the pathogenesis of multiple systems organ failure. Crit Care Clin 5: 303–314
48. Leeman M, Boeynaems JM, Degaute JP, Vincent JL, Kahn RJ (1985) Administration of dazoxiben, a selective thromboxane synthetase inhibitor, in the adult respiratory distress syndrome. Chest 87: 726–730
49. Ahmed T, Wasserman MA, Muccitelli R, Tucker S, Gazeroglu H, Marchette B (1986) Endotoxin-induced changes in pulmonary hemodynamics and respiratory mechanics: Role of lipoxygenase and cyclooxygenase products. Am Rev Respir Dis 134: 1149–1157
50. Hutcheson IR, Whittle BJ, Boughton-Smith NK (1990) Role of nitric oxide in maintaining vascular integrity in endotoxin-induced acute intestinal damage in the rat. Br J Pharmacol 101: 815–820
51. Singh S, Evans TW (1997) Nitric oxide, the biological mediator of the decade: Fact or fiction? Eur Respir J 10: 699–707

52. Frostell CG, Fratacci MD, Wain JC, Jones R, Zapol WM (1991) Inhaled nitric oxide: A selective pulmonary vasodilator reversing hypoxic pulmonary vasoconstriction. Circulation 83: 2038–2047

53. Frattaci MD, Frostell CG, Chen TY, Wain JC, Robinson DR, Zapol WM (1991) Inhaled nitric oxide: A selective pulmonary vasodilator of heparin-protamine vasoconstriction in sheep. Anaesthesiology 75: 990–999

54. Frostell CG, Blomquist H, Hedenstierna G, Lindberg J, Zapol WM (1993) Inhaled nitric oxide selectively reverses human hypoxic pulmonary vasoconstriction without causing systemic vasodilation. Anaesthesiology 78: 427–435

55. Rossaint R, Falke KJ, Lopez F, Slama K, Pison U, Zapol WM (1993) Inhaled nitric oxide for the adult respiratory distress syndrome. N Eng J Med 328: 399–405

56. Puybasset L, Rouby JJ, Mourgeon E, et al (1994) Inhaled nitric oxide in acute respiratory failure; dose response curves. Intensive Care Med 20: 319–327

57. Krafft P, Fridrich P, Fitzgerald RD, Koc D, Steltzer H (1996) Effectiveness of nitric oxide inhalation in septic ARDS. Chest 109: 486–493

58. Brett SJ, Evans TW (1995) Inhaled vasodilator therapy in acute lung injury: First, do NO harm? Thorax 50: 821–823

59. Metz C, Sibbald WJ (1991) Anti-inflammatory therapy for acute lung injury. A review of animal and clinical studies. Chest 100: 1110–1119

60. Bernard GR, Wheeler AP, Russell JA et al (1997) The effects of Ibuprofen on the physiology and survival of patients with sepsis. N Eng J Med 336, 912–918

Right Ventricular Function in ALI and ARDS

F. Brunet, A. T. Dinh-Xuan, and J. F. Dhainaut

Introduction

Severity of acute lung injury (ALI) can widely vary amongst patients, ranging from mild-to-moderate to the acute respiratory distress syndrome (ARDS) [1,2]. An abnormal inflammatory response with acute microvascular lung injury causes permeability edema and pulmonary arterial hypertension (PAH). This acute increase in pulmonary artery pressure is usually progressive and results from several mechanisms including increased vascular tone, extrinsic compression, hypoxic pulmonary vasoconstriction (HPV) and vascular microthrombi [3]. Clinical studies have demonstrated elevated pulmonary vascular resistance (PVR) persisting after correction of arterial hypoxemia [4]. The presence of PAH has been identified as a poor prognostic factor in patients with ARDS, but the relationship between PAH and outcome is still not well understood [5,6]. It is plausible that increased mortality observed in the subset of patients with PAH could be related to the effects of pulmonary hypertension on pulmonary edema formation and right ventricular (RV) performance [3,7]. We found abnormal RV performance, reflected by an increased right atrial pressure/pulmonary artery occlusive pressure ratio, was an early predictive factor of mortality in a multivariate analysis of patients with severe ARDS [8]. However, RV failure, defined as the inability to maintain adequate stroke volume, is rare in ALI/ARDS, in which RV output is usually conserved by the Frank-Starling mechanism [9–13]. RV failure occurs only when PAH is acute and severe, or when associated diseases alter RV contractile state. The effects of mechanical ventilation can also modify the RV response to PAH by aggravating loading conditions [9–14]. We discuss the RV response to PAH; the evaluation of RV function at the bedside; and the effects of therapy addressed specifically at the prevention and treatment of RV failure in ALI/ARDS.

Physiopathology of Right Ventricular Changes

A better understanding of the pathogenesis of ALI/ARDS is important if we are to expect therapeutic progress at the bedside. We will not describe the mechanisms responsible for pulmonary edema and HPV that have been extensively developed in the preceding chapter, but will focus on the consequences of PAH on RV function.

Right Ventricular Consequences of PAH

Low vascular resistance is the main characteristic of the normal pulmonary circulation and both the anatomy and physiology of the RV are appropriate for these physiological constraints. Changes of RV function in ARDS are mainly due to an increase in mean pulmonary artery pressure (MPAP) that can be considered as an increase in RV afterload, even if afterload is a more complex function dependent on other factors [15]. Both experimental and clinical studies have investigated the RV response to an increased afterload, and have permitted a better understanding of the mechanisms involved in the RV response to progressive rises in PAP and to separate them from others factors linked to patient condition and treament.

Experimental Studies: In isolated contracting intact heart preparations, acute changes in RV loading conditions can be graded and their effects studied independently from other factors found in clinical conditions.

The physiological response of the RV to PAH has been observed during acute pressure loading in dogs [16]. Frank Starling mechanisms allow the RV to maintain stroke volume when PAH is not too severe, particularly the volume overload resulting from increased venous return. This phenomenon is not fully explained by an increased segment length. Changes in RV architecture, with a more spherical end-diastolic shape allows a better mechanical effect of the contractile force [17]. Quicker relaxation when diastolic fiber length is enlarged has also been found, contributing to RV filling. In these cases of adapted response to moderate PAH, the coronary perfusion of the RV is maintained during both systole and diastole since the driving pressure remains positive, and there are no or few consequences of RV increased end-diastolic volume on left ventricular (LV) function.

Following an acute and marked onset of PAH, RV enlargment may be associated with failure, defined by a decreased stroke volume. Several factors contribute to these pathological conditions. First, failure of Frank-Starling mechanisms due to overdistension of the ventricle by excessive preload has been proposed, but this factor remains hypothetical. The existence of a descending limb of the Frank-Starling curve may result from functional tricuspid regurgitation [18]. Abnormal contractile function of the RV has also been shown in animal studies and explained as a consequence of subendocardial ischemia [19,20]. Indeed, excessive RV dilation is associated with a decrease in right coronary artery flow that changes from systolo-diastolic to diastolic at the precise time when myocardial consumption is increased [21]. Moreover, decreased systolic coronary perfusion driving pressure due to LV failure may occur concomitantly and enhance RV ischemia.

RV enlargment may also alter LV function. This concept, termed ventricular interdependence, suggests that increased RV volumes can be the source of paradoxic leftward septal shift with an alteration of geometric configuration of the left ventricle [9]. This leftward shift of the ventricular septum depends on at least 2 mechanisms: firstly competition between both ventricles inside an inextensive pericardial cavity, and secondly series interactions with a decreased LV filling due to decreased RV stroke volume. Since the absence of pericardium has been shown to have little influence in a canine model, series interactions seem to be the predominant factors [22].

Clinical Studies: Clinically, the response of the RV to an acute increase in afterload is more difficult to analyze. In patients, compensatory mechanisms are modified by other factors linked to associated diseases and to therapy.

Most clinical studies have confirmed the importance of Frank-Starling mechanisms in cases of acute increase of PAP, and showed acute PAH in ALI/ARDS to be associated with an increased RV end-diastolic volume and a decreased ejection fraction. However, stroke volume was usually maintained [7, 9, 13]. Measuring RV performance in patients with ARDS using a fast response thermistor Swan Ganz catheter, we found [13] changes in RV end-diastolic volume and ejection fraction were inversely correlated with increases in MPAP. This correlation has been reported in other clinical studies [9, 23]. Rossaint and colleagues [24], investigating the effects of pulmonary vasodilators on RV function, did not identify such a relationship perhaps because the number of patients was small and the severity of the degree of PAH rather homogeneous. Ventricular interdependence has also been assumed, but the real importance of this phenomenon is discussed in ALI/ARDS in which cardiac output, LV filling and systemic pressure are usually maintained. LV dysfunction may, however, be worsened by an associated underlying disease like chronic heart failure, coronary artery disease, acute myocarditis, or septic shock [9, 13].

Associated factors can impair the physiological response of the RV to PAH. In cases of contractile depression, as reported in patients with RV contusion associated with ARDS or RV myocardial infarction, Frank-Starling mechanisms are not sufficient to maintain RV pump function [7, 25]. Since RV oxygen consumption is difficult to measure clinically, RV ischemia has not been clearly established in clinical studies and decreased contractility due to this factor may be only advocated in extreme conditions and when coronary artery disease coexists [9]. Only a few patients with septic shock or acute viral myocarditis, unable to maintain their stroke volume as afterload was increased, are reported in clinical studies [9, 13]. Yu and colleagues [26], investigating patients with either heart failure or pulmonary hypertension, showed RV diastolic function to be frequently abnormal in both groups and that this dysfunction was not only due to elevated pulmonary artery systolic pressure.

Other Factors influencing RV Function in ALI/ARDS

As ARDS usually requires life-sustaining therapy, other factors linked to treatment cannot be separated from the mechanisms involved in RV response. A corner stone of the treatment of ALI/ARDS is mechanical ventilation with continuous positive airway pressure (CPAP) to achieve adequate alveolar recruitment. The role of mechanical ventilation on the reduction of cardiac output has been well studied [9-14].

The main effect of positive pressure ventilation (PPV) is a reduction in venous return causing a decrease in RV preload, especially marked when high levels of positive end-expiratory pressure (PEEP) were used [9–14, 27]. The resulting decrease in RV preload reduces the efficacy of Frank-Starling mechanisms facing increased afterload. Limitations in ventricular filling are mediated by a peripheral translocation of thoracic blood volume [28]. The precise mechanism of this fluid translocation has been recently revisited by Fessler et al. [29]. Since the mean systemic pressure is also increased, the pressure gradient for venous return (right atrial pressure-mean systemic pressure) is unchanged. An increase in venous resistance and a PEEP-induced right atrium waterfall upstream have been hypothesized. Decreased compliance of both ventricles has been also reported with PEEP, accentuating the decrease in venous return [30].

A second reported side effect of PPV is lung distension with high levels of PEEP that can increase PVR and RV afterload [31]. There is a close relationship between lung volume and PVR that is inversely parabolic, and which is minimal about functional residual capacity (FRC) [32]. At low pulmonary volumes, PVR is essentially due to HPV of extra-alveolar vessels and vascular endothelial injury. When high pulmonary volumes are reached with high levels of PEEP, PVR exponentially increases with volume through further compression of intra-alveolar vessels (Zone II enlargement at the expense of Zone III). This may occur even in the absence of excessive PEEP in cases of inhomogeneous lung injury which is common in ALI/ARDS [33]. In such conditions, a given level of PEEP may have no distending effects on low compliance lung units, and may promote hyperinflation in others. Lastly, from FRC, PVR is further increased by the inspiratory lung inflation [32]. The resulting increase in RV end-diastolic volume and decreased diastolic filling of the left ventricle can majorate ventricular interdependence [11, 34–36]. Concomitantly, an increase in juxtacardiac pressures may be a source of direct heart compression. These pressures depend on thoraco-pulmonary compliance and the interdependence between lungs and heart. Bein and colleagues [37] studied the effects of positioning of the patient during mechanical ventilation. They found that the right decubitus position impaired RV preload more than the other positions. Resulting from these phenomena of ventricular interdependence and direct heart compression by hyperinflated lungs, biventricular filling may be limited, inhibiting Frank Starling mechanisms from compensating for PAH.

These direct mechanical effects of CPPV can explain the observed reduction in cardiac output and the worsening of oxygen transport seen in ARDS despite improved arterial oxygenation. However, the majority of studies analyzed the effects of mechanical ventilation using high levels of airway pressures and volumes. New trends in mechanical ventilation limiting these parameters will probably reduce this phenomenon. It has been shown that optimal RV stroke volume and ejection fraction were obtained when airway pressures and volumes were limited [38]. In one study [39] comparing CPAP and mechanical ventilation with the same level of PEEP, we found CPAP decreased RV afterload and improved RV stroke volume (Fig. 1). Extracorporeal CO_2 removal with low

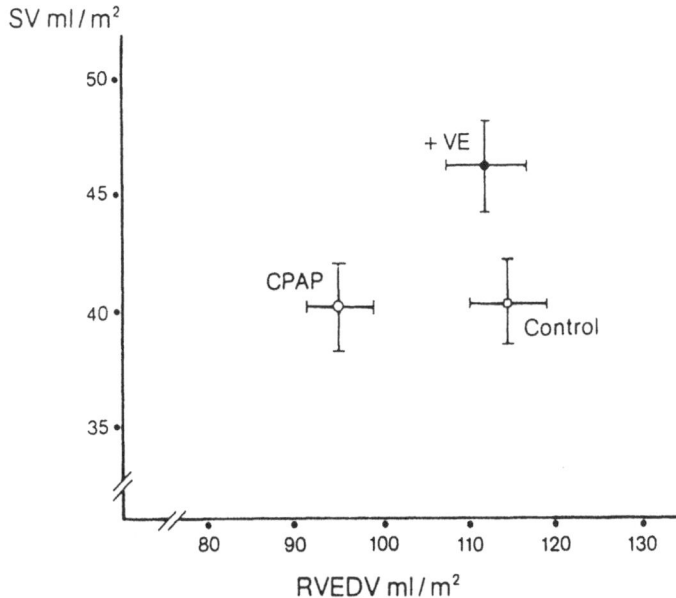

Fig. 1. Effects of decreased intrathoracic pressure by continuous positive pressure improves RV dysfunction due to positive pressure ventilation. Comparison between CPAP and mechanical ventilation (control) with the same level of PEEP showed CPAP decreased RV end-diastolic volume and improved RV stroke volume with volume expansion (+ VE). New trends in mechanical ventilation reducing insufflated volumes and pressures will probably have similar beneficial effect on RV. (Adapted from [39])

frequency PPV may provide a similar response by associating reductions in lung volume with decreased hypoxic vasoconstriction [40].

Other therapies during ALI/ARDS can also interfere with the RV response to PAH. Fluid expansion is often used to compensate for decreased venous return due to PPV or to treat associated septic shock. RV function can be either improved or worsened according to volume loading and lung water. Schulman and colleagues [27] showed the effects of PEEP on RV function depends on baseline status and are more marked in case of hypovolemia. Inotropic and vasoactive agents are often required to treat associated shock or the etiology of ARDS, and can greatly modify RV response by either reducing PVR or improving RV myocardial perfusion by maintaining systemic artery pressure [14, 27, 41].

Assessment of Right Ventricular Function

In clinical practice, the treatment of ARDS is essentially based on the application of PPV to maintain arterial oxygenation. We have seen the effects of mechanical ventilation on hemodynamics are complex and influenced by other factors. PAH can alter RV function and precipitate failure when a combination of hypercapnia, acidosis and hypoxemia promotes excessive pulmonary vasoconstriction. At the bedside, clinical evaluation of the patient's condition is often insufficient to guide the treatment and the following questions need to be addressed: What are the good variables to assess RV performance? and how and when should the evaluation of hemodynamics be realized?

What are the Good Variables to assess RV Function?

RV performance is determined by heart rate, loading conditions and myocardial contractility. RV preload can be estimated by RV end-diastolic volume and pressure [42]. On the passive RV pressure-volume (P-V) curve, optimal RV filling is near the ascending limb of the P-V relationship. The time course variation of both filling pressure or volume, and stroke volume has to be considered to appreciate in real-time the relative magnitude of RV preload. RV afterload may be estimated by MPAP and PVR [43], but assessment of contractility is clinically difficult because of the marked influence of RV afterload on ejection phase indices. This indicates the need to construct P-V lines, which seem to be minimally affected by RV loading conditions [44]. However, constructing these lines requires almost 3 or 4 points that should be obtained by changing preload [45, 46].

Obtaining a really accurate assessment of the RV performance requires a concomitant analysis of heart rate, transmural right atrial pressure, stroke volume, MPAP and RV ejection fraction, cardiac output and arterial and venous blood saturations.

Investigation Techniques of RV Function

Different techniques have been employed to assess RV function including radionuclear angiography, contrast angiography, and more recently nuclear magnetic resonance imaging. All are research tools and cannot be used at the bedside nor easily repeated [9, 13, 47, 48].

Contrast angiography was the first method proposed to investigate RV function [49]. Mathematical approximations are required to calculate RV volume which are difficult because of trabeculations, right atrial overlap and the generelly complex geometry of the ventricle. In addition, this method does not permit the measurement of all the parameters previously defined to evaluate RV function. Lastly, this investigation requires patient transfer, may cause excessive volume infusion and renal failure, and cannot be repeated easily.

Radionuclide angiography using autologous erythrocytes labelled with radionuclide agents has been used to assess RV function and remains a reference method to calculate RV volumes [9, 13]. However, technical problems and the necessity for patient transfer, the cost and the difficulty of repeating this investigation limit its use in patients with ALI/ARDS.

Bedside measurements of RV function are therefore mainly performed by right heart catheterization using a fast response thermistor catheter to evaluate

RV volumes, or two-dimensional Doppler echocardiography. The two methods can be used separately or in combination [12].

Right heart catheterization has been widely used to investigate RV function for 20 years [50]. Calculation of RV ejection fraction by thermodilution is based on the conservation of energy as measured using a fast response thermistor. Ventricular volumes are then derived from stroke volume by dividing cardiac output by heart rate. RV volume calculations and ejection fraction have been shown to be reliable in a wide range of clinical situations [45, 51]. Despite this, right heart catheterization has not been shown to improve survival [52]. However, this diagnostic procedure is often indicated in ARDS, especially at the onset of the disease and when a complication occurs. Measurements of RV parameters combined with that of PAP with calculation of vascular resistances allow the detection of RV dysfunction and the monitoring of volume expansion and drug administration to prevent RV failure [9, 13, 14]. Assessment of RV end-diastolic volume combined with right atrial pressures seems to be the best way to evaluate preload [14]. However, this technique has some limitations. In atrial fibrillation, at least 5 cold boluses should be averaged to get reliable values. As the catheter measures only the forward flow, the presence of tricuspid regurgitation may alter calculated RV volumes [53]. The use of an automatic device for serial determination of thermodilution curves synchronized to the ventilatory cycle has been proposed to limit the effects of incomplete mixing due to tricuspid regurgitation [54], but its benefits remain hypothetical. Echocardiography can detect and quantify such regurgitation, which remains a limiting factor of the thermodilution technique [12].

Two-dimensional echocardiography is a non-invasive technique that can provide reliable assessment of RV size and performance. However, this technique only estimates volume from measured areas. Despite the fact that several mathematical models have been developed, echocardiography is not considered a reference method to construct P-V volume loops. Precise calculation of RV volumes is also difficult with this technique because of modifications to RV geometry induced by mechanical ventilation in patients with ALI/ARDS [47, 48]. However, in addition to dynamic imaging, echocardiography can provide other information such as distinctive patterns between pressure and volume ventricular overload, measurements of myocardial wall thickness, heart valve morphology, diastolic function, and pericardial space investigation. The effects on RV of many events such as changes in mechanical ventilation mode, drug or fluid infusion, can be rapidly assessed using this method. When coupled with Doppler, this non-invasive method gives reliable information about PAP and cardiac output, is easily performed at the bedside, non-invasive except when transesophageal probe is used, and reproducible. However, it needs a highly trained investigator which could be a limiting factor for monitoring, and sometimes correct imaging could be difficult to obtain in patients with severe lung injury requiring mechanical ventilation. In such cases, subcostal short axis views can be the only way to get some information but does not allow complete investigation of RV function.

When is RV Function Assessment Necessary?

Whatever the method, indications for hemodynamic monitoring during the course of ARDS are not clearly defined and precise guidelines are lacking. However, it seems reasonable to propose to evaluate hemodynamic parameters at the onset of the disease to both eliminate LV failure as a cause of, or aggravating factor of pulmonary edema, and to adjust the level of PEEP. The same approach can be proposed when shock is associated with ARDS, or occurs secondarily and does not rapidly respond to fluid expansion and low dose inotropic and vasoactive agents. Lastly, administration of pulmonary vasodilators, like inhaled nitric oxide (NO) or prostacyclin, is better guided by hemodynamic monitoring.

Therapeutic Approach of RV Abnormal Function

Pulmonary hypertension reaching a level severe enough to compromise RV function leading to RV failure seldom occurs in ALI/ARDS, except if severe contractile depression of the RV coexists as previously described. In patients with severe pulmonary hypertension and RV failure, RV function has to be rapidly improved by reducing RV afterload and improving pump function to allow adequate cardiac output and oxygen transport. In other patients, abnormal loading conditions of the RV have to be analyzed to avoid inadequate therapy and to limit rapid increases in PAP. In these two situations, improvements in RV function can be achieved using a combination of non-pharmacological tools, mainly adjustment of respiratory support, and pharmacological agents, fluid expansion and inotropic and vasodilator agents. The response of the heart has to be carefully monitored when using these different approaches which are susceptible to synergistic or opposing effects.

Improvement of RV Loading Conditions

The physiological basis of therapy and the prevention of RV failure in ARDS can be schematized as follows. First, pulmonary impedance must be reduced to a minimum. This goal can be reached by several interventions. Among them sedation and muscle paralysis have been proposed to decrease body requirements and limit airway pressures during PPV. The need for hemodilution has been proposed to decrease blood viscosity, and antiaggregant and anticoagulant drugs to improve PVR [55, 56]. The role of mechanical ventilation is important in the changes of RV afterload. The optimal mode of mechanical ventilation should achieve adequate oxygenation to reduce hypoxic vasoconstriction and limit airway pressures and volume to avoid lung vessel compression. New trends in mechanical ventilation which limit airway volumes and pressures with titration of PEEP may help to achieve these goals and decrease the consequences for RV function [39, 57]. Other ventilatory support modes have been proposed in severely ill patients. Extracorporeal carbon dioxide removal with low frequency PPV decreased MPAP and improved RV function in 23 patients with severe ARDS [40]. Prone positioning, a recently proposed method to recruit atelectatic lung units by increasing regional transpulmonary pressure, improves the distribution of perfusion to ventilated lung regions and gas exchange in ARDS [58]. However, any specific effects of these different modes on RV function are not clear and they do not constitute a treatment of RV failure when occurring. This non-pharmacological approach can however be useful and enhance the effects of some pharmacological agents. Alveolar recruitment by PEEP has been proposed to optimize the beneficial effects of inhaled nitric oxide (NO) [59]. Also of interest is the possibility that the combination of prone positioning, inhaled NO and intravenous almitrine may provide even further beneficial effects on gas exchange [60].

Use of Pulmonary Vasodilators in ALI/ARDS

The rationale for using vasodilators is based on the contention that hypoxic pulmonary vasoconstriction is an important component of PAH in ALI and ARDS. The ideal response to a vasodilator should be a reduction of MPAP and calculated PVR, with a rise in cardiac output [61,62]. However, increased PVR is a locally protective mechanism which tends to reduce ventilation-perfusion (V_A/Q) mismatching [63]. Blind vasodilation of lung vessels might worsen intrapulmonary shunt whilst improving RV workload [64]. Vasodilators can also produce systemic hypotension, even when they are directly infused into the pulmonary circulation. Halmagyi and Cotes [65] considered V_A/Q mismatching as a possible explanation for worsened hypoxemia in patients receiving intravenous aminophylline.

Ideally, a pulmonary vasodilator shoud be doubly selective. Its activity must be restricted to pulmonary circulation to avoid systemic hypotension, and confined to well ventilated lung units to limit adverse effects on gas exchange. Purine nucleosides such as adenosine are considered selective vasodilators, but may adversely affect ventricular diastolic performance [66,67].

The use of inhaled NO in ARDS is based on two bodies of evidence. First, a possible physiological role for NO would be to protect the pulmonary vasculature against disproportionate vasoconstriction that might result from various chemical and physical stimuli [68]. Second, NO is rapidly inactivated by hemoglobin [69], and when given by inhalation, should be devoid of harmful effects on the systemic circulation [70]. Inhaled NO has been successfully applied in animals to reverse hypoxic and thromboxane-induced pulmonary vasoconstriction [71]. In humans, short-term inhalation of NO produces significant and selective pulmonary vasodilation in newborns, in children, and in adults with pulmonary hypertension [24,72,73]. This effect is explained in part by the effects of inhaled NO on arterial oxygenation [72], which result from a reduction of regional V_A/Q mismatching [73]. The combination of inhaled NO with infused almitrine has been proposed as almitrine reinforces hypoxic pulmonary vasoconstriction. Such a combination can enhance beneficial effects of inhaled NO on V_A/Q matching, although RV failure might occur. Together with increased arterial oxygenation, in-

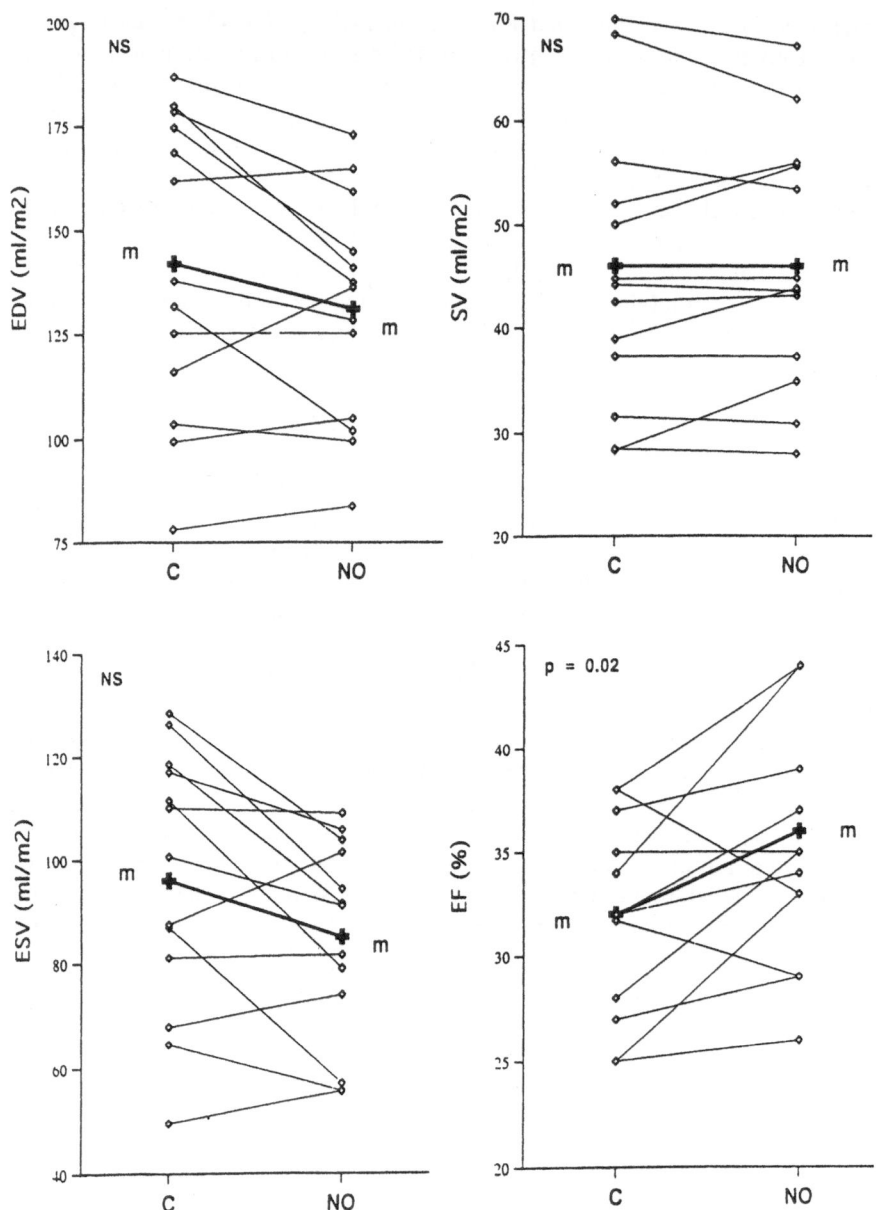

Fig. 2. Mean and individual changes in end-diastolic volumes (EDV), end-systolic volumes (ESV), stroke volume (SV) and RV ejection fraction (EF) at baseline and during inhalation of 5 ppm NO (Adapted from [74])

haled NO can also slightly decrease partial pressure of arterial carbon dioxide [74] that may contribute to the reduction of PAP [75].

The effects of inhaled NO on RV function result from these beneficial effects on gas exchange. In a series of 13 consecutive patients with ARDS [74], inhaled NO 5 ppm was associated with a significant increase of MPAP along with a significant rise in RV ejection fraction, but with no change in stroke volume (Fig. 2). Similar results were also obtained [54] in a study comparing the effects of inhaled NO with infused PGI_2 in 10 patients with ARDS, suggesting that altered RV function was not a limiting factor to cardiac output. However, in some patients such as those reported by Wisocky and colleagues [76], increased RV ejection fraction with inhaled NO can also improve cardiac index, probably more through vasodilating effects on pulmonary vessels than by improved contractility. [77] In a swine model of ARDS, inhaled NO ameliorated negative effects of hypoxic and hypercapnic vasoconstriction, and improved RV workload, but did not change intrinsic RV contractility.

Other pharmacological agents have been administered in ARDS. Intravenous administration of prostanoids led to systemic hypotension and worsening of gas exchange. Inhaled administration of these products has been proposed, in a recent study. Walmrath et al. [78, 79] comparing the effects of nebulized prostacyclin (PGI_2) with inhaled NO in a group of 16 patients with ARDS. Recent experimental data have also suggested that PGI_2 can directly affect RV contractile function through positive inotropic effects [80]. Endotracheal administration of compounds like tolazoline [81], or use of liposomal PGE_1 [82] are likely to have the same advantage and deserve to be further characterized.

Notwithstanding the numerous benefits one can get from selective pulmonary vasodilation in ALI/ARDS, some concerns remain. First, despite initial optimistic reports, some patients do not respond to inhaled NO, even at doses higher than 40 ppm [83]. Second, difficulty has been reported in weaning NO from responders who have been treated long-term. This stems from the theoretical possibility that exogenous NO could switch off endogenous production [84, 85]. Finally, due to its single unpaired electron, NO is also a free radical [86], potentially harmful to different molecular targets including: oxygen, superoxide, water, nucleotides, metalloproteins, thiols, amines, and lipids [86], necessitating the use of low doses and close monitoring for potential side effects.

Treatment of RV Failure

In RV failure associated with high levels of PAH, volume expansion and the administration of inotropic agents constitute the first steps in management. Volume expansion with macromolecules is always required to assist the physiological response of the RV to increased afterload. The quantity of fluid may vary with initial volemia, the presence of associated shock and the level of positive pressure necessary to achieve adequate gas exchange. In the absence of precise guidelines, an indexed RV end-diastolic volume higher than 100 mL/m^2 should probably be reached. Fluid expansion must be, however, cautiously performed and closely monitored using hemodynamic parameters as discussed previously, to avoid exacerbating lung injury and the induction of tricuspid regurgitation which can further decrease cardiac output [13].

Inotropic agents are required in cases of persistent cardiac failure. Several pharmacological agents are available and can be used in these circumstances [12–14]. We will not describe extensively the effects of each inotropic agent that can be prescribed in the treatment of cardiac failure associated with ALI/ARDS. The optimal choice of drug, or combination of vasoactive and inotropic agents will depend on hemodynamic status. The presence of septic shock can require specific therapy [12–14, 41]. Dopamine can reduce venous capacitance at low doses, may improve RV filling and can be used to limit fluid infusion requirements. Inotropic agents like dobutamine should be used if RV ejection fraction rapidly declines, or when cardiac output is not sufficient to meet body metabolic requirements. Combinations of these drugs, or administration of vasopressive agents like epinephrine and norepinephrine may be needed if there is a concomitant fall in systemic arterial pressure to restore adequate coronary perfusion. However, the use of epinephrine and norepinephrine should be carefully evaluated since they increase PAH and may further compromise RV function and cardiac output. In the most severe cases, treatment of RV failure often requires a combination of these therapies, needing constant adjustment on repeated evaluation of the RV response.

Conclusion

RV function remains an important factor in the prognosis and treatment of ALI/ARDS which is rarely observed, but associated with increased mortality. Abnormal RV function is mainly attributable to increased afterload, directly resulting from the acute lung injury, to sepsis, frequently associated with respiratory disease, and sometimes to inappropriate therapy. RV dysfunction must be detected by assessment of RV function and monitoring of its treatment. This approach helps the clinician to adjust mechanical ventilation and to use pulmonary vasodilators if necessary. In RV failure, inotropic agents or a combination of inotropic and vasopressive agents may be needed after adequate RV filling by fluid infusion. Lastly, pharmacologically-induced changes in pulmonary vascular tone may be optimized by use in association with new modes of ventilation, positioning of the patient and appropriate titration of PEEP to induce alveolar recruitment.

References

1. Knaus WA (1996) The ongoing mystery of ARDS. Intensive Care Med 22:517–518
2. Curzen NP, Jourdan KB, Mitchell JA (1996) Endothelial modification of pulmonary vascular tone. Intensive Care Med 22:596–607
3. Zapol WM, Snider MT (1977) Pulmonary hypertension in severe acute respiratory failure. N Engl J Med 296:476–480

4. Fox GA, Mc Cormack DG (1992) The pulmonary physician and critical care. 4. A new look at the pulmonary circulation in acute lung injury. Thorax 47 : 743-747
5. Sibbald WJ, Paterson NA, Holliday RL, Anderson RA, Lobb TR, Duff JH (1978) Pulmonary hypertension in sepsis: Measurements by the pulmonary arterial diastolic-pulmonary wedge pressure gradient and the influence of passive and active factors. Chest 73 : 583-591
6. Sturm JA, Lewis FR, Trentz O (1979) Cardiopulmonary parameters and prognosis after severe multiple trauma. J Trauma 19 : 305-318
7. Sibbald WJ, Driedger AA (1983) Right ventricular function in acute disease states: Pathophysiologic considerations. Crit Care Med 11 : 339-342
8. Brunet F, Monchi M, Renaud B, et al (1995) Multivariate analysis of survival predictive factors in the Acute Respiratory Distress Syndrome. Am J Respir Crit Care Med 151 : A 668 (Abst)
9. Sibbald WJ, Driedger AA, Myers ML, Short AIK, Wells GA (1983) Biventricular function in the adult respiratory distress syndrome. Hemodynamic and radionuclide assessment with special emphasis on right ventricular function. Chest 84 : 126-134
10. Marini JJ, Culver BH, Butler J (1981) Mechanical effect of lung distension with positive pressure on cardiac function. Am Rev Respir Dis 124 : 382-386
11. Cassidy SS, Aschenbacher WL, Robertson CH, Nixon JY, Blomquist G, Johnson JL Jr (1979) Cardiovascular effects of positive pressure ventilation in normal subjects. J Appl Physiol 47 : 453-461
12. Jardin F, Gueret P, Dubourg O, Farcot JC, Margairaz A, Bourdarias JP (1985) Right ventricular volumes by thermodilution in the Adult Respiratory Distress Syndrome. Chest 88 : 34-39
13. Brunet F, Dhainaut JF, Devaux JY, Huyghebaert MF, Villemant D, Monsallier JF (1988) Right ventricular performance in patients with acute respiratory failure. Intensive Care Med 14 : 474-477
14. Martin C, Saux P, Albanese J, Bonnery JJ, Gouin F (1992) Right ventricular function during positive end-expiratory pressure. Thermodilution evaluation and clinical application. Chest 6 : 999-1004
15. Prewitt RM, Wood LDH (1982) Effect of altered resistive load on left ventricular systolic mechanics in dogs. Anethesiology 56 : 195-202
16. Smith ER, Kingma I, Smiseth OA, et al (1985) Ventricular response to acute constriction of the pulmonary artery in conscious dogs. Am Rev Respir Dis 131 : A57 (Abst)
17. Molaug M, Geiran O, Stockland O, et al (1982) Dynamics of the interventricular septum free wall during blood volume expansion and selective right ventricular volume loading in dogs. Acta Physiol Scand 116 : 245-256
18. Tei C, Pilgrim JP, Shah PM, Ormiston JA, Wong M (1982) The tricuspid valve annulus: Study of size and motion in normal subjects and in patients with tricuspid regurgitation. Circulation 66 : 665-671
19. Vlahakes GJ, Turley K, Hoffman JI (1981) The pathophysiology of failure in acute right ventricular hypertension: Hemodynamic and biochemical correlations. Circulation 63 : 87-95
20. Laver MB, Strauss HW, Pohost GM (19-) Right and left ventricular geometry: Adjustments during acute respiratory failure. Crit Care Med 7 : 509-519
21. Romand JA, Donald FA, Suter PM (1995) Acute right ventricular failure, pathophysiology and treatment. Monaldi Arch Chest Dis 50 : 129-133
22. Calvin JE, Langlois S, Garneys G (1988) Ventricular interaction in a canine model of acute pulmonary hypertension and its modulation by vasoactive drugs. J Crit Care 3 : 43-55
23. Radermacher P, Santak B, Wust HJ, Tarnow J, Falke KJ (1990) Prostacyclin and right ventricular function in patients with pulmonary hypertension associated with ARDS. Intensive Care Med 16 : 227-232
24. Rossaint R, Falke K J, López FA, Slama K, Pison U, Zapol WM (1993) Inhaled nitric oxide for the adult respiratory distress syndrome. N Engl J Med 328 : 399-405
25. Cohn JN, Guiha NH, Broder MI, Limas CJ (1974) Right ventricular infarction. Am J Cardiol 33 : 209-214
26. Yu CM, Sanderson JE, Chan S, Yeung L, Hung YT, Woo KS (1996) Right ventricular diastolic dysfunction in heart failure. Circulation 93 : 1509-1514

27. Schulman DS, Biondi JS, Matthay RA, Barash PG, Zaret BL, Soufer R (1988) Effect of positive end-expiratory pressure on right ventricular performance. Importance of baseline right ventricular function. Am J Med 84:57–67
28. Braunwald E, Binion JT, Morgan WL, et al (1957) Alteration in central blood volume and cardiac output induced by positive pressure breathing and counteracted by metaraminol [Aramine]. Circ Res 5:670–675
29. Fessler HE, Brower RG, Wise RA, Permutt S (1991) Effects of positive end-expiratory pressure on the gradient for venous return. Am Rev Respir Dis 143:19–24
30. Santamore WP, Boye AA, Heckman JL (1984) Right and left ventricular pressure-volume response to positive end-expiratory pressure. Am J Physiol 246:H114–H119
31. Takata M, Robotham JL (1991) Ventricular external constraint by the lung and pericardium during positive end-expiratory pressure. Am Rev Respir Dis 143:872–875
32. Simmons PH, Linder CM, Miller JR, et al (1961) Relation of lung volume and pulmonary vascular resistance. Circ Res 9:465–471
33. Gattinoni L, Pesenti A, Bombono M, et al (1988) Relationship between lung tomographic density, gas exchange, and PEEP in acute respiratory failure. Anesthesiology 69:824–832
34. Jardin F, Farcot JC, Boissante LB, Curien N, Margairaz A, Bourdarias JP (1981) Influence of positive end-expiratory pressure on left ventricular performance. N Engl J Med 304:387–392
35. Sharf SM, Brown R, Saunders N, Green LH, Ingram RH Jr (1979) Changes in canine left ventricular size and configuration with positive end-expiratory pressure. Circ Res 44:672–678
36. Jardin F, Farcot JC, Guéret P, Prost JF, Ozier Y, Bourdarias JP (1984) Two-dimensional echocardiographic evaluation of left and right ventricular size and shape during continuous positive airway pressure breathing in normal subjects. J Appl Physiol 56:618–637
37. Bein Th, Metz Ch, Keyl C, Pfeifer M, Taeger K (1996) Effects of extreme lateral posture on hemodynamics and plasma atrial natriruretic peptide levels in critically ill patients. Intensive Care Med 22:651–655
38. Abraham E, Yoshihara I (1989) Cardiorespiratory effects of pressure controlled inverse ratio ventilation in severe respiratory failure. Chest 96:1356–1359
39. Dhainaut JF, Aouate P, Monsallier JF, et al (1987) Improvement of right ventricular performance by continuous positive airway pressure in Adult Respiratory Distress Syndrome. J Crit Care 2:15–21
40. Brunet F, Belghit M, Mira JP, et al (1993) ECCO$_2$R-LFPPV improves arterial oxygenation while reducing risk of pulmonary barotrauma in patients with ARDS. Chest 104:889–898
41. Dhainaut JF, Lanore JJ, de Gournay JM, et al (1988) Right ventricular dysfunction in patients with septic shock. Intensive Care Med 14:488–491
42. Brent BN, Berger HL, Matthay RA, et al (1982) Physiologic correlates of right ventricular ejection fraction in chronic obstructive pulmonary disease. A combined radionuclide and hemodynamic study. Am J Cardiol 50:255–262
43. Matthay RA, Berger HJ, Loke J (1978) Effects of aminophilline upon right and left ventricular performance in chronic obstructive pulmonary disease: Non-invasive assessment by radionuclide angiography. Am J Med 65:903–910
44. Maughan WL, Shoukas AA, Sagawa K, Weisfeldt ML (1979) Instantaneous pressure-volume relationship of the canine right ventricle. Circ Res 44:309–318
45. Dhainaut JF, Brunet F, Monsallier J, et al (1987) Bedside evaluation of RV performance using a rapid computerized thermodilution method. Crit Care Med 15:148–154
46. Reuse C, Vincent JL, Pinsky MR (1990) Measurements of right ventricular volumes during fluid challenge. Chest 96:1450–1454
47. Edelman RR, Hatabu H, Tadamura EP, Rasad WLPV (1996) Non-invasive assessment of regional ventilation in the human lung using oxygen-enhanced magnetic resonance imaging. Nature Medicine 2:1236–1239
48. Boxt LM (1996) MR imaging of pulmonary hypertension and right ventricular dysfunction. Magn Reson Imaging Clin N Am 4:307–325
49. Freis ED, Rivara GL, Gilmonte BL (1960) Estimation of residual and end-diastolic volumes of the right ventricle of men without heart disease, using the dye dilution method. Am Heart J 60:898–904

50. Swan HJ, Ganz W, Forrester J, et al (1970) Catheterization of the heart in man with used of a flow directed balloon-tipped catheter. N Engl J Med 283:447–451
51. Vincent JL, Thirion M, Brimouille S, et al (1986) Thermodilution measurement of right ventricle ejection fraction with a modified pulmonary artery catheter. Intensive Care Med 12: 33–38
52. Connors AF, Speroff T, Dawson NV, et al (1996) The effectiveness of right heart catheterization in the initial care of critically ill patients. JAMA 276:889–897
53. Kass DA, Maughan WL (1988) From Emax to pressure-volume relations: A broader view. Circulation 77:1203–1212
54. Rossaint R, Slama K, Steudel W, et al (1995) Effects of inhaled nitric oxide on right ventricular function in severe acute respiratory distress syndrome. Intensive Care Med 21:197–203
55. Agarwal JB, Paltoo R, Palmer WH (1970) Relative viscosity of blood at varying hematocrits in pulmonary circulation. J Apppl Physiol 29:866–871
56. Jacob HS, Craddock PR, Hammerschmidt DE, Moldow CF (1980) Complement induced granulocytes aggragation: An unsuspected mechanism of disease. N Engl J Med 302:789–794
57. Marini J, Kelsen A (1992) Re-targeting ventilatory objectives in adult respiratory distress syndrome. Am Rev Respir Dis 146:2–3
58. Langer M, Mascheroni D, Marcolin R, Gattinoni L (1988) The prone position in ARDS patients: A clinical study. Chest 94:103–107
59. Puybasset L, Rouby JJ, Mourgeon E, et al (1995) Factors influencing cardiopulmonary effects of inhaled nitric oxide in acute respiratory failure. Am J Respir Crit Care Med 152:318–328
60. Jolliet P, Bulpa P, Ricou B, Ritz M, Chevrolet JC (1996) Additive effects of prone position ventilation, nitric oxide and almitrine bismesylate in ARDS. Am J Respir Crit Care Med 153 (Suppl):A12 (Abst)
61. Palevsky HI, Fishman AP (1991) The management of primary pulmonary hypertension. JAMA 265:1014–1020
62. Rich S, Martinez J, Lam W, Levy PS, Rosen KM (1983) Reassessment of the effects of vasodilator drugs in primary pulmonary hypertension: Guidelines for determining a pulmonary vasodilator response. Am Heart J 105:119–127
63. Dinh-Xuan AT, Higenbottam TW (1996) Pulmonary vascular reactivity in acute respiratory failure of chronic obstructive pulmonary disease. In: Derenne JP, Whitelaw WA, Similowski T (eds) Acute respiratory failure of chronic obstructive pulmonary disease. Marcel Dekker, New York, pp 303–317
64. Dinh-Xuan AT, Brunet F, Dhainaut JF (1996) Inhaled nitric oxide: The light and shadow of a therapeutic breakthrough. In: Fink MP, Payen D (eds) Update in intensive care and emergency medicine. Vol 24. Role of nitric oxide in sepsis and ARDS. Springer-Verlag, Berlin, pp 414–425
65. Halmagyi DFJ, Cotes JE (1959) Reduction in systemic blood oxygen as a result of procedures affecting the pulmonary circulation in patients with chronic pulmonary disease. Clin Sci 18:475–481
66. Morgan JM, McCormack DG, Griffiths MJD, Morgan CJ, Barnes PJ, Evans TW (1991) Adenosine as a vasodilator in primary pulmonary hypertension. Circulation 84:1145–1149
67. Haywood GA, Sneddon JF, Bashir Y, Jennison SH, Gray HH, McKenna WJ (1992) Adenosine infusion for the reversal of pulmonary vasoconstriction in biventricular failure: A good test but a poor therapy. Circulation 86:896–902
68. Dinh-Xuan AT (1992) Endothelial modulation of pulmonary vascular tone. Eur Respir J 5: 757–762
69. Martin W, Smith JA, White DG (1986) The mechanisms by which haemoglobin inhibits the relaxation of rabbit aorta induced by nitrovasodilators, nitric oxide or bovine retractor penis inhibitory factor. Br J Pharmacol 89:563–571
70. Higenbottam TW, Pepke-Zaba J, Scott JP, Woolman P, Coutts C, Wallwork J (1988) Inhaled endothelium-derived relaxing factor in primary pulmonary hypertension. Am Rev Respir Dis 137 (Suppl):107 (Abst)
71. Frostell CG, Fratacci MD, Wain JC Jr, Jones R, Zapol WM (1991) Inhaled nitric oxide: A selective pulmonary vasodilator reversing hypoxic pulmonary vasoconstriction. Circulation 83: 2038–2047

72. Roberts JD Jr, Polaner DM, Lang P, Zapol WM (1992) Inhaled nitric oxide in persistent pulmonary hypertension of the newborn. Lancet 340:818–819
73. Rozé JC, Storme L, Zupan V, Morville P, Dinh-Xuan AT, Mercier JC (1994) Echocardiographic investigation of inhaled nitric oxide in newborn babies with severe hypoxaemia. Lancet 344:303–305
74. Fierobe L, Brunet F, Dhainaut JF, et al (1995) Effect of inhaled nitric oxide on right ventricular function in adult respiratory distress syndrome. Am J Respir Crit Care Med 151: 1414–1419
75. Viitanen A, Salmenperä M, Heinonen J (1990) Right ventricular response to hypercarbia after cardiac surgery. Anesthesiology 73:393–400
76. Wysocki M, Vignon P, Roupie E, et al (1993) Improvement in right ventricular function with inhaled nitric oxide in patients with the adult respiratory distress syndrome (ARDS) and permissive hypercapnia. Am Rev Respir Dis 147:A350 (Abst)
77. Cheifetz IM, Craig DM, Kern FH, et al (1996) Nitric oxide improves transpulmonary vascular mechanics but does not change intrinsic right ventricular contractility in an acute respiratory distress syndrome model with permissive hypercapnia. Crit Care Med 24:1554–1561
78. Walmrath D, Schneider T, Pilch J, Grimminger F, Seeger W (1993) Aerosolised prostacyclin in adult respiratory distress syndrome. Lancet 342:961–962
79. Walmrath D, Schneider T, Schermuly R, Olschewski H, Grimminger F, Seeger W (1996) Direct comparison of inhaled nitric oxide and aerosolized prostacyclin in acute respiratory distress syndrome. Am J Respir Crit Care Med 153:991–996
80. Zwissler B, Welte M, Messmer K (1995) Effects of inhaled prostacyclin as compared with inhaled nitric oxide on right ventricular performance in hypoxic pulmonary vasoconstriction. J Cardiothorac Vasc Anesth 9:283–289
81. Curtis J, O'Neill JT, Pettett G (1993) Endotracheal administration of tolazoline in hypoxia-induced pulmonary hypertension. Pediatrics 92:403–408
82. Abraham E, Park YC, Covington P, Conrad SA, Schwartz M (1996) Liposomal prostaglandin E_1 in acute respiratory distress syndrome: A placebo-controlled, randomized, double-blind, multicenter trial. Crit Care Med 24:10–15
83. Mira JP, Monchi M, Brunet F, Fierobe L, Dhainaut JF, Dinh-Xuan AT (1994) Lack of efficacy of inhaled nitric oxide in ARDS. Intensive Care Med 20:532 (Letter)
84. Buga GM, Griscavage JM, Rogers NE, Ignarro LJ (1993) Negative feedback regulation of endothelial cell function by nitric oxide. Circ Res 73:808–812
85. Gerlach H, Rossaint R, Pappert D, Falke KJ (1993) Time-course and dose-response of nitric oxide inhalation for systemic oxygenation and pulmonary hypertension in patients with adult respiratory distress syndrome. Eur J Clin Invest 23:499–502
86. Stamler JS, Singel DJ, Loscalzo J (1992) Biochemistry of nitric oxide and its redox-activated forms. Science 258:1898–1902

Systemic Circulatory Function
and Peripheral Oxygen Delivery in ALI and ARDS

J. L. Vincent and D. De Backer

Introduction

Advances in our understanding of the pathogenesis of acute respiratory distress syndrome (ARDS) and sepsis have shown the two to be intimately related. Although ARDS may develop from local lung injury, it is commonly part of the systemic inflammatory response to severe sepsis, and tissue damage in the lungs is the result of the same inflammatory mediators involved in other organ damage. Inflammatory injury to the lung microvessels is an early pathogenetic event in ARDS, and leukocytes in particular are implicated. The sequestration of neutrophils in the lungs and their activation by inflammatory mediators leads to the release of toxic substances such as lipid mediators and reactive oxygen metabolites. The result is an increase in pulmonary endothelial and epithelial permeability, and an accumulation of fluid in the pulmonary interstitial and alveolar spaces. This causes a reduced ventilated lung volume and impaired gas exchange. Hence, the same inflammatory response mechanisms take place in the lungs as in other organs leading to organ failure. Although cardiac output is normal or high and thus systemic oxygen delivery (DO_2) is well preserved, distant tissue hypoxia may thus arise. Most patients with ARDS, however, do not have tissue hypoxia, this only occurring if there is also acute circulatory failure. Poor tissue oxygenation may play a role in the development of organ failure which is often fatal. Mortality in ARDS patients is more often due to multiple organ failure than to refractory hypoxemia [1, 2], and recognition of these abnormalities is therefore vitally important. Fluid restriction aimed at limiting lung edema may also limit DO_2, and excessive restriction can result in harmful tissue hypoperfusion. These concepts thus have strong clinical relevance and application.

VO_2/DO_2 Relationships

Under normal conditions, oxygen consumption (VO_2) is independent of DO_2 because if DO_2 falls, oxygen extraction (O_2ER) by the tissues can increase, maintaining VO_2. At a particular point however, DO_2crit, O_2ER can no longer compensate sufficiently and VO_2 starts to fall. Tissue hypoxia occurs, blood lactate levels rise, and VO_2 becomes DO_2-dependent [3, 4]. The concept of pathologic VO_2/DO_2 dependency, where dependency occurs at a higher DO_2crit value due to alterations in oxygen extraction in disease, was first proposed more than 20 years ago [5]. Other studies followed supporting the presence of this phenomenon in patients with respiratory failure [6, 7] and circulatory failure and shock [8–11].

In recent years, the existence of pathological VO_2/DO_2 dependency has been challenged on the basis of methodological problems which could have created a false relationship [12, 13]. In this chapter, we will review the current situation, potential sources of error, and clinical implications of the VO_2/DO_2 relationship.

Animal Studies

VO_2/DO_2 dependency has been reported by investigators using different models and different animal species [3, 4, 14]. Several groups were able to reproduce the alterations in oxygen extraction occurring in sepsis, demonstrating an increase in DO_2crit following endotoxin administration [15, 16]. These alterations can be observed regionally as well as systemically, and the splanchnic region seems particularly sensitive [17, 18]. Sound animal data therefore exist describing both physiologic VO_2/DO_2 dependency, and pathologic dependency in septic conditions.

The effects of endotoxin on O_2ER and the DO_2/VO_2 relationship have also been investigated in models of acute lung injury. Alterations were demonstrated after smoke inhalation [19] and phorbol myristate acetate infusion [20], but not after oleic acid injury [21]. Recently in a cat model of acute lung injury, Crouser et al. [22] found no alteration in ileal VO_2/DO_2 relationships despite marked ileal endothelial damage. They suggested that factors other than an impaired DO_2, such as impaired intracellular oxygen utilization, are necessary for an alteration in the VO_2/DO_2 relationship.

Human Studies

It is rarely possible to acutely decrease DO_2 in the clinical situation but in studies in cardiopulmonary bypass patients [23] and terminally ill patients [24] where this has been done, a fall in VO_2 was observed after DO_2 fell below a critical point, supporting the findings of animal experiments. Most human studies investigating this relationship have observed the effects of increasing DO_2. Since the early descriptions of pathological VO_2/DO_2 dependency in ARDS patients by Powers et al. [5], Rhodes et al. [6] and Danek et al. [7], many other clinical studies have reported this phenomenon [8–11, 25–43]. A review of these studies is shown in Table 1. Few were able to relate the presence of pathological VO_2/DO_2 dependency to an increased mortality rate [28, 31, 32, 39], but many related its presence to impaired tissue oxygenation as indicated by raised blood lactate levels or possibly low gastric intramucosal pH (pHi) [8–11, 32, 33, 38, 40]. VO_2/DO_2 dependency may represent a transitory phenomenon associated with acute circulatory failure, as has been observed in animal studies, but which is not present in hemody-

Table 1. Studies on VO_2/DO_2 dependency in critically ill patients

Author	Ref.	Year	Total Patients	VO_2/DO_2 dependent patients	Disease	Intervention dependency associated with increased mortality
Powers et al.	[5]	1977	73	73	ARDS	Mannitol
Rhodes et al.	[6]	1978	14	13	ARDS	Mannitol
Danek et al.	[7]	1980	32	20	ARDS	PEEP
Moshenifar et al.	[25]	1983	10	10	ARDS	PEEP
Kaufman et al.	[26]	1984	8	8	Sepsis	Fluid
Kariman and Burns	[27]	1985	21	21	ARDS	PEEP
Haupt et al.	[8]	1985	14	8	Sepsis	Fluid
Gilbert et al.	[9]	1986	54	41	Sepsis	Fluid, transfusion, DB, DP
Gutierrez and Pohil	[28]	1986	30	20	Mixed	Time Yes
Wolf et al.	[29]	1987	25	17	Sepsis	Fluid, transfusion
Astiz et al.	[30]	1987	10	10	Sepsis	Fluid
Bihari et al.	[31]	1987	27	13	ARDS, Sepsis	PGI_2 Yes
Groeneveld et al.	[32]	1987	31	19	Sepsis	Fluid, transfusion, DB, DP Yes
Vincent et al.	[10]	1990	73	24	Sepsis	DB
Kruse et al.	[11]	1990	58	32	ARDS	Fluid, transfusion, PEEP
Fenwick et al.	[33]	1990	24	13	ARDS	Transfusion
Dubin et al.	[34]	1990	28	20	ARDS, Sepsis	PEEP
Pittet et al.	[35]	1990	11	11	Sepsis	PGI_2
Ronco et al.	[36]	1990	5	5	Pneumonia	Transfusion
Lorente et al.	[37]	1991	24	13	ARDS	PEEP, DB
Silverman and Tuma	[38]	1992	16	9	Sepsis	DB
Ranieri et al.	[39]	1992	18	8	ARDS, Sepsis	PEEP Yes
Esen et al.	[40]	1992	52	52	Sepsis	DB
Ruokonen et al.	[41]	1993	10	10	Sepsis	NE, DP
Spec-Marn et al.	[42]	1993	18	8	ARDS	PEEP
Krachman et al.	[43]	1994	12	8	ARDS	DB

DB: dobutamine, DP: dopamine, NE: norepinephrine, PEEP: positive end-expiratory pressure

namically stable patients. Several studies have observed that VO_2 was independent of DO_2 in patients with normal blood lactate levels [8–11, 32, 33, 44, 45], and in hemodynamically stable patients with sepsis or ARDS [8–10, 44–47]. For example, we demonstrated that dobutamine at a dose of 5 µg/kg/min increased VO_2 in patients with ARDS and high lactate levels but not in those with normal lactate

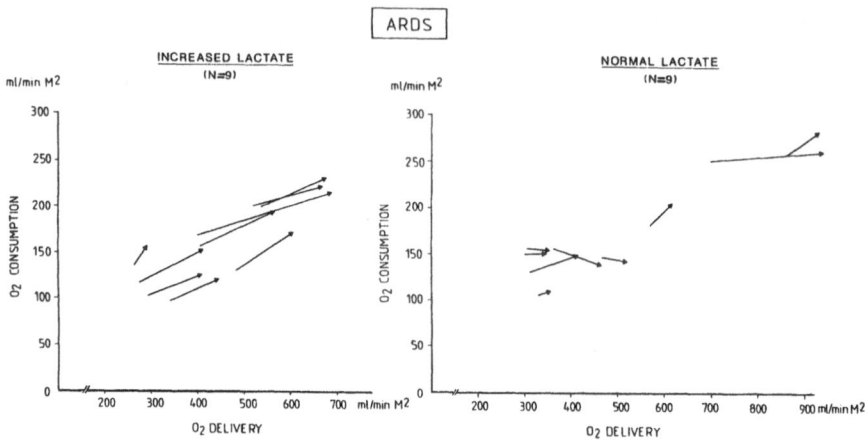

Fig. 1. Relation between VO$_2$ and DO$_2$ in patients with ARDS with high lactate levels (left panel and low lactate levels (right panel). In each case elevated lactate levels were ascribed to acute circulatory failure. (From [10] with permission)

levels (Fig. 1). Recently, Langeron et al. [48] demonstrated the presence of VO$_2$/DO$_2$ dependency in brain-dead organ donors with high blood lactate levels, but not in those with normal blood lactate levels.

For an accurate assessment of the VO$_2$/DO$_2$ relationship, the criteria for inclusion of patients in such studies are therefore crucial. Hyperlactatemia is not sufficient as it may be due to factors other than tissue hypoxia. In a study we performed [10], we stated explicitly that "in each case increased lactate levels were attributed to perfusion failure" and noted that septic and cardiac patients with elevated lactate levels had significantly lower mean arterial pressure than patients with normal lactates. This was in contrast to a study by Ronco et al. [47] who failed to show VO$_2$/DO$_2$ dependency even in patients with hyperlactatemia, but noted that in their patients "the increased lactate concentration could represent a marker of previous and resolved rather than current tissue hypoxia and anaerobic metabolism". VO$_2$/DO$_2$ dependency has also been associated with a low pHi. Silverman et al. [38] reported that VO$_2$ increased during dobutamine infusion in patients with a low pHi but not in those with a normal pHi.

Clearly, relating VO$_2$/DO$_2$ dependency to hyperlactatemia or a low pHi is overly simplistic, one needs to consider the full clinical setting. Nevertheless, on the evidence available so far, one can agree that VO$_2$ is independent of DO$_2$ in patients with ARDS or sepsis who have no signs of acute circulatory failure.

Methodological Problems

In the assessment of some of the reasons for apparently conflicting results from studies investigating the VO$_2$/DO$_2$ relationship, several methodological problems can be identified.

Change in Oxygen Demand

Under normal conditions, a change in oxygen demand is associated with a corresponding change in DO_2 so that a single plot of VO_2 against DO_2 may show an apparent dependent relationship which is in fact a normal response to altered metabolic activity. Likewise, in the critically ill patient, alterations in mechanical ventilation [49] or sedation [50, 51] can increase oxygen demand, as can routine bedside interventions [52]. These environmental factors should thus be kept as constant as possible, and the study of alterations in the DO_2/VO_2 relationship should employ techniques to acutely alter DO_2 such as fluid loading, inotropic stimulation, or application of positive end-expiratory pressure (PEEP).

Change in Oxygen Consumption by the Thermogenic Effect of Catecholamines

Catecholamines can stimulate cellular metabolism and may thus induce a thermogenic increase in tissue VO_2. Studies in healthy volunteers showing a dose-related increase in VO_2 following catecholamine administration [53–55] were used by several investigators to account for the appearance of VO_2/DO_2 dependency. However, this increase in VO_2 is much more marked in volunteers than in stable critically ill patients [10, 44, 45], and it is important to note that the increase in DO_2 was also greater in volunteers [55], so that the slope of the VO_2/DO_2 relationship was similar in volunteers and stable critically ill patients. An increase in cardiac output, by whatever means, can be associated with an increase in oxygen demand by some organs. A small slope can be observed in the independent part of the VO_2/DO_2 relationship during experimental hemorrhage [17, 56] or tamponade [14, 16], or in hemodynamically stable patients with ARDS after alteration of tidal volume [57]. An increase in VO_2 during catecholamine infusion may therefore not necessarily infer a thermogenic effect. In clinical studies, any increase in VO_2 following catecholamine administration has been shown to be small [10, 38, 44, 45, 47, 58–60] probably because these patients are already under increased sympathetic influence. This is supported by a study by Uusaro et al. [61] on healthy volunteers showing that the increase in VO_2 associated with dobutamine administration was blunted by a triple hormone infusion to reproduce the stress response. VO_2/DO_2 dependency cannot therefore merely be due to a thermogenic effect of the catecholamine.

Mathematical Coupling of Data

Mathematical coupling of data occurs when the same variable is introduced in both components of a regression analysis. Any error in this variable is thus magnified and may force a relationship between two otherwise independent factors [12, 62]. Many studies have used the same measured values of cardiac output (CO), arterial oxygen saturation, and hemoglobin concentration in their calculations of VO_2 and DO_2, and thus exposed the results to the potential problem of mathematical coupling of data. In practice the main offender is the thermodilution CO, as errors in this can reach 5–10% [63].

However, there are at least 4 reasons why observed VO_2/DO_2 dependency cannot merely be the result of mathematical coupling of data:

1) When variations in DO_2 due to therapeutic interventions are of large magnitude, the risk of mathematical coupling of data is reduced [64]

2) If any measure of CO is associated with a non-random error, it would result in a persistent over or under-estimation of the actual value. This would tend to mask any VO_2/DO_2 dependency rather than enhance it [62]. To show a spurious VO_2/DO_2 dependency, the errors in CO measurement would have to consist of an overestimation of the higher CO and/or an underestimation of the lower CO. Studies validating the thermodilution technique do not support the presence of such a phenomenon [65–67], in fact they suggest it may overestimate lower CO values in humans [68]

3) If mathematical coupling of data were indeed a problem one would expect it to affect the results of all studies similarly, but when different groups, for example those with normal and those with high lactate levels, with similar changes in CO and DO_2 were assessed, VO_2/DO_2 dependency was only shown in the subgroup with raised lactates. It is difficult to explain how mathematical coupling of data could occur in one group and not the other

4) The use of a diagram relating cardiac index to oxygen extraction can be useful in analyzing the VO_2/DO_2 relationship while avoiding any problems of mathematical coupling of data as CO and O_2ER are measured independently [69]. The calculation of O_2ER can be simplified as follows, showing its independence of hemoglobin concentration

$$O_2ER = VO_2/DO_2 = \frac{CaO_2 - CvO_2}{CaO_2}$$

$$= \frac{(Hb \times C \times SaO_2) - (Hb \times C \times SvO_2)}{(Hb \times C \times SaO_2)}$$

$$= \frac{SaO_2 - SvO_2}{SaO_2}$$

where Hb represents the hemoglobin concentration, C a constant value representing the amount of oxygen in 1 g of hemoglobin, CaO_2 and CvO_2 the arterial and mixed venous oxygen contents, and SaO_2 and SvO_2 the corresponding oxygen saturations.

The benefits of the use of the cardiac index/O_2ER relationship over VO_2/DO_2 assessment are summarized in Table 2. Studies in anemic patients and healthy volunteers have shown that the cardiac index/O_2ER relationship is indeed unaltered by the hemoglobin concentration [70] or arterial oxygen saturation [71]. If the hemoglobin remains constant, isopleths of VO_2 values can be drawn on the diagram. In a stable patient, an acute change in cardiac index by a VO_2 challenge is associated with a corresponding opposite change in O_2ER and the values will therefore move along the same isopleth. In the unstable patient, however, O_2ER

Table 2. Advantages of studying cardiac index/O$_2$ER rather than VO$_2$/DO$_2$ relationship

VO$_2$/DO$_2$	Cardiac index/O$_2$ER
Complex calculations	Simple calculations
Potential problem of mathematical coupling of data	No mathematical coupling of data
Multiplication of errors if used for continuous monitoring	Simple parameters enable continuous monitoring
Requires hemoglobin concentration	Independent of hemoglobin concentration

cannot change further and VO$_2$/DO$_2$ dependency is indicated by a move from one isopleth to another. This relationship cannot be used if there is a simultaneous alteration in the hemoglobin level, as may occur by a dilution effect during a fluid challenge with a crystalloid or albumin solution. The use of this diagram following a VO$_2$ challenge with dobutamine can reveal VO$_2$/DO$_2$ dependency in patients with high lactate levels [72] (Fig. 2).

The absence of studies showing VO$_2$/DO$_2$ dependency when VO$_2$ is determined independently from respiratory gas analysis is primarily due to study design and patient selection. The use of metabolic carts for direct measurement of VO$_2$ from respiratory gases (VO$_2$dir) is difficult in the critically ill patient, particularly those whose condition is unstable and in whom one would anticipate VO$_2$/DO$_2$ dependency, and there may thus be a selection bias in studies using this method to determine VO$_2$.

Measurements using indirect calorimetry also have their problems. Ronco et al. [13] noted that VO$_2$dir remained stable while VO$_2$ calculated from the Fick equation (VO$_2$indir) increased following blood transfusions to septic or ARDS patients. In this study, the thermodilution CO did not change during transfusion and DO$_2$ thus increased by an increase in arteriovenous oxygen difference. The

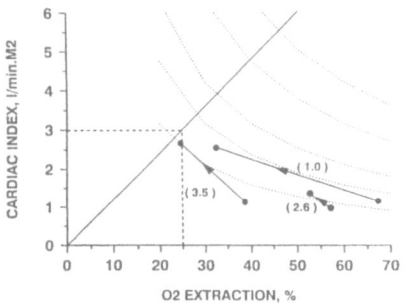
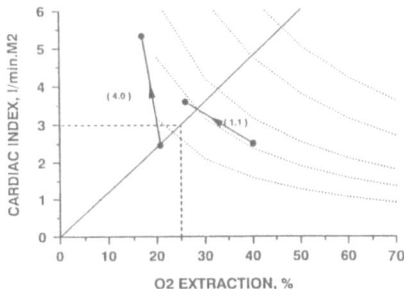

Fig. 2. Examples of the relationship between cardiac index and oxygen extraction before and during the administration of 5 mcg/kg/min of dobutamine in 3 patients with heart failure (left panel) and 2 with sepsis (right panel). The lactate level of each patient is indicated in parentheses. VO$_2$/DO$_2$ dependency (a shift from one VO$_2$ isopleth to another) is seen in the 3 patients with raised lactate levels but not in those with normal lactate levels. (From [72] with permission)

authors incriminated the thermodilution CO measurements for creating a spurious pathological VO_2/DO_2 dependency. However, if the VO_2dir measurements were correct, the increase in arteriovenous oxygen difference would imply a reduced CO, and DO_2 would therefore remain stable, invalidating the study. Alternatively, CO indeed remained unchanged so that VO_2 increased and the VO_2dir was erroneous.

Discrepancies between VO_2dir and VO_2indir may be due to various problems with the two techniques (Table 3). VO_2dir includes lung VO_2 while VO_2indir does not [73], and this may account for the common finding that VO_2dir is usually higher than VO_2indir [74], especially in acute respiratory failure. Indirect calorimetry has technical problems associated with gas leaks and poor sensitivity with high FiO_2 levels. It also requires stable pulmonary gas exchange and may be influenced by administration of inotropes or the application of PEEP. Despite these potential problems, studies have generally shown a good agreement between the two methods [40, 45, 75–79]. In a study on 12 mechanically ventilated, hemodynamically stable, septic patients [45], we observed excellent agreement between VO_2dir and VO_2indir during a dobutamine infusion (Fig. 3).

Clinical Applications

Observations that among ARDS patients survivors may have greater DO_2 values than non-survivors [80] led Shoemaker and colleagues [81] to propose maintaining DO_2 at "supranormal" levels (above 600 mL/min/m²) in all patients at risk of developing organ failure. An increase in DO_2 to "supranormal" or "optimal" lev-

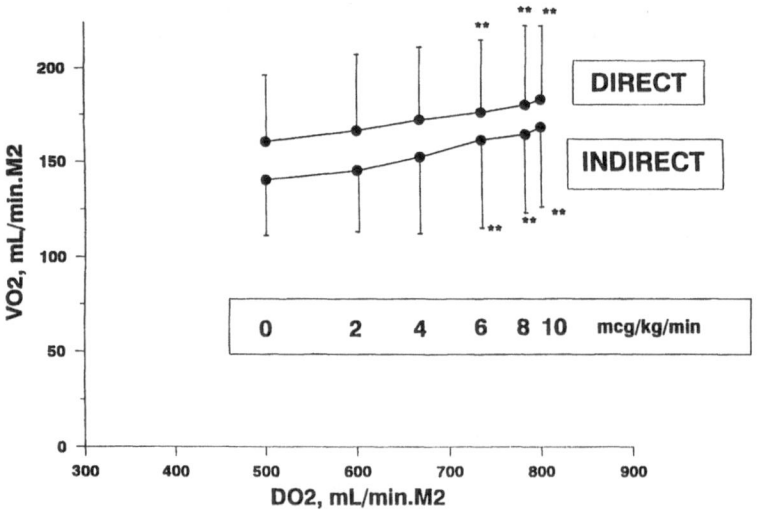

Fig. 3. Changes in VO_2 measured from respiratory gases (direct) and calculated from thermodilution (indirect) in 12 stable septic patients. (From [45] with permission)

Table 3. Potential problems associated with VO_2 measurement

Indirect VO_2 determinations (using the Fick equation)
- Errors in thermodilution cardiac output measurement
- Risk of inappropriate or uneven injection
- Inaccurate in the presence of severe tricuspid regurgitation, very low cardiac output, large fluctuations in intrathoracic pressure, shunting
- Errors in hemoglobin determination
- Errors in arterial and mixed venous saturations
- Slight underestimation of VO_2
- Physiological shunting by the bronchial veins
- Exclusion of lung VO_2

Direct VO_2 determinations (from respiratory gases)
- Requires steady state gas exchange
- Unreliable in the presence of air leaks (from chest tube, endotracheal cuff, etc.)
- Inaccurate in the presence of a high FiO_2 and influenced by changes in FiO_2
- Sensitive to humidity and moisture
- Requires meticulous calibration
- Influenced by changes in CO_2 transfer
- Change in ventilation
- Acute reduction in cardiac output (hemorrhage, arrhythmia, etc.)
- Administration of bicarbonate or hemodialysis
- Influenced by other gases (NO, anesthetics, etc.)
- Less reliable if inspiratory and expiratory gases not completely separated

els has been observed to reduce mortality and morbidity in certain groups of patients [81–84]. However, other studies have questioned the value of increasing DO_2 in all at risk patients and raised the possibility that this may in fact worsen survival [85–87].

The importance of maintaining adequate oxygen delivery in patients with ARDS and sepsis should not be underestimated. Clearly some critically ill patients benefit from supranormal DO_2 values but the definition of the "at risk" patient needs to be more specific. The degree of myocardial depression, of alteration in oxygen extraction capabilities, and of oxygen demand, can vary widely in the critically ill patient population, and a more specific evaluation of the need for supranormal DO_2 is necessary. Increasing DO_2 carries its own risks of fluid overload and side effects of excessive catecholamine administration, which can further worsen gas exchange and increase mortality rates [86] in patients who do not necessarily need such therapy.

We therefore prefer to individually titrate our therapy based on a careful clinical assessment in combination with hemodynamic and mixed venous blood gas parameters, and measures of tissue perfusion such as blood lactate levels, pHi or veno-arterial PCO_2 gradients [14, 88, 89].

SvO_2: While a normal or high SvO_2 does not guarantee adequate tissue perfusion and oxygenation, a low SvO_2 usually reflects inadequate oxygen delivery.

Blood lactate: Levels must be interpreted with caution as they reflect the balance between lactate production and elimination and may thus be protracted in liver failure. Other causes of hyperlactatemia must be eliminated but the presence of raised blood lactate levels due to circulatory failure has been associated with the VO_2/DO_2 dependency phenomenon [10]. The analysis of serial lactate levels is of particular use [90] in evaluating patient condition.

pHi: The gut mucosa may be particularly at risk of ischemia during hypoperfusion states and the measurement of pHi can reflect poor tissue perfusion. A low pHi has been associated with the presence of VO_2/DO_2 dependency [38]. Gastric mucosal PCO_2 ($PgCO_2$) may be more specific, avoiding some of the technical difficulties associated with saline tonometry, and providing an almost continuous monitoring technique. The use of blood lactate levels in combination with pHi or $PgCO_2$ may provide more information about tissue hypoperfusion than either value alone [89].

Therapeutic Applications

The identification of inadequate tissue oxygenation by the methods mentioned above, combined with clinical evaluation will indicate those patients who will benefit from increasing DO_2. DO_2 is the product of hemoglobin, arterial oxygen saturation and cardiac output and can thus, in theory, be increased by increasing any of these three components. There is an optimal hemoglobin level as a low hemoglobin is associated with a low DO_2, but a high hemoglobin leads to increased viscosity which lowers cardiac output and hence also reduces DO_2. A hemoglobin of 10–11.5 g/dL with a hematocrit of 30–33% is generally recommended in patients with ARDS and sepsis although there is limited data to support this recommendation. Interestingly, a lower hematocrit may improve tissue oxygen extraction [91]. Respiratory support should be offered to keep PaO_2 greater than 8 kPa (60 mmHg) but levels greater than this have little further effect on global DO_2 and high FiO_2 levels carry the risk of oxygen toxicity. Fluid administration is the first step to consider to increase cardiac output, even in ARDS, although increases in cardiac filling pressures can be very deleterious in this condition. If fluids alone are not sufficient, inotropic agents should be employed. Dobutamine is generally the preferred agent as it consistently increases cardiac output but does not increase cardiac filling pressures, which may be a problem with vasopressor agents.

These methods increase global DO_2 but their effect on regional DO_2 is less defined. O_2ER capabilities may vary between organs during a reduction in DO_2, and regional VO_2/DO_2 dependency may therefore occur at different DO_2crit levels [17, 92]. During sepsis, these differences may be exaggerated by blood flow redistribution, rendering certain areas, notably the splanchnic region [18], more sensitive to VO_2/DO_2 dependency and tissue hypoxia. Current interest in the role of the gut in the pathogenesis of multiple organ failure, make regional VO_2/DO_2 dependency and the influence of vasoactive drugs and other agents on regional blood flow and oxygen extraction important and exciting areas of research. We must await further results before any definite recommendations can be made regarding increasing regional DO_2 in sepsis and ARDS.

Conclusion

In most patients, VO_2 remains independent of DO_2 because oxygen extraction capabilities are not limited. However, in some patients with sepsis and ARDS, especially those with acute circulatory failure, pathological VO_2/DO_2 dependency may occur. This is probably not an all-or-none phenomenon and may occur in different regions at different times during the disease process. Regardless of the technique used, methodological problems can render the assessment of the relationship between DO_2 and VO_2 quite complex. The use of a diagram relating cardiac index to O_2ER is an easy method of studying this relationship while avoiding potential problems of mathematical coupling of data. We prefer to base our hemodynamic therapeutic strategy on individual assessment using full clinical evaluation, hemodynamic and tissue perfusion parameters, rather than randomly assigning all ëat riskí patients to receive pre-established supranormal DO_2 levels. The importance of regional DO_2 and the use of agents to increase it are areas of active current research.

References

1. Montgomery BA, Stager MA, Carrico J, et al (1985) Causes of mortality in patients with the adult respiratory distress syndrome. Am Rev Respir Dis 132:485–491
2. Ferring M, Vincent JL (1997) Is outcome from ARDS related to the severity of respiratory failure? Eur Respir J (In Press)
3. Cain SM, Adams RP (1965) Appearance of excess lactate in anesthetized dogs during anemic and hypoxic hypoxia. Am J Physiol 209:604–608
4. Bakker J, Vincent JL (1991) The oxygen supply dependency phenomenon is associated with increased blood lactate levels. J Crit Care 6:152–159
5. Powers SR, Shah D, Ryon D, et al (1977) Hypertonic mannitol in the therapy of the acute respiratory distress syndrome. Ann Surg 185:619–625
6. Rhodes GR, Newell JC, Shah D, et al (1978) Increased oxygen consumption accompanying increased oxygen delivery with hypertonic mannitol in adult respiratory distress syndrome. Surgery 84:490–497
7. Danek S, Lynch JP, Weg JG, Dantzker DR (1980) The dependence of oxygen uptake on oxygen delivery in the adult respiratory distress syndrome. Am Rev Respir Dis 122:387–395
8. Haupt MT, Gilbert EM, Carlson RW (1985) Fluid loading increases oxygen consumption in septic patients with lactic acidosis. Am Rev Respir Dis 131:912–916
9. Gilbert EM, Haupt MT, Mandanas RY, Huaringa AJ, Carlson RW (1986) The effect of fluid loading, blood transfusion and catecholamine infusion on oxygen delivery and consumption in patients with sepsis. Am Rev Respir Dis 134:873–878
10. Vincent JL, Roman A, De Backer D, Kahn RJ (1990) Oxygen uptake/supply dependency: Effects of short-term dobutamine infusion. Am Rev Respir Dis 142:2–8
11. Kruse JA, Haupt MT, Puri VK, Carlson RW (1990) Lactate levels as predictors of the relationship between oxygen delivery and consumption in ARDS. Chest 98:959–962
12. Archie J (1981) Mathematic coupling of data: A common source of error. Ann Surg 193:296–303

13. Ronco JJ, Phang PT, Walley KR, Wiggs B, Fenwick JC, Russell JA (1991) Oxygen consumption is independent of changes in oxygen delivery in severe adult respiratory distress syndrome. Am Rev Respir Dis 143:1267–1273

14. Zhang H, Vincent JL (1993) Arteriovenous differences in PCO_2 and pH are good indicators of critical hypoperfusion. Am Rev Respir Dis 148:867–871

15. Nelson DP, Beyer C, Samsel RW, Wood LDH, Schumacker PT (1987) Pathological supply dependence of O_2 uptake during bacteremia in dogs. J Appl Physiol 63:1487–1492

16. Zhang H, Vincent JL (1993) Oxygen extraction is altered by endotoxin during tamponade-induced stagnant hypoxia in the dog. Circ Shock 40:168–176

17. Nelson DP, Samsel RW, Wood LD, Schumacker PT (1988) Pathological supply dependency of systemic and intestinal O_2 uptake during endotoxemia. J Appl Physiol 64:2410–2419

18. Zhang H, Rogiers P, De Backer D, et al (1996) Regional arteriovenous differences in PCO_2 and pH are determinants of critical organ oxygen delivery during endotoxemia. Shock 5:349–356

19. Demling RH, Knox J, Youn YK, LaLonde C (1992) Oxygen consumption early postburn becomes oxygen delivery dependent with the addition of smoke inhalation injury. J Trauma 32:593–598

20. Dorinsky PM, Costello JL, Gadek JE (1988) Oxygen distribution and utilization after phorbol myrisate acetate-induced lung injury. Am Rev Respir Dis 138:1454–1463

21. Pepe PE, Culver BH (1985) Independently measured oxygen consumption during reduction of oxygen delivery by positive end-expiratory pressure. Am Rev Respir Dis 132:788–792

22. Crouser ED, Julian MW, Weisbrode SE, Dorinsky PM (1996) Acid aspiration results in ileal injury without altering ileal VO_2–DO_2 relationships. Am J Respir Crit Care Med 153:1965–1971

23. Komatsu T, Shibutani K, Okamoto K, et al (1987) Critical level of oxygen delivery after cardiopulmonary bypass. Crit Care Med 15:194–197

24. Ronco JJ, Fenwick JC, Tweeddale MG, et al (1993) Identification of the critical oxygen delivery for anaerobic metabolism in critically ill septic and non-septic humans. JAMA 270:1724–1730

25. Mohsenifar Z, Goldbach P, Tashkin DP, Campisi DJ (1983) Relationship between O_2 delivery and O_2 consumption in the adult respiratory distress syndrome. Chest 84:267–271

26. Kaufman BS, Rackow EC, Falk JL (1984) The relationship between oxygen delivery and consumption during fluid resuscitation of hypovolemic and septic shock. Chest 85:336–340

27. Kariman K, Burns SR (1985) Regulation of tissue oxygen extraction is disturbed in adult respiratory distress syndrome. Am Rev Respir Dis 132:109–114

28. Gutierrez G, Pohil RJ (1986) Oxygen consumption is linearly related to O_2 supply in critically ill patients. J Crit Care 1:45–53

29. Wolf Y, Cotev S, Perel A, Manny J (1987) Dependence of oxygen consumption on cardiac output in sepsis. Crit Care Med 15:198–203

30. Astiz ME, Rackow EC, Falk JL, Kaufman BS, Weil MH (1987) Oxygen delivery and consumption in patients with hyperdynamic septic shock. Crit Care Med 15:26–28

31. Bihari D, Smithies M, Gimson A, Tinker J (1987) The effects of vasodilation with prostacyclin on oxygen delivery and uptake in critically ill patients. N Engl J Med 317:397–403

32. Groeneveld ABJ, Kester ADM, Nauta JJP (1987) Relation of arterial blood lactate to oxygen delivery and hemodynamic variables in human shock states. Circ Shock 22:35–53

33. Fenwick JC, Dodek PM, Ronco JJ, Phang PT, Wiggs B, Russell JA (1990) Increased concentrations of plasma lactate predict pathological dependence of oxygen consumption on oxygen delivery in patients with adult respiratory distress syndrome. J Crit Care 5:81–87

34. Dubin A, Estenssoro E, Silva C, et al (1990) Different oxygen transport patterns in patients with adult respiratory distress syndrome treated with positive end-expiratory pressure. J Crit Care 5:101–107

35. Pittet JF, Lacroix JS, Gunning K, Laverriere MC, Morel DR, Suter PM (1990) Prostacyclin but not phentolamine increases oxygen consumption and skin microvascular blood flow in patients with sepsis and respiratory failure. Chest 98:1467–1472

36. Ronco JJ, Montaner JSG, Fenwick JC, Ruedy J, Russell JA (1990) Pathologic dependence of oxygen consumption on oxygen delivery in acute respiratory failure secondary to AIDS-related *Pneumocystis carinii* pneumonia. Chest 98:1463–1466

37. Lorente JA, Renes E, Gomez-Aguinaga MA, Landin L, de la Morena J, Liste D (1991) Oxygen delivery-dependent oxygen consumption in acute respiratory failure. Crit Care Med 19:770–775
38. Silverman H, Tuma P (1992) Gastric tonometry in patients with sepsis: Effects of dobutamine infusions and packed red blood cell transfusions. Chest 102:184–188
39. Ranieri VM, Giuliani R, Eissa NT, et al (1992) Oxygen delivery-consumption relationship in septic adult respiratory distress syndrome patients: The effects of positive end-expiratory pressure. J Crit Care 7:150–157
40. Esen F, Telci L, Akpri K, Kesecioglu J, Denkel T, Pembeci K (1992) Oxygen uptake/supply dependency in human sepsis: Does it increase the risk of multisystem organ failure? In: Erdmann W, Bruley DF (eds) Oxygen transport to tissue XIV, Plenum Press, New York, pp 855–861
41. Ruokonen E, Takala J, Kari A, Saxen H, Mertsola J, Hansen EJ (1993) Regional blood flow and oxygen transport in septic shock. Crit Care Med 21:1296–1303
42. Spec-Marn A, Tos L, Kremzar B, Milic-Emili J, Ranieri VM (1993) Oxygen delivery-consumption relationship in adult respiratory distress syndrome patients: The effect of sepsis. J Crit Care 8:43–50
43. Krachmann S, Lodato R, Morice R, Gutierrez G, Dantzker D (1994) Effects of dobutamine on oxygen transport and consumption in the adult respiratory distress syndrome. Intensive Care Med 20:130–137
44. De Backer D, Berré J, Zhang H, Vincent JL (1993) Relationship between oxygen uptake and oxygen delivery in septic patients: Effects of prostacyclin versus dobutamine. Crit Care Med 21:1658–1664
45. De Backer D, Moraine JJ, Berré J, Kahn RJ, Vincent JL (1994) Effects of dobutamine on oxygen consumption in septic patients: Direct versus indirect determinations. Am J Respir Crit Care Med 150:95–100
46. Annat G, Viale JP, Percival C, Froment M, Motin J (1986) Oxygen delivery and uptake in the adult respiratory distress syndrome: Lack of relationship when measured independently in patients with normal blood lactate concentrations. Am Rev Respir Dis 133:999–1001
47. Ronco JJ, Fenwick JC, Wiggs BR, Phang PT, Russell JA, Tweeddale MG (1993) Oxygen consumption is independent of increases in oxygen delivery by dobutamine in septic patients who have normal or increased plasma lactate. Am Rev Respir Dis 147:25–31
48. Langeron O, Couture P, Mateo J, Riou B, Pansard JL, Coriat P (1996) Oxygen consumption and delivery relationship in brain-dead organ donors. Br J Anaesth 76:783–789
49. El Haddad P, De Backer D, Preiser JC, Kahn RJ, Vincent JL (1994) Increase in oxygen demand during weaning from mechanical ventilation after cardiovascular surgery. Intensive Care Med 20 (Suppl 2):S133 (Abst)
50. Villar J, Slutsky AS, Hew E, Aberman A (1990) Oxygen transport and oxygen consumption in critically ill patients. Chest 98:687–692
51. Boyd O, Grounds M, Bennett D (1992) The dependency of oxygen consumption on oxygen delivery in critically ill postoperative patients is mimicked by variations in sedation. Chest 101:1619–1624
52. Weissman C, Kemper M, Damask MC, Askanazi J, Hyman AI, Kinney JM (1984) Effect of routine intensive care interactions on metabolic rate. Chest 86:815–818
53. Chioléro R, Flatt JP, Revelly JP, Jéquier E (1991) Effects of catecholamines on oxygen consumption and oxygen delivery in critically ill patients. Chest 100:1676–1684
54. Green C, Frazer R, Underhill S, Maycock P, Fairhurst J, Campbell I (1992) Metabolic effects of dobutamine in normal man. Clin Science 82:77–83
55. Bhatt SB, Hutchinson RC, Tomlinson B, Oh TE, Mak M (1992) Effect of dobutamine on oxygen supply and uptake in healthy volunteers. Br J Anaesth 69:298–303
56. Van der Linden P, Gilbert E, Engelman E, Schmartz D, Vincent JL (1991) Effects of anesthetic agents on systemic critical O_2 delivery. J Appl Physiol 71:83–93
57. Kiiski R, Takala J, Kari A, Milic-Emili J (1992) Effect of tidal volume on gas exchange and oxygen transport in the adult respiratory distress syndrome. Am Rev Respir Dis 146:1131–1135
58. Teboul JL, Annane D, Thuillez C, Depret J, Bellissant E, Richard C (1992) Effects of cardiovascular drugs on oxygen consumption/oxygen delivery relationship in patients with congestive heart failure. Chest 101:1582–1587

· 59. Teboul JL, Graini L, Boujdaria R, Berton C, Richard C (1993) Cardiac index vs oxygen-derived parameters for rational use of dobutamine in patients with congestive heart failure. Chest 103:81–85

60. Gutierrez G, Clark C, Brown SD, Price K, Ortiz L, Nelson C (1994) Effect of dobutamine on oxygen consumption and gastric mucosal pH in septic patients. Am J Respir Crit Care Med 150:324–329

61. Uusaro A, Hartikainen J, Parviainen M, Takala J (1995) Metabolic stress modifies the thermogenic effect of dobutamine in man. Crit Care Med 23:674–680

62. Moreno LF, Stratton HH, Newell JC, Feustel PJ (1986) Mathematical coupling of data: Correction of a common error for linear calculations. J Appl Physiol 60:335–343

63. Sasse SA, Chen PA, Berry RB, Sassoon CSH, Mahutte CK (1994) Variability of cardiac output over time in medical ICU patients. Crit Care Med 22:225–232

64. Stratton HH, Feustel PJ, Newell JC (1987) Regression of calculated variables in the presence of shared measurement error. J Appl Physiol 62:2083–2093

65. Forrester JS, Ganz W, Diamond G, McHugh T, Chonette DW, Swan JJ (1972) Thermodilution cardiac output determination with a single flow-directed catheter. Am Heart J 83:306–311

66. Kubo SH, Burchenal JE, Cody RJ (1987) Comparison of direct Fick and thermodilution cardiac output techniques at high flow rates. Am J Cardiol 59:384–386

67. Lipkin DP, Poole-Wilson PA (1985) Measurement of cardiac output during exercise by the thermodilution and direct Fick techniques in patients with chronic congestive heart failure. Am J Cardiol 56:321–324

68. van Grondelle A, Ditchey RV, Groves BM, Wagner WW, Reeves JT (1983) Thermodilution method overestimates low cardiac output in humans. Am J Physiol 245:H690–H692

69. Vincent JL (1996) Determination of O_2 delivery and consumption vs cardiac index vs oxygen extraction ratio. Crit Care Clinics 12:995–1006

70. Woodson RD, Wills RE, Lenfant C (1978) Effect of acute and established anemia on O_2 transport at rest, submaximal and maximal work. J Appl Physiol 44:36–43

71. Sutton JR, Reeves JT, Wagner PD, et al (1988) Operation Everest II: Oxygen transport during exercise at extreme simulated altitude. J Appl Physiol 64:1309–1321

72. Silance PG, Simon C, Vincent JL (1994) The relation between cardiac index and oxygen extraction in acutely ill patients. Chest 105:1190–1197

73. Light R (1988) Intrapulmonary oxygen consumption in experimental pneumococcal pneumonia. J Appl Physiol 64:2490–2495

74. Levinson M, Groeger J, Miodownik S, Ray C, Brennan M (1987) Indirect calorimetry in the mechanically ventilated patient. Crit Care Med 15:144–147

75. Chappell TR, Rubin LJ, Markham RV, Firth BG (1983) Independence of oxygen consumption and systemic oxygen transport in patients with either stable pulmonary hypertension or refractory left ventricular failure. Am Rev Respir Dis 128:30–33

76. Mohsenifar Z, Jasper AC, Koerner SK (1988) Relationship between oxygen uptake and oxygen delivery in patients with pulmonary hypertension. Am Rev Respir Dis 138:69–73

77. Bihari D, Smithies M, Pozniak A, Gimson A (1987) A comparison of direct and indirect measurements of oxygen delivery and consumption: The effects of prostacyclin in two human volunteers. Scand J Clin Lab Invest 47:37–45

78. Albert RK, Schrijen F, Poincelot F (1986) Oxygen consumption and transport in stable patients with chronic obstructive pulmonary disease. Am Rev Respir Dis 134:678–682

79. Iparraguirre HP, Finiger R, Garber VA, Quiroga E, Jorge MA (1988) Comparison between measured and Fick-derived values of hemodynamic and oxymetric variables in patients with acute myocardial infarction. Am J Med 85:349–352

80. Russell JA, Ronco JJ, Lockhat D, Belzberg A, Kiess M, Dodek PM (1990) Oxygen delivery and consumption and ventricular preload are greater in survivors than in non-survivors of the adult respiratory distress syndrome. Am Rev Respir Dis 141:659–665

81. Shoemaker WC, Appel PL, Kram HB, Waxman K, Lee TS (1988) Prospective trial of supranormal values of survivors as therapeutic goals in high risk surgical patients. Chest 94:1176–1186

82. Boyd O, Grounds M, Bennett ED (1993) A randomized clinical trial of the effect of deliberate perioperative increase of oxygen delivery on mortality in high risk surgical patients. JAMA 270:2699–2707

83. Tuchschmidt J, Fried J, Astiz M, Rackow E (1992) Elevation of cardiac output and oxygen delivery improves outcome in septic shock. Chest 102:216–220
84. Fleming A, Bishop M, Shoemaker W, et al (1992) Prospective trial of supranormal values as goals of resuscitation in severe trauma. Arch Surg 127:1175–1179
85. Yu M, Levy MM, Smith P, Takiguchi SA, Miyasaki A, Myers SA (1993) Effect of maximizing oxygen delivery on morbidity and mortality rates in critically ill patients: A prospective, randomized, controlled study. Crit Care Med 21:830–838
86. Hayes MA, Timmins AC, Yau EH, Palazzo M, Hinds CJ, Watson D (1994) Elevation of systemic oxygen delivery in the treatment of critically ill patients. N Engl J Med 330:1717–1722
87. Gattinoni L, Brazzi L, Pelosi P, et al (1995) A trial of goal-oriented hemodynamic therapy in critically ill patients. N Engl J Med 333:1025–1032
88. Bakker J, Vincent JL, Gris P, Leon M, Coffernils M, Kahn RJ (1992) Veno-arterial carbon dioxide gradient in human septic shock. Chest 101:509–515
89. Friedman G, Berlot G, Kahn RJ, Vincent JL (1995) Combined measurements of blood lactate concentrations and gastric intramucosal pH in patients with severe sepsis. Crit Care Med 23:1184–1193
90. Bakker J, Gris P, Coffernils M, Kahn RJ, Vincent JL (1996) Serial blood lactate levels can predict the development of multiple organ failure following septic shock. Am J Surg 171:221–226
91. Van der Linden P, Gilbert E, Paques P, Simon C, Vincent JL (1993) Influence of hematocrit on tissue O_2 extraction capabilities in anesthetized dogs during acute hemorrhage. Am J Physiol 264:H1942–H1947
92. Schlichtig R, Kramer DJ, Pinsky MR (1991) Flow redistribution during progressive hemorrhage is a determinant of critical O_2 delivery. J Appl Physiol 70:169–178

The Alveolar Epithelial Barrier

Quantifying Lung Injury in ARDS

D. P. Schuster

Introduction

Normal water homeostasis in the lung is based on a balance among the so-called "Starling" forces: a vascular-to-extravascular hydrostatic pressure gradient, a similar but directionally opposite oncotic pressure gradient, and the "leakiness" or "permeability" of the alveolo-capillary endothelial membrane to protein [1,2]. This paradigm leads to a natural and clinically relevant distinction: Pulmonary edema can be either "cardiogenic" (i.e. due to increased hydrostatic pressures) or "non-cardiogenic" (i.e. due to increased vascular permeability). The prototypical example of non-cardiogenic pulmonary edema is the acute respiratory distress syndrome (ARDS).

Despite this commonly accepted model, the diagnosis of non-cardiogenic pulmonary edema, and therefore of ARDS, is still usually made by inference: when pulmonary edema occurs in the setting of normal hydrostatic pressures (estimated either clinically or from the pulmonary artery wedge pressure), the pathogenesis is generally assumed to be non-cardiogenic (Fig. 1). Conversely, if the wedge pressure is elevated, the primary mechanism for pulmonary edema is assumed to be due to increased pulmonary hydrostatic pressures, not increased vascular permeability (Fig. 1). Importantly, patients with increased pulmonary hydrostatic pressures, regardless of other considerations, are usually excluded from clinical trials of new therapies for ARDS.

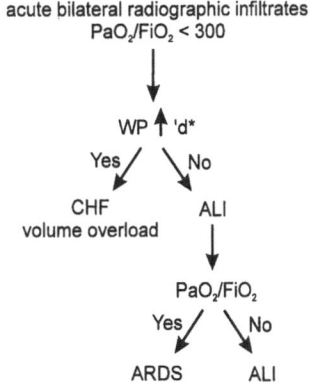

Fig. 1. Suggested algorithm, based on American Thoracic Society–European Society of Intensive Care Medicine criteria, for diagnosis of ALI or ARDS, WP = wedge pressure; CHF = congestive heart failure; * indicates that WP can be measured directly or inferred clinically. (From [4] with permission)

Table 1. Shortcomings of the current algorithm to diagnose ARDS

- excludes pulmonary edema due to lung injury and left atrial hypertension
- unable to correctly classify pulmonary edema due to pulmonary venous hypertension in absence of left atrial hypertension
- fails to provide adequate measure of severity-of-injury

Of course, there is no reason why vascular permeability and hydrostatic pressures cannot both be elevated simultaneously. Conversely, pulmonary venous hypertension (and thus pulmonary capillary hypertension) can occur without increasing the wedge pressure *per se*. And, any change in pulmonary vascular permeability from lung injury must surely cover a wide spectrum of abnormality, and not simply be "normal" or "increased". For all these reasons, a strategy in which lung injury is determined to be present only by inference and exclusion is unsatisfactory (Table 1). To fully characterize the pathogenesis of pulmonary edema, then, the relative contribution of both hydrostatic pressures and permeability should be quantified.

The importance of these issues has been recognized. In 1993, a Task Force on Research in Cardiopulmonary Dysfunction in Critical Care Medicine convened by the National Heart, Lung and Blood Institute [3] recommended "that highest priority be given to initiating clinical studies to examine the validity of definitions used in critical care medicine." Specifically mentioned were the definitions of "acute lung injury" (ALI) and "ARDS." The Task Force also recommended that additional efforts be made to "define the relationship between increased microvascular permeability and lung dysfunction ...", and that with respect to ARDS, "a descriptive definition of ARDS is needed that quantifies severity." Similar conclusions were reached by a Consensus Conference which was sponsored by the American Thoracic Society and the European Society of Intensive Care Medicine (ATS/ESICM) [4].

Vascular Permeability during ALI

Vascular permeability measurements should be important to the diagnosis and evaluation of ALI. In the ATS/ESICM report [4], the Consensus Conference committee declared that "the difficulty in determining the incidence and outcome of ARDS is largely due to the heterogeneity and lack of definitions for the underlying disease processes [and] the lack of definition for ARDS ...". In response, they recommended that ALI be defined as "a syndrome of inflammation and increasing permeability that is associated with a constellation of clinical, radiologic, and physiologic abnormalities that cannot be explained by, but may coexist with, left atrial or pulmonary capillary hypertension", and that ARDS be defined simply as a more severe form of ALI. They recommended, however, that this distinction in severity should be based solely on differences in oxygenation (Table 2) (Fig. 1). For reasons similar to those just discussed, this approach can be expected to be both non-specific and insensitive as a strategy for detecting and quantifying the severity of ALI.

At this point, it is appropriate to make a distinction between
1) the definition of a syndrome like ARDS
2) the criteria upon which that definition is based, and
3) the means or methods by which it can be determined that the criteria have been met.

Furthermore, criteria are necessarily the minimum threshold levels required for diagnosis, but a determination of severity requires some kind of continuous scale that may or may not invólve the same measures used as diagnostic criteria (Table 3).

In my opinion, since injury is central to the concept of ARDS, the definition of ARDS should link structural changes with functional abnormalities. The ATS/ESICM definition posits that ARDS is simply the most severe form of ALI, implying of course that all ALIs are similar except for degree of severity – a proposition which seems both unlikely and untrue. Instead, I suggest that ARDS be considered a specific form of lung injury, one in which structural changes are characterized pathologically as diffuse alveolar damage, and functional abnormalities are principally the result of a breakdown in the pulmonary endothelial barrier, leading first to proteinaceous alveolar edema, and then, as a consequence, to altered respiratory system mechanics and hypoxemia (Table 4).

Accordingly, ALI of the type associated with ARDS should be defined as the combination of bilateral pulmonary edema and increased pulmonary vascular permeability. Only when it is known or can reasonably be assumed that the ac-

Table 2. Criteria for ARDS, based on ATS/ESICM Consensus Conference Report

Expected	Actual
Documented inflammation	—
Elevated PMB	—
Specific clinical, radiologic, physiologic abnormalities	Acute bilateral radiographic infiltrates P/F <200
±LAH	Exclude LAH

PMB = permeability, P/F = PaO_2/FiO_2 ratio, LAH = left atrial hypertension

Table 3. Distinctions between definition of, criteria for, and measurements of severity in ARDS

Definition	a descriptive statement establishing the criteria for diagnosis
Criteria	a set of threshold values, which when exceeded qualitatively or quantitatively establish the diagnosis
Severity of injury	a quantitative scalar or set of scalars which, all else being equal, are predictive of recovery from lung injury

Table 4. Proposed definitions for ALI and ARDS

ALI	Any significant deterioration in lung function associated with characteristic pathologic abnormalities in the lungs' normal underlying structure or architecture.
ARDS	A specific form of injury in which structural changes (characterized pathologically as diffuse alveolar damage) and functional abnormalities (principally a breakdown in the pulmonary endothelial barrier) lead first to proteinaceous alveolar edema, and then (as a consequence) to altered respiratory system mechanics and hypoxemia.

companying pathology is diffuse alveolar damage should it be labeled ARDS *per se*. If pathologies other than diffuse alveolar damage can be associated with both alveolar edema and increased vascular permeability, I suggest that these should not be called ARDS but ALI due to some other cause.

These definitions clearly point to what criteria are necessary for diagnosis (Table 5) (Fig. 2): for ALI, it would only be necessary to document the presence of pulmonary edema and increased pulmonary vascular permeability. For ARDS, it would be necessary, in addition, to document that these functional abnormalities were associated with, or could be assumed to be associated with, diffuse alveolar damage. While clinically appropriate methods to identify the presence of pulmonary edema and increased vascular permeability are available, it is uncommon to determine unequivocally that diffuse alveolar damage is also present, since to do so would require obtaining tissue for histological examination. In some circumstances, it may be reasonable to assume that diffuse alveolar damage is present (for instance, ALI associated with sepsis); in others, it may not be so certain (for instance, neurogenic pulmonary edema, high altitude pulmonary edema, pulmonary edema associated with crises of pregnancy, etc). Given these uncertainties, it may be more appropriate to simply say that a patient has ALI in the setting of another specific clinical entity.

The issue of quantifying severity is yet another matter. It seems reasonable to assume that as an injury becomes more severe, recovery becomes less likely. Thus, implied in any attempt to quantify injury is really an attempt to determine prognosis, whereas the purpose of a definition and associated criteria is to determine a diagnosis. Accordingly, systems to quantify lung injury are generally judged against their ability to predict outcome. But which outcome? Typically, the outcome chosen is some global marker, such as mortality. But an index of lung in-

Table 5. Proposed citeria for ALI/ARDS

Definitive	Practical
Diffuse (bilateral) alveolar edema (EVLW >7 mL/kg with consistent CXR)	Radiographic infiltrates consistent with diffuse (bilateral) alveolar edema
Increased lung vascular permeability	Increased vascular permeability[a]
Diffuse alveolar damage pathologically	Appropriate clinical setting

[a] Until more complete information is available, a four-to fivefold increase over normal values; alternatively >2 SD from the normal population mean

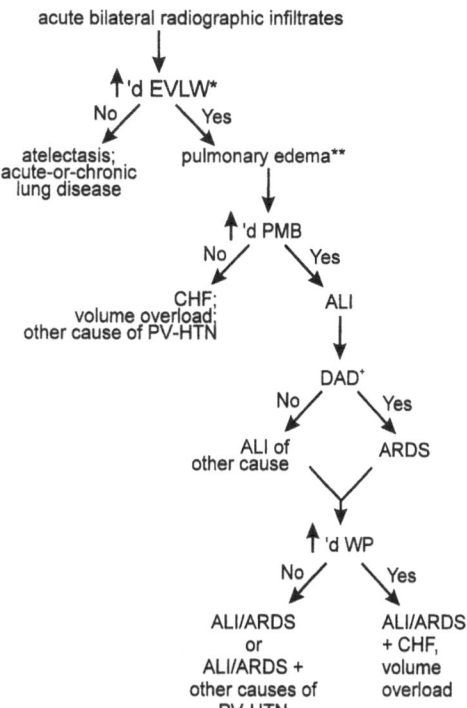

Fig 2. Alternative algorithm to determine diagnosis of ALI or ARDS. EVLW = extravascular lung water (* indicates that EVLW may be measured directly or inferred from a chest radiograph); PMB = a direct measure of vascular permeability (see text); DAD = pathologic finding of diffuse alveolar damage (+ indicates that DAD may be determined histologically, or may be assumed to be present in an appropriate clinical setting – see text); WP = wedge pressure; PV-HTN = pulmonary venous hypertension; ** indicates that alveolar hemorrhage and cellular infiltrate may also increase EVLW and appear as radiographic infiltrates while not being causes of pulmonary edema *per se*

jury *per se* should only be expected to predict recovery of lung function, all other clinical factors being equal. For instance, the "lung injury score" of Murray et al. [5] is often used to quantify "lung injury" in clinical studies of "ARDS". However, as recently reported [6], neither the PaO_2/FiO_2 ratio nor the "lung injury score" are good predictors of mortality. These observations do not necessarily mean, however, that outcome is unrelated to the severity of injury; they may only mean that the appropriate marker of lung injury or the appropriate marker of outcome (i.e. of lung recovery *per se*) have not yet been identified.

While an index of severity does not necessarily have to include the same criteria used for diagnosis, it seems natural, in the case of lung injury, to assume that measures of pulmonary edema and increased vascular permeability could be used for this purpose as well as for diagnosis. Not surprisingly, an enormous effort has been expended over many years to develop clinically appropriate methods to do just that. Of these methods, two general approaches stand out as both especially well developed and potentially clinically useful.

Quantifying Lung Injury

Quantifying increases in extravascular lung water. Although the chest X-ray is without question the most widely used method to detect the presence of pulmonary edema, generally most workers in the field do consider it a useful technique for quantifying the amount of edema accumulation in the lung. Indeed, in some circumstances (for instance, in the presence of underlying lung disease), chest radiography can be quite insensitive as a means of detecting early or mild pulmonary edema.

A wide variety of other techniques have also been evaluated for the purpose of measuring the accumulation of excess extravascular lung water (EVLW), including indicator-dilution methods, X-ray computed tomography, nuclear magnetic resonance imaging, and positron emission tomography, among others [7]. With the exception of the indicator-dilution approach, however, none of these have much chance of wide clinical implementation, because of problems with accuracy, cost, or complexity.

At the present time, the most clinically appropriate method to quantify EVLW in patients with ALI is by indicator-dilution methods. The theoretical foundation for these techniques is quite consistent, despite differences in indicators, technology, or methods of analysis. In general, temperature-time or concentration-time data are first generated in the course of determining EVLW [8–10]. These data are then analyzed by so-called "mean transit time" or "slope-volume" approaches. The former strategy is based on a rationale similar to that used to measure cardiac output by the familiar "thermodilution" method.

Two key principles underlie the mean transit time method:
1) the mean transit time of any substance (the "indicator") through a volume of fluid depends directly on the volume itself (when the volume is small, the mean transit time is short, and vice versa), and
2) the vascular and extravascular water spaces of the lung act as two separate but contiguous volumes, separated by a semi-permeable membrane.

If one indicator diffuses freely between both compartments but the other does not, the two indicators will have different mean transit times through the lung.

Although a variety of different indicators can and have been used, the most clinically applicable set of indicators are administered as cold indocyanine green dye. The temperature of the green dye is the "diffusible" indicator, distributing throughout the lung's vascular and extravascular water volume; the green dye itself is the "non-diffusible" indicator, limited to the vascular space. The dye remains within the intravascular space because it rapidly binds to serum albumin. Since the flow for both temperature and dye is the same (cardiac output), EVLW can be calculated simply as

$$EVLW = CO \cdot (MTT_{th} - MTT_{gd}) \qquad\qquad (Eq. 1)$$

where MTT_{th} and MTT_{gd} are the mean transit times of the thermal and green dye indicators, respectively. Strictly speaking, one actually measures the extravascular thermal volume (ETV), but since the extravascular water content of myocardium and non-pulmonary blood vessels is small relative to the extravascular water content of the lung, ETV and EVLW are usually considered to be equivalent.

While the theory underlying these measurements is well understood [8], commercially available equipment may have seriously biased the interpretation of performance in experimental and clinical settings. Since the early 1980s, most experimental and certainly virtually all studies involving thermodilution measurements of EVLW in the US have employed the Edwards Laboratories model 9310 Lung Water Computer®. Even though the calculation of EVLW from equation 1 is superficially straightforward, accuracy depends on corrections for baseline drift, instrument response times, proper positioning of the catheters, and recirculation artifacts (see below) [11]. For instance, the usual maximum change in temperature at the femoral artery thermistor site is about 0.25°C. Obviously, small drifts in baseline could seriously interfere with the calculation of ETV under such circumstances if not properly detected and corrected. Thus, some early reports that cardiac output could affect estimates of EVLW (which theoretically should not be true) were probably a result of the algorithms used in the Edwards Labs® computer to adjust for these problems [12, 13]. Studies which employed alternative systems did not report a similar dependency on cardiac output [10, 11, 14].

Effros [8] and Allison et al [10] have both pointed out that for accuracy the measurement of EVLW must take into account the relative transit times of the thermal indicator through red cells versus plasma, the relative specific heats of extravascular tissue versus plasma, the density of blood, and the fraction of extravascular mass represented by water. Without such corrections, EVLW should consistently overestimate EVLW by as much as 24% in normal lungs. However, as lungs become more edematous, a greater fraction of the extravascular mass becomes water, and the error introduced by ignoring these factors (which is the case with commercially available devices) actually decreases. To put such potential errors in perspective, however, a 24% error would yield an overestimate of about 72 mL if one accepts that the normal EVLW is about 5 mL/kg, or about 350 mL in a normal adult. On the other hand, clinically apparent pulmonary edema does not usually develop until EVLW increases by 50–100%, and 5-10 fold increases in EVLW have been reported in ARDS [15], yielding a dynamic range for EVLW of at least 300–3000 mL. In this context, a 24% error at the low (normal) end is probably tolerable.

Despite these many issues, many studies have shown that thermal-dye indicator dilution measurements of EVLW are usually (but not always) accurate [9, 10]. In fact, in general, there has been a tendency for EVLW to overestimate true EVLW in normal lungs, and to slightly underestimate it in edematous lungs. In addition to the correction factors discussed above, the tendency for the measured estimates of EVLW to be greater than the reference standard (gravimetric measurements) has been attributed to over-estimation of the thermal mean transit time when using monoexponential extrapolation of the descending portion of the thermal curve to correct for recirculation artifacts [16] and to the inclusion of myocardial and aortic wall water content in the EVLW calculation [16].

Overall, the correlation coefficient "r" for thermal-dye estimates of EVLW and gravimetrically-determined EVLW is usually at least 0.9, and the slope of the regression relationship usually lays between 0.9 and 1.10 [9–11]. From animal data, sensitivity has been estimated to be 88% and specificity 97%, with a coefficient of variation for repeated measurements of 4-8% [10]. However, this performance record in animals may be somewhat optimistic for the usual ICU clinical setting.

Using the Edwards computer, Laggner et al. [17] reported that most consecutive measurements were within 15% of one another, although the range was +30 to −60%. Using a newer, alternative ("COLD") system, Zeravik et al. [14] reported a coefficient of variation of only 8%.

The two commercially available systems (the Edwards® computer and the COLD® system) have also produced different results regarding the correlation of EVLW to gravimetric measurements obtained from the lungs of organ donors. Using the Edwards computer, Mihm et al. [18] reported an excellent correlation of r = 0.98, but a systematic overestimation of true EVLW by almost 4 mL/kg. In contrast, using the COLD® system, Sturm et al. [16] reported an equally strong correlation coefficient with much closer absolute agreement between methods.

In 4 studies in adults (using the Edwards® system), the average value for EVLW in normal humans has been remarkably consistent [19–22]. Average values have also been reported in patients with pulmonary edema associated with both normal and elevated wedge pressures [15, 21, 23].

The advantages of measuring EVLW by the thermal-green dye double-indicator dilution method are several: The method is (superficially) simple to implement, safe, reproducible, and repeatable. On the other hand, it is somewhat invasive (it requires central venous as well as (arterial catheterization).

Since the indicators in this technique are blood-borne the accumulation of extravascular water in any portion of lung which is "downstream" from a large vascular obstruction cannot be detected [10]. An analogous problem exists for lung regions which are poorly perfused, as a result of using positive end-expiratory pressure (PEEP) [10, 24], because of significant intravascular obstruction from emboli or in situ thrombosis (as has been documented to occur in ARDS), or because severe vasoconstriction from hypoxia is present. With vasoconstriction, the time required for full recovery of the thermal indicator from the lung may be so prolonged that recirculation artifacts are likely (see below) [10].

Vascular obstruction (from PEEP or thrombosis) may cause errors because the thermal indicator cannot equilibrate within the extravascular water space if it is not delivered sufficiently close to reach that space by diffusion. The diffusion distance of water is such that this problem probably only pertains to vessels > 500 m in size [8]. However, if PEEP levels are high enough to create regions of West's Zone I lung, estimates of EVLW can actually increase when PEEP levels are reduced, as new lung becomes reperfused, despite no actual change in EVLW *per se*. Although this phenomenon has been documented experimentally [10], its relevance to the clinical setting is unknown.

Any recirculation of indicator will interfere with the determination of the mean transit time. To avoid this, the downsloping portion of the concentration-time curves are usually extended by a mono-exponential extrapolation so that the recirculation artifact can be ignored. The mean transit time for the indicator is then calculated from these corrected data. In regions of very low perfusion, however, the cut-off point, especially for the diffusible indicator, can occur before the curve can be correctly characterized, leading to incomplete "recovery" of the diffusible indicator, and consequently, to under-estimation of the true value for EVLW.

With the American Edwards® model 9310 lung water computer, this monoexponential decay function was determined from the downsloping portion of the thermal curve between 75 and 33% of the peak value for change in temperature from baseline (manufacturer's manual). With a newer system (COLD Z-03®, Pulsion Medizintechnik, Munich, Germany), the portion of the curve used for analysis begins with the point which is 80% of the peak and continues with data until the monoexponential regression fit begins to deteriorate (representing recirculation). An alternative approach in which deconvolution algorithms are used to generate suitable transport functions for the pulmonary circulation has also been reported [25]; however, this approach has not yet been incorporated into a commercially available computer.

An alternative to the "mean transit time" approach to calculating EVLW is the so-called "slope-volume" method. Plotting the monoexponential decay of the thermodilution curve on semi-logarithmic paper will yield a straight line with a slope of V/Q where V is the volume through which the indicator is traversing and Q is the flow through that volume. For a set of volumes in series, the entity with the largest volume determines the slope [26, 27]. Thus, even though the thermal indicator traverses multiple cardiac chambers as well as the lungs, it is the lungs which determine the slope of the thermodilution curve (and, for that matter, the dye dilution curve). Therefore, EVLW can be determined by a different mathematical approach from the same set of dilution curve data, namely as the cardiac output times the difference between slope values for the two curves [26, 27]. This alternative approach has been incorporated into the COLD® computer system. It is used as a check on the calculation of EVLW by the mean transit time method, since both methods are quite sensitive to a variety of artifacts related to catheter placement and positioning [10, 11, 28].

A variation on the slope-volume method has also been reported in which the slope of the thermodilution curve measured by the pulmonary arterial catheter is compared to that detected by the femoral arterial catheter. The former set of data allows the right heart mixing volume to be calculated, which theoretically should be closely related to the pulmonary blood mixing volume [29]. As a result, it is theoretically possible to estimate EVLW from the injection of a single indicator (thermal), as cardiac output times the difference in the slope values from the femoral arterial versus pulmonary arterial dilution curves. Such an approach is very attractive since it would not be necessary to inject a second indicator (the indocyanine green dye) nor would specialized densitometry equipment be needed to detect the dye curve. Unfortunately, the only two reports of its use in the critical care setting produced conflicting results about its accuracy when compared with double indicator dilution calculations of EVLW [28, 30].

Although the use of indocyanine green dye and temperature change is the most common method of determining EVLW by the double-indicator dilution technique, other alternatives are still being evaluated. One promising possibility is to use hypertonic (3%) saline as the non-diffusible indicator, measuring changes in blood electrical conductivity instead of dye dilution [31, 32]. The obvious advantage, of course, is that one could avoid the need for using green dye.

Quantifying Increases in Pulmonary Vascular Permeability

Simply quantifying the amount of pulmonary edema does not distinguish whether the etiology represents a hydrostatic form of pulmonary edema or one due to lung injury *per se* (with its associated increase in vascular permeability). Accordingly, a quantitative measure of pulmonary edema, while a desirable component of a lung injury evaluation, cannot by itself be sufficient.

As with pulmonary edema, a number of techniques that are appropriate for clinical application have been developed to evaluate pulmonary vascular permeability. The most straightforward method is to simply sample and analyze alveolar edema fluid for its protein concentration. If the endothelial barrier is intact, the protein concentration in the fluid should be significantly less than that in plasma. With injury, the concentration of protein in the edema fluid should approach that of plasma. However, sampling errors, dilution with lavage fluid, or fluid resorption during edema resolution could all potentially affect the relationship between injury and the assessment of that injury by this simple technique.

The protein concentration of alveolar edema fluid can be determined from samples obtained (by direct aspiration from distal airways or via bronchoalveolar lavage (BAL)). In directly obtained samples, the protein concentration in the fluid should be significantly less than that in plasma if the endothelial barrier is intact and continues to truly function as a semi-permeable membrane (edema-to-plasma protein ratio < 0.65). However, with injury, the concentration of protein in the edema fluid should approach that of plasma (ratio > 0.75) [33–36]. Patients with values between 0.65–0.75 are not readily classified.

The technique for obtaining alveolar edema fluid by direct aspiration is straightforward, although not always successful. A suction catheter with a 14–18 gauge catheter attached is blindly advanced through an endotracheal tube until it reaches a "wedged" position. Fluid is collected with gentle suction, into a standard suction trap, sometimes after several attempts, and sometimes only after patient repositioning. In some instances, all maneuvers are unsuccessful and no fluid at all is obtained.

While this method is safe, quick, non-invasive, and inexpensive, it can only be performed in intubated patients. Also, it underestimates injury at times, since proteins in the alveolar space which precipitate into hyaline membranes will not be represented in the fluid sample. Furthermore, as the edema resolves, the protein concentration in the remaining fluid will increase [34]. Since edema may begin to resolve within hours of the onset of injury, the direct sampling method should lose specificity with time. In general, the measurements of protein concentration from directly sampled alveolar fluid, can only be used to differentiate hydrostatic from permeability forms of pulmonary edema when the samples are obtained within several hours of the onset of injury.

While a threshold value of 0.75 for the edema-to-plasma protein ratio may indicate that injury is present, there is no evidence that the actual value above 0.75 will correlate with the severity of injury to the alveolar-capillary membrane. However, since injury interferes with the size selectivity of the endothelial barrier, an analysis of the edema fluid composition for protein size might indicate greater injury as size selectivity was lost [37, 38]. Once again, greatest specificity would be expected at early times after the onset of pulmonary edema, since alveolar proteins are also cleared in a size-dependent fashion [39].

A modification to direct sampling is to obtain the edema fluid via BAL. With this approach, 3–5 aliquots of 30–50 mL saline are instilled either via a blindly positioned catheter [34] or via a bronchoscope positioned under direct visualization [40–42]. Although most studies report that the protein concentration in BAL fluid of ARDS patients is higher than in non-ARDS patients [40–42], the sensitivity and specificity of this approach have never been determined. It might be predicted that both would suffer because it would be nearly impossible to control for the effects of dilution caused by BAL, in different studies or patients.

Perhaps the most common clinical method of determining whether or not the integrity of the capillary endothelial barrier has been compromised is to measure the time-dependent accumulation of an intravenously administered radioactively-labeled protein tracer into lung tissue [43, 44]. Both albumin and transferrin (with approximately comparable molecular weights) have been used as protein tracers; technetium^{99m}, gallium^{68}, and indium^{113m} have been used as the radioactive labels.

After the radioactive tracer is injected intravenously, activity within lung tissue is detected and recorded for minutes to hours with one of several kinds of external radiation detection devices: probes, gamma cameras, or PET cameras have all been used successfully. Since these devices cannot distinguish whether activity within the lung tissue originates from the blood or extravascular space, similar time-activity data must be simultaneously obtained from the blood, either by measuring activity within the cardiac blood pool of the right or left ventricle with the same external detection system, or by measuring the protein activity in separately obtained blood samples [44, 45]. The blood volume within the lung tissue region-of-interest must also be determined, either by using a single protein tracer and assuming that all the protein activity at the beginning of the data collection period is intravascular (in which case one must also assume that intravascular volume does not change during the data collection period technique [46]), or by using a second tracer which can be assumed to remain intravascular (usually radioactively labeled red blood cells). The latter option is theoretically attractive since changes in intravascular volume during the data collection period can also be monitored (usually about 1–2 h) [44]. However, there is little reason to believe that intravascular volume in fact changes in a unidirectional manner during this brief period of time in clinically stable subjects.

Intuitively, as the microvascular barrier becomes more "leaky" to macromolecules like albumin, the rate of labeled albumin accumulation within the lung should increase. This intuitive notion can be made explicit by analyzing the time-activity data as if they represented the transfer of labeled tracer between vascular and extravascular compartments. The movement of tracer between these two compartments can be represented mathematically as:

$$Q(t) = [V_b Bl(t)] + [K_1 Bl(t) \cdot e^{-k_2 t}]$$

where $Q(t)$ = the time-dependent amount of activity in the lung tissue (vascular plus extravascular compartments), V_b = the blood volume in the same lung tissue region, Bl(t) = the time-dependent concentration of activity in blood within the lung tissue region, K_1 is equivalent to PS, and k_2 is the rate constant for activity moving from extravascular to vascular compartments [47, 48]. When PS is divided by the blood volume (or plasma volume, if one knows the hematocrit) within the lung region under the radiation detector [43, 47, 48], the resulting term is referred to as the "pulmonary transcapillary escape rate" (PTCER = PS/V_b) with the units of a rate constant (fractional time). PTCER can be derived by several different approaches mathematically by considering the mass balance of tracer between blood and lung tissue. After taking into account underlying assumptions, these various approaches are all essentially equivalent [43, 47, 48].

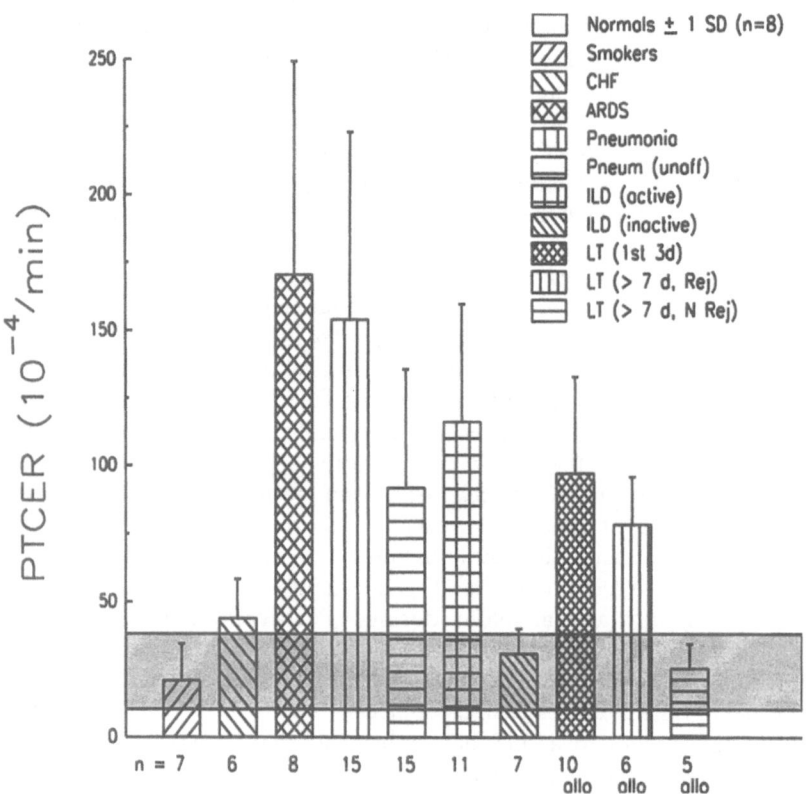

Fig. 3. The pulmonary transcapillary escape rate (PTCER), an index of vascular permeability, in a variety of patient groups. Note that PTCER is in the same range of values measured in normal subjects as in the following groups of subjects: In smokers without acute illness; clinically inactive interstitial lung disease (ILD); in lung allografts (allo) in patients without clinical rejection (Rej) post-lung transplantation (LT). PTCER is not significantly different from normal in patients with congestive heart failure (CHF). It is highest in patients with ARDS and in lung regions with lobar pneumonia. Other patient populations, including radiographically unaffected lung regions (unaff) in patients with pneumonia, have intermediate values. (From [44] with permission)

Most (but not all) experimental studies have shown that estimates of PTCER are insensitive to changes in hydrostatic pressure but are very sensitive to changes in membrane "porosity" [44, 49]. Ten fold increases in the estimate of PTCER have been measured in humans with ARDS with little or no increases detected in patients with heart failure (Fig. 3). While increased protein flux due to increased vascular permeability may be a *sine qua non* of lung injury associated with ARDS, significant increases in protein flux occur in many other conditions not necessarily characterized by pulmonary edema (Fig. 3). Nevertheless, measurements of PTCER do correlate well with morphologic indices of injury [50]. Thus, such measurements are a sensitive and probably accurate, even though non-specific, marker of injury.

Other techniques, based on indicator-dilution methods [51] or on the pulmonary uptake of an inhaled radiolabeled aerosol, are unlikely to be used extensively because of either complexity or technical artifacts which interfere with data interpretation [52].

Conclusion

The most urgent need to measure both EVLW and vascular permeability measurements is to allow a more precise definition of ARDS. Based on data shown in Fig. 3 and 4, it seems reasonable to suggest that ARDS could be defined as an EVLW >7 mL/kg with a PTCER >4–5 times the rate in normals. It would be interesting to see whether prognosis, or outcome in clinical trials, would be more easily interpreted than data using current definitions. Measurements of vascular permeability have never been incorporated into any clinical trial of therapy for pulmonary edema. It is possible that such measurements would also be more useful for prognosis since they can potentially quantify severity of injury. It is also possible that they might be used as a treatment endpoint surrogate for mortality

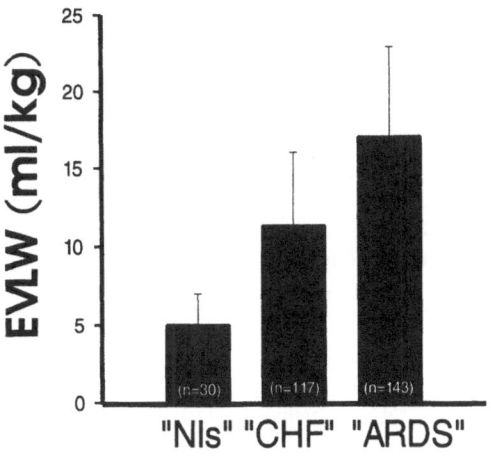

Fig. 4. Average (mean ± SD) amounts of extravascular lung water (EVLW) in patients requiring pulmonary artery catheterization without pulmonary edema (Nls), in patients with pulmonary edema and an elevated pulmonary wedge pressure (congestive heart failure, CHF), and in patients with pulmonary edema and a wedge pressure <18 mm Hg (ARDS). (Data combined from [15, 21, 23], as well as studies referred to therein)

in clinical trials. A number of studies have suggested that EVLW measurements could be used to help plan respiratory, diuretic, fluid, or other intensive care therapy [7, 15]. While logical, the actual cost versus benefit of using such measurements in patient care remains to be determined.

References

1. Staub NC (1978) The forces regulating fluid filtration in the lung. Microvasc Res 15:45–55
2. Staub N (1974) Pulmonary edema. Physiol Rev 54:678–721
3. National Heart L, and Blood Institute (NHLBI) (1994) NHLBI Task Force Report on Research in Cardiopulmonary Dysfunction in Critical Care Medicine. Bethesda, MD
4. Bernard GR, Artigas A, Grigham KL, et al (1994) The American-European Consensus conference on ARDS: Definitions, mechanisms, relevant outcomes, and clinical trial coordination. Am J Respir Crit Care Med 149:818–824
5. Murray VF, Mathay MA, Luce JM, et al (1988) Pulmonary perspectives: An expanded definition of the adult respiratory distress syndrome. Am Rev Respir Dis 138:720–723
6. Doyle RL, Szaflarski N, Modin GW, et al (1995) Identification of patients with acute lung injury: Predictors of mortality. Am J Respir Crit Care Med 152:1818–1824
7. Schuster DP (1997) The evaluation of pulmonary edema by measuring lung water. In: Tobin MJ (ed) Principles and Practice of Intensive Care Monitoring. McGraw, New York
8. Effros RM (1985) Lung water measurements with the mean transit time approach. J Appl Physiol 59:673–683
9. Sivak ED, Wiedemann HP (1986) Clinical measurement of extravascular lung water. Crit Care Clin 2:511–526
10. Allison RC, Carlile PV Jr, Gray BA (1985) Thermodilution measurement of lung water. Clin Chest Med 6:439–457
11. Pfeiffer U, Backus G, Blumel G, et al (1990) A fiberoptics based system for integrated monitoring of cardiac output, intrathoracic blood volume, extravascular lung water, O_2 saturation, and a-v differences. In: Lewis F, Pfeiffer U (eds) Practical Applications of Fiberoptics in Critical Care Monitoring. Springer Verlag, Berlin, pp 114–125
12. Wickerts CJ, Jakobsson J, Frostell C, et al (1990) Measurement of extravascular lung water by thermal-dye dilution technique: Mechanisms of cardiac output dependence. Intensive Care Med 16:115–120
13. Fallon KD, Drake RE, Laine GA, et al (1985) Effect of cardiac output on extravascular lung water estimates made with the Edwards lung water computer. Anesthesiology 62:505–508
14. Zeravik J, Borg U, Pfeiffer UJ (1990) Efficacy of pressure support ventilation dependent on extravascular lung water. Chest 97:1412–1419
15. Mitchell JP, Schuller D, Calandrino FS, et al (1992) Improved outcome based on fluid management in critically ill patients requiring pulmonary artery catheterization. Am Rev Respir Dis 145:990–998
16. Bock JC, Lewis FR (1990) Clinical relevance of lung water measurement with the thermal-dye dilution technique. J Surg Res 48:254–265
17. Laggner AN, Lenz K, Druml W, et al (1987) Reproducibility of thermal-dye lung water measurements by a lung water computer in critically ill patients. Crit Care Med 15:606–608
18. Mihm FG, Feeley TW, Jamieson SW (1987) Thermal dye double indicator dilution measurement of lung water in man: Comparison with gravimetric measurements. Thorax 42:72–76
19. Lewis FR, Elings VB, Sturm JA (1979) Bedside measurement of lung water. J Surg Res 27:250–261
20. Sivak ED, Starr NJ, Graves JW, et al (1982) Extravascular lung water values in patients undergoing coronary artery bypass surgery. Crit Care Med 10:593–596
21. Sibbald WJ, Warshawski FJ, Short AK, et al (1983) Clinical studies of measuring extravascular lung water by the thermal dye technique in critically ill patients. Chest 83:725–731

22. Gallagher JD, Moore RA, Kerns D, et al (1985) Effects of advanced age on extravascular lung water accumulation during coronary artery bypass surgery. Crit Care Med 13:68–71

23. Sibbald WJ, Short AK, Warshawski FJ, et al (1985) Thermal dye measurements of extravascular lung water in critically ill patients. Intravascular Starling forces and extravascular lung water in the adult respiratory distress syndrome. Chest 87:585–592

24. Haider M, Schad H (1990) Effect of positive end-expiratory airway pressure (PEEP) on extravascular thermal lung water estimation in the dog. In: Lewis F, Pfeiffer U (eds) Practical applications of fiberoptics in critical care monitoring. Springer Verlag, Berlin, pp 96–104

25. Bock J, Deuflhard P, Hoeft A, et al (1988) Thermal recovery after passage of the pulmonary circulation assessed by deconvolution. J Appl Physiol 64:1210–1216

26. Newman E, Merrell M, Genecin A, et al (1951) The dye dilution method for describing the central circulation. An analysis of factors shaping the time-concentration curves. Circ 4:735–746

27. Ramsey L, Puckett W, Jose A, et al (1961) Comparison of slope and mean transit time volumes by use of diffusible and non-diffusible indicators. Trans Assoc Am Physicians 74:280–289

28. Schuster DP, Calandrino FS (1991) Single versus double indicator dilution measurements of extravascular lung water. Crit Care Med 19:84–88

29. Elings VB, Lewis FR (1982) A single indicator technique to estimate extravascular lung water. J Surg Res 33:375–385

30. Baudendistel LJ, Kaminski DL, Dahms TE (1986) Evaluation of extravascular lung water by single thermal indicator. Crit Care Med 14:52–56

31. Tagawa M, Okano S, Hara Y, et al (1993) Evaluation of extravascular thermal volume in the lung in dogs with endotoxin-induced shock by double indicator dilution method using heat and sodium ions. J Vet Med Sci 55:87–91

32. Arakawa M, Kambara K, Segawa T, et al (1993) Usefulness of sodium chloride as a non-diffusible indicator in the measurement of extravascular lung thermal volume in dogs. Med Biol Eng Comput 31:S67–S72

33. Matthay MA, Eschenbacher WL, Goetzl EJ (1984) Elevated concentrations of leukotriene D4 in pulmonary edema fluid of patients with the adult respiratory distress syndrome. J Clin Immunol 4:479–483

34. Matthay MA, Wiener-Kronish JP (1990) Intact epithelial barrier function is critical for the resolution of alveolar edema in humans. Am Rev Respir Dis 142:1250–1257

35. Fein A, Grossman RF, Jones JG, et al (1979) The value of edema fluid protein measurement in patients with pulmonary edema. Am J Med 67:32–38

36. Sprung CL, Rackow EC, Fein IA, et al (1981) The spectrum of pulmonary edema: Differentiation of cardiogenic intermediate non-cardiogenic forms of pulmonary edema. Am Rev Respir Dis 124:718–722

37. Sprung CL, Long WM, Marcial EH, et al (1987) Distribution of proteins in pulmonary edema. The value of fractional concentrations. Am Rev Respir Dis 136:957–963

38. Holter JF, Weiland JE, Pacht ER, et al (1986) Protein permeability in the adult respiratory distress syndrome. Loss of size selectivity of the alveolar epithelium. J Clin Invest 78:1513–1522

39. Hastings RH, Grady M, Sakuma T, et al (1992) Clearance of different-sized proteins from the alveolar space in humans and rabbits. J Appl Physiol 73:1310–1316

40. Steinberg K, Mitchell D, Maunder R, et al (1993) Safety of bronchoalveolar lavage in patients with the adult respiratory distress syndrome. Am Rev Respir Dis 148:556–561

41. Steinberg K, Milberg J, Martin T, et al (1994) Evolution of bronchoalveolar cell populations in the adult respiratory distress syndrome. Am J Respir Crit Care Med 150:113–122

42. Clark J, Milberg J, Steinberg K, et al (1995) Type III procollagen peptide in the adult respiratory distress syndrome: Association of increased peptide levels in bronchoalveolar lavage fluid with increased risk for death. Ann Intern Med 1223:17–23

43. Roselli RJ, Riddle WR (1989) Analysis of non-invasive macromolecular transport measurements in the lung. J Appl Physiol 67:2343–2350

44. Schuster DP (1995) What is acute lung injury? What is ARDS? Chest 107:1721–1726

45. Roselli R, Harris T. (1989) Lung fluid and macromolecular transport. In: HK C, MP (eds) Respiratory physiology: An analytical approach. Marcel Dekker, New York pp 633–735

46. Schuster DP (1989) Positron emission tomography: Theory and its application to the study of lung disease. Am Rev Respir Dis 139:818–840
47. Mintun MA, Dennis DR, Welch MJ, et al (1987) Measurements of pulmonary vascular permeability with PET and gallium-68 transferrin. J Nucl Med 28:1704–1716
48. Mintun MA, Warfel TE, Schuster DP (1990) Evaluating pulmonary vascular permeability with radiolabeled proteins: An error analysis. J Appl Physiol 68:1696–1706
49. Abernathy VJ, Pou NA, Wilson TL, et al (1995) Non-invasive measurements of albumin flux into lung interstitium with increased microvascular pressure. Am J Physiol 269:H288–H296
50. Velazquez M, Weibel ER, Kuhn CD, et al (1991) PET evaluation of pulmonary vascular permeability: A structure-function correlation. J Appl Physiol 70:2206–2216
51. Dawson C, Roerig D, Linehan J (1989) Evaluation of endothelial injury in the human lung. Clin Chest Med 10:13–24
52. Peterson BT (1992) Permeability: Theory vs. practice in lung research. Am J Physiol 262:L243–L256

ALI and the Alveolar Epithelial Barrier

M. A. Matthay, B. Levin, and G. Verghese

Introduction

Until recently, the critical importance of the alveolar epithelial barrier in the pathogenesis of and recovery from severe acute lung injury had not been appreciated. However, progress in two areas has created a breakthrough in our understanding of the importance of the alveolar epithelium in ARDS. First, in the past 10 years, the mechanisms that regulate transport of fluid and protein across the normal alveolar epithelial barrier have been identified. Second, there are now new data regarding the mechanisms responsible for injury to the lung epithelial barrier and on the process of alveolar epithelial cell repair. Therefore, it is now possible to study the resolution and recovery of lung injury in both the experimental and clinical settings.

In order to relate the function of the alveolar epithelial barrier to ARDS, this chapter is divided into three parts. The first section discusses the distribution of pulmonary edema between the interstitium and airspaces of the lung, with an emphasis on the mechanisms that regulate transport of fluid and protein across the alveolar epithelial barrier. The second reviews experimental and clinical studies that have provided evidence regarding mechanisms of alveolar epithelial barrier injury. The third section reviews clinical and experimental studies that provide information on the role of the alveolar epithelial barrier in the resolution of lung injury. Some of the information contained in this chapter has been discussed in a prior publication [1].

Alveolar Fluid and Protein Transport

Physiologic and Morphologic Basis for Interstitial and Alveolar Edema

In order to appreciate the morphologic basis of the development of pulmonary edema, it is necessary to recall the normal structure of the alveolar-capillary unit. The alveolar capillaries in the lung are surrounded by an interstitial space, which is separated from the airspaces by the alveolar epithelial barrier. Under normal conditions, some fluid and a small amount of protein filters into the interstitium from the lung capillaries through small gap junctions in the endothelium [2]. The tight junctions between the cells of the normal alveolar epithelium are much tighter than the gap junctions between endothelial cells [2,3]. Thus, the alveolar epithelium offers substantial resistance to the passive movement of liquid and protein into the alveoli.

Physiologically there are two types of pulmonary edema: hydrostatic and increased permeability edema [2,4]. Hydrostatic pulmonary edema develops because of elevated pressure within the pulmonary microcirculation, usually because of left heart failure. Permeability pulmonary edema develops because of an increase in the permeability of the lung endothelial barrier leading to an abnormal extravascular accumulation of fluid. In general, these two types of pulmonary edema are distinct [4]. However, elevated pulmonary vascular pressures in the presence of increased lung vascular permeability have been shown in both experimental and clinical studies to be an important mechanism by which an increased quantity of edema fluid collects in the lung [5, 6]. Therefore, the contribution of elevated hydrostatic pressures to the development of lung injury is important in some experimental models, as well as in some clinical cases of ARDS.

In both hydrostatic and increased permeability pulmonary edema, there is a rise in the net flux of fluid from the vascular to the interstitial space of the lung. Approximately 500 mL of edema fluid can collect in the interstitium of the lung before the pressure is high enough for edema fluid to break through the epithelium and flood the airspaces [2]. Pulmonary edema fluid contains both liquid and protein. Initial samples of pulmonary edema fluid from patients with cardiac failure have a protein concentration that generally ranges from 2 to 4 g/100 mL. In patients with increased permeability pulmonary edema, the edema fluid has a protein concentration between 4 and 6 g/100 mL [4]. The distinction between hydrostatic and increased permeability mechanisms for pulmonary edema formation can usually be made by analyzing the ratio of the protein concentration in pulmonary edema fluid to the protein concentration in plasma [2, 4]. If the ratio is less than 0.65, then the edema fluid is a transudate, diagnostic of hydrostatic forces causing the extravascular accumulation of edema fluid in the lung. If the ratio is greater than 0.75, the pulmonary edema fluid reflects an increase in permeability, although as discussed below, the edema fluid must be obtained before resolution of alveolar edema has begun. If the ratio is between 0.65 and 0.75, then the type of pulmonary edema is indeterminate [7]. The cellular content of the edema fluid depends on associated conditions, such as hemorrhage or inflammation. There are always red blood cells, and usually a few monocytes and neutrophils in hydrostatic pulmonary edema; in most causes of increased permeability, the number of neutrophils is greater [8, 9].

In ARDS, there is compelling experimental and clinical evidence that there is an increase in both endothelial and epithelial permeability to protein [2, 4, 7]. However, as mentioned above, there may also be elevated pulmonary vascular pressure which contributes to the quantity of edema fluid that collects in the lung. Also, it is possible experimentally and in some clinical circumstances for markedly elevated microvascular hydrostatic pressures to actually cause a transient permeability injury to the endothelial barrier of the lung [10, 11].

What specific role does the alveolar epithelial barrier play in the development of pulmonary edema? First, because the epithelium is a much tighter barrier than the endothelial airspace, and because the extra-alveolar interstitial space can expand, pulmonary edema fluid can collect in the interstitium of the lung without flooding the airspaces [2]. However, when a critical pressure is reached, the epithelial barrier opens in response to the elevated interstitial pressure [2]. The sites or locations of airspace flooding have never been established with certainty, although some studies suggest that in some cases alveolar edema may develop from the passage of interstitial fluid through distal extra-alveolar epithelial locations with retrograde filling of the alveoli [12]. However, some severe cases of ARDS, caused by low pH gastric aspiration, sepsis, or some types of necrotizing pneumonia, can cause direct injury to the alveolar epithelial barrier with denuding of the alveolar epithelial type I cells [13]. When this type of injury develops, direct translocation of interstitial edema fluid into the alveoli occurs.

Mechanisms of Alveolar Fluid Clearance

Once the airspaces have flooded with edema fluid from the interstitium of the lung, what mechanisms are available for its removal? In order to address this issue, we instilled a protein solution (autologous serum or plasma or 5% albumin in Ringer's lactate) into the distal airspaces of sheep, and measured the removal of this fluid from the air spaces. Since protein is removed from the airspaces of the lung very slowly because of the normally tight alveolar epithelial barrier [14], we were able to use the concentration of protein in the airspaces as an indicator of alveolar fluid clearance. Interestingly, the concentration of protein in the air spaces progressively increased to levels well above those of plasma [15, 16]. Over time, the alveolar protein concentration increased in proportion to the removal of the liquid volume from the air spaces and the lung as a whole (Table 1). These observations in sheep led us to propose that the process of alveolar fluid clearance required an active ion transport process [15]. In subsequent clinical studies, we found the same pattern of protein concentration during the resolution of pulmonary edema in patients (Table 2) [4].

Subsequent *in vivo* studies from our own and other laboratories have confirmed that the process of alveolar fluid reabsorption requires an active process

Table 1. Alveolar liquid clearance in sheep as reflected by progressive concentrations of protein in the air spaces of the lung

Time (h)	Alveolar protein concentration (g/100 mL)		Lung liquid clearance (% of instilled)
	Initial*	Final*	
>4	6.3 ± 0.6	8.4 ± 0.6	33
>12	5.9 ± 0.4	10.2 ± 1.2[a]	59[a]
>24	6.4 ± 0.6	12.9 ± 1.9[a]	76[a]

Data as mean ± SD – [a] p < 0.05 compared to other groups (From [15, 16] with permission)

and does not depend on lung inflationor transpulmonary pressure. For example, in studies in both sheep and dogs, the mode of ventilation (positive pressure or spontaneous) did not alter the rate of alveolar liquid clearance [15, 16, 17]. In addition, even the removal of all ventilatory support did not alter the rate of clearance [18]. In order to provide direct evidence for the role of sodium transport in the process of alveolar fluid reabsorption *in vivo*, we found that alveolar fluid reabsorption in sheep [19] and rabbits [20] could be inhibited with amiloride, an inhibitor of apical sodium channel uptake, as well as by ouabain, an inhibitor of Na,K-ATPase enzyme activity [18]. *In vitro* studies of alveolar epithelial type II cells in monolayers as well as studies in Ussing chambers have demonstrated that these cells actively transport sodium from the apical to the basal surface [21, 22, 23]. Thus, current evidence indicates that the process of alveolar fluid reabsorption depends on sodium uptake into channels on the apical membrane of alveolar type II cells with subsequent active extrusion of the sodium to the basolateral interstitial space by the Na, K-ATPase pump [24, 25]. Chloride moves from the alveolar to the interstitial space to maintain electrical neutrality by as yet incompletely identified transcellular pathways [24]. Water crosses the alveolar barrier to maintain isoosmolar conditions, probably by specific proteinacious water transporters (CHIP 28) that have recently been identified [26] and described in the alveolar epithelium [27].

It is important to also emphasize that several experimental studies from our own and other laboratories have indicated that basal alveolar fluid clearance can be accelerated by β adrenergic agonist therapy. We have found an impressive increase in alveolar liquid clearance in our *in vivo* studies in sheep [28], dogs [17], and rats [29], although rabbits do not respond [20]. Other investigators have also found an impressive increase in sodium transport in isolated, alveolar type II cells [30] as well as in the isolated perfused rat lung [31]. Our most recent work indicates that β adrenergic agonist therapy increases alveolar liquid clearance in the isolated human lung [32], suggesting that basal clearance can be accelerated.

Mechanisms of Alveolar Protein Clearance

What are the mechanisms available for the removal of the excess protein in the airspaces of the lung? After flooding of the airspaces in hydrostatic pulmonary

Table 2. Resolution of alveolar edema in patients with acute pulmonary edema

Classification of edema	No.	Total protein concentration (g/100 mL)	
		Initial	Final
Hydrostatic	15	3.3 ± 1.0	4.8 ± 2.3[a]
Increased permeability	9	4.7 ± 0.9	6.8 ± 1.6[a]

Data as mean ± SD – [a] $p < 0.05$ – Data collected from [4]

edema, a considerable quantity of protein needs to be removed. Experimental studies from our laboratory have indicated that soluble protein is removed from the air spaces primarily by diffusion between alveolar epithelial cells [33]. Evidence for this conclusion is based in part on the clearance of molecules across the epithelium at a rate inversely related to molecular size [34]. There is undoubtedly some endocytosis and transcytosis of protein by alveolar epithelial cells, although most of our *in vivo* studies indicate that this mechanism cannot account for the majority of alveolar protein clearance when large quantities have entered the airspaces [33, 34]. Mucociliary clearance is a minor pathway, as is protein degradation and macrophage engulfment, at least in the uninjured lung [33]. However, in the setting of lung injury in which precipitation of protein occurs in the alveoli, the mechanism for removal of excess protein may include a more important role for alveolar macrophage engulfment and protein degradation.

Mechanisms of Alveolar Epithelial Injury

Experimental Data: Until recently, there was very little data concerning the pathogenesis of alveolar epithelial injury under experimental conditions simulating clinical ARDS. In fact, several studies from our laboratory indicated that the alveolar epithelial barrier is much more resistant to injury than the pulmonary vascular endothelium. For example, intravenous endotoxin causes significant injury to the lung endothelial barrier, but the combination of alveolar and intravenous endotoxin did not injure the alveolar epithelial barrier, based on physiologic and morphologic studies [35]. Also, the administration of an i.v. bolus of high dose live bacteria (*P. aeruginosa*) was not sufficient to cause injury to the alveolar epithelium despite the development of moderate pulmonary edema restricted to the interstitial space [36]. However, after maximizing the injury caused by live bacteria to the lung by administering a continuous infusion of live *P. aeruginosa* over 8 h in anesthetized sheep, 30% of the bacteremic animals developed an alveolar epithelial injury that correlated with the severity of systemic injury from sepsis [37]. Finally, preliminary data from our laboratory indicate that the alveolar epithelium is not injured during the ischemic phase of hemorrhagic shock in anesthetized rats [38]. In fact, we found that the development of septic or hemorrhagic shock was associated with an upregulation of the fluid clearance across the alveolar epithelium secondary to the release of endogenous catecholamines induced by low systemic arterial pressure [36, 38]. This effect was mediated through the activation of β adrenergic receptors situated on the alveolar epithelium, and was dependent on an augmented uptake of sodium by lung epithelial cells. Since our recent study indicated that β adrenergic agonist therapy stimulated epithelial liquid clearance in isolated human lung [32], the findings of these experimental studies strongly suggest that the endogenous release of epinephrine in human septic shock or in other pathological conditions, such as cardiogenic or traumatic shock, may result in an increase in the capacity of the lung epithelial barrier to remove excess alveolar fluid, a novel previously unrecognized mechanism promoting the clearance of alveolar edema.

By contrast, instillation of live bacteria (*P. aeruginosa*) into the airspaces caused injury to the lung epithelial barrier (Table 3). The results of these studies indicated that part of the mechanism for injury depends on specific extracellular products, such as exoenzyme S and phospholipase A [39]. Also, Dr. Folkesson and colleagues [40] recently reported that aspiration of hydrochloric acid into the distal airspaces of the lung caused a limited injury to the endothelial and epithelial barriers of the lung, resulting in the release of interleukin-8 (IL-8) by epithelial cells and by alveolar macrophages. Interestingly, the release of this chemokine resulted in a major amplification of the lung injury through the recruitment and activation of neutrophils in the pulmonary circulation. Finally, work from Dr. Jayr and colleagues [41] suggests that hyperoxia in rats exposed to over 40 h 100% oxygen causes injury to the alveolar epithelial barrier. Part of the mechanism for this effect may depend on toxic products of oxygen metabolism, as illustrated by the results of *in vitro* studies [42, 43].

Experimentally and clinically, neutrophils alone, recruited to the lung by specific chemotactic factors such as leukotriene B_4 (LTB_4), do not cause alveolar epithelial injury [16, 44]. However, in the presence of lung injury from blood-borne sepsis, primary pneumonia, or gastric aspiration, there may be a cumulative effect from recruitment of neutrophils to the airspaces of the lung and injury from the degranulation and release of neutrophil intracellular products into the airspaces [45, 46]. Future studies will be needed to work out the specific step by step mechanisms by which this injury occurs, although several clinical studies described below indicate that a pro-inflammatory milieu certainly exists in the airspaces of patients in whom lung injury has occurred (see next section).

Clinical Studies: Almost a decade ago, clinical studies from our group indicated that there were markedly elevated levels of leukotriene D_4 (LTD_4), a vasoconstrictor and bronchoconstrictor in patients with ARDS compared to control patients with hydrostatic pulmonary edema (Table 4) [10]. This observation was confirmed by other investigators who used bronchoalveolar lavage (BAL) to sample the distal air spaces of the lung [47]. However, LTD_4 levels did not correlate with or predict the severity of lung injury or a poor outcome [10]. In some patients, LTB_4 was el-

Table 3. Effect of alveolar *E. coli* endotoxin and *P. aeuroginosa* on bidirectional protein permeability across the alveolar epithelial barrier in sheep over 24 h

Condition	No	^{125}I-albumin in lung (% of instilled)	^{125}I-albumin in blood (% of instilled)	Alveolar fluid/plasma ^{131}I-albumin
Control sheep Serum alone	4	74±9	8±3	0.32±0.10
Group 4 (alv endo)	6	74±8	8±2	0.26±0.13
Group 6 (alv pseudo)	4	65±2[a]	12±1[a]	0.47±0.14[a]

Data as mean ± SD – [a] p < 0.05 – Data collected from [35]

evated, but this was not a uniform finding (Table 4). Recently, studies from our own unit have indicated that patients with ARDS have higher levels of some neuropeptides such as substance P in their alveolar edema fluid compared again with cardiogenic pulmonary edema controls (Table 4) [48]. Although it is unlikely that substance P is a primary cause of lung injury, it may be an important pro-inflammatory factor in the setting of ALI.

Finally, we have recently studied the concentrations and biologic activity of cytokines in the airspaces of the lung in order to correlate their presence with injury severity and outcome. IL-8 was markedly elevated in the undiluted alveolar edema fluid as well as in BAL from patients with ARDS compared to appropriate controls (Table 4) [49]. In addition, there was a tendency for IL-8 levels to be higher in patients who did not survive. It is not clear whether the higher IL-8 levels were a marker of inflammation in the lung or simply contributed to the severity of lung injury. Subsequently, other investigators have found additional clinical evidence for the importance of IL-8 in ARDS. For example, IL-8 concentrations in BAL were high in ARDS patients compared to controls [50] and in patients at risk for ARDS, IL-8 concentrations in BAL were higher in those who later developed ARDS than in those who did not [51].

Also, recent studies of IL-6 levels in patients with sepsis and ARDS showed elevated levels in the plasma and alveolar fluid of some patients [1]. There were also elevated concentrations of tumor necrosis factor (TNF) in the alveolar fluid of patients with ARDS, but there was considerable overlap with the values in patients with hydrostatic pulmonary edema (Table 4) [1]. These clinical studies at our institution provide a descriptive picture of several chemotactic and pro-inflammatory factors that are present in the airspaces of the lung (Table 4).

Other investigators have presented evidence for the presence of neutrophil elastase and other potentially injurious substances [52]. In addition, there may be important toxic concentrations of metabolites of oxygen radical metabolism that may cause lung injury, but measuring these compounds in the air spaces of the lung is very difficult. The specific role of these factors in injuring the alveolar epithelial barrier in patients with ALI will need to be examined systematically in experimental studies.

Table 4. Concentration of pro-inflammatory factors in pulmonary edema fluid from patients with hydrostatic and permeability pulmonary edema

Potential mediators of ALI	Alveolar edema fluid		Ref
	Hydrostatic	Permeability	
Leukotriene B_4, pmoles/mL	5.8 ± 4.6	10.2 ± 7.1	[10]
Leukotriene D_4, pmoles/mL	4.4 ± 1.1	18.5 ± 6.8[a]	[10]
Substance P, nmoles/mL	0.18 ± 0.09	0.57 ± 0.29[a]	[48]
TNF-α, μ/mL	8.9 ± 4.7	16.7 ± 14.6	[66]
IL-8, ng/mL	17 ± 34	73 ± 72[a]	[49]

Data as mean ± SD – [a] $p < 0.5$ compared to hydrostatic controls. Data collected from [1]

In summary, the mechanism for damage to the alveolar epithelial barrier may be specific to the type of injury. For example, injury to the alveolar epithelial barrier from a primary pneumonia may depend on extracellular products of the infecting organism rather than necessarily the products of neutrophils or macrophages [39]. In the case of gastric aspiration, some of the alveolar epithelial barrier injury probably occurs from the direct effects of gastric acid aspiration, though some may be mediated by inflammatory products of epithelial cells and macrophages, such as IL-8, that are subsequently recruited to the airspaces of the lung. The mechanism of blood-borne non-pulmonary sepsis-induced injury to the epithelial barrier is still not clear, though it may involve a cascade of mediators that in most cases depend on neutrophil-dependent mechanisms. Other factors may contribute to alveolar epithelial injury including the degree of alveolar distension from positive pressure ventilation, although the specific contribution of this potential mechanism in the setting of experimental and clinical ARDS needs further study [53].

Recovery and Repair in ALI

Because of our increased understanding of the role of the alveolar epithelial barrier in regulating fluid and protein balance under normal and abnormal conditions, it was possible to develop methods to monitor the function of the alveolar epithelial barrier. Two well described properties of the alveolar epithelial barrier that can be monitored experimentally are:
1) its relative impermeability to the bidirectional movement of protein, and
2) its capacity to remove excess alveolar fluid from the airspaces of the lung.

In several of our experimental studies, alveolar epithelial injury has been quantified by the degree of bidirectional or protein flux across the epithelial barrier; also, the net capacity of the alveolar epithelial barrier to remove excess alveolar fluid has been used as a marker of its overall function [28, 35]. Logically, in order to remove excess alveolar fluid, a significant fraction of the alveolar epithelial barrier must be sufficiently intact with normal tight junctions and a functioning sodium transport system.

For example, after severe oleic acid-induced pulmonary edema in sheep, the initial concentration of protein in edema fluid was equal to that in plasma, indicating a marked increase in protein permeability of both the lung endothelial and alveolar epithelial barriers [54]. In these studies, in spite of the early increase in epithelial permeability following administration of intravenous oleic acid, there was evidence that the epithelial barrier was beginning to recover between 5 and 8 h after the oleic acid was given. Alveolar protein concentration had risen to 30% above plasma protein concentration and there was a parallel decline in extravascular lung water, indicating that the epithelial barrier was capable of recovering soon after severe injury. Similar data is available from our recent studies in which rats were exposed to 100% oxygen for 40 h, resulting in a 30% increase in extravascular lung water and a modest increase in epithelial permeability to protein

[41]. However, when fluid was instilled into the airspaces of these rat lungs, it was removed normally and the rats even responded to an exogenous β adrenergic agonist (terbutaline) with an increase in the rate of alveolar liquid clearance. Thus, in the setting of mild to moderate lung injury or following severe injury, the alveolar epithelial barrier is apparently capable of removing fluid and providing a barrier to further alveolar flooding. This was also true in a study carried out in sheep over 24 h in which *P. aeruginosa* pneumonia caused a marked increase in epithelial permeability to protein, but after 24 h the epithelial barrier had recovered and net alveolar fluid clearance had occurred [35]. In recent studies in rats, we have found that TNF-α can up-regulate alveolar fluid clearance 24 h after the onset of Gram-negative pneumonia [55].

Our clinical studies have been designed to assess the function of the alveolar epithelial barrier in the first 12–24 h after the onset of ARDS. By measuring sequential concentrations of protein in alveolar fluid in such patients, it is possible to determine if fluid is being removed from the air spaces of the lung in spite of the presence of acute respiratory failure. In our initial study, we found that approximately 40% of patients with ARDS and increased permeability pulmonary edema were capable of removing some of their excess alveolar fluid within the first 12 h after injury [4]. This finding indicated that the epithelial barrier was functional and intact, at least to some degree. Interestingly, these patients had a lower mortality and a more rapid recovery than those who showed no evidence of alveolar fluid clearance in the first 12 h after onset. In that study, the patients who showed evidence of alveolar fluid reabsorption, displayed no significant difference in pulmonary arterial wedge pressure, levels of positive end-expiratory pressure (PEEP) and other indices of mechanical ventilation when compared to patients who had no evidence of alveolar fluid reabsorption. These results suggested that the patients who had no evidence of alveolar fluid protein concentration in the first 12 h had endothelial and/or epithelial injury sufficiently severe so that net alveolar fluid clearance could not occur. By contrast, patients who were able to concentrate their alveolar protein had evidence of net alveolar fluid reabsorption and a functionally intact and recovering alveolar barrier. In that same study, there was evidence of some improvement radiographically in the patients who had a rise in alveolar fluid protein concentration. Thus, this index of alveolar barrier function may be clinically useful as a prognostic index [55]. It is inexpensive, non-invasive, and independent of changes in the tidal volume or PEEP, interventions that may improve oxygenation, but not necessarily change the distribution of alveolar edema fluid or the total quantity of pulmonary edema in the lung. Also, it may be useful in several types of lung injury, as we recently reported in a case of salt water near-drowning [56].

The critical role of the alveolar epithelial type II cell in regenerating an intact alveolar wall in ARDS has been established in both experimental and clinical studies *in vivo* [57]. Although alveolar type II cells cover less than 5% of the total lung surface area, they are responsible for forming a new epithelial barrier following alveolar epithelial type I cell necrosis [13, 57]. The factors that promote alveolar wall regeneration are largely unknown. However, recent studies regarding the mechanisms of wound healing in non-pulmonary epithelial and endothelial cells have demonstrated the importance of extracellular matrix molecules, interaction of cell adhesion molecules and the autocrine and paracrine actions of growth factors in the lung [53].

In order to understand the basic function of the alveolar epithelial type II cell in wound healing, we recently developed an experimental *in vitro* model in which this phenomenon can be studied quantitatively [59]. The results indicate that the process of wound healing can be accelerated with transforming growth factor (TGF)-α, a growth factor that is present in the alveolar fluid of patients with ARDS [59]. The results also indicate that soluble and insoluble fibronectin accelerates wound healing [60].

In summary, it is likely that interaction of growth factors, cytokines, and extracellular matrix are important in determining the ability of the alveolar epithelial barrier to recover from lung injury [60-63]. More work is needed to determine the basic mechanisms of repair, as well as to identify why in some patients the process of repair is complicated by a destructive fibrosing alveolitis that results in obliteration of functional airspaces and a loss of vascular supply to the lung [64].

Conclusion

The central importance of the alveolar epithelial barrier in the pathogenesis and recovery from ALI has only recently been appreciated. Considerable progress has been made in understanding the basic mechanisms that regulate alveolar epithelial fluid clearance under normal and pathologic conditions. The alveolar epithelium is more resistant than the lung endothelium, particularly after blood-borne injury. The mechanisms that cause injury to the alveolar barrier are just beginning to be explored in different experimental models of lung injury. Also, recent *in vitro* work on mechanisms of alveolar epithelial repair after lung injury has provided new insights into its recovery.

Acknowledgment: This work was supported in part by NIH Grant HL51854 and HL5186.

References

1. Matthay MA, Folkesson HG, Campagna A, et al (1993) The alveolar epithelial barrier and acute lung injury. New Horizons 1:613–622
2. Matthay MA (1985) Pathophysiology of pulmonary edema. Clin Chest Med 6:301–314
3. Schneeberger-Keeley EE, Karnovsky MJ (1971) The influence of intravascular fluid volume on the permeability of the newborn and adult mouse lungs to ultrastructural protein tracers. J Cell Biol 49:319–327
4. Matthay MA, Wiener-Kronish JP (1990) Intact epithelial barrier function is critical for the resolution of alveolar edema in humans. Am Rev Respir Dis 142:1250–1257
5. Ohkuda K, Nakahara K, Binder A, et al (1981) Venous air emboli in sheep; reversible increase in lung microvascular permeability. J Appl Physiol 51:887–894
6. Unger KM, Shibel EM, Moser KM (1975) Detection of left ventricular failure in patients with the adult respiratory distress syndrome. Chest 67:8–13

7. Matthay MA, Eschenbacher WL, Goetzl EJ (1984) Elevated concentrations of leukotriene D4 in pulmonary edema fluid of patients with the adult respiratory distress syndrome. J Clin Immunol 4:479–483
8. Ratnoff WD, Matthay MA, Wong MYS (1988) Sulfidopeptide-leukotriene peptidases in pulmonary edema fluid from patients with the adult respiratory distress syndrome. J Clin Immunol 8:250–258
9. Cohen AB, Stevens MD, Miller EJ, et al (1993) Neutrophil-activating peptide-2 in patients with pulmonary edema from congestive heart failure or ARDS. Am J Physiol 264:L490–L495
10. Bachofen H, Schurch S, Wiebell ER (1993) Experimental hydrostatic pulmonary edema in rabbit lungs. Am Rev Respir Dis 147:997–1004
11. Colice GI, Matthay MA, Bass E, et al (1984) Neurogenic pulmonary edema. Am Rev Resp Dis 130:941–948
12. Gee MH, Williams DO (1979) Effect of lung inflation on perivascular cuff fluid volume in isolated dog lung lobes. Microvasc Res 19:209–216
13. Bachofen M, Weibel ER (1977) Alterations of the gas exchange apparatus in adult respiratory insufficiency associated with septicemia. Am Rev Respir Dis 116:589–615
14. Gorin AB, Stewart PA (1979) Differential permeability of the endothelial and epithelial barriers to albumin flux. J Appl Physiol 47:1315–1324
15. Matthay MA, Landolt CC, Staub NC (1982) Differential liquid and protein clearance from the alveoli of anesthetized sheep. J Appl Physiol 53:96–104
16. Matthay MA, Berthiaume Y, Staub NC (1985) Long-term clearance of liquid and protein from the lungs of unanesthetized sheep. J Appl Physiol 59:928–934
17. Berthiaume Y, Broaddus VC, Gropper MA, et al (1988) Alveolar liquid and protein clearance from normal dog lungs. J Appl Physiol 65:585–593
18. Sakuma T, Pittet JF, Jayr C, et al (1993) Alveolar liquid and protein clearance in the absence of blood flow or ventilation in sheep. J Appl Physiol 74:176–185
19. Matthay MA (1985) Resolution of pulmonary edema: Mechanisms of liquid, protein, and cellular clearance from the lung. Clin Chest Med 6:521–545
20. Smedira N, Gates L, Hastings R, et al (1991) Alveolar and lung liquid clearance in anesthetized rabbits. J Appl Physiol 70:1827–1835
21. Mason RJ, William MC, Widdecombe JH, et al (1982) Transepithelial transport by pulmonary alveolar type II cells in primary culture. Proc Natl Acad Sci USA 79:6033–6037
22. Goodman BE, Crandall ED (1982) Dome formation in primary cultured monolayers of alveolar epithelial cells. Am J Physiol 243:C96–C100
23. Cheek K, Kim KJ, Crandall ED (1989) Tight monolayers of rat alveolar epithelial cells: Bioelectric properties and active sodium transport. Am J Physiol 256:C688–C693
24. Saumon G, Basset G (1993) Electrolyte and fluid transport across the mature alveolar epithelium. J Appl Physiol 74:1–15
25. Matalon S (1991) Mechanisms and regulation of ion transport in adult mammalian alveolar type II pneumocytes. Am J Physiol 261:C727–738
26. Verkman AS (1992) Water channels in cell membranes. Ann Rev Physiol 54:97–108
27. Folkesson HG, Matthay MA, Hasegawa H, et al (1994) Transcellular water transport in lung alveolar epithelium through mercurial-sensitive water channels. Proc Natl Acad Sci USA 91:4970–4974
28. Berthiaume Y, Staub NC, Matthay MA (1987) Beta-adrenergic agonists increase lung liquid clearance in anesthetized sheep. J Clin Invest 79:335–343
29. Jayr C, Garat C, Meignan C, et al (1994) Alveolar liquid and protein clearance in anesthetized, ventilated rats. J Appl Physiol 76:2636–2642
30. Goodman BE, Fleischer RS, Crandall ED (1983) Evidence for active Na^+ transport by cultured monolayers of pulmonary alveolar epithelial cells. Am J Physiol 245:C78–C83
31. Crandall E, Heming RA, Palombo RL, et al (1986) Effects of terbutaline on sodium transport in isolated perfused rat lung. J Appl Physiol 60:289–294
32. Sakuma OG, Nakada T, Nishimura T, et al (1994) Alveolar fluid clearance in the resected human lung. Am J Respir Crit Care Med 150:305–10
33. Berthiaume Y, Albertine KH, Grady M, et al (1989) Protein clearance from the air spaces and lungs of unanesthetized sheep over 144 h. J Appl Physiol 67:1887–1897

34. Hastings RH, Grady M, Sakuma T, et al (1992) Clearance of different-sized proteins from the alveolar space in humans and rabbits. J Appl Physiol 73:1310–1316
35. Wiener-Kronish JP, Albertine KH, Matthay MA (1991) Differential responses of the endothelial and epithelial barriers of the lung in sheep to *Escherichia coli* endotoxin. J Clin Invest 88:864–875
36. Pittet JF, Wiener-Kronish JP, McElroy M, et al (1994) Stimulation of alveolar epithelial liquid clearance by endogenous release of catecholamines in septic shock. J Clin Invest 94:663–671
37. Pittet JF, Wiener-Kronish JP, Serikov V, et al (1995) Resistance of the alveolar epithelium to injury from septic shock in sheep. Am J Respir Crit Care Med 151:1093–1100
38. Pittet JF, Brenner T, Modelska K, Matthay MA (1996) Alveolar liquid clearance is increased by endogenous catecholamines in hemorrhagic shock in rats. J Appl Physiol 81:830–837
39. Wiener-Kronish JP, Sakuma T, Kudoh I, et al (1993) Alveolar epithelial injury and pleural empyema in acute *P. aeruginosa* pneumonia in anesthetized rabbits. J Appl Physiol 75:1661–1669
40. Folkesson HF, Matthay MA, Hebert C, et al (1995) Acid aspiration induced-lung injury in rabbits is mediated by IL-8 dependent mechanisms. J Clin Invest 96:107–116
41. Garat C, Meignan M, Matthay M, et al (1997) Alveolar epithelial fluid clearance mechanisms are intact after moderate hyperoxic lung injury in rats. Chest (In press)
42. Kim KJ, Suh DJ (1993) Asymmetric effects of H_2O_2 on alveolar epithelial barrier properties. Am J Physiol 264:L308–L315
43. Bauer ML, Beckman JS, Bridges RJ, et al (1992) Peroxynitrite inhibits sodium uptake in rat colonic membrane vesicles. Biochem Biophys Acta 1104:87–94
44. Martin T, Pistorese B, Chi EY, et al (1984) The effect of leukotriene instilled into the airspaces of the human lung. J Clin Invest 84:1609–1619
45. Tate RM, Repine JE (1991) Neutrophils and the adult respiratory distress syndrome. Am Rev Respir Dis 144:251–252
46. Martin TM, Pistorese BP, Hudson LD, et al (1991) The function of lung and blood neutrophils in patients with the adult respiratory distress syndrome. Am Rev Resp Dis 144:254–262
47. Fowler AA, Hyers TM. Fisher B, et al (1987) The adult respiratory distress syndrome: cell populations and soluble mediators in the air spaces of patients at high risk. Am Rev Resp Dis 136:1225–1231
48. Espiritu RF, Pittet JF, Matthay MA, et al (1992) Neuropeptides in pulmonary edema fluid of adult respiratory distress syndrome. Inflammation 16:509–517
49. Miller EJ, Cohen AB, Nagao S, et al (1992) Elevated levels of NAP-1/Interleukin-8 are present in the airspaces of patients with the adult respiratory distress syndrome and are associated with increased mortality. Am Rev Respir Dis 146:427–432
50. Chollet-Martin S, Montravers P, Gilbert C, et al (1993) High levels of interleukin-8 in the blood and alveolar spaces of patients with pneumonia and adult respiratory distress syndrome. Infect Immun 61:4553–4559
51. Donnelly SC, Strieter RM, Kunkel SL, et al (1993) Interleukin-8 and development of adult respiratory distress syndrome in at risk patients groups. Lancet 341:643–647
52. Wiener-Kronish, JP, Gropper M, Matthay MA (1990) The adult respiratory distress syndrome: Definition and prognosis, pathogensis and treatment. Br J Anaesth 65:107–129
53. Matthay MA (1989) New modes of mechanical ventilation for ARDS: How should they be evaluated? Chest 95:1175–1177
54. Wiener-Kronish JP, Broaddus VC, Albertine KH, et al (1988) Relationship of pleural effusions to increased permeability pulmonary edema in anesthetized sheep. J Clin Invest 82:1422–1429
55. Rezaiguia S, Garat C, Delclaux C, et al (1997) Acute bacterial pneumonia in rats increases alveolar epithelial fluid clearance by a tumor necrosis factor-alpha-dependent mechanism. J Clin Invest 99:325–335
56. Cohen DS, Matthay MA, Cogan MG, et al (1992) Acute lung injury associated with salt water drowning: New insights. Am Rev Respir Dis 146:794–796
57. Adamson IY, Bowden DH (1974) The type II cell as progenitor of alveolar epithelial regeneration: A cytodynamic study in mice after exposure to oxygen. Lab Invest 30:35–42

58. Barrandon Y, Green H (1987) Cell migration is essential for sustained growth of keratinocytes colonies: The role of TGF-α and EGF. Cell Vol 50:1131–1137
59. Kheradmand F, Folkesson HG, Shum L, Derynck R, Pytela R, Matthay MA (1994) Transforming growth factor-α (TGF-α) enhances alveolar epithelial cell repair in a new *in vitro* model. Am J Physiol 267:L728–L738
60. Garat C, Kheradmand F, Albertine KH, et al (1996) Soluble and insoluble fibronectin increases alveolar epithelial wound healing *in vitro*. Am J Physiol 271 (Lung Cell Mol Physiol) 15:L844–L853
61. Chestnutt AN, Kheradmand F, Folkesson HG, et al (1997) Soluble transforming growth factor-α is present in the pulmonary edema of patients with acute lung injury. Chest 111: 652–656
62. Strandjord TP, Clark JG, Hodson WA, et al (1993) Expression of transforming growth factor alpha in mid-gestation human fetal lung. Am J Resp Cell Mol Biol 8:266–272
63. Matthay MA (1995) Fibrosing alveolitis in the adult respiratory distress syndrome. Ann Int Med 122:65–66
64. Raaberg L, Nexo E, Buckley S, et al (1992) Epidermal growth factor transcription, translation and signal transduction by rat type II pneumocytes in culture. Am J Resp Cell Mol Biol 6: 44–49
65. Pittet JF, Mackersie RC, Martin TR, et al. (1997) Biological markers of acute lung injury: Prognostic and pathogenetic significance. Am J Respir Crit Care Med 155:1187–1205
66. Matthay MA, Wiener-Kronish JP, Mathison J, et al (1991) Biologically active tumor necrosis factor in the pulmonary fluid of patients with either hydrostatic or increased permeability edema. Am Rev Resp Dis 143:A804 (abstract)

Mechanical Ventilation

Pressure-Volume Relationship in the Injured Lung

V. M. Ranieri, C. Tortorella, and S. Grasso

Introduction

Acute lung injury (ALI) is known to be associated with abnormal mechanical properties of the respiratory system with hallmark features of a reduction in functional residual capacity (FRC) and a reduction in static compliance of the respiratory system [1]. Measurements of the inspiratory pressure-volume (P-V) curves of the respiratory system have been hence used in mechanically ventilated patients with ALI as a means of assessing their status and progress [1] and to optimize the use of positive end-expiratory pressure (PEEP) [2] and of mechanical ventilation [3–8]. However, although FRC and static compliance of the respiratory system are known to be reduced in patients with ALI [4], the question remains whether this simply reflects the downward displacement along the P-V relationship described in normal humans [9] or an overall change of the characteristic P-V relationship of the respiratory system [10].

The aims of this chapter are
1) to review the basic physiology of the P-V relationship of the respiratory system in patients with ALI;
2) to describe the methodology to assess the P-V relationship in the clinical setting; and
3) to discuss the potential role of chest wall mechanics in the alteration of the elastic properties of the respiratory system in patients with ALI.

The Volume-Pressure Diagram

Physiology

The elastic properties of the respiratory system, lungs and chest wall have been described in terms of volume-pressure relationship since the pioneering work of Rohrer and the classic analysis by Rahn and colleagues (Fig. 1) [11]. Although a single P-V relationship can actually describe the relation between changes in volume and changes in pressure in some simple solid such as an elastic balloon, it may be surprising that a single P-V diagram can also describe the elastic properties of the total respiratory system. Indeed, the respiratory system is a complex set of solid structures, namely the lungs and airways plus rib cage, abdomen, and res-

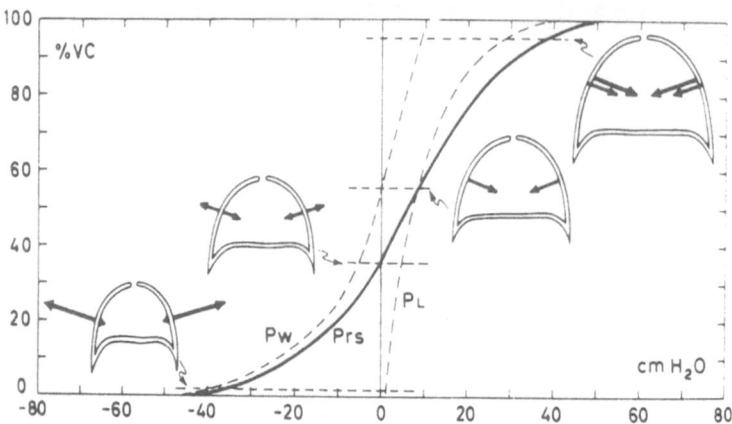

Fig. 1. Static volume-pressure curves of the lung (PL), chest wall (PW) and total respiratory system (Prs) during relaxation in normal humans in sitting posture. Large arrows: static forces of the lung and chest wall; horizontal broken line: volume for each drawing; VC: vital capacity. (From [8] with permission)

piratory muscles. Solid structures, unlike fluids, have a proper shape and react with inhomogeneously distributed opposing forces to deformations. In the respiratory system, there are structures with remarkable different degrees of stiffness. In a hypothetical scale of stiffness, the rib cage would be at one extreme (the farthest from fluids) and the lungs at the other extreme (closer to fluid-like behavior) with the diaphragm in between depending from the degree of contraction. Due to the enormous amount of variables describing elastic changes of solid structures having complex form and internal inhomogeneity, there can be little doubt that only few and extremely motivated experts would have continued to investigate the mechanical properties of the respiratory system in health and disease using the complex equations of mechanics in three dimensions. Fortunately for the development of knowledge in clinical respiratory physiology, it has been shown that, accepting a reasonable degree of simplification, a single P-V diagram may be adapted to describe the elastic behavior of the respiratory system [9].

If isolated lungs are inflated from residual volume (RV) to total lung capacity (TLC) with stepwise increasing levels of pressure, it is difficult to observe any rough deformation in the overall shape. In contrast, the rib cage diaphragm compartment is made of structures with different degree of stiffness. Indeed, plotting changes in volume against changes in diameter, the breathing movements describe circles and not lines, indicating that the shape of the rib cage changes from inspiration to expiration [12]. At any lung volume, during the breathing cycle, there are two thoracic shapes, one for inspiration and one for expiration. This difference increases during resistive loaded breathing. It has been attributed to the inhomogeneous distribution of inspiratory muscle force during contraction [12]. If respiratory muscles are relaxed, the degree of chest wall anysothropism is much lower and the relation between changes in volume and changes in pressure can be described by a single P-V relationship also for the chest wall [9, 12]. In other words, the changes of shape which are likely to occur have small influence on lung volumes. Therefore, the single P-V relationship seems adequate to describe the elastic behavior of the total respiratory system, i.e. the relation between changes in volume and changes in pressure, at least for the vast majority of clinical conditions.

Fig. 1 shows the static P-V relationship of the respiratory system, chest wall and lung in normal human beings. The chest wall and the lung are mechanically in series; thus the sum of the pressure exerted by the chest wall (PcW) and by the lung (PL) equals the pressure of the respiratory system (Prs):

$$PcW + PL + Prs,$$

whereas the change of volume (ΔV) of each part must be equal (except for shifts of blood volume) and equal to that of the respiratory system

$$\Delta VcW = \Delta VL = \Delta vrs$$

FRC represents the equilibrium volume of the respiratory system (Vr) as determined by the opposing elastic forces of the lungs and the chest wall. It is identified by the crossing of the P-V curve of the respiratory system with the zero pressure line. Under normal circumstances, FRC corresponds to the amount of gas in the lungs and the airways at the end of a tidal expiration. This suggested the use of two parameters: FRC, as the volume at the end of tidal expiration and; Vr, as the relaxation volume of the respiratory system. In normal subject, FRC and Vr corresponds to the end-expiratory lung volume (EELV), and the static pressure developed by the lungs and chest wall are equal and opposite. The PW (estimated from the esophagus) is about -5 cmH$_2$O, PL is about $+5$ cmH$_2$O and Prs is 0 (Fig. 1). The resting volume of the lung is at about 55% VC. Above this volume, both the chest wall and lung recoil inwards, and below this volume, the chest wall recoils outward; Hence the lung and the chest wall behave like two opposing springs. In the midrange of volume, the two structures contribute about equally to the change in static pressure with change in the volume of the total respiratory system. At the maximal inspiratory level (100% VC), the lung is farthest from its resting state, and at a minimal volume (0% VC) the chest wall is farthest from its resting state. As the extremes of volumes are approached, static pressures increase rapidly with further volume change; At high volume, this is due to the lung, at low volume to the chest wall.

The Elastic Properties of the Respiratory System during ALI

Representative P-V curves of mechanically ventilated patient with ALI are shown in Fig. 2. A common characteristic of this kind of patients is the reduced range of volume excursion due to the reduction in the ventilating units, and hence a smaller change in volume for unit of change in pressure. In a significant number of pa-

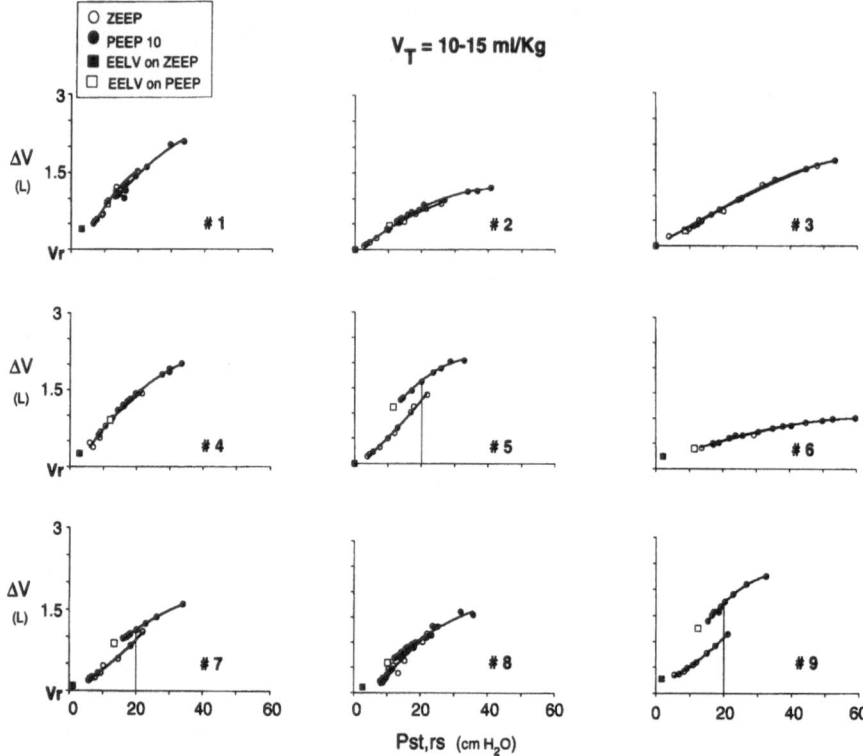

Fig. 2. Static inflation volume-pressure relationships of the total respiratory system in nine patients with ALI during mechanical ventilation with VT 10–15 ml/kg during ZEEP (open circles)
and 10 cmH₂O of PEEP (closed circles). ΔV: changes in lung volume relative to the elastic equilibrium point of the respiratory system (Vr); Pst, rs: static elastic recoil pressure. Total PEEP (intrinsic PEEP + externally applied PEEP) values and the corresponding increase in end-expiratory lung volume relative to Vr (EELV) are indicated on ZEEP (closed squares) and on 10 cmH₂O
of applied PEEP (open squares). (From [8] with permission)

tients, the initial part of the P-V curve, at the very low lung volume, is remarkably
even flatter than the rest of the curve with a so called "lower inflection point"
(Pinf) separating a lower compliance from an optimal compliance. Following
this, an upper inflection point (UIP) may be present where the P-V curve flattens
at lower values of VT (VT) than normal subjects (Fig. 3) [13, 14], representing the
point where elastance starts to increase, and hence represents the volume at
which stretching and overdistension of at least some alveolar structures occurs
[3]. Similarly, Pinf is thought to represent the average critical pressure required to
re-open previously closed peripheral airways and/or alveoli [3–5, 8, 15, 16].

Lower Inflection Point (Pinf): Lungs excised from the chest and allowed to deflate freely do not exhale all their air. Some gas (minimal volume) remains trapped because of 1) closure of small airways, and 2) the resistance of the alveoli to col-

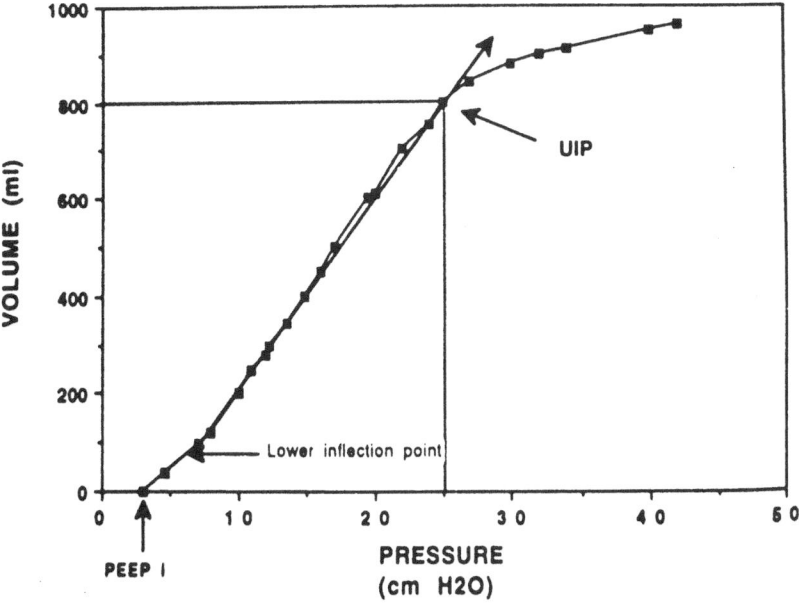

Fig. 3. Pressure-volume curve of the respiratory system obtained in one representative patient. Intrinsic PEEP (PEEPi), present during the course of mechanical ventilation, represents the starting point of the curve. The lower and upper inflection points are indicated. (From [3] with permission)

lapse. The minimum lung volume is below 0% of VC, i.e. the residual volume in the intact thorax is greater than the minimum volume. When excised lungs are inflated, an opening pressure, necessary to re-expand the collapsed alveoli, appears on the P-V curve [17]. Gas-free lungs occur in all newborn mammals before their first breath, and it is well known that the first breath requires a much higher inspiratory pressure than successive breaths. Also the P-V curve, below 0% VC, measured by Cavagna, et al. [18] in experimental animals, showed that the lowest part of the curve had an expanded hysteresis. A similar event occurs in parts of expanded lungs that have had occlusion of their bronchial connection. In this case, the gas trapped behind the occlusion is absorbed into the pulmonary circulation because of the subatmospheric gas pressure of venous blood. Cavagna, et al. [18] indicated that alveoli resist complete approximation of their wall with a pressure of -5 to -15 cmH$_2$O. This pressure is not exerted thereafter; in other words, atelectatic alveoli do not re-expand spontaneously, but a greater positive pressure is required to re-expand the atelectatic alveoli. In this lowest volume range, the hysteresis is expanded too. The significant change in static mechanical characteristic of gas-free lungs compared with partially expanded lungs is the appearance of a minimum opening pressure described by Lindskog and Bradshaw [19] for adult animal lungs, and by Wilson and Farber [20] and Gruenwald [21] in newborn infants. These authors observed that until a certain pressure was reached, no gas entered gas-free lungs. If the pressure was increased slowly above the initial opening pressure, the lungs filled irregularly until complete expansion of the lung had occurred. This property of a minimum opening pressure before expansion begins may be readily observed in living animals when atelectasis has been produced artificially [22], and it stands in sharp contrast to the elastic behavior of lungs expanded with physiologic salt solution [17]. In adult humans, opening pressure, i.e. the transpulmonary pressure able to recruit collapsed alveoli, amounts roughly to 20 cmH$_2$O [17]. Alveolar dimension is correlated to the amount of opening pressure in a sense that larger alveolar radius corresponds to lower opening pressure values [17].

Mancebo reviewed the data concerning the measurement of the opening pressure in ALI patients, reporting values ranging between 8–12 cmH$_2$O and indicating that this pressure should represent the PEEP level able to recruit [23]. Some discrepancies appear therefore between clinical [23] and physiologic [17] data regarding the minimal opening pressure value able to recruit collapsed alveoli. As discussed above, in gas-free preparations, the opening pressure, i.e. the transpulmonary pressure able to recruit collapsed alveoli, in adult humans amounts roughly to 20 cmH$_2$O [17]. The gravitational gradient in pleural [24] and alveolar expanding pressure [25] may solve this discrepancy between values of critical opening pressure in clinical and physiologic settings [26]. ALI is highly asymmetric along the vertical axis in a sense that a healthy "non-dependent" lung zone lean on an atelectatic "dependent" lung region [27]. In between, a "poorly inflated" area was described [28]. Elastic pressure of the respiratory system (Pel, rs) represents the sum of elastic pressures of the lungs (Pel, l) and of the chest wall (Pel, cw) according to the formula [9]:

$$Pel, rs = Pel, l + Pel, cw.$$

It has been shown that a vertical gradient exists in intrathoracic pressure [24]. When the percentage of lung height is plotted against the pleural surface pressure at the resting volume of the respiratory system, a negative curvilinear relationship is found [24]. In the supine position and at the 100% of lung height ("non-dependent" zone), pleural pressure ranged from −5 to −3 cmH$_2$O, while at the 0% of lung height ("dependent" zone), pleural pressure is equal to 0 cmH$_2$O. At the 50% of the lung height ("poorly inflated" zone), pleural pressure ranged between −3 and −2 cmH$_2$O [23]. The increased lung weight due to the gravitational distribution of edema observed in the lungs of ALI patients [27] may enhance the relative amount of the vertical gradient in intrathoracic pressure. The elastic pressure that must be applied to the respiratory system to reach the opening pressure value in the "poorly inflated" zone is hence lower than in the "dependent" area because of the relative contribution of pleural pressure. Besides, in such "poorly inflated" area, alveoli have a radius larger than the alveoli in the "dependent" area, because of the vertical gradient of alveolar expansion [25]. All these phenomena may therefore explain that a pressure level of 8–12 cmH$_2$O is able to re-open collapsed alveoli only in the "poorly inflated" area but not in the "non-dependent" lung region. Higher pressure levels must be applied to recruit permanently alveoli in the "dependent " region. However, such pressure levels may enhance a "regional" risk of barotrauma in the normal "non-dependent" area and in the recruited alveoli of the "poorly aerated" zone [23].

Upper Inflection Point (UIP): In normal subjects, the UIP of the P-V curve is obtained at a lung volume approximately 85 to 90% of total lung capacity [29]. In patients with ALI, a flattening of the P-V curve occurs at much lower volume than in normal patients, as reported in some early studies of ALI [14]. Any further increase of pressure above the UIP, via augmentation of VT or PEEP, or both, provides less increase in volume, indicating that maximal stretching of at least some alveolar structures has been reached, exposing them to overdistension [3]. In a recent study, Roupie and co-workers [3] showed that patients with ALI had a UIP at low airway pressure (26 ± 6 cmH$_2$O) and lung volumes (850 ± 200 mL) indicating that the presence of a severe restrictive process. In Roupie's study, the mean UIP corresponded to a transpulmonary pressure of about 23 cmH$_2$O. These levels of airway or transpulmonary pressure are much lower than those expected to cause overdistension-induced injury in normal animals [30–37].

Functional Residual Capacity

Although measurement of absolute lung volume is a complicated procedure in mechanically ventilated patients and is not a common practice in the intensive care unit (ICU), several studies have documented that FRC is markedly lower than normal (from 20 to 40% of predicted values) in patients with ALI [4, 15, 38–41]. It is thought that the reduction in FRC is the result of the reduction in the amount of ventilating alveoli due to terminal airspace flooding and collapse, rather than the consequence of increased lung recoil with normal chest wall mechanics [42, 43]. Gas dilution studies showed that as little as one third to one half of the total lung volume at FRC is air filled during the acute phase of injury [39, 44] and this small amount of functional tissue must bear the entire burden of gas exchange. That the reduction of FRC in ALI is the consequence of a reduction in ventilating lung tissue has been supported also by computer tomography (CT) scan numbers distribution which was displaced toward areas of densities, rather than being concentrated in areas with normal ventilation, compared to healthy lungs [4], with a significant, positive correlation between absolute FRC measured with the helium dilution techniques and the amount of normally aerated areas, computed by the CT scan numbers distribution [4]. It has been suggested that the injured lung should be considered a "baby lung" rather than a "stiff lung" [4].

Hysteresis

Hysteresis may be defined as the "failure of a system to follow identical paths of response upon application or withdrawal of a forcing agent" [9]. Static elastic hysteresis is a common phenomenon exhibited by the various structural tissues of the body [45] and by some non-biological materials as rigid metals and rubber. The degree of hysteresis is comparatively small in the respiratory system. In the physiologic range of VT and respiratory frequency, static hysteresis is negligible [9].

Three mechanisms accounting for volume-pressure hysteresis may be involved for normal lungs:
1) surface tension changes [46, 47];
2) stress relaxation [48]; and
3) alveolar recruitment [49].

The latter is clearly of major importance when the lungs are collapsed. Under these conditions, the opening pressure must be exceeded, thus at equal pressures, the number of alveolar units open is much greater during deflation than during inflation, as shown by experimental preparations of collapsed lungs [49, 50].

Similar results may be obtained when terminal airway, rather than alveoli are collapsed [45]. In physiological conditions, it appears likely that in quantitative terms, recruitment is not a major factor in static hysteresis observed at FRC [17]. It is evident from diffusion and inert gas washout studies, that the difference in compliance between inspiration and expiration during quite breathing of normal subjects is primarily due to hysteresis of surfaces forces and the related phenomenon of a difference in tissue configuration [51]. On the contrary, when the reduction in volume induces lung collapse, closing of alveoli (alveolar atelectasis) or of alveolar sacs, ducts and terminal small airways (alveolar collapse), alveolar recruitment becomes a more important factor causing hysteresis [51]. With ALI, the changes in inspiratory and expiratory resting compliance, observed in animal models [50, 52, 53] and in patients [54, 55], are therefore caused by progressive inspiratory alveolar recruitment and expiratory derecruitment. On the contrary, a depletion of alveolar surfactant, described in patients with ALI [56, 57], should not increase hysteresis, since it has been demonstrated that static P-V curves of animals in whom surfactant was depleted by alveolar lavage with saline solution did not show any hysteresis [58].

P-V Curve to set Mechanical Ventilation

In an attempt to limit the lung injury caused by ventilation at high lung volumes, it has been suggested that one should limit VT to maintain the end-inspiratory volume less than UIP [3–5]. The concept is that UIP represents the point where elastance starts to increase and hence represents the volume at which stretching and overdistension of at least some alveolar structures occurs [3]. Similarly, it has been suggested that ventilation should occur above Pinf [1–5, 13, 14, 16] to ensure recruitment of the lung, since Pinf is thought to represent the average critical pressure required to re-open previously closed peripheral airways and/or alveoli. Animal studies showed that, even at lower airway pressures, mechanical ventilation can damage and aggravate lung function in previously injured lungs [30–37]. Fu and colleagues [59] demonstrated that endothelial and epithelial injury, which the authors call "stress failure", increased when lung volume was increased from a transpulmonary pressure of 5 to only 20 cmH_2O. Hernandez and co-workers [36] demonstrated that mechanical ventilation with peak airway pressure of 25 cmH_2O was deleterious to rat lungs injured by oleic acid infusion. In patients with ALI, peak alveolar pressure as low as 25 cmH_2O may also be harmful. In normal subjects, the static transpulmonary pressure measured at total lung capacity may vary from 24 to 36 cmH_2O, depending on age and sex [29]; even if compliance of the aerated lung is close to normal in ALI [43], such pressures are likely to place the aerated lung areas close to maximal stretching. Amato and co-workers [60] recently compared the conventional approach to mechanical ventilation (VT of 10–15 mL/kg, minimum PEEP guided by FiO_2 and hemodynamics and normal $PaCO_2$) with an alternative approach consisting of maintenance of end-expiratory pressure above Pinf, VT <6 mL/kg, peak pressure <40 cmH_2O, permissive hypercapnia and stepwise utilization of pressure-limited modes of ventilation. Amato, et al. found that such new approach to the ventilatory management of patients with ALI markedly improved lung function, increasing the chances of early weaning and lung recovery during mechanical ventilation [60]. Valenza and co-workers [61] examined the hypothesis that particular ventilatory strategies can promote lung injury by causing release of pro-inflammatory mediators. P-V curves were obtained in the isolated lungs of 9 rats. Then, the animals were randomly assigned to three ventilatory strategies: Control (VT = 7 mL, PEEP = 5 cmH_2O), high volume-high PEEP (VT = 15 mL, PEEP = 15 cmH_2O), and high volume-low PEEP (VT = 15 mL, PEEP = 0 cmH_2O). They found that after 100 min of mechanical ventilation, high volume-low PEEP ventilation caused a decreased in compliance together with a rightward shift of P-V curve and a 23-fold increase in the cytokine concentration [61]. These experimental and clinical data therefore seem to suggest the hypothesis that ventilatory strategies not based on the morphology of the inspiratory P-V curve may promote and/or sustain the pulmonary inflammatory reaction in patients with ALI. This implies that ventilator settings causing "ventilatory stress" as defined by the occurrence of tidal ventilation below the Pinf and/or above the UIP may cause a "ventilator-induced secondary lung injury" directly related to the incorrect ventilator settings.

Methods to Assess P-V Curve

The Super-syringe Technique

To detect these aspects at the bedside, and to assess the status and progress of patients with ALI [62, 63], optimising the clinical use of PEEP [2, 15], the super-syringe technique has been proposed to measure the static inflation P-V curve (Fig. 4) [15, 63]. Briefly, when the super-syringe method is used to assess the status of the elastic properties of the respiratory system, mechanically ventilated ALI patients are placed in supine position while being sedated and paralysed to permit the slow inflation of the lung with a predetermined gas volume. Pulmonary

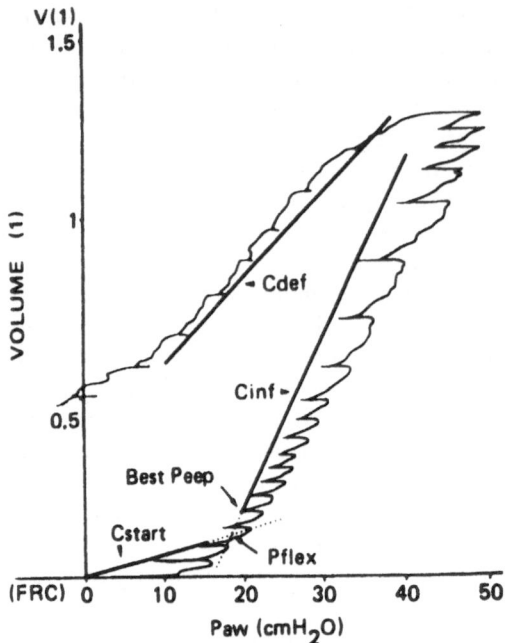

Fig. 4. A typical P-V curve obtained in a patients with ALI using the super-syringe technique. Paw: airway opening pressure, V: lung volume above relaxed equilibrium volume of the respiratory system, Cdef: deflection compliance, Cinf: inflation compliance, Cstart: starting compliance, Pinf: pressure at the lower inflection point. (From [4] with permission)

secretions are carefully aspirated and the air-tightness of the cuff is checked. Inspiratory FiO_2 is increased up to 100% and the ventilators is set to deliver a single deep breath up to total lung capacity. The patient is then disconnected from the ventilator and, at the end of a prolonged expiration to Vr, is connected to the super-syringe. The procedure begins with inflation of 100–200 ml of gas (the syringe should be filled with pure oxygen) using the syringe. Once this volume has been inflated, the plunger of the syringe stops for 2 or 3 sec in order to measure the elastic recoil of the respiratory system (Pst, rs). Then the respiratory system is inflated with intermittent pause until a volume of 25 mL/kg is introduced into the lung or an airway pressure of 40 cmH$_2$O is reached. When this occurs, deflation begun by slowly aspirating with the syringe using the same pauses and changes in volume as during inflation. Two P-V loops are inscribed one after the other, separated by a brief connection to the ventilator. These loops should be identical, if not the maneuver should be repeated (Table 1) [64–66].

Using the super-syringe technique, Matamis and co-workers [15] found that alterations of pulmonary mechanics, assessed by P-V curves, paralleled rather closely the natural history and evolution of ALI in man. Indeed, they found that early alveolar flooding was indicated by increased hysteresis, whereas reduced compliance, defined as the slope of the P-V curve during deflation, indicated late

Table 1. Different techniques to assess the pressure-volume relationship of the respiratory system in patients with ALI

Super-syringe technique
- Methods: Initial inflation of 100–200 mL of gas using the syringe filled with O_2. The syringe stops for 2–3 sec. Then the respiratory system is inflated with intermittent pause until a volume of 25 mL/kg or an airway pressure of 40 cmH$_2$O are reached
- Pro: It allows easy detection of the lower and upper inflection points
- Con: Requires sedation and paralysis, disconnection of the patient from the ventilator and special equipment. It is influenced by continuous gas exchange. Reflects a volume history characterized by prolonged expiration and deep inspiration with pure oxygen and hence different from the one of the patient connected to the ventilator

Rapid airway occlusion technique
- Methods: It is based on single-breath occlusions at different inflation during mechanical ventilation. Different inflation volumes are achieved by changing the respiratory frequency of the ventilator while keeping the inspiratory flow constant. Each occlusion is maintained until an apparent plateau in airway opening pressure is observed. This plateau pressure represents the static recoil pressure of the total respiratory system. The static inflation V-P curve is then constructed by plotting the different inflation volumes against the corresponding values of pressure
- Pro: The volume history preceding the measurements corresponds to the actual ventilatory pattern of the patient. Effects of continuous gas exchange are negligible because measurements are rapid. There is no need to disconnect the patient from the ventilator. The measurements do not require special devices
- Con: Requires sedation and paralysis. Results are not immediately available at the bedside. It may be difficult to identify a distinct lower and upper inflection points.

Constant flow technique
- Methods: Elastic properties may be determined from the airway opening pressure-time curve obtained during mechanical ventilation with constant inspiratory flow, based on the assumption that the rate of change of airway opening pressure is related to the elastance of the respiratory system
- Pro: The volume history preceding the measurements is fixed and corresponds to the actual ventilatory pattern of the patient in the clinical setting. There is no need to disconnect the patient from the ventilator. The measurements do not require special devices and is available, on line, at the bedside
- Con: Requires sedation and paralysis. It is difficult to identify a distinct lower and upper inflection points. May be affected by patient's and endotracheal tube resistance.

interstitial disease, and was correlated with the interstitial process quantified through the analysis of the chest X-ray film. In contrast, alveolar opacities were correlated with an increased hysteresis and an inflection point on the inspiratory part of the static P-V curve. The lower inflection point was first documented by Cook, et al. [22] in dogs with pulmonary edema. In studies on excised lungs, Glaister and co-workers [67–68] demonstrated that this inflection point on the inspiratory P-V curve was explained on the basis of re-opening of the units closed during the deflation. This phenomenon has likewise been found by Slustky, et al. [50] in oleic acid-induced edema. On these basis, Matamis and co-workers [40] concluded that, if this inflection point pressure corresponds to an opening airway pressure, the level of PEEP should be preferably set above that pressure, in order to prevent distal airway collapse at the end of expiration.

The measurements of the P-V curve with the super-syringe technique is relatively long and the results can therefore be influenced by continuing gas exchange on lung volume [4, 64]. In paralysed subjects, the rate of decrease in thoracic volume due to continuing gas exchange should amount to 110 ± 64 mL/min, involving a 50% over-estimation of the area of the hysteresis loop of the respiratory system using the super-syringe method [64]. Trying to overcome these limitations, Gattinoni and co-workers [4] proposed a complex algorithm to correct the measurement of the super-syringe P-V curve, taking into consideration gas exchange, temperature, humidity and gas compression. However, despite these correction factors, when the P-V curves is obtained with methods that do not require disconnection of the patients from the ventilator, and are not affected by volume leak due to gas exchange, the degree of hysteresis in mechanically ventilated ALI patients is minimal [66, 69]. Second, the super-syringe method involves disconnection from the ventilator and a prolonged expiration after deep inspiration with pure oxygen. This may affect the quantification of the opening pressure values in ALI patients through several mechanisms. The mechanical properties of the respiratory system depends on the volume history of the actual tidal ventilation [51]. At variance, the elastic properties assessed by the super-syringe technique reflects a volume history characterized by prolonged expiration and deep inspiration with pure oxygen [15]. Under these circumstances, in conditions of high alveolar instability, the disconnection from the ventilator may allow the collapse of alveolar units that are otherwise ventilated during mechanical tidal breathing. Besides, ventilation with pure oxygen may per se affect the morphology of the initial part of the inspiratory P-V curve causing the development of further atelectasis. An additional source of errors in the measurement of the alveolar opening pressure (i.e. the inflection point of the inspiratory P-V curve) with the super-syringe technique is the chest wall. As previously mentioned, in awake, normal, young and supine individuals, the inflection point on the inspiratory P-V curve of the total respiratory system, reflects a stiffer chest wall at low lung volume [9]. In older individuals, small airway closure may contribute to allow total respiratory system compliance at lung volumes close to supine FRC [70]. To the extent that the FRC is reduced in ALI patients, the change in total respiratory system compliance with increasing lung volume observed above the inflection point of the inspiratory P-V curve of ALI patients may in part therefore reflect decreased chest wall compliance with increasing volume [9].

The Rapid Airway Occlusion Method

To gather a better view of the elastic properties of the respiratory system and to assess the effects of PEEP on alveolar recruitment, possibly avoiding some of the methodological problems related to the super-syringe method, the rapid airway occlusion method has been developed [6–8, 71]. Briefly, this method is based on single breath occlusions at different inflation volumes within EELV and baseline VT during the clinically set mechanical ventilation of the patients. Different inflation volumes may be achieved by changing the respiratory frequency of the ventilator while keeping the inspiratory flow at baseline level. Each occlusion is maintained until an apparent plateau in airway opening pressure is observed. This plateau pressure, which is usually reached in about 3 sec, represents the static recoil pressure of the total respiratory system (Pst, rs). After each test breath, baseline ventilation may be resumed until the value of pressure recorded at the airway opening (Pao) returned to its pre-test configuration (usually in less than 4 breaths) (Fig. 5). The static inflation P-V curves (static P-V curve) is then constructed by plotting the different inflation volumes against the corresponding values of Pst, rs (Fig. 6) [6]. Compared with the super-syringe, the "rapid airway occlusion" technique is a method for determining the static volume-pressure relationship in which:

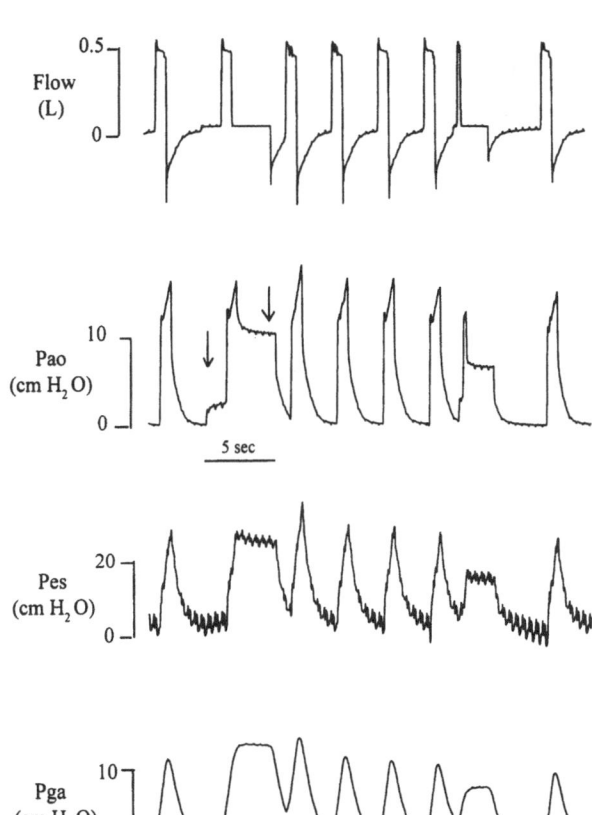

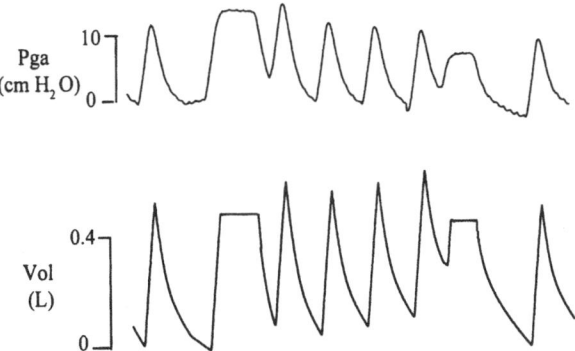

Fig. 5. Experimental record illustrating the test breaths performed to obtained the static P-V curve using the interrupter technique. From top to bottom, flow, airway opening (Pao), esophageal (Pes) and gastric (Pga) pressures and volume (Vol). Arrows indicate end-expiratory and end-inspiratory occlusions. (Modified from [82] with permission)

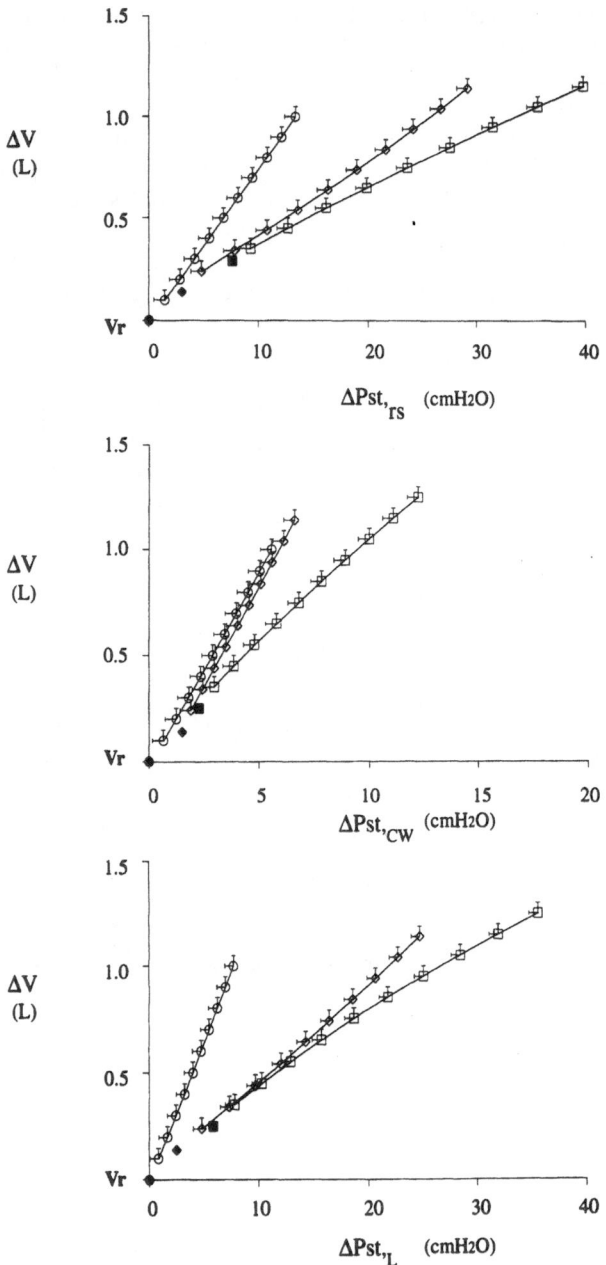

Fig. 6. Mean static inflation volume-pressure curves of the respiratory system (rs), chest wall (CW) and lung (L) in pre-operative cardiac surgery (open circle), surgical ALI (open square), and medical ALI patients (open diamond). Intrinsic PEEP and the corresponding increase in end-expiratory lung volume relative to the elastic equilibrium volume of the respiratory system (Vr) are indicated on the volume-pressure curves (closed signs). ΔV: changes in lung volume relative to Vr. (Modified from [82] with permission)

1) The volume history preceding the measurements of Pst, rs is fixed and corresponds to the actual ventilatory pattern of the patient in the clinical setting;
2) The individual measurements of Pst, rs are rapid and, hence, the effects of continuing gas exchange on lung volume are negligible;
3) There is no need to disconnect the patient from the ventilator; and
4) measurements do not require special devices (Table 1) [71].

Using the rapid airway occlusion method, the elastic properties of the respiratory system were studied in ALI patients [3, 6–8, 72]. In these studies, changes in lung volume with mechanical ventilation and PEEP were referred to the elastic equilibrium volume of the respiratory system, known by allowing the patient to breath out till Vr during a prolonged expiration (Fig. 7). Therefore, it was possible to quantify the alveolar volume recruited by PEEP as the shift along the volume axis at a fixed value of Pst, rs of the P-V curve on PEEP referred to the P-V curve on zero end-expiratory pressure (ZEEP). We observed that on ZEEP some patients showed an upward concavity of the static inflation P-V curve, i.e. there was a progressive increase with compliance as inflating volume increased. In contrast, in other patients, the static inflation P-V curve on ZEEP was characterized by an upward convexity and a progressive reduction in compliance as volume increase (Fig. 2).

A progressive increase in compliance with inflation volume (as reflected by a P-V curve concave toward the volume axis) means that a progressive alveolar recruitment is obtained within end-expiratory lung volume and VT. These findings are apparently in contrast with the concept that only PEEP greater than the inflection point of the inspiratory P-V curve is able to recruit [15]. Beside, a close inspection of Fig. 2 reveals that an inflection point on the inspiratory P-V curve is not always evident, and often below the tidal end-expiratory lung volume [72]. These experimental evidences suggest that in some ALI patients the inflation up to VT is already able to recruit some alveolar units. In these patients application of PEEP produced a further recruitment as evidenced by the shift of the P-V curves on ZEEP referred to the initial P-V curve on ZEEP. The fact that application of PEEP caused a further recruitment changing the elastic properties of the respiratory system (as evidenced by the change in shape and position of the P-V curve) may reflect the fact that the recruited alveoli with PEEP have a totally different elastic behavior compared to the alveoli normally ventilated. In line with these considerations, it was found that in some patients the volume recruited with PEEP increased the concavity of the inspiratory P-V curve, i.e. the new alveoli recruited to the tidal ventilation improved the elastic characteristic of the respiratory system, while in other patients the recruited alveoli caused a worsening in the elastic properties of the respiratory system as reflected by the fact that PEEP made the inspiratory P-V curve convex rather than concave toward the volume axis. In the patients who had an inspiratory P-V curve with a progressive reduction in compliance as volume inflated the lung, the application of PEEP caused a volume displacement along the P-V curve obtained on ZEEP. This indicates that the increase in FRC induced by PEEP did not result in recruitment of previously collapsed alveoli but caused the hyperinflation of the normal, already ventilated alveoli.

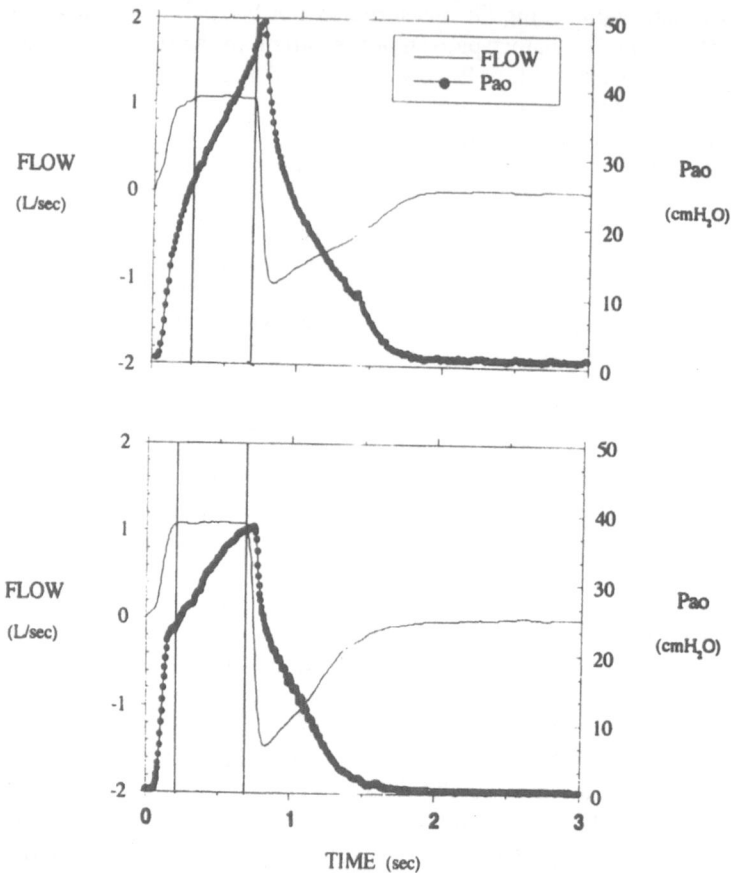

Fig. 7. Records of flow (right axis) and airway opening pressure (Pao) (left axis) in two patients with ALI. Vertical line indicate the steady-state portion of the pressure-time curve when inspiratory flow was constant. An upward concavity of the pressure-time profile during constant flow (top) indicates the progressive decrease in compliance with tidal inflation due to alveolar overdistension; a downward concavity (bottom) indicates a progressive increase in compliance compliance with tidal inflation due to alveolar recruitment. (From [7] with permission)

The Constant Flow Methods

In order to overcome the need for intermittent airway occlusions, the "constant flow inflation" or "pulse" method [73] has been proposed. Simply stated, static compliance of the respiratory system may be determined from the slope of the linear aspect of the P-V curve obtained during passive mechanical ventilation during constant inspiratory flow (dynamic P-V curve). This method is based on the assumption that when inspiratory flow is constant during passive inflation of the relaxed respiratory system, the rate of change of airway opening pressure (Pao) is related to the elastance of the respiratory system [73]. Using this method,

Suratt, et al [74] computed static compliance of the respiratory system (Cst, rs) in 9 mechanically ventilated patients with acute respiratory failure (ARF) of different etiologies. They found that the values of Cst, rs, measured with the "constant flow" method, closely correlated with the Cst, rs measured with the "rapid airway occlusion" technique. These results were later confirmed by Rossi, et al in some but not in all patients included in his study [75].

We recently showed [7] that, in mechanically ventilated patients with ALI, the pattern observed in the dynamic P-V curve was similar to the one observed in the static P-V curve obtained with the rapid occlusion technique. The shape of the P-V curves were assessed by fitting a second order polynomial equation that was fitted to the experimental points for both static and dynamic P-V curves [76]:

$$\Delta V = a + b\ Pst, rs + c\ Pst, rs^2 \qquad\qquad (Eq.\ 1)$$

$$and \quad \Delta V = a + b\ Pao + c\ Pao^2 \qquad\qquad (Eq.\ 2)$$

A highly significant correlation between static (Eq. 1) and dynamic (Eq. 2) non-linear coefficients was found, the regression lines not being significantly different from the line of identity. In patients who had a dynamic P-V curve on ZEEP with a convex shape (negative value of the non-linear coefficient in Eq. 2, and in whom compliance decreased with inflating volume (hyperinflation) [77], the application of PEEP resulted in a volume displacement along the dynamic P-V curve on ZEEP without any alveolar recruitment. On the contrary, in patients who had a dynamic P-V curve on ZEEP with a progressive increase in compliance during inflation (i.e. a concave shape and a positive value of the non-linear coefficient in Eq. 2), application of PEEP resulted in a shift along the volume axis of the dynamic P-V curve, indicating recruitment of previously collapsed alveoli. The effects of PEEP on cardiac index, shunt, O_2 delivery and PaO_2 were significantly more pronounced in patients who had a concave shape of the dynamic P-V curve than in patients who had a convex shape of the dynamic P-V curve on ZEEP. As a consequence, the shape of the dynamic P-V curve on ZEEP was able to predict the effects of PEEP on alveolar recruitment, gas exchange and hemodynamics as well as the static P-V curve. These results indicate that the simple observation of the dynamic P-V curve on ZEEP (i.e. pressure-time curve) makes it possible to predict the effects of PEEP on alveolar recruitment, hemodynamics and gas-exchange (Fig. 7) [77].

On a theoretical basis, the time course of applied pressure during constant flow inflation should be characterized by an immediate step change in Pao due to the resistive components of the respiratory system, abruptly followed by a progressive increase in Pao (steady-state portion of the dynamic P-V curve), reflecting the elastance of the respiratory system [73, 75]. However, this may not always be present in patients (Fig. 1, top) [75]. This discrepancy between theoretical [73] and clinical application of the "pulse" or "constant flow" technique [75] may be due to pendelluft (i.e. the time required to achieve a steady-state in flow to each respiratory unit with different time constants) [73] and/or viscoelasticity [78]. Another element that limits our analysis to the steady-state portion of the dynamic P-V curve is the fact that the ventilator used in our present study (Siemens 900C) is incapable of providing a constant flow from the very onset of inspiration. All these elements preclude analysis of the initial pressure and volume events, although analysis under the subsequent steady-state portion of the dynamic P-V curve remains valid. Several ventilators are actually equipped with monitoring system providing the dynamic P-V curve continuously, non-invasively and at the bedside. Our physiological data show that the shape of the dynamic P-V curve ("constant flow inflation" method) provides information regarding the elastic properties of the respiratory system and may be considered as an alternative to the static P-V curve ("rapid airway occlusion" technique). We may therefore conclude that inspection of the shape of the dynamic P-V curve, represents a simple and non-invasive clinical tool that allows to detect hyperinflation and predicts the effects of PEEP on alveolar recruitment, hemodynamics and gas exchange (Table 1).

Role of Altered Mechanics of The Chest Wall

Given the underlying pulmonary injury that is present in patients with ALI, the increase in static elastance is thought to reflect mainly alterations of the elastic properties of the lung rather than of the chest wall [15]. However, a number of studies have also reported an increase in chest wall elastance in mechanically ventilated patients with ALI [79, 80]. Mutoh and co-workers [81] showed in an animal model that abdominal distension markedly altered respiratory mechanics by its effect on the elastic properties of the chest wall. Based on these results, the increase in chest wall elastance found in patients with ALI was ascribed to abdominal distension [80]. However, the specific role played by abdominal distension in the impairment of the elastic properties of the respiratory system has never been assessed in patients with ALI.

Recently, we [82] partitioned chest wall and lung mechanics, assessed the role of abdominal distension and verified whether the underlying disease responsible for ALI may affect the impairment of respiratory mechanics. The P-V relationship of the respiratory system and lung in 9 patients with ALI due to major abdominal surgery showed an upward convexity and a P-V relationship of the chest wall that was shifted to the right and flattened (Fig. 6). In the medical ALI patients, the P-V relationship of the respiratory system and lung showed an upward concavity and the P-V relationship of the chest wall was superimposable with the one observed in the control group (Fig. 6). In addition, in the patients with medical ALI, values of end-inspiratory abdominal pressure (Pst, abd) were not statistically different from those of the control group whereas, in patients with surgical ALI, values of Pst, abd were about 4 times greater than the values observed in the controls ($p < 0.0001$). Consistent with these findings, the static inflation P-V curve of the abdomen in patients with medical ALI was superimposable to the one measured in the control group, while a rightward shift was observed in patients with surgical ALI (Fig. 6). These data therefore indicate that when the underlying disease responsible for ALI is an abdominal pathological process requiring major abdominal surgery, abdominal distension may occur and alteration of the elastic properties of the chest wall may contribute to the derangement of respiratory mechanics.

Increased abdominal pressure which can occur in a variety of clinical situations such as tense ascites, abdominal hemorrhage, abdominal obstruction, laparoscopy, large abdominal tumors, and peritoneal dialysis, all of which can adversely affect respiratory, cardiac, renal, and metabolic functions [83–86]. Elevations in intra-abdominal pressure will occur when the distensible components of the peritoneal cavity (peritoneum, abdominal muscles, and diaphragm) become less compliant due to increased intra-abdominal volume (i.e. ascites, abdominal hemorrhage). Under these circumstances, direct compression of the abdominal contents occurs, venous return from the lower extremities is impaired, and intra-abdominal pressure is transmitted via the diaphragm to the thoracic cavity [87]. The respiratory system may be partitioned into two compartments: The chest wall and the lung. Although the diaphragm forms the caudal boundary of the chest cavity, the diaphragm is mechanically coupled to the abdominal wall and contents. Any increase in abdominal pressure may therefore affect lung mechanics by increasing the propensity for the development of atelectasis and by decreasing FRC [81–85] which may also indirectly alter chest wall mechanics by shifting the P-V curve of the chest wall to a lower lung volume [89]. Abdominal distension may also directly impact on chest wall mechanics by affecting chest wall configuration, and/or changing in the interaction at the zone at which the lungs are opposed to the lateral surface of the diaphragm, and/or causing inhomogeneity in the displacement among different parts of the chest wall [86]. Mutoh and co-workers [81] studied the effects of abdominal distension on lung and chest wall mechanics in anesthetized, paralyzed and mechanically ventilated pigs. Abdominal distension was induced by inflating a liquid-filled balloon placed in the abdominal cavity. During baseline conditions, Pst, abd was 2.8 ± 1.0 cmH$_2$O and increased up 15.2 ± 1.5 cmH$_2$O after inflation of the abdominal balloon. Abdominal distension caused a rightward and downward shift of the static P-V curves of the respiratory system, chest wall, lung and abdomen. Consequently, compliance of the respiratory system, chest wall, and lung was reduced by 47, 48, and 39%, respectively, after abdominal distension. FRC decreased by 54% from control values. In patients with ALI following major abdominal surgery, we found values of Pst, abd that were markedly higher than those found in patients undergoing general anesthesia for cardiac surgery and patients with medical ALI. In 5 of our surgical ALI patients, a reduction in static end-inspiratory pressure of the abdomen ($69 \pm 4\%$), respiratory system ($30 \pm 3\%$), chest wall ($41 \pm 2\%$), and lung ($27 \pm 3\%$) was observed after abdominal decompression for acute bleeding [82]. These data seem to suggest that interpretation of the elastic properties of the respiratory system requires assessment of both lung and chest wall mechanics, and may vary with the underlying disease responsible for ALI. Besides, the flattening of the P-V curve at high pressures observed in some patients with ARDS may be due to increase in chest wall elastance related to abdominal distension.

Conclusion

Assessment of the P-V relationship of the respiratory system in patients with ALI is widely accepted in the clinical practice to minimize side effects and optimize therapeutic benefits of mechanical ventilation. Experimental data and preliminary clinical observations support the notion that putting the lung under mechanical stress by setting VT below the lower inflection point and/or above the upper inflection point of the inspiratory P-V curve may determine a primary injury in normal lung or induce a secondary lung injury to the primitive ALI. However, consensus on techniques and on interpretative algorithms of the P-V relationship in patients with ALI has not been reached by the clinical and scientific community.

Acknowledgement: This chapter was supported by Consiglio Nazionale delle Ricerche, grant 95. 00934. CT04. The authors thank Professors A. Brienza, S. Antonaci, T. Fiore and F. Bruno for the support they provide to this work.

References

1. Marini JJ (1990) Lung mechanics in the adult respiratory distress syndrome. Clin Chest Med 11:673–690
2. Benito S, Lemaire F (1990) Pulmonary pressure-volume relationship in acute respiratory distress syndrome: Role of positive end-expiratory pressure. J Crit Care 1:27–34
3. Roupie E, Dambrosio M, Servillo G, et al (1995) Titration of VT and induced hypercapnia in acute respiratory distress syndrome. Am J Respir Crit Care Med 152:121–128
4. Gattinoni L, Pesenti A, Avalli L, et al (1987) Pressure volume curve of total respiratory system in acure respiratory failure. Am Rev Respir Dis 136:730–736
5. Brunet F, Jeanbourquin D, Monchi M, et al. (1995) Should mechanical ventilation be optimized to blood gases, lung mechanics, or thoracic CT scan ? Am J Respir Crit Care Med 152:524–530
6. Ranieri VM, Eissa NT, Corbeil C, et al (1991) Effect of PEEP on alveolar recruitment and gas exchange in ARDS patients. Am Rev Respir Dis 144:544–551
7. Ranieri VM, Giuliani R, Dambrosio M, et al (1994) Volume-pressure curve of the respiratory system predicts effects of PEEP in ARDS patients: "Occlusion" vs "constant flow" technique. Am Rev Respir Dis 149:19–27
8. Ranieri VM, Mascia L, Fiore T, et al (1995) Cardiorespiratory effects of positive end-expiratory pressure during progressive VT reduction (permissive hypercapnia) in patients with acute respiratory distress syndrome. Anesthesiology 83:710–720
9. Agostoni E, Mead J (1964) Statics of the respiratory system. In: Fenn WO, and Rahn H (eds) Handbook of Physiology. Respiration, Vol 1. Am Physiol Soc, Bethesda, MD, pp 387–409
10. Rossi A, Ranieri VM (1994) Positive end-expiratory pressure. In: Tobin MJ (ed) Principle and practice of mechanical ventilation. McGraw-Hill, New York, NY, pp 259–303
11. Rahn H, Otis AB, Chadwick E, et al (1946) The pressure-volume diagram of the thorax and lung. Am J Physiol 146:161–178
12. Agostoni E (1970) Volume-pressure relations of the respiratory system during relaxation. In: Campbell EJM, Agostoni E, Newsom Davis J (eds) The Respiratory Muscles. London; Lloyd-Luke, pp 48–79
13. Muscedere JG, Mullen JB, Gan K, Slutsky AS (1994) Tidal ventilation at low airways pressures can augment lung injury. Am J Respir Crit Care Med 149:1327–1334
14. Suter PM, Fairley HB, Isenberg MD (1978) Effect of VT and end-expiratory pressure on compliance during mechanical ventilation. Chest 73:158–162

15. Matamis D, Lemaire F, Hart A, et al (1984) Total respiratory pressure-volume curves in the adult respiratory distress syndrome. Chest 86:58–66
16. Lachmann B, Robertson B, Vogel J (1980) *In vivo* lung lavage as an experimental model of respiratory distress syndrome. Acta Anaesth Scand 24:231–236
17. Radford EP Jr (1970) Static mechanical properties of mammalian lungs. In: Fenn WO, Rahn H (eds) Handbook of physiology: Respiration (Vol I). Am Physiol Soc, Washington, DC, pp 429–449
18. Cavagna GA, Stemmler EJ, Dubois AB (1967) Alveolar resistance to atelectasis. J Appl Physiol 22:441–452
19. Lindskog GE, HH Bradshaw (1934) The reinflation of atelectatic lung. J Thoracic Surg 3:333–340
20. Wilson JL, Farber S (1933) Pathogenesis of atelectasis of newborn child. Am J Dis Child 46:590–603
21. Gruenwald P (1947) Surface tension as a factor in the resistance of neonatal lungs to aeration. Am J Obstet Gynecol 53:996–1007
22. Cook CD, Mead J, Schreiner GL, et al (1959) Pulmonary mechanic during induced edema in anesthetized dogs. J Appl Physiol 14:177–186
23. Mancebo J (1992) PEEP, ARDS and alveolar recruitment. Intensive Care Med 18:383–385
24. Agostoni E (1972) Mechanics of the pleural space. Physiol Rev 52:57–128
25. Kaneko K, Milic-Emili J, Dolovich MB, et al (1966) Regional distribution of ventilation and perfusion as a function of body position. J Appl Physiol 21:767–777
26. Ranieri VM, Giuliani R (1994) PEEP, ARDS and alveolar recruitment, the physiologist point of view. Intensive Care Med 20:82–84
27. Gattinoni L, Pesenti A, Bombino M, et al (1988) Relationship between lung computed tomographic density gas-exchange and PEEP in acute respiratory failure. Anesthesiology 69:824–832
28. Gattinoni L, Pesenti A (1987) The non-homogeneous lung: Facts and hypothesis. Crit Care Dig 6:1–4
29. Knudson RJ, Clark DF, Kennedy, et al (1997) Effect of aging alone on mechanical properties of the normal adult human lung. J Appl Physiol 43:1054–1062
30. Dreyfuss D, Basset G, Soler P, et al (1985) Intermittent positive-end expiratory pressure hyperventilation with high inflation pressures produces pulmonary microvascular injury in rats. Am Rev Respir Dis 132:880–884
31. Dreyfuss D, Soler P, Basset G, et al (1988) High inflation pressure pulmonary edema. Respective effects of high airway pressure, high VT, and positive end-expiratory pressure. Am Rev Respir Dis 137:1159–1164
32. Kolobow T, Moretti MP, Fumagalli R, et al (1987) Severe impairment in lung function induced by high peak airway pressure during mechanical ventilation. Am Rev Respir Dis 135:312–315
33. Tsuno K, Prato P, Kolobow T (1990) Acute lung injury from mechanical ventilation at moderately high airway pressures. J Appl Physiol 69:956–961
34. Parker JC, Hernandez GL, Longnecker GL (1990) Lung edema caused by high peak inspiratory pressures in dogs: Role of increased microvascular filtration pressure and permeability. Am Rev Respir Dis 114:321–328
35. Coker PJ, Hernandez LA, Peevy KJ, et al (1992) Increased sensitivity to mechanical ventilation after surfactant inactivation in young rabbit lung. Crit Care Med 20:635–640
36. Hernandez LA, Coker PJ, May S, et al (1990) Mechanical ventilation increases microvascular permeability in oleic acid-injured lungs. J Appl Physiol 69:2057–2061
37. Dreyfuss D, Saumon G (1993) Role of VT, FRC and end-inspiratory volume in the development of pulmonary edema following mechanical ventilation. Am Rev Respir Dis 48:1184–1203
38. Suter PM, Fairley HB, Isenberg MD (1975) Optimum end-expiratory airway pressure in patients with acute pulmonary failure. N Engl J Med 292:284–289
39. Suter PM, Scholobohm RM (1974) Determination of functional residual capacity during mechanical ventilation. Anesthesiology 41:605–607
40. Suter PM (1985) Assessment of respiratory mechanics in ARDS. In: Zapol M, Kalke KJ (eds) Acute respiratory failure. Marcell Dekker, New York, Basel, pp 507–519

41. Lemaire F, Beydon L, Jonson B (1991) Lung mechanics in ARDS. Compliance and pressure-volume curves. In: Zapol WM, Lemaire F (eds) Adult respiratory distress syndrome. Marcel Dekker, New York, pp 139-161
42. Lamy M, Fallat RJ, Koeniger E, et al (1976) Pathologic features and mechanisms of hypoxemia in adult respiratory distress syndrome. Am Rev Respir Dis 114:267-284
43. Gattinoni L, D'Andrea L, Pelosi P, et al (1993) Regional effects and mechanisms of positive end-expiratory pressure in early adult respiratory distress syndrome. JAMA 16:2122-2127
44. Ramanchandran PR, Fairley HP (1970) Changes in functional residual capacity during respiratory failure. Can Anaesth Soc J 17:359-369
45. Bernstein L (1957) The elastic pressure-volume curves of the lungs and thorax of the living rabbit. J Physiol (London) 138:473-487
46. Mead J, Whittenberger JL, Radford EP Jr (1957) Surface tension as a factor in pulmonary volume-pressure hysteresis. J Appl Physiol 10:191-196
47. Bachofen H, Schurch S, Urbinelli M, et al (1987) Relations among alveolar surface tension, surface area, volume and recoil pressure. J Appl Physiol 62:1878-1887
48. D'Angelo E, Calderini E, Torri G, et al (1989) Respiratory mechanics in anesthetized paralyzed humans: Effects of flow, volume, and time. J Appl Physiol 67:2556-2564
49. Glaister DH, Schroter RC, Sudlow MF, et al (1973) Transpulmonary pressure gradient and ventilation in excised lung. Respir Physiol 17:365-386
50. Slutsky AS, Scharf SM, Brown R, et al (1980) The effect of oleic acid-induced pulmonary edema on pulmonary and chest wall mechanics in dogs. Am Rev Respir Dis 121:91-96
51. Mead J, Collier C (1959) Relation of volume history of lungs to respiratory mechanics in anesthetized dogs. J Appl Physiol 14:669-678
52. Cook CD, Mead J, Schreiner GL, et al (1959) Pulmonary mechanic during induced edema in anesthetized dogs. J Appl Physiol 14:177-186
53. Blanch L, Roussos C, Brotherton S, et al (1992) Effect of VT and PEEP in ethchlorvynol-induced asymmetric lung injury. J Appl Physiol 72:108-116
54. Valta P, Takala J, Eissa NT, et al (1993) Does alveolar recruitment occur with positive end-expiratory pressure in adult respiratory distress syndrome. J Crit Care 1:34-43
55. Mancebo J, Benito S, Martìn M, et al (1988) Value of static pulmonary compliance in predicting mortality in patients with acute respiratory failure. Intensive Care Med 14:110-114
56. Petty TL, Reiss OK Paul GW, et al (1977) Characteristics of pulmonary surfactant in adult respiratory distress syndrome with trauma and shock. Am Rev Respir Dis 115:531-536
57. Petty TL Silvers GW, Paul GW, et al (1979) Abnormalities in lung elastic properties and surfactant function in adult respiratory distress syndrome. Chest 5:571-574
58. Goerke J, Clements JA (1986) Alveolar surface tension and lung surfactant. In: Macklem PT, Mead J (eds) Handbook of physiology. Sect 3, Vol III. Am Physiol Soc, Bethesda, MD, pp 247-261
59. Fu Z, Costello ML, Tsukimoto K, et al (1992) High volume increases stress failure in pulmonary capillaries. J Appl Physiol 73:123-133
60. Amato MBP, Barbas CSV, Medeiros DM, et al (1995) Beneficial effects of the "open lung approach" with low distending pressures in acute respiratory distress syndrome. Am J Respir Crit Care Med 152:1835-1846
61. Tremblay L, Valenza F, Slutsky AS, et al (1997) Injurious ventilatory strategies increased cytokines and c-fos mRNA expression in an isolated rat lung model. J Clin Invest 99:944-952
62. Eissa N., Milic-Emili J (1991) Modern concepts in monitoring and management of respiratory failure. Anesth Clin N Am 9:199-218
63. Mancebo J, Benito S, Martìn M, et al (1988) Value of static pulmonary compliance in predicting mortality in patients with acute respiratory failure. Intensive Care Med 14:110-114
64. Dall'Ava-Santucci J, Armaganidis A, Brunet F, et al (1988) Causes of error of respiratory pressure-volume curves in paralyzed subjects. J Appl Physiol 1:42-49
65. Gattinoni L, Mascheroni D, Basilico E, et al (1987) Volume/pressure curve of total respiratory system in paralyzed patients: Artefacts and correction factors. Intensive Care Med 13:19-25
66. Sydow M, Burchardi H, Zinserling J, et al (1991) Improved determination of static compliance by automated single volume steps in ventilated patients. Intensive Care Med 17:108-114

67. Glaister DH, Schroter RC, Sudlow MF, et al (1973) Bulk elastic properties of excised lungs and the effect of a transpulmonary pressure gradient. Respir Physiol 17:347–364

68. Glaister DH, Schroter RC, Sudlow MF, et al (1973) Transpulmonary pressure gradient and ventilation in excised lung. Respir Physiol 17:365–386

69. Valta P, Lavoie A, Corbeil C, et al (1993) Quasi-static hysteresis during tidal breathing in mechanically ventilated ARDS patients. Am Rev Respir Dis 4:A352 (Abst)

70. Leblanc P, Ruff F, Milic-Emili J (1970) Effects of age and body position on "airway closure" in man. J Appl Physiol 28:448–451

71. Levy P, Similowski T, Corbeil C, et al (1989) A method for studying the static volume-pressure curves of the respiratory system during mechanical ventilation. J Crit Care 4:83–89

72. Broseghini C, Brandolese R, Poggi R, et al (1988) Respiratory mechanics during the first day of mechanical ventilation in patients with pulmonary edema and chronic airway obstruction. Am Rev Respir Dis 138:355–361

73. Bates JHT, Rossi A, Milic-Emili J (1985) Analysis of the behavior of the respiratory system with constant inspiratory flow. J Appl Physiol 58:1840–1848

74. Suratt PM, Owens DH (1981) A pulse method of measuring respiratory system compliance in ventilated patients. Chest 80:34–38

75. Rossi A, Gottfried SB, Higgs BD, et al (1985) Respiratory mechanics in mechanically ventilated patients with respiratory failure. J Appl Physiol 58:1849–1858

76. Murphy BG, Engel LA (1978) Models of the pressure-volume relationship of the the human lung. Respir Physiol 32:183–194

77. Milic-Emili J, Ploysongsang Y (1986) Respiratory mechanics in the adult respiratory distress syndrome. Crit Care Clin 3:573–584

78. Eissa NT, Ranieri VM, Chasse M, et al (1991) Analysis of the behaviour of the respiratory system in ARDS patients: Effects of flow, volume and time. J Appl Physiol 70:2719–2729

79. Katz JA, Sellin SE, Ozanne GM, et al (1981) Pulmonary, chest wall and lung-thorax elastances in acute respiratory failure. Chest 80:304–311

80. Pelosi P, Cereda P, Foti G, et al (1995) Alterations of lung and chest wall mechanics in patients with acute lung injury: Effects of positive end-expiratory pressure. Am J Respir Crit Care Med 152:531–537

81. Mutoh T, Wayne J, Lamm E, et al. (1991) Abdominal distension alters regional pleural pressures and chest wall mechanics in pigs *in vivo*. J Appl Physiol 70:2611–2618

82. Ranieri VM, Brienza N, Santostasi S, et al (1997) Impairment of lung and chest wall mechanics in patients with acute respiratory distress syndrome: Role of abdominal distension. Am J Respir Crit Care Med (In press)

83. Kron IL, Harman PK, Nolan SP (1984) The measurement of intra-abdominal pressure as a criterion for abdominal re-exploration. Ann Surg 199:28–30

84. Iberti TJ, Lieber CE, Benjamin E (1989) Determination of intra-abdominal pressure using a transurethral bladder catheter: Clinical validation of the technique. Anesthesiology 70:47–50

85. Richardson JD, Trinkle JK (1976) Hemodynamic and respiratory alterations with increased intra-abdominal pressure. J Surg Res 20:401–404

86. Fahy BG, Barnas GM, Flowers JL, et al (1995) The effects of increased abdominal pressure on lung and chest wall mechanics during laparoscopic surgery. Anesth Analg 81:744–750

87. Robotham JL, Wise RA, Bromberger-Barnea B (1985) Effects of changes in abdominal pressure on left ventricular performance and regional blood flow. Crit Care Med 13:803–809

88. Richardson JD, Trinkle JK (1976) Hemodynamic and respiratory alterations with increased intra-abdominal pressure. J Surg Res 20:401–404

89. Gilroy RJ, Lavietes MH, Loring SH, et al (1985) Respiratory mechanical effects of abdominal distension. J Appl Physiol 58:1997–2003

Lung Recruitment During ARDS

J. J. Marini and M. B. Amato

Introduction

Accomplishing the lung's primary function of gas exchange requires close contact between gas and blood across the extensive alveolar surface. Because of non-uniform regional and local forces, certain lung units are naturally predisposed to closure, even in the healthy lung. Extensive airway or parenchymal disease greatly accentuates this tendency.

The consequences of lung unit de- recruitment depend not only on its prevalence and duration, but also on the anatomic level at which collapse occurs. Although unrelieved airway occlusion reduces aerated volume when trapped gas is absorbed without being replenished, tidally "phasic expiratory" closure of central and small airways may lead to gas trapping without loss of volume, as in severe emphysema. Collapse at the alveolar level, however, not only causes volume loss with hypoxemia to the extent allowed by hypoxic vasoconstriction, but also predisposes to pulmonary infection and lung injury during mechanical ventilation with high cycling pressures.

Depriving normal lung tissue from gas contact is not invariably deleterious; sustained closure of otherwise normal alveoli ventilated at low tidal pressures is not associated with lasting adverse consequences; atelectasis occurs routinely in proximity to a pleural effusion or pneumothorax and generally resolves without sequelae when the pleural collection of fluid or air drains. As another example, dependent lung units tend to collapse in the supine anesthetized adult during routine surgery [1]. Any temporarily impaired gas exchange that results is typically countered easily by supplemental inspired oxygen and reversed by simple measures that maintain or periodically restore overall lung volume. Microcollapse resolves quickly and uneventfully once the patient regains full consciousness.

In the setting of acute respiratory distress syndrome (ARDS), however, airway closure and alveolar collapse may be less innocuous. The topic of lung collapse and recruitment has assumed particular importance in recent years because of concerns regarding the impact of regional lung collapse on the ability of the lung to initiate healing and withstand the rigors of mechanical ventilation [2–4]. Our purpose is to describe the lung mechanics bearing on recruitment and to examine the clinical implications arising from those considerations in the setting of ARDS. We also develop the rationale for a practical bedside approach that seeks to minimize adverse affects of inadequate recruitment.

Collapse, Recruitment, and the Ventilatory Cycle

When interpreting laboratory studies that address mechanisms of ventilator-induced lung injury, emphasis generally has been placed on the detrimental effects of over-stretching fragile lung units with high airway pressure [5–7]. Whereas high tidal pressures are necessary to injure the lungs of a previously normal laboratory animal, there is increasing experimental evidence that collapse-persistent or phasic collapse of edematous, inflamed, or surfactant-depleted lung tissue can inflict further damage, encourage fibrosis, or retard healing. These adverse effects occur most commonly (but not exclusively) when high tidal pressures are used [8, 9].

The relative importance of persistent collapse and tidally phasic collapse and re-opening is not known. Both may be contributory. "Persistent" contact of denuded epithelial surfaces is theorized to provoke inflammation [10], stimulate the ingrowth of granulation tissue, or initiate neovascular cross bridges between them. Subjecting collapsed units to high tidal stresses and/or allowing "tidal closure and re-opening" under high pressure potentially may damage structural elements directly, induce capillary stress fracture, or simply provide the requisite mechanical signal for inflammation.

Collapse is also concerning when it occurs at the bronchiolar (rather than alveolar) level. Small airways unsupported by cartilage sustain damage when exposed to high tidal airway pressures without sufficient positive end-expiratory pressure (-PEEP) [11]. Such changes resemble bronchopulmonary dysplasia resulting from high pressure ventilation of the premature lung and are thought responsible for cyst formation, poor secretion clearance, and predisposition to infection [12].

Mechanisms of Recruitment

Forces Encouraging Closure

Gas-filled lung units have an innate tendency to collapse, due to tissue elastic recoil, surface tension, and disproportionate absorption of oxygen by blood flowing past poorly ventilated lung units. Tissue elastic forces reach maximal intensity at high lung volumes, whereas surface forces increase as the lung deflates to its functional residual capacity. Whereas both phenomena contribute to the total recoil tendency, surface forces normally predominate throughout the usual tidal range of lung volume, especially when surfactant is depleted or inactivated [13, 14]. Adding to these closure tendencies is the potential for absorptive collapse to occur when ventilation is disproportionately reduced with respect to perfusion, especially when the subject breathes high inspired fractions of oxygen.

Forces Opposing Closure

Several defenses oppose this tendency for collapse. Lung units are mutually interdependent, linked through a meshwork of shared alveolar, interstitial, and connective tissues. Each alveolus is tethered to others, so that heightened distending forces are brought to bear on any individual lung unit tending to collapse. The magnitude of these forces was estimated theoretically by Mead and colleagues [15] who reasoned that stresses would be greatly amplified in the wall shared by the collapsed alveolus with surrounding freely expandable units. From their work, the approximate magnitude of those forces can be estimated using the following equation:

$$P_{eff} \approx P_{app} \times (V/V_O)^{2/3}$$

Arguing from a purely geometrical standpoint and assuming that the relative volumes of expanded (V) and collapsed (V_O) units might approximate $\approx 10:1$, Mead et al. estimated that tissue tensions equivalent to an effective pressure (P_{eff}) of 140 cmH$_2$O would act on a collapsing unit completely enveloped by others expanded by an applied pressure (P_{app}) of 30 cmH$_2$O [15]. This elastic interdependence, coupled with the surfactant system that operates to reduce surface forces at low lung volumes, stabilizes the normal lung. Any tendency for absorptive collapse is countered by collateral ventilation and by the subject's ability to increase ventilation to oppose the absorptive tendency. The effectiveness of collateral ventilation is species-dependent; it is negligible in the pig, extensive in the dog, and questionably important in the human adult [16].

When lung units collapse despite these protective mechanisms, lung volume can be raised both to reduce the importance of surface forces and to amplify elastic interdependence. Thus, periodic lung stretching to total lung capacity (deep sighing) tends to recruit recently collapsed, disadvantaged units [1, 17]. These maneuvers also stimulate surfactant production and improve its effectiveness [14]. A sustained deep breath is more effective than a breath of the same depth only briefly held.

Site of Collapse

The gas channel that links the airway opening with the alveolus can close for varying portions of the tidal cycle at any point along the path – proximally or distally – with different pathophysiologic consequences. When high airway pressures are applied to a bronchus closed at any anatomic level, no pressure dissipates against flow resistance, so that with each inflation cycle, a high proportion of the peak inflation pressure impacts all sites proximal to the point of occlusion. Such forces are not likely to cause major structural problems in proximal airways, which are reinforced to withstand them. Yet, similar pressures in distal airways unsupported by cartilage can lead to airway dilatation, distortion, cyst formation, and mucosal trauma secondary to shearing forces [11, 12]. The resulting bronchopulmonary damage encourages infection and impairs gas exchange. Given that the critically ill patient with ARDS often receives >30000 tidal cycles each day, such repetitive shear stresses have the potential to extend damage and retard healing.

Hypoxemia is the immediate physiologic consequence of extensive collapse occuring at the alveolar level. In the setting of high tidal pressures or prior lung injury, however, a growing body of experimental and clinical data indicate that inflammation, hemorrhage and other pathological alterations occur as well (see below).

Opening and Closing Pressures

The pressures required to open the collapsed airway are a function of the site of closure and the duration over which the pressure is held. It is important to understand that the pressures under discussion are trans-structural (trans-bronchial and trans-alveolar) pressures, which can be loosely approximated as the difference between the local airway and local pleural pressures. This pragmatic convention is an over-simplification, as the pressures that surround bronchi and alveoli undoubtedly differ on a microscopic scale [18]. The pressure that actually surrounds an alveolus or bronchus may be considerably lower or higher than that suggested by an estimate of local pleural pressure [13]. Peribronchial pressures are believed to be lower centrally than peripherally (helping to account for the migration of gas to the mediastinum that occurs after alveolar disruption). Therefore, assuming an airway already cleared of mucus and debris, lower pressures will generally be required to open a collapsed central bronchus than are needed to open a distal bronchiole or collapsed alveolus, particularly if surfactant is depleted.

Collapse, Reopening, and Volume History

Liquid-filled lungs open and close at very similar pressures. During gas breathing, however, the pressures required to open the airway and alveolus exceed those required to prevent closure, due to surfactant-mediated differential surface forces at the gas-tissue boundary [14, 19]. The extent of this difference must vary for airways lined with fluids of different viscosities and is almost certain to be influenced by the site of closure. Once opened, interdependent forces act to keep the alveolus open; once closed, surface forces favor continued collapse.

Recent volume history powerfully impacts the pressure-volume (P-V) relationship. After all closed but potentially patent units are recruited, it is generally possible to maintain a higher average volume in this fully "opened" lung at a reduced distending pressure. ("P-V hysteresis"). Moreover, because additional lung units are available to accept gas once recruitment has occurred, the same tidal volume (VT) requires less tidal pressure to achieve it. These phenomena are easily demonstrated experimentally in surfactant depletion models of lung injury [20, 21].

Whether similar principles apply to most adult patients with acute lung injury (ALI) is much less clear. Although frequently evident during the edematous phase, P-V hysteresis and reduced compliance at low inflation volumes may be undetectable in the later stages of ARDS [22–24]. Even at an early stage, differential inspiratory-expiratory compliance characteristics are not always observed.

Hysteresis implies both recruitment during the inflation maneuver and a significant difference between opening and closing pressures. The extent of hysteresis, therefore, is generally diminished by using sufficient PEEP to hold most lung units open during the tidal cycle. It must be clearly understood however, that the absence of hysteresis does not mean the absence of recruitment during lung inflation or imply the non-utility of PEEP. The absence of hysteresis means only that, on average, the opening and closing pressures of lung units that inflate at some point in the tidal cycle are equivalent.

During ARDS, for example, little hysteresis may be evident unless sufficient pressure is sustained long enough to reach the "yield point" of the recruitable airways (Fig. 1). Therefore, over time PEEP could help re-establish patency of initially dormant but eventually recruitable alveoli, provided that peak tidal pressure rises above some critical threshold. Alternatively, the absence of hysteresis might reflect extreme deficiency of surfactant and the futility of PEEP, but this is not known with certainty until a trial of PEEP application is conducted with an ample P-V following vigorous recruiting efforts (see below).

Time Course of Opening and Closure

Just as the lung's mechanical characteristics differ by site, volume history, and phase of the tidal cycle, differences may also exist regarding the time course of lung unit opening and closure [25–27]. It is generally accepted that airways open more slowly than they collapse, and this discrepancy has implications for the times allotted to inspiration and expiration during the tidal cycle. An unchanging

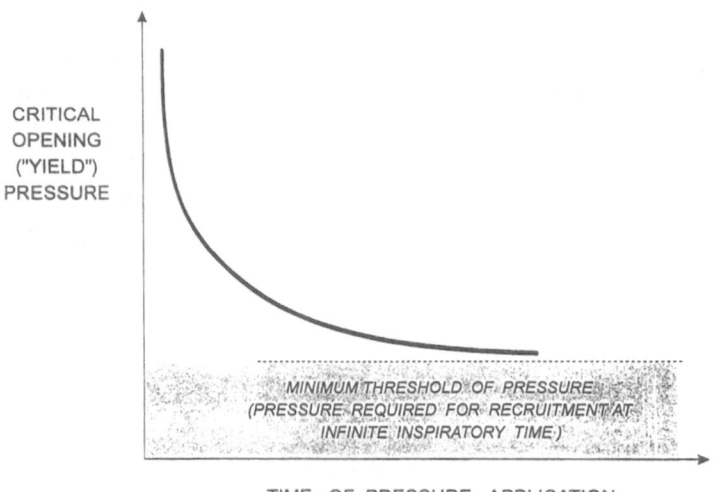

Fig. 1. Theoretical curve representing the "yield" (opening) pressures for a hypothetical lung unit. The minimum threshold (gray zone) of pressure is determined by the surface tension of the liquid/air interface, whereas time dependence is a function of the viscosity of the fluid and secretions which seal the air space

tidal pattern may only succeed in opening the airway over the course of multiple ventilatory cycles, so that the recruitment consequent to certain combinations of P-V and PEEP may not be completed for many breaths after its initiation (Fig. 2) [28]. Although central airways tend to open with the first few cycles, de-gassed alveoli may require much longer.

The mechanism for this time dependence is multifactorial and not precisely determined. It is reasonable, however, to assume that at any given pressure, interdependent forces are augmented by the added traction of each newly recruited unit, creating an "avalanche" effect. Because peak alveolar pressure tends to decline as lung units open progressively at a fixed P-V, gradual recruitment might be somewhat more sustained or effective if a constant tidal "pressure" (as opposed to a constant tidal "volume" that initially achieves the same pressure) were used to make the step change in peak alveolar pressure [29]. The ability to consolidate any gain in resting lung volume resulting from a recruiting maneuver may depend critically on the P-V employed or the interval between inflation cycles; a small P-V or a lengthy expiratory period may encourage gradual recurrence of microcollapse (Fig. 2) [17, 30].

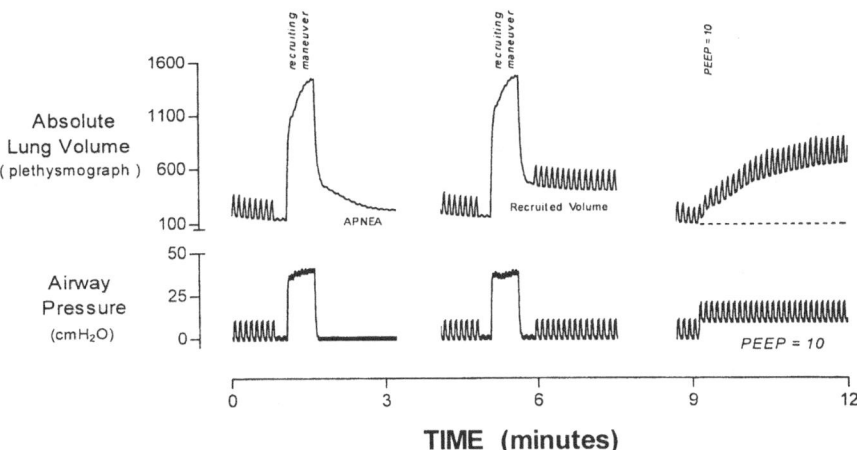

TIME (minutes)

Fig. 2. *Upper:* Changes in lung volume occuring after recruiting maneuvers which were followed by different strategies to maintain recruited volume (preparation: pigs after saline lung lavage). In the first tracing, a recruiting maneuver (CPAP of 40 cmH₂O applied for 30 sec) was followed by 90 sec of apnea (CPAP = 0). All volume gained during the recruiting maneuver was gradually lost over the ensuing minute. *Lower:* In the second tracing, the recruiting maneuver was followed by tidal ventilation with pressure control of 12 cmH₂O and 0 PEEP. Although somewhat better sustained, all recruited volume was lost within 15 min. (A recruiting maneuver followed by pressure controlled ventilation of 20 cmH₂O (PEEP = 0) maintained recruitment intact for more than 20 min of observation (data not shown)). C. In the third tracing, sudden application of 10 cmH₂O PEEP was followed by a progressive gain in lung volume. The functional residual capacity (FRC) stabilized only after 10 min (total gain of lung volume: 700 mL). For the same driving pressure, the amplitude of P-V excursions progressively increased, indicating improving lung compliance as new lung units were progressively recruited

Implications of Mechanical Heterogeneity

Vertical Heterogeneity

That pleural and transpulmonary pressures normally extend along opposing hydrostatic gradients has been well documented [31, 32]. The vertical gradient of transpulmonary pressure allows dependent airways to seal in conditions such as chronic obstructive pulmonary disease (COPD) and asthma [33]. For alveoli in ARDS that are not liquid filled, a similar but intensified vertical gradient of transpulmonary pressure accentuates the tendency for collapse in dependent regions [32, 34]. The pleural pressure gradient in ALI is accentuated by the altered mechanics of this condition. The weight of the edematous lung exerts forces that raise pleural pressures in dorsal areas as they attenuate pressures in ventral areas. The nature of these pleural pressure gradients is position dependent; dorsal regions may expand dramatically as the prone position is assumed [35].

Chest Wall Compliance

Regional forces exerted by the chest wall determine lung shape and volume distribution. In the supine position, abdominal hydrostatic forces curve the diaphragm more sharply in dorsal than in the ventral areas, and changes of position influence local pleural pressures and regional lung volumes [36]. Apart from variations in position, relatively little has been done clinically to modify the contribution of the chest wall to transpulmonary pressure. Yet, regional mass loading of the chest wall or external pneumatic compression can alter regional chest wall compliance, transpulmonary pressure distribution, and local recruitment. Finally, even within the same hydrostatic plane within the chest, there is almost certain to be a proximal to distal gradient of transpulmonary pressure that affects alveolar size, regional ventilation, and the tendency for collapse [37]. The importance of these forces in relation to the vertical gradient of transpulmonary pressure has not been adequately explored.

De-Recruitment, Amplified Tissue Stresses, and Capillary Disruption

Interesting work has been conducted by West and colleagues [38–41] exploring the tendency for capillary stress fracture to occur in a variety of animal species. Capillary tensile strength is insufficient to withstand transmural pressures that vary from approximately 40 mmHg in small, immature animals (e.g. rabbit) to ≈ 100 mmHg in large, mature animals (e.g. dog) [40]. The incidence of stress fractures is accentuated at high trans-alveolar pressures and volumes. Although intraluminal pressures of the required magnitude are virtually never encountered in the clinical setting, extramural forces exerting traction on the capillary could conceivably reach sufficient magnitude to allow stress fractures and eventual rupture. Such forces may account for the hemorrhagic changes observed in animal models of ALI and ventilator-induced lung trauma. No adequate analysis of the tractive forces engendered by different patterns of lung inflation has been attempted for the setting of ARDS; however, it seems clear that such extramural forces should be amplified at high transalveolar pressures. Extrapolating from the theoretical work of Mead et al. already discussed, we speculate that tissue tensions at the junctions of expanding and collapsed lung units conceivably might be of the magnitude required. High surface tension would tend to protect capillaries embedded in the alveolar walls from rupture.

In large animal models of ventilator-induced lung trauma, hemorrhagic changes tend to prevail in dependent regions [42, 43]. This distribution could be explained by intensified regional atelectasis at the bases and amplified tissue stresses resulting from heterogeneity in those areas. This contention, however, is hardly proven; both blood flow and vascular pressures are highest in dependent regions, and recent experiments emphasize the importance of perfusion to the manifestations of ventilator-induced lung injury [44].

Requirements of a Lung Protective Strategy

When all scientific evidence is considered, reversal of lung collapse emerges as central to a lung-protection strategy of mechanical ventilation. Achieving optimal recruitment of the lung demands a peak airway pressure high enough to open all recruitable lung units and an end-expiratory pressure sufficient to prevent their re-closure. In the clinical setting, the peak inflation and end-expiratory alveolar pressures have traditionally been determined by selecting a P-V and PEEP combination that results in clinically adequate arterial blood gases and hemodynamics. A smaller number of practitioners select P-V according to a customary guideline (e.g. 10 mL/kg), but adjust PEEP on the basis of computations of tidal (chord) compliance.

Excessive tidal pressures and insufficient end-expiratory pressures both inflict parenchymal damage in experimental animals. Although not yet proven unequivocally, it is logical to expect that similar events might be observed in the clinical arena as well. Thus, according to current thinking, there is a need to track events that jeopardize lung tissue either by overstretching fragile alveolar units or by allowing their extensive de-recruitment. At present, it remains uncertain whether the key problem is persistent collapse of injured or inflamed tissue, or whether tidal opening and collapse of lung units proves the most damaging [45, 46].

That collapse of injured tissue should not be allowed to persist is suggested by observations from the clinical literature of high frequency ventilation. Data from the neonatal high frequency oscillation (HIFI) trial indicate an unchanging incidence of barotrauma in infants ventilated with insufficient end-expiratory lung pressures, despite the trivial P-Vs and modest peak inflation pressures of high frequency oscillation [47]. Moreover, later comparisons using higher PEEP indicated a clear advantage for the oscillation technique [48]. Data corroborating the importance of reversing alveolar collapse is available from the experimental laboratory. Changes suggesting lung damage are observed when the excised lungs of surfactant depleted animals are ventilated with low tidal peak pressures and end-expiratory pressures below those needed to prevent extensive atelectasis [8, 49].

Indirect evidence for the importance of a strategy centered on lung recruitment is now emerging in the adult literature as well. Improvements in compliance, hemodynamics, and mortality were observed in patients for whom maximizing lung recruitment was the central element of the ventilation strategy [50]. Conversely, at least two recently completed multicenter trials in which PEEP did not vary between test groups failed to show benefit of reducing inflation pressures and P-V (Laurent Brochard and Thomas Stewart, personal communications).

Mechanical ventilation fails to damage normal lung tissue unless high peak tidal pressures are used. However, excessive tidal pressures severely damage the lung, unless sufficient end-expiratory airway pressure is used, or the pleural pressure gradient is adequately modified. Thus, in the early studies of Webb and Tierney [51], modest tidal inflation pressures without PEEP did not injure the lungs of normal rats. Brief application of high peak tidal pressures without PEEP, however, produced severe hemorrhagic damage. Modest PEEP prevented the severe lung injury incurred by the same peak tidal pressures. It is tempting to speculate that high tidal pressures without PEEP increased endothelial and epithelial permeability, allowing edema that encouraged collapse. Failure to use sufficient PEEP increased injury by permitting persistent collapse of damaged units or tidal opening or closure of lung units with each respiratory cycle. The latter interpretation is consistent with the work of Gattinoni and colleagues [52] who demonstrated differences in gas/tissue ratios at end-expiration and end-inspiration by CT densitometry in patients with ARDS. Their tidal differences in gas/tissue ratios were nearly obliterated by using sufficient end-expiratory pressure. Thus, available experimental and clinical data strongly suggest the importance of reversing atelectasis in the setting of ALI, both because persisting collapse may itself be damaging, and because reversal of atelectasis minimizes the tissue stresses encountered during tidal breathing.

P-V Curves and Recruitment

In managing ARDS, it is an intimidating clinical problem to select an optimal combination of P-V and end-expiratory pressure that simultaneously ensures lung recruitment and avoids lung damage while accomplishing adequate gas exchange and oxygen delivery. In this setting of heterogeneous regional mechanics, difficulty arises largely because it is the transmural pressure – not simply the airway pressure – which is the important determinant of alveolar distention. The practical need is for the capability to easily and accurately assess the conditions that jeopardize the lung (overstretch and de-recruitment) using the pressures and flows accessible at the airway opening. Although airway and alveolar pressures can be estimated readily, local pleural pressures cannot be measured for every hydrostatic level. The static P-V curve of the respiratory system has been used primarily in a research context to provide such information [23, 53]. By studying the contours (tangential compliance) of these curves, the wisdom of applying a PEEP or P-V increment could theoretically be determined, even if absolute lung size and the actual numbers of open lung units are unknown.

Conceptual Problems with P-V Curve Assessment

Although static P-V curves have been used effectively in scientific work, numerous problems arise when attempting to use them to guide selections of P-V and PEEP at the bedside. In the majority of patients, only airway pressure is routinely available, and this pressure is influenced jointly by the characteristics of the chest wall as well as lung. In fact, the shaping characteristics (inflection regions) of the P-V curve may be determined primarily by chest wall distensibility in some patients. Each loop is comprised of two limbs – inspiratory and expiratory – and each curve pools information coming simultaneously from all lung regions (Fig. 3). Some lung units remain collapsed at airway pressures that over-distend others. Moreover, because the volumes recorded in the clinical setting are measured spirometrically, they are referenced to the equilibrium position of the lung, and do not reflect absolute gas volumes. The curve inscribed, therefore, is a function of volume history and may not be entirely relevant to tidal ventilation.

As P-V curves are classically constructed, applied static airway pressures (plotted on the horizontal axis) extend from 0 to 30–45 cmH$_2$O, a range that usually – but not invariably – suffices to approximate total lung capacity, depending on lung and chest wall compliances. The inflation limb of the P-V curve may depart significantly from the expiratory limb of the same curve, owing to the differences in opening and closing pressures of the lungs. (However, the magnitude of "tidal" hysteresis for the patient with ARDS remains seriously in doubt, especially at small P-Vs and moderate to high levels of PEEP [22, 24, 54, 55].) The completed P-V curve is the "outer envelope" of all possibilities that might pertain to tidal breathing; most often, the actual tidal P-V loop resides somewhere within its interior (Fig. 4). Whether the patient is ventilated in close proximity to the inspiratory limb, the expiratory limb, or somewhere in the interior of the P-V envelope is a function of volume history and key characteristics of the tidal breathing pattern itself: Peak inspiratory and end-expiratory pressures, duty cycle, expiratory time.

Characteristics of the P-V Curve

Inspiratory Limb: The inspiratory limb of the P-V curve is comprised of several portions, not all of which may be present or well demarcated (Fig. 3). Although the processes of airway and alveolar recruitment, normal elastic expansion, and non-elastic overdistention probably occur to varying and overlapping extents in most patients, the recorded P-V relationship is a composite of all such phenomena.

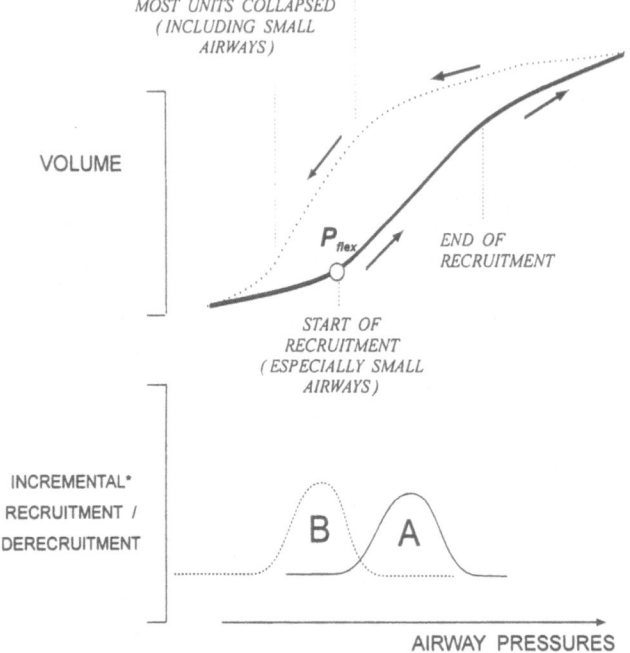

A: Frequency distribution of opening pressures (inspiration)
B: Frequency distribution of closing pressures (expiration)
(*: incremental recruitment = number of units opening at a certain pressure)

Fig. 3. Theoretical P-V loop with its expiratory (dotted) and inspiratory (solid) limbs. In this curve, phases 2, 3, and 4 of inspiration (see text and figure 5) are merged, due to a wide distribution of opening pressures. Therefore, overdistention of elastic elements in many units that are already patent occurs at the same airway pressures at which a relatively small number of units are still being recruited. Despite the wide distributions of critical pressures across the parenchyma, the opening pressures are substantially higher than the closing pressures

Therefore, curves from different individuals might be interpreted to display as few as two (linear and overdistention) or as many as the four phases described below.

As pressure and volume build from the origin, poor compliance is observed initially because relatively high pressure increments are needed to ventilate the relatively small volume of tissue ("baby lung") that is aeratable when many lung units are consolidated, liquid-filled, or collapsed (Fig. 5) [56]. The compliance of this first segment can be very poor if alveolar (as opposed to airway) collapse and

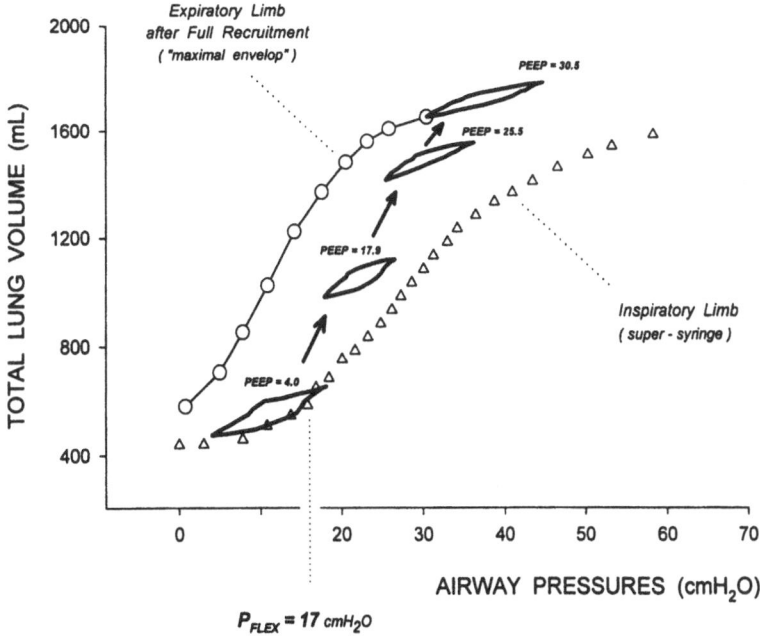

Fig. 4. The "maximal P-V envelope". These curves were obtained in a dog subjected to lung injury caused by oleic acid infusion. The inspiratory limb was constructed with a super syringe using 50 mL steps. Absolute lung volume measured with a constant pressure body plethysmograph eliminated artifacts caused by gas trapping and thoracic blood displacement. The expiratory limb ("maximal envelop") was constructed by plotting FRC at decreasing PEEP levels, after full recruitment obtained by ventilating the animal with PEEP = 30 cmH$_2$O and plateau pressures of 50 cmH$_2$O for 2 min. The closed loops represent tidal ventilation at a fixed VT = 200 mL during progressive increments in PEEP. The closed tidal loops are progressively displaced toward the maximum envelope at each PEEP step; therefore, the inspiratory limb does not represent the P-V "track" after PEEP use. Furthermore, the expiratory portion of the maximal envelope was reached only after using a PEEP of 30.5 cmH$_2$O, well above the lower P$_{flex}$, indicating that even at PEEP greater than P$_{flex}$, maximal recruitment was not obtained during tidal breathing. Finally, after full recruitment (using PEEP = 30.5 cmH$_2$O) a PEEP level slightly above P$_{flex}$ was enough to maintain lung volume considerably higher than before recruitment

flooding predominate, and relatively few gas channels are patent along their entire length.

A rather abrupt upward inflection often marks a transition into the second segment of the P-V curve (Fig. 5). In a patient with a normal chest wall, this usually occurs in the range of 10–15 cmH$_2$O$_2$, a pressure more compatible with airway opening than with the generally higher pressures required to open the alveoli of a de-gassed lung. In many patients, therefore, improving compliance as the P$_{flex}$ zone is crossed may signify more in the way of units coming on line due to airway opening, as opposed to the popping open of adhesed alveolar walls. As this transitional "P$_{flex}$" zone is crossed, compliance steadily improves and then stabilizes as it reaches its zenith [23]. (It should be understood that the sharpness of

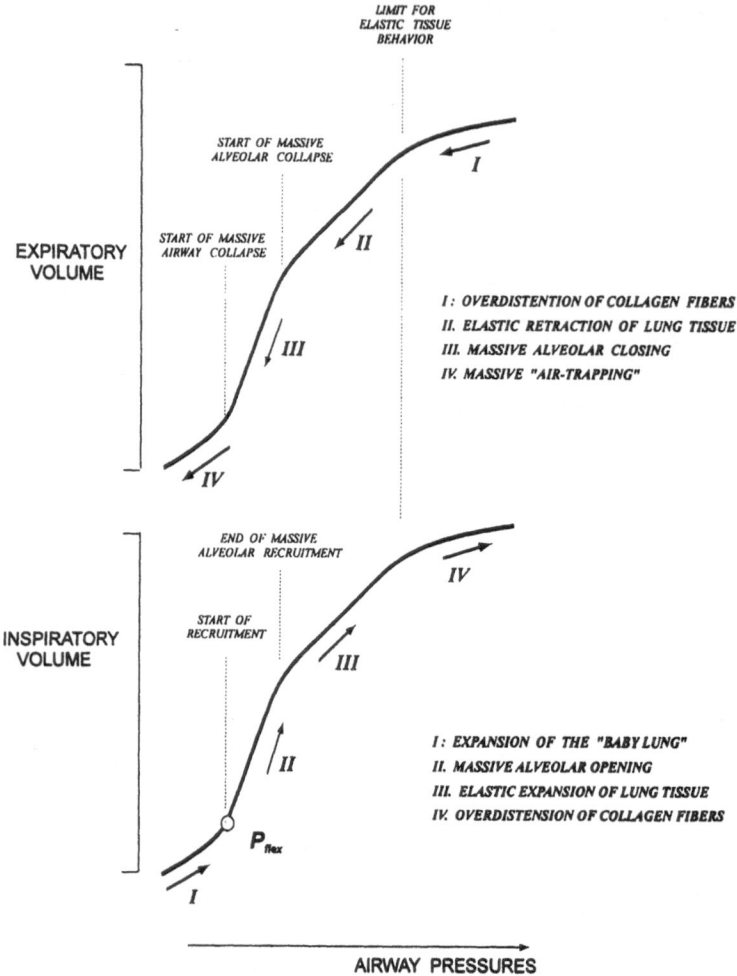

Fig. 5. Theoretical curves for the expiratory and inspiratory limbs of the P-V relationship. Each limb may be comprised of as many as four distinct segments; however, different phases overlap in most clinical situations-blurring sharp transitions of slope

the compliance transition depends on the distribution of opening pressures. A lung with a disproportionate number of recruitable units that open at similar pressures will evoke a distinct P_{flex}; one whose recuitable units are more evenly distributed among those easily opened and those more refractory, will not.) Over this high compliance "phase 2" segment, pressure increments simultaneously redistribute luminal fluids, expand units already open and recruit units which achieve patency once their critical opening pressures are applied for the requisite time. (Chest wall compliance generally remains unchanging in this middle segment.) Many of these newly opened units – perhaps a majority – are located in dependent regions. It should be noted that although the slope of the P-V relationship may appear linear, this linearity does not imply uniformity throughout the lungs – an unchanging slope may be the resultant of the offsetting effects of recruitment (often disproportionately from dependent regions) and overdistension (often disproportionately in non-dependent regions) (Fig. 3)[57].

A third phase may then be entered wherein the great majority of recruitable units are already "on line" (aerated), so that this segment of the curve displays the elastic properties of open units in various stages of distention (Fig. 5). In the final segment of the inflation curve, there is extensive over-distention of lung units, many of which are located in non-dependent regions. Over this range, the preserved integrity of the alveolus depends on the tensile strength of the lung's collagen fibroskeleton.

Expiratory Limb: The expiratory limb of the P-V curve also may display a variable number of distinct sub-sections; depending on the nature and extent of the pathology as well as the maximum distending pressure applied to the respiratory system. Like their inspiratory counterparts, expiratory curves from different individuals might be interpreted to display as few as two (linear and overdistention) or as many as four phases.

In the first expiratory segment, overstretching of many units is relieved as pressures descend from those corresponding to total lung capacity (Fig. 5). The second phase of the deflation curve (like the third phase of its inspiratory counterpart) primarily reflects the elastic retraction properties of patent lung tissue. Relatively few units – those that are most unstable – reach their critical closing pressures in this upper range. In the third phase of expiration, however, the rate of closure progressively increases in tandem with deflation of open units (Fig. 3). When a sharp transition into phase 3 (the "expiratory" deflection point) can be identified, this "earliest closure" point often occurs at a pressure that approximates the inspiratory P_{flex} zone (Fig. 3 and 4). In the fourth and final phase, there is extensive airway (as opposed to alveolar) closure and gas trapping.

Potential Clinical Applications of the P-V Curve

Having described the potential complexities of the P-V relationship, two logical questions to pose are these:
1) Which sement of the P-V envelope is most relevant to tidal ventilation?, and
2) To what extent do inspiratory and expiratory curves differ?

The answers to these questions are likely to vary with the models of disease examined, the stage of ALI under consideration, the tidal breathing pattern in use, and the precise technique by which the P-V curve is constructed. In the laboratory setting, clear differences between the inspiratory and expiratory phases of the P-V relationship characterize surfactant depletion and the earliest edematous stage of ALI. For these models, tidal ventilation tends to occur on the "expiratory" limb of the P-V envelope, provided that a volume recruiting maneuver has been undertaken recently [21]. Similar principles may well apply to the clinical setting of the infant respiratory distress syndrome. There is less agreement on the efficacy of periodic recruitment maneuvers in displacing the tidal breath onto the expiratory limb of the P-V curve in adult patients – particularly those who are in the later phases of ARDS. As already noted, several excellent investigative groups have reported that the inspiratory and expiratory P-V curves differ minimally when they are constructed with care to avoid artifacts [22, 24, 54, 55].

According to current thinking, tidal ventilation within the optimal compliance region of the inspiratory P-V curve (phase 2 or 3) is the pattern least likely to allow extensive collapse, overdistention, and a tidal recruitment/de-recruitment cycle. Although P_{flex} may occasionally exceed the least PEEP necessary to prevent widespread airway closure, P_{flex} seldom exceeds the early deflection point of the "expiratory" limb by more than a few cmH_2O. Moreover, when care is taken simultaneously to avoid tidal excursions into the upper deflection zone of the inspiratory segment, the risk of widespread alveolar overdistention should be low. Even if P_{flex} gives acceptable guidance for PEEP selection and the upper deflection point of the inspiratory curve identifies the maximum target for tidal alveolar pressure acceptably well, it should be understood that recruitment maneuvers still may be practically worthwhile if they restore "continuing" patency of substantial numbers of persistently collapsed or unstable units.

Alternative Methods for P-V Construction, Practical Problems, and Precautions

As already noted, the technique selected for constructing the P-V curve may have questionable relevance to tidal breathing. All methods for delineating the static P-V relationship require the patient to remain passive. Traditionally, the P-V curve has been constructed by disconnecting the patient's airway from the mechanical ventilator and using a "super syringe" to administer and withdraw small volume increments in stepwise fashion as pressure is recorded. This research technique may not be completely relevant to selecting PEEP in the clinical setting; care must be taken to insure a standardized volume history before data recording.

Because volume cumulates for an extended period, construction of the entire P-V curve in a single procedure is itself a recruitment maneuver. Therefore, at any given inspiratory limb pressure, the number of aerated lung units may be substantially greater than exist at the end of tidal inflation to the same pressure without PEEP. Conversely, the recruiting effects of PEEP during tidal ventilation displace the tidal loop to the interior of the envelope, with the highest PEEP values enabling an approach to the expiratory limb (Fig. 4).

In constructing the P-V curve, PEEP is released immediately after ventilator disconnection, a maneuver which may alter the characteristics of the lung or put the patient at risk for hypoxemia or airway flooding. Ongoing gas absorption and/or gas trapping behind closed airways near end-expiration gives rise to important artifacts [58]. A second method for constructing the inspiratory limb is to administer a very slow rate of constant flow, recording pressure continuously under these "quasi static" conditions over a wide range. Similar concerns regarding gas absorption and recruitment artifacts apply to this technique as well. Other approaches more relevant to tidal ventilation involve selecting a given PEEP level and varying P-V [59], or conversely, fixing P-V and varying PEEP [60]. These latter methods offer the advantages of evading gas absorption artifacts, being somewhat easier to perform safely, and avoiding the disruption of tidal ventilation. The lower inflection zone crucial to selecting PEEP, however, may be less easily identified.

PEEP, P-V, and Recruitment

In the acutely injured lung, differences in the opening and closing pressures of small airways and alveoli give rise to an interdependence between P-V, PEEP, and the calculated compliance of the respiratory system. When compliance is judged as the quotient of P-V and the difference of static pressures required to achieve it, no unique value of PEEP corresponds to optimal recruitment for all P-Vs (Fig. 6) [60, 61]. Moreover, the same combination of PEEP and P-V can result in markedly different levels of recruitment, depending on volume history and stage of disease, as already indicated.

The static (alveolar plateau) pressure achieved at end-inspiration determines the number of lung units open at that juncture. Similarly, total PEEP (the sum of PEEP and auto-PEEP) determines the number of lung units open at the end of expiration. The compliance values calculated at these points reflect this difference. Therefore, high compliance can be recorded when using a large P-V and low PEEP, even though many lung units that close at pressures within the tidal range are excluded from participating in gas exchange at the end of expiration. The clear potential exists for a large P-V with low PEEP to initiate a tidal recruitment and collapse cycle that exposes many regions of the heterogeneous lung to stresses that could extend or perpetuate lung injury. Whereas it is theoretically possible for a large P-V and low PEEP to result in an "open lung" without end-expiratory collapse, this is seldom the case; PEEP is generally needed to preserve arterial oxygenation. Failure to provide PEEP allows oxygenation to deteriorate, even when tidal compliance of the respiratory system appears well preserved.

Recruiting Maneuvers and the Time-Dependence of PEEP

It must be remembered that to open the airway, adequate pressure must be applied for a long enough period, and that the inflation "pressure-time product" that results from the combination of PEEP with a low P-V may not be sufficient to recruit all units potentially available. Periodic recruiting maneuvers – the sustained application of pressure sufficient to approach total lung capacity (trans-alveolar pressures $\approx 30–35$ cmH$_2$O)-may help offset the tendency for progressive collapse that occurs when small P-V are used. In the clinical setting, choosing the appropriate recruiting pressure and duration is something of an empirical exercise. The pressure needed to achieve full recruitment may be an inverse function

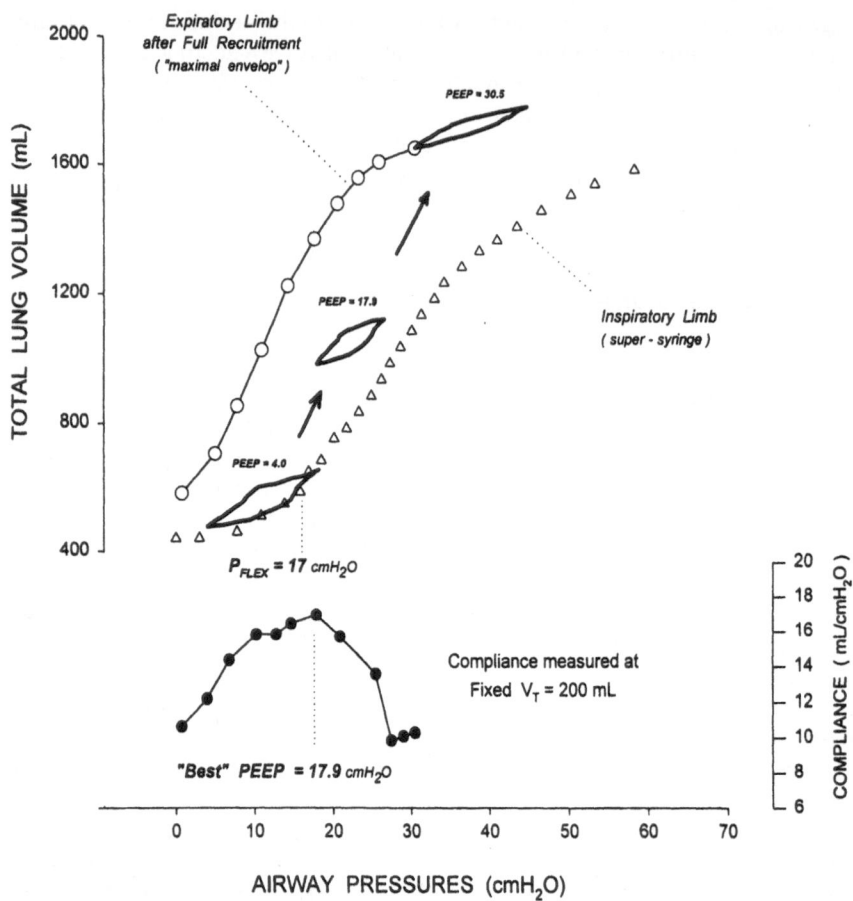

Fig. 6. Relationship between pulmonary compliance and lung recruitment. Observe that the best compliance was obtained at PEEP levels close to P_{flex} as long as low P-V are used in compliance calculations (approximately 4–6 mL/kg). Nevertheless, this coincidence is empirical, and the concordance is not always precise. Compliance values are the combined result of recruitment (increasing the compliance values) and overdistention (decreasing the compliance values). Full recruitment was only obtained at PEEP levels of 30.5 cmH$_2$O, but overdistention of many units at these high pressures depressed overall tidal compliance

of its application time and will reflect the compliance of the respiratory system. A typical recruiting protocol might apply continuous positive airway pressure (CPAP) of $\approx$ 35–45 cmH$_2$O for 30 sec, if tolerated hemodynamically, but the optimal pressures and duration would vary with the characteristics of the problem at hand. Finally, although currently out of favor, there might yet be a place for extended or multiple sighs used in conjunction with PEEP and modest P-V in the treatment of ARDS.

In the experimental setting of ALI, the P-V relationship inscribed after a sustained recruitment maneuver typically shows upward displacement along the to-

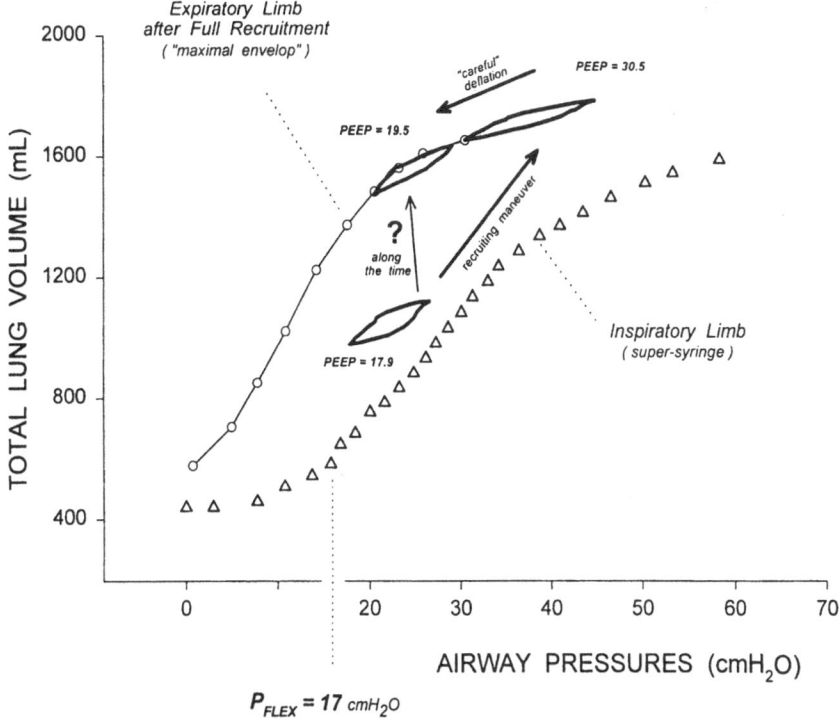

Fig. 7. Effects of a recruiting maneuver and sustaining end-expiratory pressure on lung volume and recruitment. Stepwise definition of the P-V curve by the super-syringe technique does not achieve full recruitment, as the expiratory limb defined after a sustained recruiting maneuver or after applying a high level of PEEP (30.5 cmH₂O) is displaced upward along the absolute (total) volume axis. (Oleic acid-ALI in dog.) Although not tested in this experiment, sustained application of sufficient PEEP might also succeed in approaching the expiratory "maximal envelope"

tal lung volume axis when compared to the P-V curve that preceded it (Fig. 7). (In other words, the highest pressures used during a standard P-V curve determination are not applied long enough to achieve full recruitment.) Moreover, the continued application of a PEEP and P-V combination high enough to exceed the yield threshold of refractory units can gradually move the tidal loop closer to the expiratory P-V envelope, but this process may require many hours to complete, as suggested by the time dependence of airway pressure release [62, 63].

Conclusion

For reasons outlined earlier, most investigators exploring the implications of ventilatory management in ARDS agree that it is desirable to assure recruitment of all available units at pressures that do not overdistend those already open. Unfortunately, even though many approaches have been advocated, fulfillment of this objective remains elusive. The relative emphasis on recruitment (versus avoidance of overdistention) should be relaxed after the first 72–96 h of ventilation, after which time the risks of overdistention begin to outweigh those of under-recruitment. Not enough data are currently at hand to decide the wisdom of advocating any specific combination of PEEP, P-V, and recruiting maneuvers that would be universally applicable. In the absence of convincing data, we believe that pressure and volume information provides the best guidance. Although a good rationale exists for undertaking the construction of P-V curves at the bed-side, this maneuver can often be difficult to undertake safely, even by experienced investigators. We do not believe it is advisable to advocate the routine clinical use of P-V curves until this process can be undertaken safely, quickly, and reproducibly. In the future, this may be possible with automated equipment. For the present time, we believe that it is reasonable to suggest the following – currently unproven – guidelines to optimize recruitment at safe distending pressures:

1. Consider the use of the prone position early in the course of ventilatory management.
2. Assuming good hemodynamic tolerance, perform a recruiting maneuver before undertaking any manipulation of PEEP and P-V. The process of PEEP and P-V selection requires a well sedated and passive subject.
3. Utilize relatively small P-V (4–6 mL/kg) to limit the end-inspiratory stress applied to non-recruited tissue and to patent alveoli surrounded by the most negative pleural pressures. (P-V bears no independent relationship to PaO_2; the plateau pressure achieved at end-inspiration does.)
4. Starting from a PEEP value of ≈ 8 cmH_2O and using a fixed P-V in the flow controlled volume-cycled mode, PEEP should be stepped upward in 2 cmH_2O increments, waiting approximately 2 min (>20 cycles) between PEEP steps. An end-inspiratory pause of approximately 1 sec is applied to the last tidal cycle of each PEEP step, and the plateau pressure is recorded along with the PEEP increment applied. The pause is removed after this recording is made.
5. PEEP steps are continued until the change in plateau pressure exceeds the change in PEEP by >1 cmH_2O in each of 2 successive steps, hemodynamic deterioration occurs, or the plateau pressure exceeds 40 cmH_2O (in a passive patient with a normal chest wall.) A second recruiting maneuver should be attempted in those with good hemodynamic tolerance (Fig. 7).
6. PEEP is then dropped back one step and used as the "optimal PEEP value" for ventilation with the selected P-V. Gradual deterioration of arterial oxygenation suggests that the addition of sighs to reach closer to the expiratory limb of the maximal envelope, periodic recruiting maneuvers, or even reconstruction of the entire P-V curve at a slightly higher P-V should be considered.

This evaluation procedure should take no longer than 20 min to complete and should be repeated daily (or whenever clinically significant deterioration or improvement has been encountered). After the first 72–96 h of ventilation, attempts to deliberately withdraw PEEP (in stepwise fashion, as tolerated) should begin in patients with stable or improving oxygen exchange. Although clearly a suboptimal compromise, such a practical regimen may have value in standardizing the ventilatory management of ARDS while adhering to lung protection principles, as they are currently understood.

References

1. Hedenstierna G, McCarthy G, Bergstrom M (1976) Airway closure during mechanical ventilation. Anesthesiology 44:114-123
2. Lachmann B (1992) Open up the lung and keep the lung open. Intensive Care Med 18:319-321
3. Dreyfuss D, Saumon G (1994) Should the lung be rested or recruited? The charybdis and scylla of ventilator management. Am J Respir Crit Care Med 149:1066-1068
4. Slutsky AS (1993) Barotrauma and alveolar recruitment (editorial). Intensive Care Med 19:369-371
5. Tsuno K, Prato P, Kolobow T (1990) Acute lung injury from mechanical ventilation at moderately high airway pressures. J Appl Physiol 69:956-961
6. Parker JC, Hernandex LA, Peeby KJ (1993) Mechanisms of ventilator-induced lung injury. Crit Care Med 21:131-143
7. Dreyfuss D, Soler P, Basset G, et al (1988) High inflation pressure pulmonary edema. Respective effects of high airway pressure, high P-V, and positive end-expiratory pressure. Am Rev Respir Dis 137:1159-1164
8. Muscedere JG, Mullen JB, Gan K, et al (1994) Tidal ventilation at low airway pressures can augment lung injury. Am J Respir Crit Care Med 149:1327-1334
9. Bryan AC, Froese AB (1991) Reflections on the HIFI trial. Pediatrics 87:565-567
10. Sugiura M, McCulloch PR, Wren S, Dawson RH, Froese AB (1994) Ventilator pattern influences neutrophil influx and activation in atelectasis-prone rabbit lung. J Appl Physiol 77:1355-1365
11. Rouby JJ, Lherm T, Martin de Lassale E (1993) Histologic aspects of pulmonary barotrauma in critically ill patients with acute respiratory failure. Intensive Care Med 19:383-389
12. Bancalari E, Gerhardt T (1986) Bronchopulmonary dysplasia. Ped Clin N Amer 33:1-23
13. Stamenovic D (1990) Micromechanical foundations of pulmonary elasticity. Physiol Rev 70:1117-1134
14. Lewis JF, Jobe AH (1993) Surfactant and the adult respiratory distress syndrome. Am Rev Respir Dis 147:218-233
15. Mead J, Takishima T, Leith D (1970) Stress distribution in lungs: A model of pulmonary elasticity. J Appl Physiol 28:596-608
16. Terry PB, Traystman RJ, Newball HH, Batra G, Menkes HA (1978) Collateral ventilation in man. N Engl J Med 298:10-15
17. Bendixen H H, Hedley-Whyte J, Laver M B (1963) Impaired oxygenation in surgical patients during general anesthesia with controlled ventilation. N Engl J Med 269:991-997
18. Lai-Fook SJ (1991) Stress distribution. In: Crystal RG, West JB, et al (eds) The Lung. Scientific Foundations. New York, pp 829-837
19. Stamenovic D, Wilson TA (1992) Parenchymal stability. J Appl Physiol 73:596-602
20. Kolton M, Cattran CB, Kent G, et al (1982) Oxygenation during high-frequency ventilation compared with conventional mechanical ventilation in two models of lung injury. Anesth Analg 61:323-332
21. Rimensberger P, Cox P, Bryan AC, et al (1995) Inverse ratio ventilation: Simply an alternative or something more? Crit Care Med 23:1786-1789
22. Benito S, Lemaire F (1990) Pulmonary P-V relationship in acute respiratory distress syndrome in adults: Role of positive end-expiratory pressure. J Crit Care 5:27-34
23. Matamis D, Lemire F, Harf A, Brun-Buisson C, Ansquer JC, Atlan G (1984) Total respiratory pressure volume curves in the adult respiratory distress syndrome. Chest 86:58-66
24. Valta P, Takala J, Eissa, NT, et al (1993) Does alveolar recruitment occur with positive end-expiratory pressure in adult respiratory distress syndrome patients? J Crit Care 8:34-42

25. Yap DYK, Liebkemann WD, Solway J, et al (1994) Influences of parenchymal tethering on the reopening of closed pulmonary airways. J Appl Physiol 76:2095–2105
26. Gaver DP, Samsel RW, Solway J (1990) Effects of surface tension and viscosity on airway opening. J Appl Physiol 69:74–85
27. Naureckas ET, Dawson CA, Gerber BS, et al (1994) Airway reopening pressure in isolated rat lungs. J Appl Physiol 76:1372–1377
28. Katz JA, Ozanne GM, Zinn SE, Fairley HB (1981) Time course and mechanisms of lung volume increase with PEEP in acute pulmonary failure. Anesthesiology 54:9–16.
29. Cereda M, Foti G, Musch G, Sparcino ME, Pesenti A (1996) PEEP prevents the loss of respiratory compliance during low P-V ventilation in acute lung injury patients. Chest 109:480–485
30. Bond DM, McAllon J, Froese AB (1994) Sustained inflations improve respiratory compliance during high-frequency oscillatory ventilation but not during large P-V positive-pressure ventilation in rabbits. Crit Care Med 22:1269–1277
31. Pelosi P, D'Andrea L, Vitale G, Pesenti A, Gattinoni L (1994) Vertical gradient of regional lung inflation in adult respiratory distress syndrome. Am J Respir Crit Care Med 149:8–13
32. Gattinoni L, D'Andrea L, Pelosi P, et al (1993) Regional effects and mechanism of positive end-expiratory pressure in early respiratory distress syndrome. JAMA 269:2122–2127
33. Shim C, Chun KJ, Williams MH Jr, Blaufox MD (1986) Positional effects on distribution of ventilation in chronic obstructive pulmonary disease. Ann Internal Med 105:346–350
34. Gattinoni L, Pesenti A, Bombino M (1988) Relationships between lung computed tomographic density, gas exchange, and PEEP in acute respiratory failure. Anesthesiology 69:824–832
35. Lamm WJE, Graham MM, Albert RK (1994) Mechanism by which the prone position improves oxygenation in acute lung injury. Am J Respir Crit Care Med 150:184–193
36. Froese AB, Bryan AC (1974) Effects of anesthesia and paralysis on diaphragmatic mechanics in man. Anesthesiology 41:242–255
37. Rehder K, Sessler AD, Rodarte JR (1977) Regional intrapulmonary gas distribution in awake and anesthetized paralyzed man. J Appl Physiol 42:391–402
38. West JB, Mathieu-Costello O (1992) Stress failure of pulmonary capillaries: Role in lung and heart disease. Lancet 340:762–767
39. Fu Z, Costello ML, Tsukimoto K, et al (1992) High lung volume increases stress failure in pulmonary capillaries. J Appl Physiol 73:123–133
40. Mathieu-Costello O, Willford DC, Fu Z, et al (1995) Pulmonary capillaries are more resistant to stress failure in dogs than in rabbits. J Appl Physiol 79:908–917
41. Namba Y, Kurdak S, Fu Z, et al (1995) Effect of reducing alveolar surface tension on stress failure in pulmonary capillaries. J Appl Physiol 79:2114–2121
42. Ravenscraft SA, Shapiro RS, Adams AB, Marini JJ (1995) Dependent damage in ventilator-induced lung injury. Am J Respir Crit Care Med 151:A551 (Abst)
43. Broccard AF, Shapiro RS, Schmitz LL, Ravenscraft SA, Marini JJ (1997) Influence of prone position on the extent and distribution of lung injury in a high P-V oleic acid model of acute respiratory distress syndrome. Crit Care Med 25:16–27
44. Broccard AF, Hotchkiss JR, Kuwayama N, Wangensteen OD, Marini JJ (1996) Effects of blood flow on lung injury induced by mechanical ventilation in an isolated perfused rabbit lung model. Am Rev Respir Dis 153:A378 (Abst)
45. Marini JJ (1996) PEEP, P-V, and barotrauma: An open and shut case? Chest 109:302–304
46. Marini JJ (1996) Evolving concepts in the ventilatory management of ARDS. Clin Chest Med 17:555–575
47. The HIFI Study Group (1989) High-frequency oscillatory ventilation compared with conventional mechanical ventilation in the treatment of respiratory failure in preterm infants. N Engl J Med 370:88–95
48. Clark RH, Gerstman DR, Null DM, deLemos RA (1992) Prospective randomized trial of high frequency oscillatory and cnventional ventilation in respiratory distress syndrome. Pediatrics 89:5–12.
49. McCulloch PR, Forkert GEK, Froese AB (1988) Lung volume maintenance prevents lung injury during high frequency oscillatory ventilation in surfactant-deficient rabbits. Am Rev Respir Dis 137:1185–1192

50. Amato MB, Barbas CS, MedeirosDM, et al (1995) Beneficial effects of the open lung approach with low distending pressures in acute respiratory distress syndrome. Am J Respir Crit Care Med 152:1835–1846
51. Webb HH, Tierney DF (1974) Experimental pulmonary edema due to intermittent positive pressure ventilation with high inflation pressures. Protection by positive end-expiratory pressure. Am Rev Respir Dis 110:556–565
52. Gattinoni L, Pelosi P, Crotti S, Valenza F (1995) Effects of positive end-expiratory pressure on regional distribution of tidal volume and recruitment in adult respiratory distress syndrome. Am J Respir Crit Care Med 151:1807–1814
53. Beydon L, Lamaire F, Jonson B (1991) Lung mechanics in ARDS. In: Zapol WM, Lemaire F (eds) Adult Respiratory Distress Syndrome. Vol 50. Lung Biology in Health and Disease. Dekker, New York, pp 139–160
54. Ranieri VM, Mascia L, Fiore T, Bruno F, Brienza A, Giuliani R (1995) Cardiorespiratory effects of positive end-expiratory pressure during progressive tidal volume reduction (permissive hypercapnia) in patients with acute respiratory distress syndrome Anesthesiology 83:710–720
55. Sydow M, Burchardi H, Zinserling J, Ische H, Crozier TA, Weyland W (1991) Improved determination of static compliance by automated single volume steps in ventilated patients. Intensive Care Med 17:108–114
56. Gattinoni L, Pesenti A, Avalli L, et al (1987) Pressure-volume curve of total respiratory system in acute respiratory failure. Am Rev Respir Dis 136:730–736
57. Pesenti A, Pelosi P, Gattinoni L (1990) Lung mechanics in ARDS. In: Vincent JL (ed) Yearbook of Intensive Care and Emergency Medicine. Springer Verlag, Berlin, pp 231–238
58. Gattinoni L, Mascheroni D, Basilico E, et al (1987) Volume/pressure curve of total respiratory system in paralysed patients: Artifacts and correction factors. Intensive Care Med 13:19–25
59. Levy P, Similowski T, Corbeil C, et al (1989) A method for studying volume-pressure curves of the respiratory system during mechanical ventilation. J Crit Care 4:83–89
60. Amato MBP, Barbas CSV, Meyer EC, et al (1995) Setting the "best PEEP" in ARDS: Limitations of choosing the PEEP according to the "best compliance". Am J Resp Crit Care Med 151:A550 (Abst)
61. Suter P, Fairley HB, Isenberg MD (1978) Effect of tidal volume and positive end-expiratory pressure on compliance during mechanical ventilation. Chest 73:158–162
62. Sydow M, Burchardi H (1993) Influence of time on alveolar recruitment in acute lung injury. In: Vincent JL (ed) Yearbook of Intensive Care and Emergency Medicine. Springer Verlag, Berlin, pp 127–140
63. Sydow M, Burchardi H, Ephraim E, Zielmann S, Crozier TA (1994) Long term effects of two different ventilatory modes on oxygenation in acute lung injury. Comparison of airway pressure release ventilation and volume controlled inverse ratio ventilation. Am J Respir Crit Care Med 149:1550–1556

Permissive Hypercapnia

M. B. Amato

Introduction

Permissive hypercapnia (PH) is becoming a widely accepted strategy for decreasing ventilator-induced lung injury [1-13]. It is not a therapeutic endpoint, but rather the penalty we have to pay for decreasing alveolar ventilation when we give priority to the limitation of lung overdistension. Its rationale is the assumption that transitory effects of hypercapnia are less deleterious than the lung damage produced by conventional attempts to keep a target $PaCO_2$ around 40 mmHg [13-15].

Initially used only in asthmatic patients [1-3], permissive hypercapnia has now been included as part of a "lung-protective-strategy" in recent clinical studies on acute respiratory distress syndrome (ARDS). The results were encouraging [4, 5, 9-12]. Hickling and coworkers obtained an improved survival in their ARDS population, when compared with historical series and APACHE II scores [4, 5]. Six recent studies on asthmatic patients exhibited a lower mortality (0-4%) and morbidity [2, 16-20] than equivalent studies published in the same period but not using PH (reported mortality = 2-23%) [21-24]. Lewandowski and coworkers [25, 26] obtained a very low mortality rate in severe ARDS patients when using an integrated approach which included PH, prone position and inhalation of nitric oxide (mortality around 20%). Uncontrolled studies have also reported good tolerance to the procedure in trauma [9, 11, 12] and pediatric patients with ARDS [27] or burns [28]. Multicenter retrospective studies have observed a lower incidence of bronchopulmonary dysplasia in infants receiving mechanical ventilation with $PaCO_2$ levels above the physiologic range (> 50 mmHg) [29].

And very recently, in a prospective and randomized experience with permissive hypercapnia, the investigators [10] demonstrated an improved lung function and better chances of weaning when using a combined approach of PH plus high positive end-expiratory pressure (PEEP) levels ($PEEP_{ideal}$) in severe ARDS. Further continuation of this study revealed an unquestionable improvement in overall survival [30].

Rationale for Implementation

PH is usually the direct consequence of a deliberated change in ventilatory parameters, normally leading to some decrement in alveolar ventilation with impairment of carbon dioxide (CO_2) removal. For instance, in an ARDS population with moderate/severe lung injury, Roupie and coworkers [31] observed that subtle reductions of tidal volume (VT) from 10 down to $\cong$ 8 mL/kg (maintaining an usual respiratory rate = 14–24 cycles/min) frequently resulted in considerable hypercapnia ($PaCO_2 \cong 70$ mmHg). Concerned with the recent recommendations of the Consensus Conference [32], many physicians today focus their attention on plateau pressure (P_{plat}) measurements, decreasing VT until obtaining a P_{plat} ≤ 35 cmH$_2$O. Mild hypercapnia usually ensues during these attempts. One could say that PH has been basically used as a "P_{plat}-sparing" agent.

Nevertheless, we have to remember that, although a high P_{plat} may be one important marker of an imminent lung injury, there are other conditions also associated to an increased risk. For instance, if we translate the study of Bshouty and Younes [33] to a human scenario, we can expect that the beneficial effect of a reduction of $\cong$ 9 cmH$_2$O in P_{plat} would be nullified by a concomitant increment in breathing frequency from 20 to 30 cycles/min. Although the increased frequency might attenuate the raise in $PaCO_2$, these opposite changes would result in persisting injury if taken together.

Such antagonistic changes can be frequently observed during our bedside experience with synchronized intermitent mandatory ventilation (SIMV). This mode usually represents a safe alternative for installing permissive hypercapnia, since a minimum ventilation is guaranteed at the same time that any additional breath required by the patient could still be supported. This facility usually decreases the need for curarization. But the problem appears when, concerned about the observation of high P_{plat} values, one attempts to simply decrease the volume or pressure of mandatory breaths. Under this condition, as the central stimulation of hypercapnia is very strong, small increments in $PaCO_2$ commonly have a dramatic excitatory effect in the young ARDS patient, resulting in an immediate increment in respiratory drive and rate. The initial raise in $PaCO_2$ might be attenuated. But the important issue is that this "compensatory" maneuver cannot be endorsed as safe at all. Indeed, high transpulmonary pressures during spontaneous efforts have resulted in experimental lesions as severe as those produced by positive pressure ventilation – and sometimes even worse, due to the increased venous return and a consequently increased lung edema [34–36]. Very likely, the reiteration of these pernicious forces at a faster rate would be troublesome.

Accordingly, the passive observation of some increment in respiratory rate after PH attempts is unwise, since unpredictable risks may be associated to this practice. We have to remember that the whole rationale for PH usage was extrapolated from experimental data and, therefore, we have to be cautious about any maneuver already reported as detrimental in the lab setting. Other examples of contradictory maneuvers can be observed in our daily clinical experience. In the following sections we will be talking about the paradox of alveolar collapse with persisting lung injury potentially associated to PH. It will be a good opportunity to stress that PH is not a synonym of VT or P_{plat} reductions. Sometimes, the priority should be given to more important maneuvers, as PEEP increments or deeper sedation of patients under spontaneous or pressure support breaths.

There are two particular problems concerning the use of pressure support ventilation (PSV) during PH. The first is related to the fact that usual attempts to decrease inspiratory airway pressures commonly result in tiny changes in VT. The reason is that the patient substitutes the machine work by his own muscle work, as long as he is strongly stimulated by high CO_2 levels. Although the airway pressures may be reduced in this situation, the high transpulmonary pressures will be maintained. Whatever the source of work for inflating the lung, the stress on lung tissues will be quite the same in both situations. As a practical example, consider a patient under PSV of 5 cmH_2O with a static lung compliance of 20 mL/cmH_2O: he must generate more than 15 cmH_2O of negative pleural pressure in order to obtain VT as low as 400 mL. The resultant transpulmonary pressure (20 cmH_2O) would be equivalent to that generated by a relaxed inflation with more than 23 cmH_2O of positive airway pressure. In other words, underestimation of "true" transpulmonary pressures is common during PSV, although this variable is probably the most important component in the ventilator-induced lung injury process [36, 37].

Another issue is the hazards of sedation during PSV. As stated above, the only way to control respiratory rate during PH is heavy sedation, especially through opioid infusions. But two practical problems commonly emerge. The limit between apnea and an adequate respiratory rate is not easy, requiring careful monitoring and titration of opioid doses. The use of some back-up ventilation should be strongly recommended. The second problem is that some patients reduce their respiratory rates in response to opioids, but not the inspiratory effort per breath. Indeed, deeper inspirations at a lower rate can be sometimes observed, with potentially detrimental consequences. In this condition, partial or total paralysis with institution of some controlled or combined mode (volume-assured pressure support – VAPS [38] or pressure-regulated volume control – PRVC [39]) could be advised.

Summing up, the manner we produce PH is very important and must be based on good rationale. As PH is always a compromise between high CO_2 versus lung injury, there is a natural tendency to counterbalance an "excessive" $PaCO_2$ with a respiratory maneuver judged to be "less likely to produce lung injury" and capable of attenuating the raise in CO_2. But according to the considerations made above, we have to be very cautious, never focusing our attention only on peak/plateau airway pressures. The global adjustment of ventilatory parameters should always be considered as a complex compromise: a composition of many potentially dangerous maneuvers.

But despite this complexity, there are some general rules and useful concepts to be used at the bedside. As a reasonable starting point, one could consider that reductions of minute ventilation usually result in decreased lung injury [33]. Sometimes, the best way to reduce minute ventilation is evident. This would be the case of a patient with moderate P_{plat} values (25–30 cmH_2O), under volume controlled ventilation, and with clear signals of insufficient PEEP levels (high shunt values and mechanical signals of tidal volume recruitment) (Fig. 1). In this case, some increment in PEEP levels, the maintenance of respiratory rate, and some attempt to keep P_{plat} at similar-to-lower values (by decreasing VT and driving pressure accordingly) would be the best rational solution [36, 40–47].

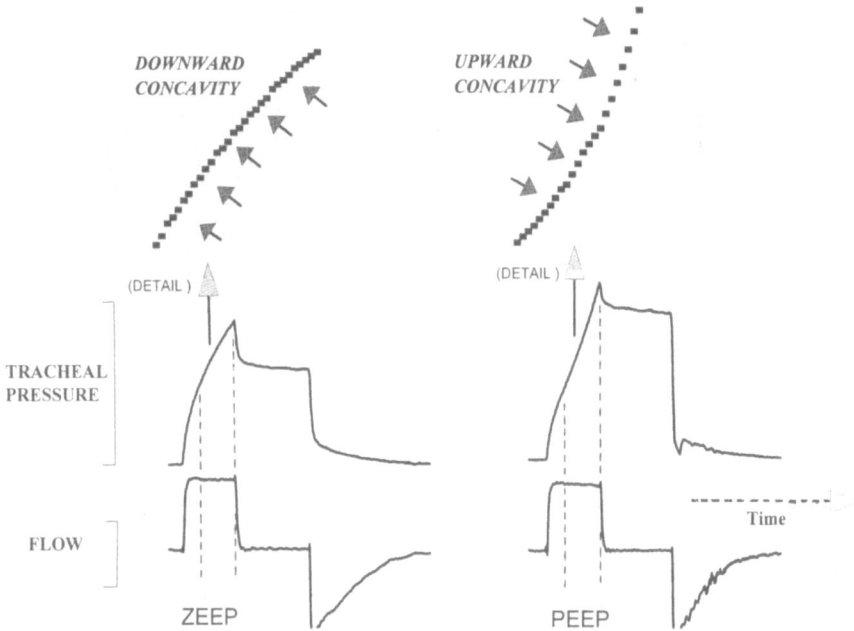

Fig. 1. Tracings representing airway pressure monitoring. The tracing on the left illustrates the ventilation of an ARDS patient under ZEEP (zero-PEEP), during constant (square wave) inspiratory flow and volume controlled ventilation. The downward concavity of pressure-time curve represents lung recruitment during tidal inflation, with a progressive gain in compliance. Higher PEEP levels should be strongly recommended in this situation. The tracing on the right represents the situation of the same patient under PEEP (16 cmH$_2$O). The upward concavity in this case represents loss of compliance during tidal inflation. An excessive stretch of collagen structures is probably responsible for this response and, in this case, one cannot guarantee that further increments in PEEP will result in additional benefit

Unfortunately, there are many other situations in which the best solution is not obvious. For instance, if the patient above had signals of adequate PEEP levels, should we try first a reduction in respiratory rate or a reduction in P$_{plat}$? Or should we maintain the same settings, after considering that the risks of hypercapnia would be greater than the benefits of a reduced lung stress (considering that P$_{plat}$ was not so high in this patient)?

Much work has to be done in the future. The relative role of each respiratory maneuver – its potential to produce lesions – shall be established and quantified. A rational choice should be based on a calculated sum of many positive and negative interactions, including all the systemic effects associated to hypercapnia as well as the toxic effects associated to high FiO$_2$.

Meanwhile, our decisions have to be based on the best bedside clinical judgment, after considering two major points: 1) potentially harmful effects of hypercapnia, and 2) some maneuvers that minimize hypercapnia with low chances of producing lung injury.

Consequences of Hypercapnia

Systemic Circulation

The hemodynamic effects of hypercapnia are clinically relevant, being the consequence of 2 basic phenomena:
1) sympathetic nervous activity with enhanced catecholamine secretion [6, 7, 48], and
2) the direct depressant properties of CO_2 on cardiac contractility and systemic arteriolar tone [49–51].

The sympathetic stimulation can normally overcome the depressant effects on cardiac performance, being helped by some decrement in afterload to left ventricle (due to the direct vasodilator effects of CO_2 on systemic vessels [49, 52]) and by some increment in preload (the peripheral veno-constriction of capacitance vessels enhances the venous return and frequently results in elevations of right and left atrial pressures [49, 53, 54]). The net result is usually predictable:
1) increased cardiac output mainly due to an increased heart rate
2) maintained or slightly increased stroke volume
3) maintained or slightly increased arterial blood pressure

Oxygen delivery increases as a direct consequence of increased cardiac output [52, 55–57]. Besides, the central venous PO_2 markedly increases due to the sum of two phenomena: increased oxygen delivery in the context of maintained oxygen consumption; and a rightward shift of the oxygen dissociation curve [6, 7, 52, 55, 57].

The consequences of this hyperdynamic state to the kidney and gastrointestinal tract have received some attention [55, 58, 59]. Up to know, we can say that, as long as the arterial oxygenation is well preserved, commonly tolerated levels of hypercapnia ($PaCO_2 \cong 80$ mmHg) do not alter renal function. Also, the risk for gastric hemorrhage seems not to be increased [7]. Indeed, some studies showed an increased splanchnic perfusion [59] and a fall in lactate levels [52, 55, 56, 60]. Although hypercapnia might affect respiratory muscle contractility [7], no relevant muscle dysfunction has been described.

Pulmonary Circulation

The most striking hemodynamic effect of hypercapnia is pulmonary hypertension [52, 55, 57, 60–64]. This phenomenon seems to be the net result of:
1) overflow
2) increased downstream pressure
3) increased pulmonary vascular resistance

As shown in Fig. 2, the overflow condition is caused by an increased cardiac output. The increments in downstream pressures (wedge pressures) are probably the necessary result of increased left atrial pressures produced by veno-constriction

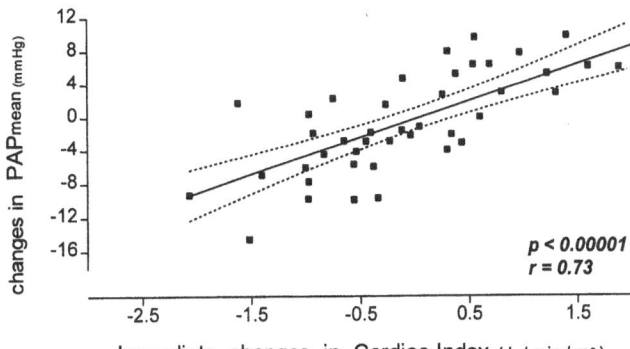

Fig. 2. Immediate changes of pulmonary arterial pressure after the installation of PH in patients with ARDS. As shown in this picture, there is a clear correlation between cardiac output and pulmonary arterial pressures: the higher the increment in cardiac output, the higher the increment in pulmonary vascular pressures, suggesting a simple system with linear resistance: the higher the flow, the higher the dissipation of pressures (From [60] with permission)

of capacitance vessels with increased effective volemia (Fig. 3) [53, 54]. Finally, the increased pulmonary vascular resistance (PVR) is a controversial topic in view of the marked influence of airway pressures on PVR. As demonstrated many years ago, PVR is usually a "J-shaped" function of mean airway pressures, especially during acute lung injury (ALI), what means that there is an optimal lung volume for blood flow where PVR is minimal [65, 66]. At this optimal lung volume, a large population of capillaries from previously collapsed zones can be recruited and the cross sectional area of the vascular bed is increased. On the oth-

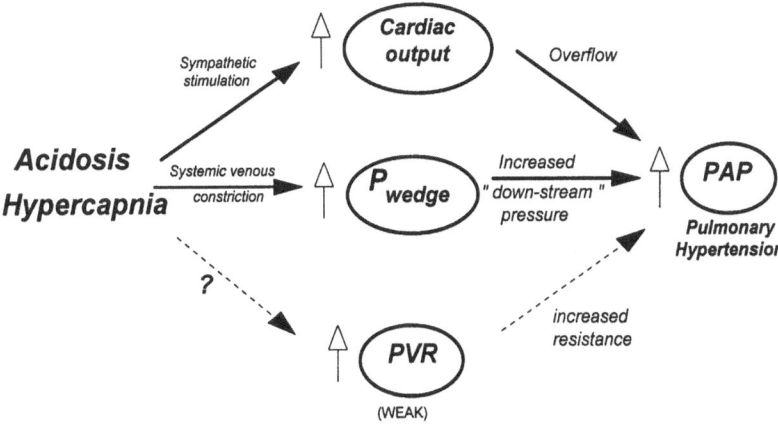

Fig. 3. Suggested mechanisms for pulmonary hypertension observed during PH. PVR = pulmonary vascular resistance; PAP = pulmonary arterial pressure; Pwedge = pulmonary arterial wedge pressure

er hand, any further increment of airway pressures to beyond this optimal volume might compress an excessive amount of small intra-alveolar vessels, straying the PVR from its minimum. Therefore, investigators provoking hypercapnia by simply reducing minute ventilation (and consequently reducing the operating lung volume) have reported an increased PVR associated to hypercapnia [57]. On the contrary, investigators producing hypercapnia with a simultaneous increment in the PEEP level (maintaining or even increasing operating lung volume) have reported an unchanged PVR in response to hypercapnia [55, 60].

Whatever its mechanism, pulmonary hypertension is the most preoccupying alteration of hypercapnia in the context of this chapter. Theoretically, we can expect that all three alterations mentioned above may produce an increased filtration pressure in the lung capillary bed, increasing the lung edema. Besides the well-known effect of raised wedge pressures on pulmonary edema formation [67], we know today that pulmonary overflow frequently alter the longitudinal distribution of pulmonary resistance, increasing disproportionally the venous resistance and the effective pressures at the filtration site [68]. Also, despite the controversial effect of CO_2 on pulmonary vascular resistance, we do not know yet if this "constrictor" effect is caused by a predominant arteriolar effect (what would be the least deleterious to lung edema formation) or by a dangerous venous constriction [69, 70].

This subject deserves further investigation. We have evidences today suggesting that the net effect of PH is beneficial to lung function and compliance [10]. Very probably, the lower distending pressure during PH can avoid excessive generation of negative interstitial pressures, decreasing so the transmural capillary pressures [42, 71, 72]. This beneficial tendency could overcome the opposite effect caused by pulmonary hypertension/overflow, with a reasonable net result.

However, we can still suppose that the protective effects of hypercapnia would be even better, had the pulmonary hypertension been avoided in the studies above. In this context, the associated use of nitric oxide [57, 70, 73] or alkalinizing agents to attenuate pulmonary hypertension [62] might be good theoretical alternatives.

Cardiac Stress

Pulmonary hypertension and tachycardia usually result in some stress to the heart, specially the right ventricle. Nevertheless, clinical signs of right ventricular dysfunction or arrhythmia have not been reported during PH [4–8, 10, 52]. The patients normally make use of their cardiac reserve, keeping the stroke volume despite an increased afterload to the right ventricle [52, 56, 60]. The situation of the left ventricle is less critical, since the systemic vasodilatation attenuates the increments in left cardiac work.

It should be noticed that most clinical studies on PH dealt with a population of young patients. This situation could well be different in the presence of previous cardiac or coronary disease. Increased heart rate and right ventricular overload could be of harmful consequences to an ischemic myocardium.

Intracranial Pressure

Besides the well-known vasodilator effects of hypercapnia on the brain vessels [7, 74], there are two additional reasons for expecting marked intracranial hypertension during PH: increased venous pressures due to increased right atrial pressures [53, 54]; and increased intrathoracic venous resistance due to an eventual association with high PEEP levels [75, 76].

Taking into account these risky alterations, the management of polytrauma patients should always receive special attention. Careful monitoring of intracranial pressures and cerebral perfusion would be essential for a safe installation of permissive hypercapnia.

But as long as these monitoring procedures are available, head trauma should no longer be considered as an absolute contraindication to PH. We have observed that whenever simple measures to minimize intracranial hypertension are concomitantly applied (straight neck position, slight head elevation, control of hyperthermia, pain and agitation, avoidance of cough, gentle aspiration of secretions under sedation or rapid paralysis, and judicious use of mannitol and barbiturates) hypercapnia may be well tolerated, even in the presence of severe head injury [12].

As a word of caution, marked fluctuations of intracranial pressure in the last hours and a reduced cerebral compliance should be considered as warning signals, suggesting the need for a very gradual installation of PH (or even its avoidance).

We would like to call attention to the special cases of patients with a previous cardiac arrest and risk of cerebral hypoxic injury. This situation is not rare when dealing with asthmatic patients admitted to the ICU. The hypoxic injury is commonly followed by marked cerebral edema in the following 2–3 days, and intracranial pressure monitoring is a wise procedure in this situation. There is a crucial dilemma in these cases. On one hand, marked hypercapnia commonly aggravates intracranial hypertension, by producing intracerebral arteriolar vasodilatation. On the other hand, by increasing minute ventilation, we commonly produce dynamic hyperinflation with increments in airway pressures and jugular pressures, impairing so the venous return and increasing intracranial pressures. The clinician has to balance the difficult compromise between these two opposite tendencies.

Minimization of Hypercapnia

Associated Use of PEEP

Although the concept of alveolar dead-space is usually regarded as representing wasted ventilation, it should be remembered that marked pulmonary shunt also produces important physiological dead space [77]. In this context, the associated use of PEEP, specially when resulting in a remarkable reduction of shunt values (what is usually accomplished by setting it above the lower P_{flex}) may have a theoretical additive effect [77–81], allowing the minimization of hypercapnia during reductions of VT (Fig. 4).

Use of Inverse-Ratio Pressure-Controlled Ventilation (PC-IRV)

Independently of reductions in shunt fraction, inverse ratio ventilation usually results in significant reductions of physiological dead space [82–85]. Except for some small degree of cardiovascular depression, the use of PC-IRV *per se* has not been associated to an increased lung injury, as long as some limitation of excessive P_{plat} is observed. On the contrary, some studies suggest a beneficial effect on lung recruitment along the time (12–48 h) [86, 87]. Therefore, this mode represents an attractive alternative during situations of very low lung compliance, decreasing minute volume requirements for the same $PaCO_2$.

General Measures to Decrease CO_2 Production

Frequently forgotten, the minimization of IV infusions of glucose and the use of high fat diets can be responsible for a reduction of 56% in carbon dioxide production [88]. This might represent an enormous reduction of minute volume requirements – approximately down to its half – for the same $PaCO_2$ [81].

If some doubts remain concerning the effects of IV lipid infusions on the lung [89], the simple suspension of IV glucose infusions during critical periods [90]

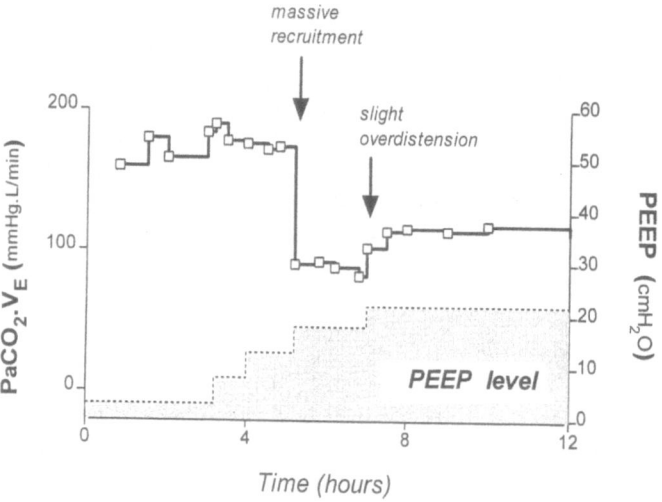

Fig. 4. Influence of PEEP on physiological dead-space. The progressive increment in PEEP resulted in a sudden drop in dead-space (represented in the figure as the product $PaCO_2$ times minute ventilation). Further increment in PEEP probably resulted in overdistension with subsequent raise in dead-space

and the use of enteral nutrition with low glucose contents should be considered as compelling alternatives.

Obviously – but not less importantly – rigorous control of temperature and anxiety, and the minimization of work of breathing are essential during permissive hypercapnia [91, 92].

Artificial Measures to Improve CO_2 Removal

The use of IVOX [93–97], tracheal gas insufflation (TGI) [98–105], and the associated use of chest wall vibration [106] can be considered as adjunctive measures to minimize hypercapnia. We call attention for the indication of these procedures only after the observance of easier general procedures discussed above. The clinical experience with TGI taught us an important lesson: those patients requiring high values of minute ventilation to keep moderately elevated CO_2 levels – and especially when high gradients between arterial versus end-tidal PCO_2 can be demonstrated [105] – are those less likely to benefit from TGI. Under this situation, the priority should be the use of simple maneuvers to decrease the alveolar dead-space (using optimal PEEP, for instance [77, 78, 80]), or to decrease CO_2 production (avoiding fever or high carbohydrate loads).

Risks of Under-Recruitment

The hazards of under-recruitment during mechanical ventilation have been recognized in the last years [36, 41, 45, 47, 107]. There is increasing experimental evidence that collapse – persistent or phasic – of edematous, inflamed or surfactant-depleted lung tissue can inflict further damage or retard lung healing. The ability of the lung to withstand the rigors of mechanical ventilation would be markedly impaired in the presence of atelectasis [108, 109]. In many experiments, the magnitude of the damage associated to airspace collapse was more impressive than the injury associated to parenchyma overdistention. Amplified septal/capillary stress at the boundary of the atelectatic regions [110, 111] and the shear forces produced at the wall of a collapsed airway (especially at the small airway unsupported by cartilage and located just above the site of closure [112–117]) have been implicated in this injuring process.

In this context, a preoccupying consequence of PH can be anticipated. Our daily clinical experience show us that the use of low VT (≤ 8 mL/kg) frequently result in some loss of lung recruitment with deterioration of arterial oxygenation along the time [118, 119]. This phenomenon is certainly exacerbated in the presence of ALI with alveolar instability. Which are the implications of this silent and progressive alveolar collapse during our attempts to reduce overdistention?

One of the major mechanisms responsible for the maintenance of alveolar patency during high-VT–low-PEEP ventilation seems to be small airway closure [120]. Accordingly, the bulk of refreshed air entering the alveoli at end-inspiration can be repeatedly "trapped" by small airway closure at end-expiration, keeping alveolar patency until the next breath. The airway pressures during inspiration have just to be slightly above the critical "yield" pressures of closed airways, refreshing the trapped units. A reasonable degree of lung recruitment and arterial oxygenation can usually be accomplished with this strategy. But were the inspiratory pressures a little bit lower in the following breaths, this cyclic "refreshment" of air could be impaired. Airway pressures constantly bellow the critical "yield" pressure of the small airway would permit a progressive reabsorption of the trapped air behind it, with ultimate alveolar collapse. This is the current explanation for the progressive deterioration of compliance and oxygenation along the time, after institution of small VT ventilation [118].

Therefore, it is not difficult to understand why the simple reduction of VT (to avoid high P_{plat} values) can be troublesome in many situations. Although Hickling and coworkers have reported good results with permissive hypercapnia associated with simple VT reductions [4, 5], Cereda et al. [118] showed that PEEP levels of at least 15 cmH$_2$O would be necessary to counterbalance the strong collapsing tendency associated to the use of low VT in mild ARDS patients. When one considers the probable mechanisms involved in the ventilator-induced lung injury and the striking relevance of alveolar collapse, it seems a logical strategy the use of recruiting maneuvers plus high PEEP levels associated to PH – whenever the presence of alveolar collapse can be inferred. In most circumstances, when enough PEEP is added, the plateau pressures needed to keep lung recruitment are frequently lower than those required at a lower PEEP level [10]. The presumed explanation is that, by preventing airspace collapse at end-expiration, the surface tension forces at the bronchiolar level are minimized – because the air/liquid interface is now displaced towards the alveolar sac with a larger radius – and lower inspiratory pressures are then required to "refresh" unstable units, maintaining alveolar patency.

In conclusion, besides the obvious effects on arterial oxygenation, by keeping an optimal lung recruitment one could prevent further lung injury during PH, as suggested by many clinical and experimental evidences. The studies on high-frequency ventilation have already demonstrated the hazards of under-recruitment – even when very low "pressure-swings" are applied [121]. In a recent retrospective analysis of ARDS patients submitted to PH, the investigators came to the conclusion that, among the maneuvers adopted to reduce driving pressures/VT, the increments in PEEP were at least as important (if not more important) as the reductions in P_{plat} for obtaining some improvement in lung function, reduction in clinically detectable barotrauma [122], and improvement in overall survival [30]. Thus, the possibility of massive alveolar collapse is crucial during PH especially in the context of an ALI/ARDS. A special care with PEEP levels would be essential in this situation.

Management of Severe Respiratory Acidosis

The correction of PH-associated respiratory acidosis with sodium bicarbonate is very controversial. However, we have observed that this maneuver may be very useful when the cardiovascular effects of PH are excessive (for instance, the presence of very high heart rates accompanied by high wedge pressures and marked pulmonary hypertension). In this situation, the partial correction of acidosis seems to attenuate the excessive sympathetic stimulation, especially in young patients.

Also, the partial correction of acidosis – even in the presence of a maintained hypercapnia – attenuates the stimulation of ventilatory drive, facilitating the intended hypoventilation during assisted or spontaneous modes. Lower dosages of opioid agents will be required. Obviously, patients with impaired renal function usually need an increased amount of bicarbonate reposition.

Whenever administration of sodium bicarbonate is required (we have not advocated the correction of respiratory acidosis based on fixed arbitrary numbers, but only after judging that the consequences of sympathetic stimulation are excessive), we have used slow infusions lasting for 4–6 h, with careful monitoring of $PaCO_2$ levels. The major problem associated with bicarbonate infusion is a temporary increase in $PaCO_2$ levels. As a rule of thumb, 250 mEq of sodium bicarbonate commonly result in an increase in $PaCO_2$ of 30%, if administered over 1 h, and an increase about 5 % when administered over 6 h (considering a constant alveolar ventilation and constant body CO_2 production during this period).

The Pace of Installation of PH

In a recent study enrolling more than 50 patients with ARDS, the installation of PH – from a $PaCO_2$ close to 35 mmHg up to 60–80 mmHg – was immediate and without serious adverse consequences [30]. The cardiovascular tolerance to this maneuver was very adequate [60]. Therefore, except for situations of previous heart and/or neurological disease, the progressive and gradual installation of hypercapnia seems to be an unwise procedure, consisting indeed in a harmful waste of time. The experimental evidence [45, 123] and at least one clinical study [10] suggest that the ventilator-induced lung injury process is very fast, evolving in minutes or few hours. Accordingly, the initial ventilatory approach adopted in the first 24–48 h may have dramatic consequences to lung recovery and survival [30, 122]. In our current understanding, the immediate avoidance of lung injury should have priority over the potential cardiovascular effects of PH.

References

1. Menitove SM, Goldring RM (1983) Combined ventilator and bicarbonate strategy in the management of status asthmaticus. Am J Med 74:898–901
2. Darioli R, Perret C (1984) Mechanical controlled hypoventilation in status asthmaticus. Am Rev Respir Dis 129:385–387
3. Perret C, Feihl F (1992) Respiratory failure in asthma: management of the mechanically ventilated patient. In: Vincent JL (ed) Update in Intensive Care Medicine. Springer-Verlag, Berlin, pp 364–371
4. Hickling KG, Henderson SJ, Jackson R (1990) Low mortality associated with low volume pressure limited ventilation with permissive hypercapnea in severe adult respiratory distress syndrome. Intensive Care Med 16:372–377

5. Hickling KG, Walsh J, Henderson S, Jackson R (1994) Low mortality rate in adult respiratory distress syndrome using low-volume, pressure-limited ventilation with permissive hypercapnia: a prospective study. Crit Care Med 22: 1568–1578
6. Bidani A, Tzouanakis AE, Cardenas VJ Jr, Zwischenberger JB (1994) Permissive hypercapnia in acute respiratory failure. JAMA 272: 957–962
7. Feihl F, Perret C (1994) Permissive hypercapnia. How permissive should we be? Am J Respir Crit Care Med 150: 1722–1737
8. Tuxen DV (1994) Permissive hypercapnia. In: Tobin MJ (ed) Principles and Practice of Mechanical Ventilation. McGraw Hill, New York, pp 371–392
9. McIntyre RC, Haenel JV, Moore FA, Read RR, Burch JM, Moore EE (1994) Cardiopulmonary effects of permissive hypercapnia in the management of adult respiratory distress syndrome. J Trauma 37: 433–438
10. Amato MBP, Barbas CSV, Medeiros DM, et al (1995) Beneficial effects of the "open lung approach" with low distending pressures in ARDS: A prospective randomized study on mechanical ventilation. Am J Respir Crit Care Med 152: 1835–1846
11. Simon RJ, Mawilmada S, Ivatury RR (1994) Hypercapnia: Is there a cause for concern? J Trauma 37: 74–81
12. Gentilello LM, Anardi D, Mock C, Arreola-Risa C, Maier RV (1995) Permissive hypercapnia in trauma patients. J Trauma 39: 846–853
13. Pesenti A (1990) Target blood gases during ARDS ventilatory management. Intensive Care Med 16: 349–351
14. Rahn H (1976) Why are pH of 7.4 and $PaCO_2$ of 40 mmHg normal values for man? Bull Eur Physiopathol Res 12: 5–12
15. Rahn H, Reeves RB, Howell BJ (1975) Hydrogen ion regulation, temperature and evolution. Am Rev Respir Dis 112: 165–172
16. Braman SS, Kaemmerlen JT (1990) Intensive care of status asthmaticus. A 10–year experience. JAMA 264: 366–368
17. Sydow M, Burchardi H (1991) Intensive care management of life-threatening status asthmaticus. In: Vincent JL (ed) Update in Intensive Care and Emergency Medicine. Springer-Verlag, Berlin, pp 313–323
18. Henderson A, Wright M (1992) Status asthmaticus: experience of 100 consecutive admissions to an intensive care unit. Clin Intensive Care 3: 148–152
19. Williams TJ, Tuxen DV, Scheinkestel CD, Czarny D, Bowes G (1992) Risk factors for morbidity in mechanically ventilated patients with acute vere asthma. Am Rev Respir Dis 146: 607–615
20. Bellomo R, McLaughlin P, Tai E, Parkin G (1994) Asthma requiring mechanical ventilation. A low morbidity approach. Chest 105: 891–896
21. Picado C, Montserrat JM, Roca J, et al. (1983) Mechanical ventilation in severe exacerbation of asthma. Eur J Respir Dis 64: 102–107
22. Higgins B, Greening AP, Crompton GK (1986) Assisted ventilation in severe acute asthma. Thorax 41: 464–467
23. Mansel JK, Stegner SW, Petrini MF, Norman JR (1990) Mechanical ventilation in patients with acute severe asthma. Am J Med 89: 42–48
24. Luksza A, Smith P, Coakley J, Gordan IJ, Atherton ST (1986) Acute severe asthma treated by mechanical ventilation: 10 years' experience from a district general hospital. Thorax 41: 459–463
25. Lewandowski K, Slama K, Falke KJ (1992) Approaches to improve survival in severe ARDS. In: Vincent JL (ed) Update of Intensive Care and Emergency Medicine. Springer-Verlag, Berlin, pp 372–383
26. Lewandowski K, Pappert D, Gerlach H, Rossaint R, Kuhlen R, Falke KJ (1995) Permissive hypercapnia in the treatment of ARDS. Am J Respir Crit Care Med 151: A79 (Abst)
27. Reynolds EM, Ryan DP, Doody DP (1993) Permissive hypercapnia and pressure-controlled ventilation as treatment of severe adult respiratory distress syndrome in a pediatric burn patient. Crit Care Med 21: 944–947

28. Sheridan RL, Kacmarek RM, McEttrick MM, et al (1995) Permissive hypercapnia as a ventilatory strategy in burned children: Effect on barotrauma, pneumonia and mortality. J Trauma 39:854–859

29. Kraybill EN, Runyan DK, Bose CL, Khan JH (1989) Risk factors for chronic lung disease in infants with birth weights of 751 to 1000 grams. J Pediatr 115:155–170

30. Amato MBP, Barbas CSV, Medeiros D, et al (1996) Improved survival in ARDS: Beneficial effects of a lung protective strategy. Am J Respir Crit Care Med 153:A531 (Abst)

31. Roupie E, Dambrosio M, Servillo G, et al (1995) Titration of tidal volume and induced hypercapnia in acute respiratory distress syndrome. Am J Respir Crit Care Med 152:121–128

32. Slutsky AS (1993) ACCP Consensus Conference. Mechanical Ventilation. Chest 104:1833–1859

33. Bshouty Z, Younes M (1992) Effect of breathing pattern and level of ventilation on pulmonary fluid filtration in dog lung. Am Rev Respir Dis 145:372–376

34. Stalcup SA, Mellins RB (1977) Mechanical forces producing pulmonary edema in acute asthma. N Engl J Med 297:592–596

35. Mascheroni D, Kolobow T, Fumagalli R, Moretti MP, Buckhold D (1988) Acute respiratory failure following pharmacologically induced hyperventilation: an experimental study. Intensive Care Med 15:8–14

36. Dreyfuss D, Soler P, Basset G, Saumon G (1988) High inflation pressure pulmonary edema. Respective effects of high airway pressure, high tidal volume and positive end-expiratory pressure. Am Rev Respir Dis 137:1159–1164

37. Hernandez LA, Peevy KJ, Moise AA, Parker JC (1989) Chest wall restriction limits high airway pressure-induced lung injury in young rabbits. J Appl Physiol 66:2364–2368

38. Amato MBP, Barbas CSV, Bonassa J, Saldiva PHN, Zin WA, Carvalho CRR (1992) Volume-assured pressure support ventilation (VAPSV). A new approach for reducing muscle workload during acute respiratory failure. Chest 102:1225–1234

39. Andersen JB (1992) Introducing pressure regulated volume control (PRVC) and volume support (VS). In: Improved Care for the Critically Ill – Siemens – Life Support Systems (divulging material), Copenhagen, pp 5–20

40. Webb HH, Tierney DF (1974) Experimental pulmonary edema due to intermittent positive pressure ventilation with high inflation pressures: protection by positive end-expiratory pressure. Am Rev Respir Dis 110:556–565

41. Argiras EP, Blakeley CR, Dunnill MS, Otremski S, Sykes MK (1987) High PEEP decreases hyaline membrane formation in surfactant deficient lungs. Br J Anaesth 59:1278–1285

42. Snyder JV (1987) Pulmonary physiology. In: Snyder JV, Pinsky MR (eds) Oxygen Transport in the Critically Ill. Year Book Medical Publishers, pp 295–317

43. Sandhar BK, Niblett DJ, Argiras EP, Dunnill MS, Sykes MK (1988) Effects of positive end-expiratory pressure on hyaline membrane formation in a rabbit model of the neonatal respiratory distress syndrome. Intensive Care Med 14:538–546

44. Bshouty Z, Younes M (1988) Effect of tidal volume and PEEP on rate of edema formation in in situ perfused canine lobes. J Appl Physiol 64:1900–1907

45. Corbridge TC, Wood LDH, Crawford GP, Chudoba MJ, Yanos J, Sznadjer JI (1990) Adverse effects of large tidal volume and low PEEP in canine acid aspiration. Am Rev Respir Dis 142:311–315

46. Dreyfuss D, Saumon G (1994) Should the lung be rested or recruited? The charybdis and scylla of ventilator management. Am J Respir Crit Care Med 149:1066–1068

47. Muscedere JG, Mullen JBM, Slutsky AS (1994) Tidal ventilation at low airway pressures can augment lung injury. Am J Respir Crit Care Med 149:1327–1334

48. Sechzer PH, Egbert LD, Linde HW, Cooper DY, Dripps RD, Price HL (1960) Effect of CO_2 inhalation on arterial pressure, ECG and plasma catecholamines and 17-OH corticosteroids in normal man. J Appl Physiol 15:454–458

49. Walley KR, Lewis TH, Wood LDH (1990) Acute respiratory acidosis decreases left ventricular contractility but increases cardiac output in dogs. Circ Res 67:628–635

50. Wexels JC, Mjos OD (1987) Effects of carbon dioxide and pH on myocardial function in dogs with acute left ventricular failure. Crit Care Med 15:1116–1120

51. Tang W, Weil MH, Gazmuri RJ, Bisera J, Rackow EC (1991) Reversible impairment of myocardial contractility due to hypercarbic acidosis in the isolated perfused rat heart. Crit Care Med 19:218–224
52. Thorens JB, Jolliet P, Ritz M, Chevrolet JC (1996) Effects of rapid permissive hypercapnia on hemodynamics, gas exchange, and oxygen transport and consumption during mechanical ventilation for the acute respiratory distress syndrome. 22:182–119
53. Rothe CF, Stein PM, MacAnespie CL, Gaddis ML (1985) Vascular capacitance responses to severe systemic hypercapnia and hypoxia in dogs. Am J Physiol 249:H1061–1069
54. Gaddis ML, MacAnesoie CL, Rothe CF (1986) Vascular capacitance responses to hypercapnia of the vascularly isolated head. Am J Physiol 251:H164–170
55. Amato MBP, Barbas CSV, Medeiros DM, et al (1994) Hemodynamic effects of permissive hypercapnia with high PEEP and low tidal volume in ARDS. Am J Respir Crit Care Med 149:A75 (Abst)
56. Thorens JB, Chopard P, Jolliet P, Chevrolet JC (1994) Effect of permissive hypercapnia on tissue oxygenation in acute respiratory failure. Am J Respir Crit Care Med 149:A68 (Abst)
57. Puybasset L, Stewart T, Rouby JJ, et al (1994) Inhaled nitric oxide reverses the increase in pulmonary vascular resistance induced by permissive hypercapnia in patients with ARDS. Anesthesiology 80:1254–1267
58. Anderson RJ, Rose CE, Berns AS, Erickson AL, Arnold PE (1980) Mechanism of effect of hypercapnic acidosis on renin secretion in the dog. Am J Physiol 238:F119–F125
59. Nguyen PJ, Tao W, Zwischenberger T, et al (1994) Effect of rapid permissive hypercapnia on carotid, renal and mesenteric blood flows in an ovine model. Am J Respir Crit Care Med 149:A69 (Abst)
60. Carvalho CRR, Barbas CSV, Medeiros DM, et al (1997) Temporal hemodynamic effects of permissive hypercapnia associated with "ideal PEEP" in ARDS (In press)
61. Vittanen A, Salmenperä M, Heinonen J, Hynynen M (1989) Pulmonary vascular resistance before and after cardiopulmonary bypass. The effect of $PaCO_2$. Chest 95:773–778
62. Chang AC, Zucker HA, Hickey PR, Wessel DL (1995) Pulmonary vascular resistance in infants after cardiac surgery: Role of carbon dioxide and hidrogen ion. Crit Care Med 23:568–574
63. Baudouin SV, Evans TW (1993) Action of carbon dioxide on hypoxic pulmonary vasoconstriction in the rat lung: evidence against specific endothelium-derived relaxing factor-mediated vasodilation. Crit Care Med 21:740–746
64. Malik AB, Kidd BSL (1973) Independent effects of changes in H^+ and CO_2 concentrations on hypoxic pulmonary vasoconstriction. J Appl Physiol 34:318–323
65. Leeman M, Lejeune P, Closset J, Vachiéry JL, Mélot C, Naeije R (1990) Effects of PEEP on pulmonary hemodynamics in intact dogs with oleic acid pulmonary edema. J Appl Physiol 69:2190–2196
66. Canada E, Benumof JL, Tousdale FR (1982) Pulmonary vascular resistance correlates in intact normal and abnormal canine lungs. Crit Care Med 10:719–723
67. Prewitt RM, McCarthy J, Wood LDH (1981) Treatment of acute low pressure pulmonary edema in dogs. Relative effects of hydrostatic and oncotic pressure, nitroprusside, and positive end-expiratory pressure. J Clin Invest 67:409–418
68. Younes M, Bshouty Z, Ali J (1987) Longitudinal distribution of pulmonary vascular resistance with very high pulmonary blood flow. J Appl Physiol 62:344–358
69. Collee GG, Lynch KE, Hill RD, Zapol WM (1987) Bedside measurement of pulmonary capillary pressure in patients with acute respiratory failure. Anesthesiology 66:614–620
70. Benzing A, Bräutigam P, Geiger K, Loop T, Beyer U, Moser E (1995) Inhaled nitric oxide reduces pulmonary transvascular albumin flux in patients with acute lung injury. Anesthesiology 83:1153–1161
71. Hida W, Hildebrandt J (1984) Alveolar surface tension, lung inflation, and hydration affect interstitial pressure [Px(f)]. J Appl Physiol 57:262–270
72. Inoue H, Inoue C, Hildebrandt J (1980) Vascular and airway pressures, and interstitial edema affect peribronchial fluid pressure. J Appl Physiol 48:177–185

73. Frostell CG (1994) Acute lung injury and inhaled NO. The reduction of pulmonary capillary pressure has implications for lung fluid balance. Acta Anaesthesiol Scand 38:623–624

74. Oyesiku NM, Amacher AL (1990) Intracraneal pressure. In: Oyesiku NM, Amacher AL (eds) Patient Care in Neurosurgery, third ed. Little, Brown and Co, Boston, Toronto, London, pp 25–59

75. Fessler HE, Brwer RG, Shapiro EP, Permutt S (1993) Effects of positive end-expiratory pressure and body position on pressure in the thoracic great veins. Am Rev Respir Dis 148: 1657–1664

76. Nanas S, Magder S (1992) Adaptations of the peripheral circulation to PEEP. Am Rev Respir Dis 146:688–693

77. Fletcher R (1989) Relationship between alveolar dead space and arterial oxygenation in children with congenital cardiac disease. Br J Anaesth 62:168–176

78. Blanch L, Fern·ndez R, Benito S, Mancebo J, Net A (1987) Effect of PEEP on the arterial minus end-tidal carbon dioxide gradient. Chest 92:451–454

79. Murray IP, Modell JH, Gallagher TJ, Banner MJ (1984) Titration of PEEP by the arterial minus end-tidal carbon dioxide gradient. Chest 85:100–104

80. Coffey RL, Albert RK, Robertson HT (1983) Mechanisms of physiological dead space response to PEEP after acute oleic acid during lung injury. J Appl Physiol 55:1550–1557

81. Selecky PA, Wasserman K, Klein M, Ziment I (1978) A graphic approach to assessing interrelationships among minute ventilation, arterial carbon dioxide tension, and ratio of physiologic dead space to tidal volume in patients on respirators. Am Rev Respir Dis 117: 181–184

82. Cole AGH, Weller SF, Sykes MK (1984) Inverse ratio ventilation compared with PEEP in adult respiratory failure. Intensive Care Med 10:227–232

83. Lichtwarck-Aschof M, Nielsen JB, Sjostrand UH, Edgren EL (1992) An experimental randomized study of five different ventilatory modes in a piglet model of severe respiratory distress. Intensive Care Med 18:339–347

84. Lachmann B, Haendly H, Schultz H, Jonson B (1980) Improved arterial oxygenation, PaCO$_2$ elimination, compliance and barotrauma following changes of volume-generated PEEP ventilation with inspiratory/expiratory (I/E) ratio of 1:2 to pressure-generated ventilation with I:E ratio of 4:1 in patients with severe adult respiratory distress syndrome (ARDS). Intensive Care Med 6:64–76

85. Gattinoni L, Mascheroni D, Borelli M, Basilico E, Pesenti A (1991) Ventilation in severe ARDS: Inverted ratio ventilation and CO$_2$ removal. In: Lemaire F (ed) Mechanical Ventilation. Springer-Verlag, Berlin, pp 129–145

86. Sydow M, Burchardi H, Ephraim E, Zielmann S, Crozier TA (1994) Long-term effects of two different ventilatory modes on oxygenation in acute lung injury. Comparison of airway pressure release ventilation and volume-controlled inverse ratio ventilation. Am J Respir Crit Care Med 149:1550–1556

87. Marini JJ (1994) Ventilation of the acute respiratory distress syndrome. Looking for Mr. Goodmode. Anesthesiology 80:972–975

88. Al-Saady NM (1994) Does dietary manipulation influence weaning from artificial ventilation? Intensive Care Med 20:463–465

89. Venus B, Smith RA, Patel C, Sandoval E (1989) Hemodynamics and gas exchange alterations during intralipid infusion in patients with adult respiratort distress syndrome. Chest 95:1278–1281

90. Askanazi J, Elwyn DH, Silverberg PA, Rosebaum SH, Kinney JM (1980) Respiratory distress syndrome secondary to a high carbohydrate load. Surgery 87:596–598

91. Tobin MJ, Fahey PJ (1994) Management of the patient who is "fighting the ventilator". In: Tobin MJ (ed) Principles and Practice of Mechanical Ventilation. McGraw Hill, New York, pp 1149–1162

92. Manthous CA, Hall JB, Kushner R, Schmidt GA, Russo G, Wood LDH (1995) The effect of mechanical ventilation on oxygen consumption in critically ill patients. Am J Respir Crit Care Med 151:210–214

93. Zwischenberger JB, Nguyen TT, Tao W, et al (1994) IVOX with gradual permissive hypercapnia: a new management technique for respiratory failure. J Surg Research 57:99–105

94. Zwischenberger JB, Cardenas VJ Jr, Tao W, Niranjan SC, Clark JW, Bidani A (1994) Intravascular membrane oxygenation and carbon dioxide removal with IVOX: can improved design and permissive hypercapnia achieve adequate respiratory support during severe respiratory failure? Artif Organs 18:833–839

95. Tao W, Zwischenberger JB, Nguyen TT, et al (1994) Performance of an intravenous gas exchanger (IVOX) in a venovenous bypass circuit. Ann Thorac Surg 57:1484–1491

96. Brunet F, Mira JP, Cerf C, et al (1994) Permissive hypercapnia and intravascular oxygenator in the treatment of patients with ARDS. Artif Organs 18:826–832

97. Mira JP, Brunet F, Belghith M, et al (1995) Reduction of ventilator settings allowed by intravenous oxygenator (IVOX) in ARDS patients. Intensive Care Med 21:11–17

98. Nahum A, Ravenskraft SA, Nakos G, et al (1992) Tracheal gas insufflation during pressure-control ventilation. Effect of catheter position, diameter, and flow rate. Am Rev Respir Dis 146:1411–1418

99. Nahum A, Burke WC, Ravenskraft SA, et al (1992) Lung Mechanics and gas exchange during pressure control ventilation in dogs: augmentation of CO_2 elimination by an intratracheal catheter. Am Rev Respir Dis 146:965–973

100. Nahum A, Ravenscraft SA, Nakos G, Adams AB, Burke WC, Marini JJ (1993) Effect of catheter flow direction on CO_2 removal during tracheal gas insufflation in dogs. J Appl Physiol 75:1238–1246

101. Ravenscraft SA, Burke WC, Nahum A, et al (1993) Intratracheal gas insufflation augments CO_2 clearance during mechanical ventilation. Am Rev Respir Dis 148:345–351

102. Nakos G, Zakinthinos S, Kotanidou A, Tsagaris H, Roussos C (1994) Tracheal gas insufflation reduces tidal volume while $PaCO_2$ is maintained constant. Intensive Care Med 20:407–413

103. Burke WC, Nahum A, Ravenscraft SA et al (1993) Modes of tracheal gas insufflation. Comparison of continuous and phase-specific gas injection in normal dogs. Am Rev Respir Dis 148:562–568

104. Nahum A, Shapiro RS, Ravenscraft SA, Adams AB, Marini JJ (1995) Efficacy of expiratory tracheal gas insufflation in a canine model of lung injury. Am J Respir Crit Care Med 152:489–495

105. Kuo PH, Wu HD, Yu CJ, Yang SC, Lai YL (1996) Efficacy of tracheal gas insufflation in acute respiratory distress syndrome with permissive hypercapnia. Am J Respir Crit Care Med 154:612–616

106. Eckmann DM, Gavriely N (1996) Chest vibration redistributes intra-airway CO_2 during tracheal insufflation in ventilatory failure. Crit Care Med 24:451–457

107. Sandhar BK, Niblett DJ, Argiras EP, Dunnill MS, Sykes MK (1988) Effects of positive end-expiratory pressure on hyaline membrane formation in a rabbit model of the neonatal respiratory distress syndrome. Intensive Care Med 14:538–546

108. Egan EA (1982) Lung inflation, lung solute permeability, and alveolar edema. J Appl Physiol 53:121–125

109. Egan EA (1980) Response of alveolar epithelial solute permeability to changes in lung inflation. J Appl Physiol 49:1032–1036

110. Macklem PT, Murphy B (1974) The forces applied to the lung in health and disease. Am J Med 57:371–377

111. Mead J, Takishima T, Leith D (1970) Stress distribution in lungs: A model of pulmonary elasticity. J Appl Physiol 28:596–608

112. Avery ME, Tooley WH, Keller JB, et al (1987) Is chronic lung disease in low birth weight infants preventable? Pediatrics 79:26–30

113. Van Marter LJ, Pagano M, Allred EN, Leviton A, Kuban KCK (1992) Rate of bronchopulmonary dysplasia as a function of neonatal intensive care practices. J Pediatr 120:938–946

114. Enhorning G, Robertson B (1972) Lung expansion in the premature rabbit fetus after tracheal deposition of surfactant. Pediatrics 50:58–66

115. Snyder JV, Froese A (1987) Respirator lung. In: Snyder JV, Pinsky MR (eds) Oxigen Transport in the Critically Ill. Year Book Medical Publishers, pp 358–373

116. Berg TJ, Pagtakhan RD, Reed MH, Langston C, Chernick V (1975) Bronchopulmonary dysplasia and lung rupture in hyaline membrane disease: influence of continuous distending pressure. Pediatrics 55:51–54
117. Nilsson R, Grossmann G, Robertson B (1980) Bronchiolar epithelial lesions induced in the premature rabbit neonate by short periods of artificial ventilation. Acta Path Microbiol Scand 88:359–367
118. Cereda M, Foti G, Musch G, Sparacino ME, Pesenti A (1996) Positive end-expiratory pressure prevents the loss of respiratory compliance during low tidal volume ventilation in acute lung injury patients. Chest 109:480–485
119. Blanch L, Fernandez R, Valles J, Sol'e J, Roussos C, Artigas A (1994) Effect of two tidal volumes on oxygenation and respiratory system mechanics during the early stage of adult respiratory distress syndrome. J Crit Care 9:151–158
120. Hoppin FG, Hildebrandt J (1977) Mechanical properties of the lung. In: West JB (ed) Bioengineering Aspects of the Lung. Marcel Dekker, New York and Basel, pp 83–162
121. McCulloch PR, Forkert PG, Froese AB (1988) Lung volume maintenance prevents lung injury during high frequency oscillatory ventilation in surfactant-deficient rabbits. Am Rev Respir Dis 137:1185–1192
122. Amato MBP, Barbas CSV, Pastore L, Grunauer MA, Magaldi RB, Carvalho CRR (1996) Minimizing barotrauma in ARDS: Protective effects of PEEP and the hazards of driving and plateau pressures. Am J Respir Crit Care Med 153:A375 (Abst)
123. Dreyfuss D, Saumon G (1993) Role of tidal volume, FRC and end-inspiratory volume in the development of pulmonary edema following mechanical ventilation. Am Rev Respir Dis 148:1194–1203

Low versus High Tidal Volumes

L. Brochard

Introduction

In the last 5 to 10 years, considerable attention has been paid to the ventilatory strategies used in the acute respiratory distress syndrome (ARDS) because ventilation could act not only as a symptomactic support but could also have an important impact on lung injury itself. Two general ideas are supporting this view. The first one is that mechanical ventilation by itself has the potential to induce lethal lesions of the alveolo-capillary membrane [1]. The severe evolution of some patients ventilated in the intensive care unit could be a result of inappropriate ventilatory settings. Up to now, it is extremely difficult to apply the experimental findings of different animal models to patients. Results are so impressive, however, that this concern became rapidly a rule and deliberate reduction in pressure or volume have been proposed as almost mandatory settings [2]. The second concern is the necessity to open up the collapsed zones of the lung and to keep them open [3]. The ventilatory settings producing these effects and enhancing what is referred to as alveolar recruitment, have been studied in details in patients by means of computed tomography (CT) scan [4–6]. Keeping the lung open necessitates to maintain a positive end-expiratory pressure (PEEP) which, in addition to obvious symptomatic improvement in oxygenation, has been found to be potentially important for the evolution of the disease in animal studies [7, 8]. One of the important aspect seems to avoid the opening collapse phenomenon which necessarily occurs when the lung is allowed to collapse at end expiration [9, 10].

These findings have generated the basis for two ventilatory strategies: maintaining a sufficient level of end-expiratory lung volume, including recruited volume, and minimizing the lung stretch at end-inflation. These two strategies interact together and may be sometimes contradictory [11]. Increasing end-expiratory lung volume or pressure on the one hand, and reducing end-inspiratory lung volume or pressure on the other hand, both result in reducing the tidal volume delivered to the patient. Reducing tidal volume has thus been specifically tested in patients.

Importance of the PEEP Setting on Tidal Volume

Gattinoni and coworkers [6] quantified the amount of recruitment by means of CT scan. These authors measured the recruitment both at end-expiration and at end-inspiration with increasing levels of PEEP (0, 5, 10, 15 and 20 cmH$_2$O). Interestingly, the total amount of recruitment at end-inspiration was not substantially modified from define zero-PEEP to the highest level of PEEP. What was essentially changed was the re-opening-collapsing tissue, i.e. the amount of lung tissue recruited at end-inflation which collapsed with PEEP. The recruitment process was thus essentially made by tidal volume (VT), while PEEP acted to keep the recruited lung units open. Of note, this factor has long been viewed as crucial for the treatment of ARDS and for minimizing the risk of ventilator-induced injury [3, 12, 13]. In a study applying some of the modern concepts of ventilatory strategy, Ranieri et al. [11] emphasized the importance of the volume history on the amount of recruited volume with PEEP. Specifically, they compared recruitment obtained with PEEP adjusted on small (6 mL/kg) versus high (10–12 mL/kg) define VT. They found a striking difference suggesting a much larger recruitable volume when PEEP was added to small VT than to already large VT. The greatest value of oxygenation and static compliance were obtained during application of PEEP with low VT. In line with previous older studies showing the importance of volume history on lung mechanics [14–16] and with more recent data [17], this study was of particular relevance to illustrate the inter-relationship between the level of PEEP and VT selected during mechanical ventilation in ARDS.

In some of the studies discussed below, this inter-relationship was not taken into account. It is possible, although not clearly proven, that reduction of VT should be "coupled" with an increase in the PEEP level to always optimize alveolar recruitment, which magnitude is probably very dependent on the end-inspiratory lung volume [16].

Physiological Studies Suggesting to Reduce Tidal Volume in Patients

Because of major concerns in ventilating patients with high volume-high pressure ventilation and the subsequent risk of alveolar trauma, many authors proposed to adapt a deliberate reduction of ventilation [18–25]. Because no obvious limit could be obtained from experimental animal studies where airway pressure as low as 30 cmH$_2$O was shown to induce lung damage [26, 27], it was suggested to use the upper inflection point on the pressure-volume (P-V) curve as an upper limit for titration of VT [23, 28, 29]. In 42 patients with acute respiratory failure or ARDS, Roupie et al. [23] tried to determine the presence or absence of an upper inflection point (UIP), either by eye or by automatic curve fitting, hypothetizing the presence of a linear part on all curves. Such an upper inflection point was found only in the group of patients with ARDS in the range of volume studied, again confirming the restrictive nature of this disease. The mean pressure value for this UIP was only 26 cmH$_2$O. When patients were ventilated with an upper limit of VT set at this point, hypercapnia ensued in all patients. It is noteworthy than the individual value of the UIP ranged from 18 to 40 cmH$_2$O. Roupie et al. excluded patients with chest wall abnormalities and checked in a few patients that the shape of the curve, i.e. the presence of an inflection at high volume, was not influenced by chest wall mechanical properties. In patients, however, it is always a problem to rely only on airway pressure without partitioning lung and chest wall mechanics. Indeed, many authors have previously shown that patients with severe lung failure frequently have chest wall stiffness, especially in case of sepsis and systemic capillary leakage [30–32].

Studies in Patients with ARDS

Hickling and coworkers [18, 20] in two large studies suggested that low VT limited pressure ventilation could improve survival in ARDS patients. Comparing their observed mortality to the predicted mortality based on several severity scores, they convincingly shown a reduction in mortality in patients treated with the "permissive hypercapnia" technique. Obviously these are important and interesting findings. Unfortunately their interpretation is limited by the retrospective nature of these studies and by the methodology used. Indeed, several interpretations are possible. One is that the indices used to predict mortality are not well adapted to the sample of population studied. Another is that it is the general care of the patients which resulted in improved outcome, having only little to do with the ventilatory strategy. The same question apply to other studies showing a consistent decrease in mortality over the last years [33].

Other authors demonstrated on small clinical studies [21] or on well-done physiological studies that reducing VT with the same PEEP level was safe, well tolerated or even potentially beneficial on oxygen delivery to the tissues [22, 24, 25, 34]. Oxygen delivery was found to be improved by deliberate reduction of VT, essentially because of the major increase in cardiac output [22, 24, 25, 35]. Also, the marked shift to the right of the oxyhemoglobin dissociation curve under the effects of respiratory acidosis can potentially favor oxygen delivery to tissue [25]. Negative aspects concerned arterial oxygenation or content which was found consistently decreased in some studies [25, 35, 36] but not in others [23]. Abrupt increase in pulmonary hypertension have also been described, reversible under nitric oxide (NO) administration [35]. Lastly, of great concern but only poorly studied, is the risk of alveolar instability and of progressive occurrence of alveolar collapse. This was suggested by Cereda and coworkers [37] who found a progressive fall in compliance with low VT ventilation.

Randomized Studies in ARDS

The first study showing beneficial effects of a new ventilatory approach in a randomized study was published by Amato and coworkers [38], who recently presented preliminary results showing an improved mortality [39]. These results are presented and discussed elsewhere in this book. It is important to note, however, that many aspects of ventilatory management differed between the two groups (PEEP level, VT, ventilatory mode), as well as general management (sedation, suctioning) and it is thus difficult to conclude which is the main factor explaining an improved outcome.

We underwent a multicenter randomized study to assess the impact of VT reduction during mechanical ventilation of patients with ARDS [40]. This study has been only presented in the abstract format. 108 patients were included with a Lung Injury Score (LIS) above 2.5 [41] with no other organ dysfunction on admission, as defined by Knaus [42] and were randomized between two groups. In one arm (limited VT) the goal was to maintain the end-inspiratory plateau pressure to 25 cmH_2O. In the other group, VT was 10 mL/kg or higher to maintain $PaCO_2$ between 38 and 42 mmHg except when the peak airway pressure reached 60 cmH_2O. The same PEEP level was used in both groups. The two groups were similar both on admisssion and at inclusion in the study. The end-point was mortality at day 60. No significant difference could be found between the two groups in terms or mortality at day 60 (41% in the standard treatment group versus 48% in the low VT group, p = 0.49), nor on the survival curve with a Log-Rank analysis. Secondary variables were not different between the two groups, including occurrence of secondary multiple organ failure (44 versus 43%), occurrence of pneumothorax (13 versus 15%) or duration of mechanical ventilation. Therefore, it seems that a systematic reduction of VT to limit the plateau pressure to 25 cmH_2O does not appear to be of any benefit in the mechanical ventilation of patients with ARDS. It should be noted, however, that the standard group was treated with a relatively "reasonable" VT between 10 and 11 mL/kg of ideal body weight. This differs from many other series of ARDS patients or from the Amato study. The relationship between the risk of alveolar trauma and the pressure reached is probably not linear and below "reasonable" values, there may little benefit of varying VT and the alveolar pressure. Also, an important aspect is the absence of individual titration of VT. When the same "average" limit for plateau pressure was applied in this multicentric study to search for a reduction in mortality with the "permissive hypercapnia" approach, no benefit was found over a more conventional approach. Wheter the absence of individual titration ot the ventilatory settings on the P-V curve explains the lack of difference between the two groups is an attractive hypothesis which need to be studied.

Using simple technique such as the low flow inflation method may help for future investigations in this direction [43].

References

1. Dreyfuss D, Saumon G (1994) Ventilation-induced injury. In: Tobin MJ (ed) Principles and practice of mechanical ventilation. Mac Graw Hill, New York, pp 793–811
2. Slutsky A (1994) Mechanical Ventilation (Consensus Conference) Intensive Care Med 20: 64–79 and 150–162.
3. Lachmann B (1992) Open the lung and keep the lung open. Intensive Care Med 18:319–321
4. Gattinoni L, Pesenti A (1991) Computed tomography scanning in acute respiratory failure. In: Zapol WM, Lemaire F (eds) Adult respiratory distress syndrome. Marcel Dekker, New York, pp 199–221
5. Gattinoni L, D'Andrea L, Pelosi P, Vitale G, Pesenti A, Fumagalli R (1993) Regional effects and mechanisms of positive end-expiratory pressure in early adult respiratory distress syndrome. JAMA 269:2122–2135

6. Gattinoni L, Pelosi P, Crotti S, Valenza F (1995) Effects of positive end-expiratory pressure on regional distribution of tidal volume and recrutement in adult respiratory distress syndrome. Am J Respir Crit Care Med 151:1807–1814
7. Corbridge TC, Wood LDH, Crawford GP, Chudoba MJ, Yanos J, Sznajder JI (1990) Adverse effects of large tidal volume and low PEEP in canine acid aspiration. Am Rev Respir Dis 142: 311–315
8. Muscedere JG, Mullen JBM, Gari K, Bryan AC, Slutsky AS (1994) Tidal ventilation at low airway pressures can augment lung injury. Am J Respir Crit Care Med 149:1327–1334
9. Taskar V, John J, Evander E, Wollmer P, Robertson B, Jonson B (1995) Healthy lungs tolerate repetitive collapse and reopening during short periods of mechanical ventilation. Acta Anaesthesiol Scand 39:370–376
10. Taskar V, John J, Evander E, Robertson B, Jonson B (1997) Surfactant dysfunction makes lung vulnerable to repetitive collapse and reexpansion. Am J Respir Crit Care 155:313–320
11. Ranieri VM, Mascia L, Fiore T, Bruno F, Brienza A, Giuliani R (1995) Cardiorespiratory effects of positive end-expiratory pressure during progressive tidal volume reduction (permissive hypercapnia) in patients with acute respiratory distress syndrome. Anesthesiology 83:710–720
12. Lachmann B, Jonson B, Lindroth M, Robertson B (1982) Modes of artificial ventilation in severe respiratory distress syndrome. Crit Care Med 10:724–732
13. Slutsky AS (1993) Barotrauma and alveolar recruitment. Intensive Care Med 19:369–371
14. Glaister DH, Schroter RC, Sudlow MF, Milic-Emili J (1973) Bulk elastic properties of excised lungs and the effect of a transpulmonary pressure gradient. Respir Physiol 17:347–364
15. Salmon RB, Primiano Jr FP, Saidel GM, Niewoehner DE (1981) Human lung pressure-volume relationships: Alveolar collapse and airway closure. J Appl Physiol 51:353–362
16. Benito S, Lemaire F, Mankikian B, Harf A (1985) Total respiratory compliance as a function of lung volume in patients with mechanical ventilation. Intensive Care Med 11:76–79
17. Benito S, Lemaire F (1990) Pulmonary pressure-volume relationship in acute respiratory distress syndrome in adults: Role of positive end-expiratory pressure. J Crit Care 5:27–34
18. Hickling KG, Henderson SJ, Jackson R (1990) Low mortality associated with low volume pressure limited ventilation with permissive hypercapnia in severe adult respiratory distress syndrome. Intensive Care Med 16:372–377
19. Hickling KG (1990) Ventilatory management of ARDS: Can it affect the outcome? Intensive Care Med 16:219–226
20. Hickling KG, Walsh J, Henderson SJ, Jackson R (1994) Low mortality rate in adult respiratory distress syndrome using low-volume, pressure-limited ventilation with permissive hypercapnia: A prospective study. Crit Care Med 22:1568–1578
21. Lee CT, Fein AM, Lipmann M, Holtzman H, Kimbel P, Weinbaum G (1981) Elastase activity in pulmonary lavage fluid from patients with adult respiratory distress syndrome. N Engl J Med 304:192–196
22. Kiiski R, Takala J, Kari A, Milic-Emili J (1992) The effect of tidal volume on gas exchange and oxygen transport in ARDS. Am Rev Respir Dis 146:1131–1135
23. Roupie E, Dambrosio M, Servillo G, et al (1995) Titration of tidal volume and induced hypercapnia in acute respiratory distress syndrome. Am J Respir Crit Care Med 152:121–128
24. Kiiski R, Kaitainen S, Karppi R, Takala J (1996) Physiological effects of reduced tidal volume at constant minute ventilation and inspiratory flow rate in acute respiratory distress syndrome. Intensive Care Med 22:192–198
25. Thorens JB, Jolliet P, Ritz M, Chevrolet JC (1996) Effects of rapid permissive hypercapnia on hemodynamics, gas exchange, and oxygen transport and consumption during mechanical ventilation for the acute respiratory distress syndrome. Intensive Care Med 22:182–192
26. Tsuno K, Prato P, Kolobow T (1990) Acute lung injury from mechanical ventilation at moderately high airway pressures. J Appl Physiol 69:956–961
27. Hernandez L, Coker PJ, May S, Thompson AL, Parker JC (1990) Mechanical ventilation increases microvascular permeability in oleic acid-injured lungs. J Appl Physiol 69:2057–2061
28. Milic-Emili J, Tantucci C, Chassé M, Corbeil C (1991) Introduction with special reference to ventilator-associated barotrauma. In: Benito S, Net A (eds) Pulmonary function in mechanically ventilated patients. Berlin, Springer Verlag, pp 1–8

29. Brunet F, Jeanbourquin D, Monchi M, et al (1995) Should mechanical ventilation be optimized to blood gases, lung mechanics, or thoracic CT scan ? Am J Respir Crit Care Med 152:524–530
30. Jardin F, Genevray B, Brun-Ney D, Bourdarias JP (1985) Influence of lung and chest wall compliances on transmission of airway pressure to the pleural space in critically ill patients. Chest 88:653–658
31. Katz JA, Zinn SE, Ozanne GM, Fairley HV (1981) Pulmonary, chest wall, and lung-thorax elastances in acute respiratory failure. Chest 80:304–311
32. Pelosi P, Cereda M, Foti G, Giacomini M, Pesenti A (1995) Alterations in lung and chest wall mechanics in patients with acute lung injury: Effects of positive end-expiratory pressure. Am J Respir Crit Care Med 152:531–537
33. Milberg JA, Davis DR, Steinberg KP, Hudson LD (1995) Improved survival of patients with acute respiratory distress syndrome (ARDS):1983–1993. JAMA 273:306–309
34. Feihl F, Perret C (1994) Permissive hypercapnia. How permissive should we be ? Am J Respir Crit Care Med 150:1722–1737
35. Puybasset L, Stewart T, Rouby JJ, et al (1994) Inhaled nitric oxide reverses the increase in pulmonary vascular resistance induced by permissive hypercapnia in patients with acute respiratory distress syndrome. Anesthesiology 80:1254–1267
36. Blanch L, Fernandez R, Vallés J, Solé J, Roussos C, Artigas A (1994) Effect of two tidal volumes on oxygenation and respiratory system mechanics during the early stage of adult respiratory distress syndrome. J Crit Care 9:151–158
37. Cereda M, Foti G, Musch G, Sparacino ME, Pesenti A (1996) Positive end-expiratory pressure prevents the loss of respiratory compliance during low tidal volume ventilation in acute lung injury patients. Chest 109:480–485
38. Amato MBP, Barbas CSV, Medeiros DM, et al (1995) Beneficial effects of the "Open lung approach" with low distending pressures in acute respiratory distress syndrome: A prospective randomized study on mechanical ventilation. Am J Respir Crit Care Med 152:1835–1846
39. Amato MBP, Barbas CSV, Medeiros DM, et al (1996) Improved survival in ARDS: Beneficial effects of a lung protective strategy. Am J Respir Crit Care Med 153:A531 (Abst)
40. Brochard L, Roudot-Thoraval F, and the collaborative groupe on VT reduction (1997) Tidal volume (VT) reduction in acute respiratory distress syndrome (ARDS): A multicenter randomized study. Am J Respir Crit Care Med (In press) (Abst)
41. Murray JF, Matthay MA, Luce JM, Flick MR (1988) An expanded definition of the adult respiratory distress syndrome. Am Rev Resp Dis 138:720–723
42. Knaus WA, Drager EA, Wagner DP, Zimmerman JE (1985) Prognosis in acute organ system failure. Ann Surg 292:685–693
43. Servillo G, Svantesson C, Beydon L, et al (1997) Pressure-volume curves in acute respiratory failure. "Automated low flow inflation" vs "occlusion". Am J Resp Crit Care Med (In press)

Respiratory Muscle Fatigue and Weaning

M. J. Tobin, A. Jubran, and F. Laghi

Introduction

This chapter focuses on patients with acute lung injury (ALI) and/or acute respiratory distress syndrome (ARDS). Patients with these disorders usually receive mechanical ventilation for several days or weeks, and every critical care physician can recall a patient with ARDS who experienced difficulty when attempting to resume spontaneous ventilation. Yet, research that specifically focuses on the problems of discontinuing ventilator support in patients with ALI and/or ARDS does not exist. In reporting research on weaning, investigators have not indicated that patients with ARDS exhibit unique behavior that makes them different from other patients being weaned from mechanical ventilation. Accordingly, this review is based on data obtained in patients recovering from acute respiratory failure due to a variety of causes and not exclusively from ARDS.

Pathophysiological Determinants of Ventilator Dependency

Difficulties with discontinuation of mechanical ventilation can result from three major problems: hypoxemia, psychological problems, and problems with the respiratory muscles [1, 2]. In the acute phase of ARDS, patients exhibit major abnormalities in pulmonary gas exchange, with severe hypoxemia largely due to shunt and a smaller contribution from ventilation/perfusion mismatch. Weaning is not even contemplated at this stage of the illness. Attempts to discontinue mechanical ventilation are not initiated until the patient exhibits reasonable recovery from lung injury, as signalled by an arterial oxygen tension (PaO_2) of greater than 60 torr with a fractional inspired oxygen concentration of 0.40. During a reduction in the level of ventilator support (especially with cessation of positive end-expiratory pressure (PEEP)) or a switch to spontaneous breathing, patients can develop hypoxemia [3]. Such hypoxemia may be more common in patients recovering from ARDS (consequent to alveolar instability) than from other causes of respiratory failure, although this possible distinction has not been investigated systematically. Psychological problems can contribute to weaning difficulty in any patient who has required prolonged ventilator support [4], but there is no reason to believe that the prevalence or nature of these problems are different in patients recovering from ARDS than in other patients. Problems with respiratory muscle function are the major source of difficulty with weaning from mechanical ventilation, and this constitutes the primary focus of this chapter. Impaired performance of the respiratory muscle pump may arise from decreased respiratory center output, decreased respiratory muscle strength, a mechanical load that exceeds the capabilities of the respiratory muscles, and/or the development of respiratory muscle fatigue.

Respiratory Center Output

A decrease in respiratory center output in patients recovering from ARDS could arise from a genetic predisposition, a consequence of drugs such as sedatives or analgesics, alterations in the metabolic milieu, or down-regulation of neuronal activity in response to the underlying disease or ventilator management. Patients who fail a weaning trial, however, typically display heightened respiratory center output, as reflected by airway occlusion pressure or mean inspiratory flow [5, 6]. Moreover, patients exhibit a further increase in respiratory drive as alveolar hypoventilation progressively develops during an unsuccessful trial of spontaneous breathing [5]. Thus, it is doubtful that abnormalities in respiratory center function are primarily responsible for weaning failure in patients recovering from ARDS.

Respiratory Muscle Strength

There are no data to indicate that patients recovering from ARDS are more prone to respiratory muscle weakness than other ventilator-supported patients. However, the recent notion that corticosteroids are helpful in patients exhibiting a slow recovery from ARDS could aggravate respiratory muscle weakness. In patients with chronic obstructive pulmonary disease (COPD), an average daily dose of 14 mg of prednisone given over extended periods has been shown to induce severe histological abnormalities in the respiratory muscles associated with decreases in respiratory muscle strength [7].

Measurement of maximum static inspiratory pressures (Pi_{max}) during forceful efforts against an occluded airway reflects global inspiratory muscle strength. Reported values of Pi_{max} may underestimate true inspiratory muscle strength, because the measurements are extremely dependent on the technique of measurement, and patient cooperation and motivation. Since the pressure generated by the respiratory muscles is highly dependent on muscle length, Pi_{max} should be recorded at residual volume or functional residual capacity (FRC). In an attempt to improve the reliability of Pi_{max} measurements in ventilator-supported patients, a two-step modification in the technique has been introduced [8]. This involves a one-way valve that permits expiration (ensuring that measurements are made at a low lung volume) and maintaining the occlusion for 20 sec. Values of Pi_{max} are about one-third more negative using this technique than without it. When performed by a single investigator, values of Pi_{max} with this technique have a coefficient of variation of 12%, but when the measurement is performed by different investigators the coefficient of variation increases to 42% [9]. The reliability of

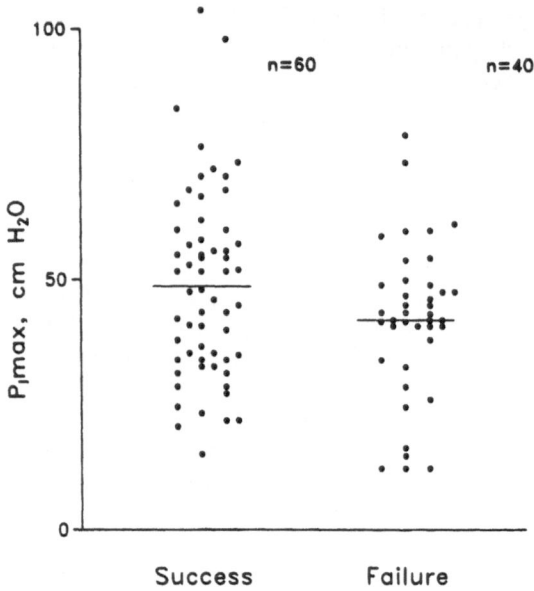

Fig. 1. Measurements of maximal inspiratory pressure (Pi_{max}) in 60 patients who were successfully weaned from mechanical ventilation and extubated, and 40 patients who failed a weaning trial and required the reinstitution of mechanical ventilation. (From [12] with permission)

the Pi_{max} can be enhanced by stimulation of conjuction with the one-way valve method. It has been generally assumed that obtaining reproducible values of Pi_{max} ($< 5\%$ variation) indicates that a patient is truly making maximal efforts. However, in a recent study of Pi_{max} measurements, the coefficient of variation of maximal efforts was not different than the coefficient of variation of submaximal attempts [10].

In many ways, Pi_{max} is easier to measure in ventilator-supported patients than in non-intubated patients, because obtaining a good seal between the instrumentation and the patient's airway is less of a problem. Pi_{max} is one of the standard measurements used to determine a patient's readiness for discontinuation of mechanical ventilation [11]. If Pi_{max} is very small, i.e. less negative than -20 cm H_2O, a patient is generally incapable of sustaining spontaneous ventilation. However, more negative values of Pi_{max} do not guarantee weaning success, and in most studies it has been found to be an unreliable predictor of weaning outcome (Fig. 1) [1, 2, 12, 13]. The poor predictive power of Pi_{max} may be due to the fact that it is measured under static conditions, and the recorded value is probably very different than the value available to patients who fail a weaning trial. Moreover, the patient's maximal respiratory effort must be interpreted alongside the ventilatory demand for power output. Patients who fail a weaning trial are tachypneic, have rapid flow rates, and often display dynamic hyperinflation [5] – all of which decrease the proportion of Pi_{max} that is available for force generation [14].

Respiratory Mechanics

From Fig. 1, it is apparent that some patients with a very low Pi_{max} can tolerate discontinuation of mechanical ventilation while other patients with a high Pi_{max} cannot successfully sustain spontaneous ventilation. One of the major factors that determines this apparent discrepancy is the work load encountered during spontaneous breathing. Relatively few investigators have systematically examined changes in respiratory mechanics in patients who are attempting to resume spontaneous breathing following a period of mechanical ventilation.

We [15, 16] recently obtained such measurements in 17 patients with COPD who developed severe distress during a trial of spontaneous breathing lasting 45 ± 8 min, and in a control group of 14 patients with COPD who tolerated the trial and were extubated after 45 ± 3 min. The pathophysiology of COPD is obviously different from that of ARDS, but since equivalent data have not been obtained in patients recovering from ARDS we believe that these data are nevertheless instructive. At the onset (2nd min) of the trial of spontaneous breathing, inspiratory pulmonary resistance was not statistically different in the failure and success groups, 9.0 ± 1.7 (SE) and 5.8 ± 1.1 cmH$_2$O/L/sec, respectively (Fig. 2). At the end of the trial, resistance increased to 14.8 ± 2.0 cmH$_2$O/L/sec in the failure group, whereas it remained unchanged from the start of the trial in the failure group. The increase in resistance in the failure group could have resulted from several mechanisms:

1) an increase in flow, but this is unlikely since flow increased by the same extent over the course of the trial in the success group;
2) a decrease in lung volume, but this is unlikely since the failure group also developed an increase in auto-PEEP (vide infra);
3) accumulation of secretions, but the airways of all patients were suctioned before the trial; and/or
4) development of bronchoconstriction, since patients with COPD are known to exhibit heightened airway reactivity [17].

At the start of the spontaneous breathing trial, dynamic lung elastance was higher in the failure group than in the success group, 21.2 ± 3.4 and 9.9 ± 1.7 cmH$_2$O/L, respectively (Fig. 2). At the end of the trial, elastance was more than two-fold higher in the failure group than in the success group, 34.1 ± 4 and 14.0 ± 2.0 cmH$_2$O/L, respectively. The mechanism of the increase in dynamic elastance in the failure group is unknown, and it may reflect dynamic hyperinflation [8].

Auto-PEEP was higher in the failure group than in the success group at the onset of the spontaneous breathing trial, 2.0 ± 0.5 and 0.7 ± 0.1 cmH$_2$O, respectively. At the end of the trial, auto-PEEP increased to 4.1 ± 0.8 cmH$_2$O in the failure group and it increased slightly in the success group (1.1 ± 0.2 cmH$_2$O). The progressive increase in auto-PEEP in the failure group may be due to dynamic hyperinflation, and this possibility is supported by the fact that 85% of the variance in auto-PEEP was accounted for by inspiratory resistance, respiratory frequency and tidal volume.

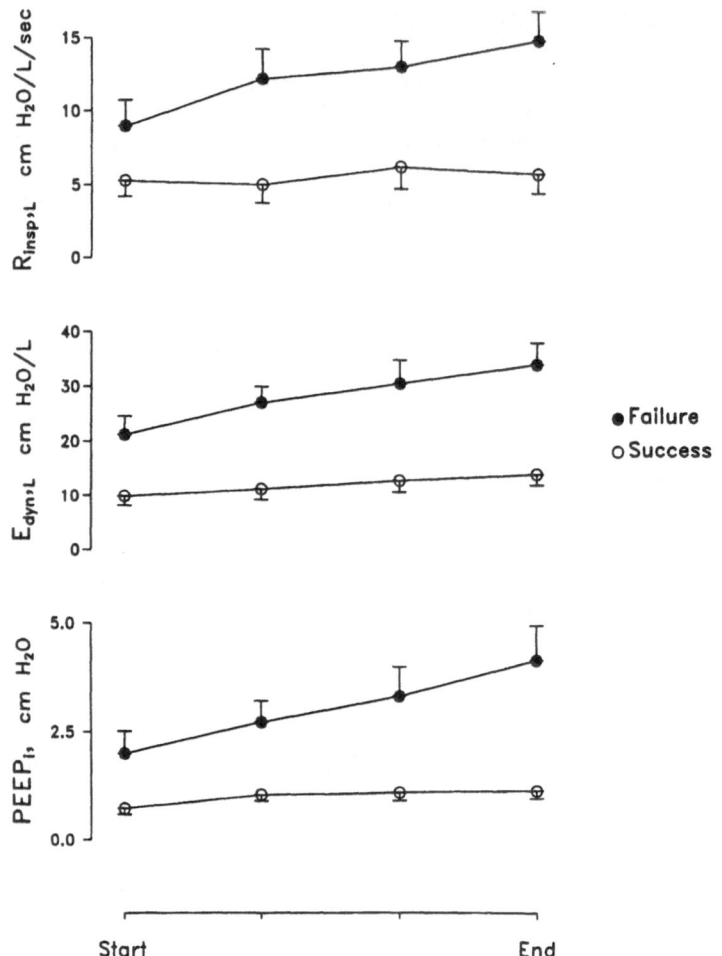

Fig. 2. Inspiratory resistance of the lung (Rinsp, L), dynamic lung elastance (Edyn, L), and intrinsic positive end-expiratory pressure (PEEPi) during a trial of spontaneous breathing in patients with COPD who succeeded and failed such a trial. Between the onset and the end of the trial, increases in Rinsp, L ($p < 0.009$), Edyn, L ($p < 0.0001$) and PEEPi ($p < 0.0001$) occurred in the failure group, and increases in Edyn, L ($p < 0.0006$) and PEEPi ($p < 0.02$) occurred in the success group. Over the course of the trial, the failure group had higher values of Rinsp, L ($p < 0.003$), Edyn, L ($p < 0.0006$) and PEEPi ($p < 0.0009$) than the success group. Bars represent $\pm$ SE (From [15] with permission)

From Fig. 2, it is apparent that the patients who failed the trial of spontaneous breathing experienced progressive worsening of their respiratory mechanics over the course of the trial. Respiratory muscle energy expenditure was quantitated in terms of pressure-time product per minute rather than mechanical work of breathing. At the onset of the trial, pressure-time product was not significantly different in the two patient groups, but by the end of the trial, it was almost twice as high in the failure group than in the success group, 388 ± 68 and 205 ± 25 cmH$_2$O · s/min, respectively.

Respiratory Muscle Fatigue

Patients who fail a trial of weaning from mechanical ventilation often have a decreased respiratory muscle strength (Fig. 1) and an increased respiratory load (Fig. 2). Such an imbalance is the perfect set-up for the development of respiratory muscle fatigue, a condition in which there is a loss in the capacity for developing force resulting from activity under load and is reversible by rest [9]. The development of respiratory muscle fatigue has long been suspected in patients experiencing acute progressive ventilatory failure, although unequivocal evidence of contractile fatigue has not been demonstrated.

In one of the first studies to use weaning failure as a model of acute ventilatory failure, Cohen et al. [20] observed a shift in the power spectrum of the diaphragmatic electromyogram (EMG), which they considered to signify fatigue. In-

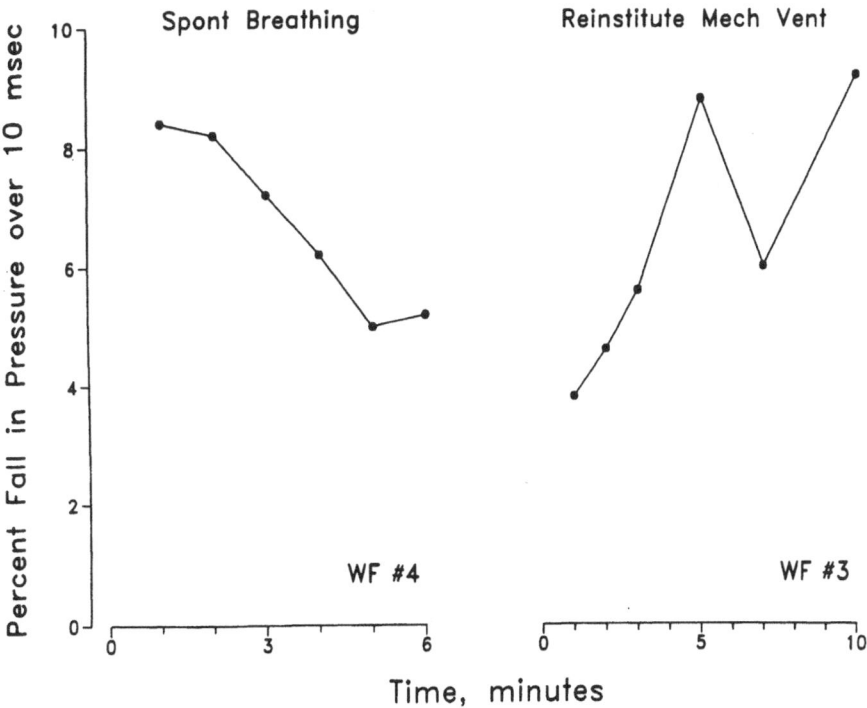

Fig. 3. Maximum relaxation rate (MRR) calculated from transdiaphragmatic pressure tracings obtained during the first 6 min of spontaneous breathing in a patient who failed a weaning trial (WF #4) (*left*). MRR during the first 10 min following the reinstitution of mechanical ventilation in another patient (WF #3) who failed a trial of spontaneous breathing (*right*). MRR is expressed as the percent fall in pressure over 10 milliseconds. (Adapted from [21])

itially, this interpretation was readily and widely accepted because it is hard to conceive of a group of patients who are at greater risk of respiratory muscle fatigue than patients who fail a weaning trial. It is now recognized however that the EMG power spectrum is influenced by several factors and does not necessarily signify impaired muscle contractility.

In 5 patients who failed a weaning trial, Goldstone et al. [21] observed a 44% decrease in the maximal relaxation rate measured from the decay portion of the transdiaphragmatic.pressure signal. When mechanical ventilation was re-instituted, the maximum relaxation rate recovered within 10 min (Fig. 3). In contrast, 4 patients who were successfully weaned showed no change in their relaxation rate. Slowing of the maximum relaxation rate has been interpreted as evidence of respiratory muscle fatigue [22]. However, like changes in the EMG power spectrum, the maximum relaxation rate changes very early in a fatiguing process and is not necessarily associated with a decrease in contractile force. As such, it is more closely related to an increased load on the respiratory system rather than a direct reflection of neuromechanical uncoupling.

In contrast to the reports of Cohen et al. [20] and Goldstone et al. [21], other data cast doubts on the importance of respiratory muscle fatigue as a primary mechanism of weaning failure. Swartz and Marino [23] measured transdiaphragmatic pressure in 9 patients who failed a weaning trial, 7 of whom developed hypercapnia. Swings in transdiaphragmatic pressure increased significantly over the period of the weaning trial despite the development of CO_2 retention, leading the investigators to conclude that the unsuccessful weaning outcome was not due to failure of the diaphragm as a pressure generator. However, they did not measure maximal transdiaphragmatic pressure, and thus one cannot exclude the development of fatigue.

The question of whether or not weaning failure in an individual patient is due to respiratory muscle fatigue, which in part is due to structural damage in the muscles, is of crucial importance for several reasons. Rest is the only means of reversing fatigue, and for the respiratory muscles this means mechanical ventilation. If a patient develops respiratory muscle fatigue during the course of an unsuccessful attempt to discontinue ventilator support, it is likely that the new structural injury to the muscles will impair the patient's performance and represent an additional medical complication for this patient. Trying to minimize the risk of fatigue by postponing attempts at weaning places the patient at risk for the many complications associated with mechanical ventilation. Moreover, excessive muscle rest can cause muscle atrophy [24, 25], thus initiating a vicious circle. These issues are compounded by the lack of simple, reliable means of detecting respiratory muscle fatigue in critically ill patients. Measurement of Pi_{max} provides information on the strength of the respiratory muscles but it does not quantitate a patient's susceptibility to fatigue nor indicate whether fatigue is present or not. Many of the approaches employed in conducting research on fatigue in healthy volunteers, such as ability to maintain a target pressure over time, do not serve as satisfactory diagnostic or monitoring tools in critically ill patients because of their dependence on patient motivation and cooperation.

Tension-Time Index

The major determinants of inspiratory muscle fatigue are inspiratory muscle strength, mean inspiratory pressure, and the duration of inspiratory effort. These factors can be combined as follows into a tension-time index (TTI):

$$TTI = mean \; Pbr/P_{max} \times TI/TTOT$$

where Pbr is the pressure per breath, P_{max} is the respiratory pressure during a maximum static maneuver, and TI/TTOT is the fractional inspiratory time or duty cycle. When TTI was calculated using transdiaphragmatic pressure data, Bellemare and Grassino [26] found that diaphragmatic fatigue became inevitable when TTI exceeded 0.15 in healthy volunteers breathing against large external mechanical loads.

In our study of patients with COPD who failed and succeeded in trials of spontaneous breathing, we calculated TTI from measurements of esophageal pressure. At the onset of the trial, TTI was 0.06 ± 0.01 and 0.05 ± 0.01 in the failure and success groups, respectively (Fig. 4). By the end of the trial, TTI increased to 0.10 ± 0.01 in the failure group, while it did not change in the success group. Five of the patients in the failure group developed a TTI above 0.15, all but one of whom exhibited increases in arterial carbon dioxide of 20–30 torr; no success patient showed such a change.

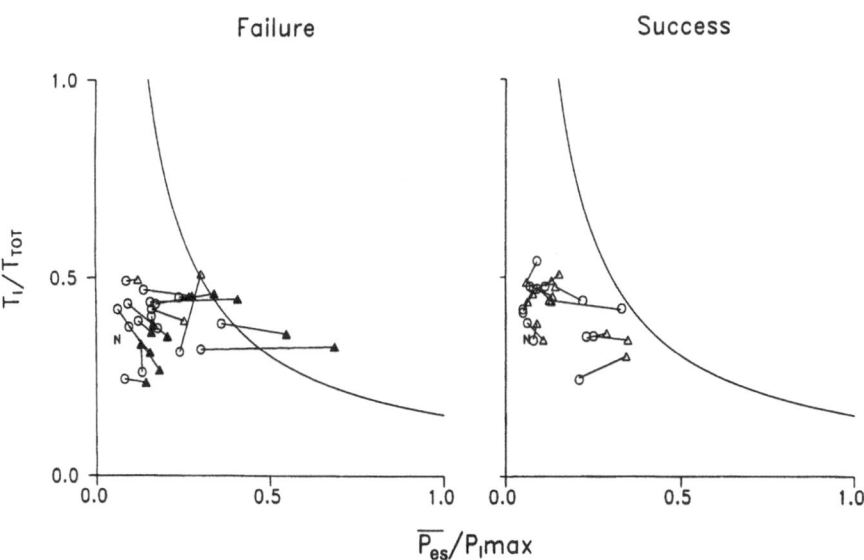

Fig. 4. The relationship between mean esophageal pressure/maximum inspiratory pressure ratio ($\overline{P}es/Pi_{max}$) and duty cycle (TI/TTOT) in patients who failed and succeeded in a trial of spontaneous breathing. Circles and triangles represent values at the start and end of the trial, respectively; closed symbols indicate patients who developed an increase in $PaCO_2$ during the trial. Five of the 17 patients in the failure group developed a tension time index (TTI) of >0.15 (indicated by the isopleth). N represents value in a normal subject. (From [15] with permission)

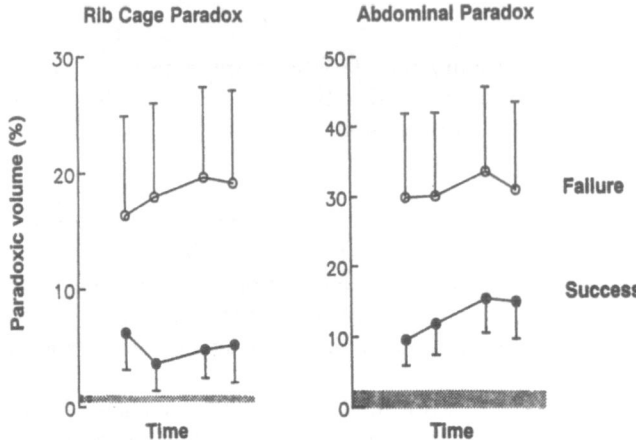

Fig. 5. Paradoxic volume of the rib cage and abdomen during inspiration in patients who were successfully weaned and in patients who failed a trial of weaning. Measurements were obtained at 4 consecutive time blocks during the weaning trial. The paradoxic volumes were greater in the failure group (p < 0.003 for both compartments) (From [31] with permission)

On the surface, these data suggest that some of the patients who failed the weaning trial developed respiratory muscle fatigue. However, interpretation of TTI is confounded by several caveats:

1) In their original study Bellemare and Grassino [26] employed a controlled square-wave breathing pattern during inspiratory resistive loading. This results in a very low flow rate and minimal velocity of muscle shortening in contrast to the tachypneic pattern commonly observed in critically ill patients [27, 28].

2) Bellemare and Grassino [26] related the threshold of 0.15 to "task failure", i.e. the inability to maintain a target inspiratory pressure, which may be a late manifestation of a progressive fatiguing process. In subjects performing voluntary hyperpnea, Babcock et al. [29] observed significant fatigue (~ 30% decrease in the response of Pdi to phrenic nerve stimulation) without evidence of task failure.

3) Abnormalities in the lung parenchyma in critically ill patients will increase the level of hypercapnia for a given decrease in respiratory muscle function.

4) Critically ill patients commonly develop dynamic hyperinflation, which will increase pressure-generating capacity as a result of inspiratory muscle shortening [30].

5) TTI does not take into account impaired performance that results from asynchronous and paradoxic motion of the rib cage and abdomen. In a study where we employed the Konno-Mead method of analysis to assess rib cage-abdominal motion, we found that patients who failed a weaning trial displayed significantly greater asynchrony and paradox than patients who were successfully weaned (Fig. 5) [31]. Such a manner of breathing is extremely inefficient and results in a marked increase in the energy costs for a given level of ventilation [32].

Central Fatigue

In addition to alterations in muscle contractility, decreased muscle force may result from a reduction in neuronal activation. Indeed the response of the respiratory control system to the development of acute progressive respiratory failure has aroused considerable interest [33]. If ventilation is defended by an increase in controller output, respiratory muscle fatigue is ultimately inevitable. Alternatively, the controller may decrease its output and such disfacilitation is termed central fatigue [34]. Although hypercapnia necessarily ensues, a decrease in controller output is considered an appropriate response, since it reduces the risk of long-lasting structural injury [35]. Despite its theoretical attraction, there is no evidence that patients respond in this manner, and, indeed, conscious humans are very intolerant of acute increases in $PaCO_2$ [36, 37]. In healthy volunteers, respiratory motor output is preserved or increased following the induction of respiratory muscle fatigue [38, 39]. These studies however deal with the control of breathing following removal of a fatiguing load, and they do not exclude a decrease in muscle activation while a load is in place.

Proponents of the central wisdom hypothesis have postulated that patients who fail a weaning trial display a decrease in pressure-time product [33]. On the contrary, the weaning failure group in our study developed a >40% increase in pressure-time product between the onset and end of the trial, with only 1 patient displaying a small decrease. Since many patients developed hypercapnia, one could argue that pressure-time product should have increased to an even greater extent than the observed amount; nevertheless, the data indicate that a decrease in pressure-time product was not primarily responsible for the ventilatory failure. This observation is in agreement with our previous study [5], in which no patient exhibited a decrease in respiratory drive as weaning failure progressed. Taken together, it is evident that most patients failing a weaning trial do not reduce respiratory muscle activation, despite theoretical advantages of so doing.

Detecting Contractile Fatigue

The reference standard for demonstrating the presence of peripheral muscle fatigue is to externally stimulate the motor nerve and demonstrate a reduction in contractile force. For the respiratory system, this basically means stimulating the phrenic nerves at increasing frequencies (typically 1, 10, 20, 50 and 100 Hz) and measuring the change in transdiaphragmatic pressure. Once maximal activation has been achieved (as indicated by monitoring the compound motor action potential), the intensity of the stimulus is increased by a further 25% to ensure supramaximal stimulation. However, at stimulation frequencies above 35 Hz, it is extremely difficult to maintain a maximal stimulus due to cathode displacement. This results from contraction of the underlying scalene muscles and movement of the arm and shoulder due to activation of the brachial plexus [40]. Accordingly, a full force-frequency curve is very difficult to obtain in healthy volunteers and completely unsuited to research in critically ill patients. As a result of this problem, increasing attention has been focused on measuring the contractile response to single supramaximal nerve stimulations – so called, twitch stimulation. At a Workshop on respiratory muscle fatigue sponsored by the National Institutes of Health, it was considered that "information obtained from bilateral transcutaneous supramaximal phrenic nerve twitch stimulation had the best potential of becoming a diagnostic test."

Twitch pressure responses have been shown to provide a reliable means of detecting and tracking low-frequency fatigue [29, 41] – the type of fatigue that has greatest clinical implications. Twitch stimulation achieved by electrical stimulation of both phrenic nerves has been successfully employed in healthy volunteers [29] and patients [42]. Although much easier to perform than force-frequency curves, electrical stimulation for elicitation of twitch pressures has several limitations. In particular, locating the phrenic nerves can be challenging in patients with underlying respiratory disease and maintaining a constant symmetrical maximal stimulus can be difficult. Consequently, repetitive stimulations are commonly required, which in turn lead to twitch potentiation, which confound data interpretation.

A new technique of stimulating the phrenic nerves, magnetic stimulation, overcomes many of these problems [43]. With this technique, a circular coil placed over the back of the patient's neck generates a brief intense magnetic field which reaches and stimulates both phrenic nerves. Unlike electrical stimulation, there is no difficulty in locating the phrenic nerves, and the technique is considerably less uncomfortable than electrical stimulation. The transdiaphragmatic twitch pressures achieved by magnetic stimulation are almost 20% greater than those with electrical stimulation. We recently investigated the mechanism of the difference in twitch pressures elicited by the two techniques [44]. Whereas electrical stimulation almost solely activated the diaphragm, magnetic stimulation also recruited the sternomastoid, trapezius, parasternal and pectoral muscles. The two stimulation techniques were examined in terms of their ability to detect changes in diaphragmatic contractility after induction of fatigue. Despite the differences in muscle activation patterns, the decreases in twitch Pdi detected with the two techniques were closely correlated ($r = 0.96$) (Fig. 6), indicating that the relative non-selectivity of magnetic stimulation does not undermine its ability to detect diaphragmatic fatigue.

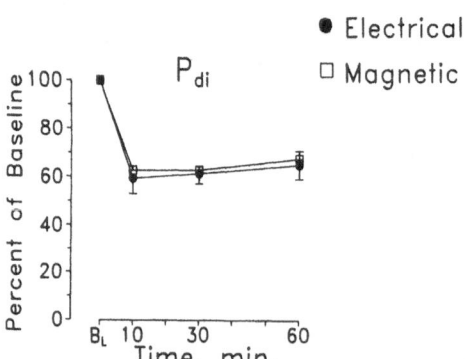

Fig. 6. Transdiaphragmatic twitch pressure at baseline and the percentage decrease at 10, 30 and 60 min after induction of diaphragmatic fatigue. The decreases were similar for magnetic (□) and electrical (●) stimulation of the phrenic nerves. (From [44] with permission)

The feasibility of employing magnetic stimulation in ventilator-supported patients has yet to be demonstrated. However, experience to date suggests that this should be feasible. If this promise is fulfilled, it should at last be possible to definitively answer the question of whether or not contractile muscle fatigue is an important mechanism of ventilator-dependency and failure to wean.

Timing of the Weaning Process

One of the major challenges in the management of mechanically ventilated patients is deciding when is the best time to wean a patient [1, 2, 10]. If a physician is too conservative and postpones weaning onset, the patient is placed at an increased risk of life-threatening, ventilator-induced complications. If weaning is commenced prematurely, the patient may suffer severe cardiopulmonary and/or psychological decompensation, which sets the patient back in his/her clinical course. In a patient with ARDS, it is essential that the underlying parenchymal pulmonary process has resolved sufficiently before attempting to discontinue ventilator-support. Careful clinical assessment is necessary in deciding when to discontinue mechanical ventilation, but this alone is not sufficient as demonstrated by Stroetz and Hubmayr [45]. They studied 31 patients being weaned by gradual reductions in the level of pressure support. The physician in charge of each patient was asked to predict a patient's ability to sustain unassisted breathing without distress for one hour. Of 22 patients whom the physicians thought likely to fail a weaning trial, 11 were successfully weaned; of 9 patients thought likely to be successfully weaned, 3 failed the trial. Clearly, objective tests are needed to guide physicians in predicting a patient's ability to sustain spontaneous ventilation.

Functional tests used in guiding the weaning process include measurements of the gas exchange properties of the lung (e.g. arterial O_2 tension >60 torr with inspired oxygen concentration of less than 0.40) and ventilatory demands (e.g. a minute ventilation of <10 L/min is desirable) [1]. Considering the important role played by respiratory muscle dysfunction in the pathophysiology of weaning failure, it is not surprising that measures of respiratory muscle performance are commonly used to decide if mechanical ventilation can be safely discontinued. A global measurement of inspiratory muscle strength, maximal inspiratory pressure, is a classic weaning predictor [10], but, as discussed above, it is often unreliable.

One of the most accurate predictors of weaning outcome is derived from simple measurements of respiratory frequency (f) and tidal volume (VT) during one minute of spontaneous breathing. These measurements can be combined into an index of rapid shallow breathing, the f/VT ratio [11]. Values of f/VT above 100 breaths/min/L suggest that a patient is likely to fail a weaning trial, and *vice versa*. In a study of 100 patients, the f/VT ratio had positive and negative predictive values of 0.78 and 0.95, respectively, which were the highest values noted for 10 different predictive indices evaluated in the study [11].

Weaning Techniques

Four different methods of weaning have been described. According to common wisdom, it has been widely accepted that patients recovering from an episode of respiratory failure cannot tolerate sudden discontinuation of mechanical ventilation. Instead, the workload imposed on the respiratory muscles is progressively increased by a gradual reduction in the level of ventilator assistance – as implied by the term "weaning". The oldest approach is to perform T-tube trials several times a day [1, 10]. During these trials, the patient is disconnected from the ventilator and he/she breathes an oxygen-enriched gas mixture. The trials are initially very brief (~ 5 min) and their duration is gradually increased in accordance with a patient's performance as assessed by clinical examination. The optimal duration of rest between the trials has never been defined, but commonly is as little as 1 to 3 h. When the patient is able to sustain spontaneous ventilation for some fixed time, such as 1–2 h, extubation is performed. This technique has been superseded by intermittent mandatory ventilation [46] and pressure support [47], which are now the most popular weaning techniques. These ventilator modes provide partial assistance, albeit in a different manner. By adjusting the ventilator settings, it is believed that the load imposed on the respiratory muscles can be altered gradually, and that this in itself will facilitate the successful resumption of spontaneous breathing.

A fourth approach to weaning has recently been described, consisting of a trial of spontaneous breathing performed once a day through a T-tube circuit [48]. If the patient sustains spontaneous ventilation for 2 h without undue distress, he/she is extubated. If the patient develops signs of distress on physical examination, the trial is stopped and mechanical ventilation is re-instituted for at least 24 h. This contrasts with other techniques where reductions in ventilator assistance are made several times a day and the period of respiratory muscle rest following a failed trial is relatively brief. The rationale behind the once-daily approach is that respiratory muscles require a prolonged period of rest in order to allow recovery from stressful efforts (Fig. 7) [35].

Two rigorously controlled, prospective studies [48, 49] were recently published comparing the relative efficacy of different weaning strategies in the subgroup of patients who are difficult to wean. In both studies, intermittent mandatory ventilation was found to delay the weaning process. In the study of Brochard et al. [49], pressure support was found to result in faster weaning than T-tube trials, whereas in the study of Esteban et al. [48], a once-daily trial of spontaneous breathing was found to achieve a two-fold increase in the rate of successful weaning and extubation compared with pressure support. Although readers may focus on the different outcomes in these studies, both studies are consistent on a very important point: patient outcome is very much influenced by the selection of a weaning technique. The different outcomes in the studies is probably due to the specific criteria employed at different stages of the weaning process.

The insight gained from these studies was recently extended in a randomized, controlled study by Ely et al. [50], who investigated whether predictive indices combined with a trial of spontaneous breathing would hasten the pace of wean-

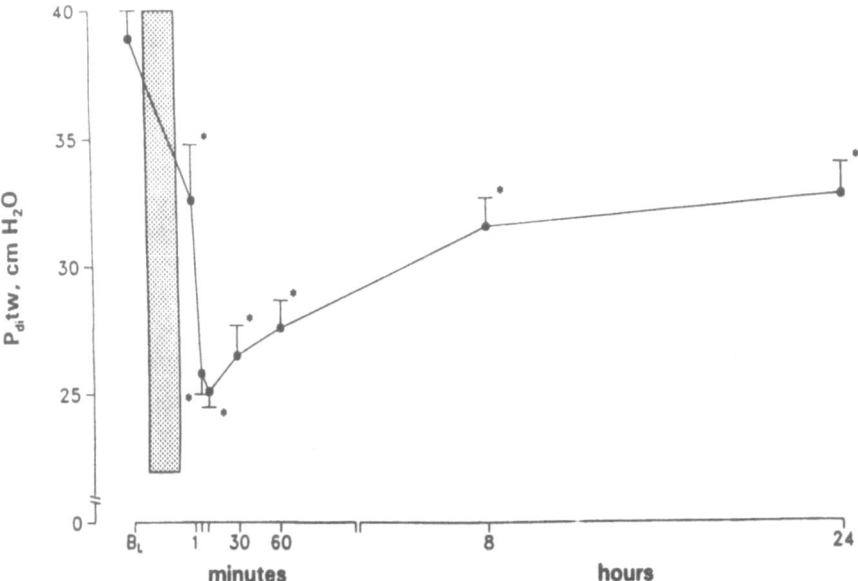

Fig. 7. Induction of diaphragmatic fatigue (stippled bar) produced a significant fall in trans-diaphragmatic pressure (Pdi) elicited by twitch stimulation of both phrenic nerves. Significant recovery of transdiaphragmatic twitch pressure was noted in the first 8 h following completion of the fatigue protocol, but no further change was observed between 8 and 24 h; the 24-h value was significantly lower than baseline. The delay in reaching the nadir of twitch transdiaphragmatic pressure probably resulted from twitch potentiation, induced by repeated contractions, which was present at termination of the protocol. Values are means ± SE. * Significant difference compared with baseline value, $p < 0.01$. (From [35] with permission)

ing. The patients were screened each morning for 5 factors: PaO_2/FiO_2 ratio > 200; PEEP ≤ 5 cmH$_2$O; f/VT ≤ 105 br/min/L; intact cough on suctioning; and absence of infusions of sedative or vasopressor agents. Patients in the intervention group (n = 149) who met all 5 criteria underwent a 2-h trial of spontaneous breathing that same morning. If the patient did not develop clinical signs of distress – employing the criteria of the studies of Brochard et al. [49] and Esteban et al. [48] – the trial was considered successful, and the patient's physician was notified of this result. The control group (n = 151) had daily screening but did not undergo the spontaneous breathing trial. Although patients in the intervention group had more severe disease, with higher APACHE II and acute lung injury scores, their median duration of mechanical ventilation was 1.5 days less than the control group (p = 0.003), and they had lower rates of complications (p = 0.001) and re-intubation (p = 0.04), and lower ICU charges (p = 0.03).

Conclusion

While the preceding discussion is based on data obtained in patients recovering from different causes of acute respiratory failure, little reason exists to believe that patients with ARDS behave differently. Attempts to discontinue ventilator-support cannot be made until the underlying lung injury has recovered to the extent that hazardous hypoxemia is no longer a likelihood. At this time, inability of the respiratory muscles to cope with the abnormal pulmonary mechanics is the major factor deciding continued ventilator dependency. To decide whether a patient can tolerate the discontinuation of mechanical ventilation, it is necessary to perform simple objective physiological measurements; bedside clinical examination is not sufficient to guide this decision. In our view, the measurement of predictive indices combined with a trial of spontaneous breathing is the most successful method of expediting the weaning process [11, 48, 50].

References

1. Tobin, MJ, Alex CG (1994) Discontinuation of mechanical ventilation. In: Tobin MJ (ed) Principles and Practice of Mechanical Ventilation. McGraw Hill, New York, pp 1177–1206
2. Lessard MR, Brochard LJ (1996) Weaning from ventilatory support. Clinics Chest Med 17: 475–489
3. Rodriguez-Roisin R (1994) Effect of mechanical ventilation on gas exchange. In: Tobin MJ (ed) Principles of Mechanical Ventilation. McGraw Hill, New York, pp 673–693
4. Criner GJ, Isaac L (1994) Psychological problems in the ventilator-dependent patient. In: Tobin MJ (ed) Principles and Practice of Mechanical Ventilation. McGraw Hill, New York, pp 1163–1175
5. Tobin MJ, Perez W, Guenther SM, et al (1986) The pattern of breathing during successful and unsuccessful trials of weaning from mechanical ventilation. Am Rev Respir Dis 134: 1111–1118
6. Sassoon CSH, Mahutte CK (1993) Airway occlusion pressure and breathing pattern as predictors of weaning outcome. Am Rev Respir Dis 148:860–866
7. Decramer M, de Bock V, Dom R (1996) Functional and histologic picture of steroid-induced myopathy in chronic obstructive pulmonary disease. Am J Respir Crit Care Med 153: 1958–1964
8. Marini JJ, Smith TC, Lamb V (1986) Estimation of inspiratory muscle strength in mechanically ventilated patients: The measurement of maximal inspiratory pressure. J Crit Care 1: 32–38
9. Multz AS, Aldrich TK, Prezant DJ, Karpel JP, Hendler JM (1990) Maximal inspiratory pressure is not a reliable test of inspiratory muscle strength in mechanically ventilated patients. Am Rev Respir Dis 142:529–532
10. Aldrich TK, Spiro P (1995) Maximal inspiratory pressure: Does reproducibility indicate full effort? Thorax 50:40–43
11. Sahn SA, Lashminarayan S (1973) Bedside criteria for discontinuation of mechanical ventilation. Chest 63:1002–1005
12. Yang KL, Tobin MJ (1991) A prospective study of indexes predicting the outcome of trials of weaning from mechanical ventilation. N Engl J Med 324:1445–1450
13. Tobin, MJ, Jubran A (1994) Pathophysiology of failure to wean from mechanical ventilation. Schweiz Med Wochenschr 124:2139–2145
14. Tobin MJ (1988) Respiratory muscles in disease. Clinics Chest Med 9:263–286
15. Jubran A, Tobin MJ (1997) Pathophysiological basis of acute respiratory distress in patients who fail a trial of weaning from mechanical ventilation. Am J Respir Crit Care Med 155: 906–915

16. Jubran A, Tobin MJ (1997) Passive mechanics of lung and chest wall in patients who failed or succeeded in trials of weaning. Am J Respir Crit Care Med 155:916–921
17. Ramsdell JW, Nachtwey FS, Moser KM (1982) Bronchial hyperactivity in chronic obstructive bronchitis. Am Rev Respir Dis 126:829–832
18. Woolcock AJ, Vincent NJ, Macklem PT (1969) Frequency dependence of compliance as a test for obstruction in the small airways. J Clin Invest 48:1097–1106
19. NHLBI Workshop Summary (1990) Respiratory muscle fatigue: Report of the respiratory muscle fatigue workshop group. Am Rev Respir Dis 42:474–480
20. Cohen C, Zagelbaum G, Gross D, Roussos C, Macklem PT (1982) Clinical manifestations of inspiratory muscle fatigue. Am J Med 73:308–316
21. Goldstone JC, Green M, Moxham J (1994) Maximum relaxation rate of the diaphragm during weaning from mechanical ventilation. Thorax 49:54–60
22. Esau SA, Bye PTP, Pardy RL (1983) Change in rate of relaxation of sniffs with diaphragmatic fatigue in humans. J Appl Physiol 55:731–735
23. Swartz MA, Marino PL (1985) Diaphragmatic strength during weaning from mechanical ventilation. Chest 85:736–739
24. Le Bourdelles G, Viires N, Boczkowski J, et al (1994) Effects of mechanical ventilation on diaphragmatic contractile properties in rats. Am J Respir Crit Care Med 149:1539–1544
25. Anzueto A, Peters JT, Tobin MJ, et al (1997) Effects of prolonged mechanical ventilation on diaphragmatic function in healthy adults. Crit Care Med (In press)
26. Bellemare F, Grassino A (1982) Effect of pressure and timing of contraction of the human diaphragm fatigue. J Appl Physiol 53:1190–1195
27. McCool FD, McCann DR, Leith DE, Hoppin FG (1986) Pressure-flow effects on endurance of inspiratory muscles. J Appl Physiol 60:299–301
28. Clanton TL, Dixon GF, Drake J, Gadek JE (1985) Effects of breathing pattern on inspiratory muscle endurance in humans. J Appl Physiol 59:1834–1841
29. Babcock MA, Pegelow DR, McClaran SR, Suman OE, Dempsey JA (1995) Contribution of diaphragmatic power output to exercise-induced diaphragm fatigue. J Appl Physiol 78:1710–1719
30. Leblanc P, Summers E, Inman MD, Jones NL, Campbell EJM, Killian KJ (1988) Inspiratory muscles during exercise: A problem of supply and demand. J Appl Physiol 64:2482–2489
31. Tobin MJ, Guenther SM, Perez W, et al (1987) Konno-Mead analysis of ribcage-abdominal motion during successful and unsuccessful trials of weaning from mechanical ventilation. Am Rev Respir Dis 135:1320–1328
32. Goldman MD, Grimby G, Mead J (1976) Mechanical work of breathing derived from rib cage and abdominal V-P partitioning. J Appl Physiol 41:752–763
33. Roussos, C, Moxham J, Bellemare F (1995) Respiratory muscle fatigue. In: Roussos C (ed) The Thorax (2nd ed) Marcel Dekker, New York, pp 1405–1461
34. Bellemare F, Bigland-Ritchie B (1987) Central components of diaphragmatic fatigue assessed by phrenic nerve stimulation. J Appl Physiol 62:1307–1316
35. Laghi F, D'Alfonso N, Tobin MJ (1995) Pattern of recovery from diaphragmatic fatigue over 24 hours. J Appl Physiol 79:539–546
36. Banzett, RB, Lansing RW, Reid MB, Adams L, Brown R (1989) "Air hunger" arising from increased PCO_2 in mechanically ventilated quadriplegics. Resp Physiol 76:53–68
37. Dunn WF, Nelson SB, Hubmayr RD (1991) The control of breathing during weaning from mechanical ventilation. Chest 100:754–761
38. Mador MJ, Tobin MJ (1992) The effect of inspiratory muscle fatigue on breathing pattern and ventilatory response to CO_2. J Physiol (Lond) 455:17–31
39. Yan, S, Sliwinski P, Gauthier AP, Lichros I, Zakynthinos S, Macklem PT (1993) Effect of global inspiratory muscle fatigue on ventilatory and respiratory muscle responses to CO_2. J Appl Physiol 75:1371–1377
40. Bellemare F, Bigland-Ritchie B, Woods JJ (1986) Contractile properties of the human diaphragm in vivo. J Appl Physiol 61:1153–1161
41. Ferguson GT (1994) Use of twitch pressure to assess diaphragmatic function and central drive. J Appl Physiol 77:1705–1715
42. Similowski T, Yan S, Gauthier AP, Macklem PT, Bellemare F (1991) Contractile properties of the human diaphragm during chronic hyperinflation. N Engl J Med 325:917–923

43. Similowski T, Fleury B, Launois S, Cathala HP, Bouche P, Derenne JP (1989) Cervical magnetic stimulation: A new painless method of bilateral phrenic nerve stimulation in conscious humans. J Appl Physiol 67:13311–1318

44. Laghi F, Harrison MJ, Tobin MJ (1996) Comparison of magnetic and electrical phrenic nerve stimulation in assessment of diaphragmatic contractility. J Appl Physiol 80:1731–1742

45. Stroetz RW, Hubmayr RD (1995) Tidal volume maintenance during weaning with pressure support. Am J Respir Crit Care Med 152:1034–1040

46. Sassoon CSH (1994) Intermittent mandatory ventilation. In: Tobin MJ (ed) Principles and Practice of Mechanical Ventilation. McGraw Hill, New York, pp 221–237

47. Brochard L (1994) Pressure support ventilation. In: Tobin MJ (ed) Principles and Practice of Mechanical Ventilation. McGraw Hill, New York, pp 239–257

48. Esteban A, Frutos F, Tobin MJ, et al (1995) A comparison of four methods of weaning patients from mechanical ventilation. N Engl J Med 332:345–350

49. Brochard L, Rauss A, Benito S, et al (1994) Comparison of three methods of gradual withdrawal from ventilatory support during weaning from mechanical ventilation. Am J Respir Crit Care Med 150:896–903

50. Ely EW, Baker AM, Dunagan DP, et al (1996) Effect of the duration of mechanical ventilation of identifying patients capable of breathing spontaneously. N Engl J Med 335:1864–1869

Liquid Ventilation

Perfluorocarbon Liquid Ventilation in Pediatric ALI

B. P. Fuhrman

Introduction

The response of infants and children to pulmonary injury or inflammatory stimulation, like that of the adult, triggers a final common pathway that has come to be known as acute lung injury (ALI). If sufficiently severe, the disorder has been termed acute respiratory distress syndrome (ARDS). In ALI, capillary permeability to water and large molecules increases. Water and protein leak from pulmonary capillary to lung interstitium. The alveolar basement membrane is less permeable to these substances than is the capillary basement membrane, so fluid accumulates in the interstitium of the lung. Pulmonary lymphatics drain the interstitium, and can substantially increase their intrinsic flow rates, but, if this is not sufficient to limit interstitial fluid accumulation, the dam bursts, and interstitial fluid and protein begin to leak into alveoli. This liquid impairs surfactant function, raising alveolar surface tension.

ALI is not homogeneous. Some alveolar segments are worse affected than others. Those of relatively high surface tension and poor compliance may resist inflation, and be poorly responsive to positive end-expiratory pressure (PEEP). Other, less affected segments, may be PEEP responsive, and become overdistended. This sets the stage for maldistribution of ventilation, volutrauma and hypoxemia. Perfusion of the lung is most dramatically regulated locally, at the alveolar capillary unit. Those segments that are exposed to high alveolar pressures during the application of positive airway pressure will be compressed. This sets the stage for redistribution, often maldistribution, of perfusion, high V/Q mismatch, and hypercarbia.

There are also specific pathways of pathophysiology in ALI that assume special importance when the appropriate triggering event occurs. For example, chest trauma directly injures the lung, causing hemorrhage into the parenchyma; inhalation of hot smoke causes airway burns and may be associated with copious secretions; and infection may cause consolidation and hepatization of lung. The presence of these specific disturbances further complicates the already complex function of the affected lung.

Ventilation-perfusion (V-P) mismatch is the principal impediment to gas exchange in ALI, though extensive absolute intrapulmonary shunt also occurs. Until quite recently, the intensivist could only force air into non-receptive lungs and hope that this strategy would improve V/Q matching, but in the past decade, new approaches that modify lung function and improve V/Q matching have been developed. Perfluorocarbon liquid ventilation is one such approach.

Partial Liquid Ventilation and Perfluorocarbon Associated Gas Exchange

A recent innovation variously termed perfluorocarbon-associated gas exchange (PAGE) or partial liquid ventilation (PLV) has simplified the technical aspects of using perfluorocarbons in the lung. It has been shown possible to fill the functional residual capacity (FRC) of the lungs with perfluorocarbon liquid, and to "bubble oxygenate" the liquid *in situ* (*in vivo*) using a conventional gas ventilator [1]. This technique, gas ventilation of the fluid filled lung, allows liquid to be used to recruit atelectatic lung and reduce surface tension at the alveolar lining. In expiration, the liquid FRC represents an incompressible reservoir of oxygen, occupying alveoli that would otherwise collapse and permit intrapulmonary shunting. In inspiration, tidal volumes of gas purge that reservoir of carbon dioxide and replenish the supply of dissolved oxygen after the fashion of a very efficient bubble oxygenator.

In normal piglets, PLV provides excellent gas exchange. The airway pressure excursion required to deliver a fixed tidal volume of gas to the perfluorocarbon-filled lung is no greater than that required to ventilate the dry lung [1]. It has only recently been appreciated that there is a small but consistent decline in oxygenation when the normal lung is filled with perfluorocarbon. Hernan et al. [2] have shown that this reduction in arterial oxygen tension is probably related in part to a diffusion barrier imposed by the perfluorocarbon liquid itself. This implies a limit to the theoretically achievable paO_2 during PLV. It also suggests that the alveolar lining is exposed to less oxygen when ventilated across a layer of perfluorocarbon than when ventilated "dry".

In larger animals such as sheep, oxygenation is affected by hydraulic factors as well. It has been shown that arterial oxygenation is tidal volume (VT)-dependent in the large lung [3]. This reflects the tendency of gas to gravitate to non-dependent regions of fluid-filled lung when small tidal volumes and low peak airway pressures are used. In the large lung, gas exchange is often greatly enhanced by a slight increase in peak inflation pressure and VT [4]. Hydraulic issues appear to be important in the large lung but not in the small lung. In the large lung, hydraulic effects cannot be readily distinguished from consequences of lung stiffness, both of which elevate end-inspiratory airway pressure. Measurements of compliance do not reflect stiffness alone in the large lung during PLV.

It has been show in animal models that PLV is effective over prolonged treatment periods [5, 6], and that recovery to gas breathing is readily accomplished.

Use of Perflubron for Partial Liquid Ventilation

Toxicologic evidence from prolonged studies supports the suitability of perfluorooctylbromide (perflubron or LiquiVenttm, Alliance Pharmaceutical Corp, San Diego, CA) for PLV in patients. Perflubron has important physical properties that enhance its use for PLV. It is not metabolized. Its solubility in water is very low and it is virtually immiscible with aqueous solutions. Its absorption from the respiratory system into the blood is negligible. Perflubron has a surface tension of about 18 dynes/cm, lower than saline (approximately 70 dynes/cm) and lower than the presumed surface tension of normal lung at total lung capacity (believed to be about 30 dynes/cm), but greater than the estimated normal surface tension of the alveolar lining at full expiration (less than 2 dynes/cm). The surface tension of a perflubron-aqueous interface is substantially reduced by the presence of even small amounts of surfactant and is felt to be physiologically inconsequential. Because of its surface tension characteristics, perflubron tends to spread over biological surfaces rather than bead. This may be an important determinant of its spreading properties in the lung.

The vapor pressure of perflubron at body temperature is 10.5 torr, substantially lower than most other perfluorocarbons that have been used for PLV or tidal liquid ventilation. This reduces evaporative losses. Rates of evaporation in infant models of lung disease are about 2–3 mL/kg/h, and it is this quantity of liquid that must be replaced over prolonged treatment periods.

PLV in Models of Lung Disease

Tutuncu et al. [7] have shown that rabbit lungs lavaged with saline to induce surfactant deficiency exchange gas more efficiently during PLV than during conventional gas ventilation. Leach et al. [8] have shown this also to be the case in premature lambs with hyaline membrane disease, and that PLV is compatible with exogenous surfactant therapy [9]. Wilcox et al. [10] have studied lambs with surgically induced congenital left diaphragmatic hernia, and has shown that this lesion (which is complicated by surfactant deficiency) is amenable to treatment by PLV. In all of these models, lung compliance was improved by the presence of perflubron within the lung. Clearly, surfactant deficiency is highly responsive to PLV.

PLV has also been applied to piglets after intratracheal instillation of meconium [11]. In this model, oxygenation and 6-h survival were both substantially improved, but improvement in gas exchange was less striking and less rapid than in models of surfactant deficiency. Though meconium is thought to impair surfactant function, it is also known to obstruct distal airways. This mechanical issue contributed to the difficulty of rescuing animals after meconium instillation.

Several models of ALI and ARDS have been studied. Papo et al [12] have shown that lung injury induced by intravenous oleic acid infusion is ameliorated by PLV. Nesti et al. [13] have shown that gastric aspiration induced ARDS benefits from PLV with perflubron, and Hernan et al. [8] have demonstrated amelioration of acid-induced ARDS in large sheep. Improvement in histology was seen in Nesti and Papo's studies. Hirschl et al. [14] have also documented improved histology in an oleic acid injury model treated by tidal liquid ventilation.

When the efficacy data for PLV in various models of lung disease is plotted on a single bar graph, a striking observation emerges. Arterial pO_2 falls by about 100 torr when the normal lung is filled with perfluorocarbon. In surfactant deficiency, oxygenation improves after instillation of perfluorocarbon and the lung generates oxygenation comparable to the normal liquid filled lung. PLV with perflubron makes the surfactant deficient lung function almost as though it were normal. But surprisingly, several inflammatory models also behave as though the lung were made to function normally after perflubron instillation. The combination of near normal oxygenation and near normal histology in Nesti's study of aspiration ARDS suggests that perflubron may have anti-inflammatory effects distinct from the beneficial effects of PLV on lung function.

Anti-inflammatory Effects of Perflubron

Smith et al. [15] have shown that endotoxin-stimulated alveolar macrophages generate fewer free radicals and less hydrogen peroxide after exposure to perflubron. Perflubron also reduces neutrophil infiltration in the acutely injured lung [16]. It reduces phagocytosis but not killing by alveolar macrophages [17], and reduces nitric oxide production by alveolar macrophages *in vitro* [18]. Electron micrographs of alveolar macrophages exposed to perflubron *in vivo* reveal vesicles that probably represent ingested perflubron. This is compatible with pinocytosis of the liquid, which might be expected to internalize receptor sites (as vesicle membrane) that are normally bound to the cell surface. It is also possible that perflubron dissolves in the macrophage's cell membrane much like a volatile anesthetic, altering membrane function. Many volatile anesthetics alter inflammation, though their predominant effect is clearly to alter neuronal surface membrane function.

The clinical significance of these anti-inflammatory effects is not yet clear. There might well be concern that perfluorocarbons might make the lung susceptible to nosocomial infection. Findings of Steinhorn and Sajan contradict this [19].

Surfactant Production

Perfluorocarbons are not miscible with aqueous solutions or gels. Surfactant is not readily soluble in perflubron. Moreover, during PLV, perfluorocarbon leaves the lung by evaporation, a route not possible for non-volatile phospholipid surfactants. It is not likely that PLV would deplete the lung of phospholipid. Steinhorn et al. [20] have shown that, to the contrary, PLV with perflubron increases de novo synthesis of surfactant by normal lung. Similar findings apply to the immature lung studied by Leach et al [21]. It has been hypothesized that lung stretch mediates these increases in surfactant synthesis.

Management of Secretions

Secretions are not miscible in perfluorochemicals. Early clinical experience suggested that this might be a problem during PLV. Subsequent laboratory experience has shown that secretions may be effectively debrided from the lung by saline lavage during PLV (Fuhrman, unpublished results). This may, if fact, prove to be a beneficial effect of the treatment.

Clinical Trials of PLV in Infants and Children

PLV is an investigational technique using an investigational liquid (LiquiVen[ttm]) now in clinical trials for FDA approval. Results in infants with ARDS have been published [22] as well as preliminary findings in children [23]. These trials document mortality rates lower than historic controls and show physiologic improvements in gas exchange and lung compliance. However, they lack companion control populations.

In the first of these trials, 13 premature infants were studied. Patients were viable gestation and birth weight, near birth (to avoid pretreatment volutrauma), surfactant deficient, surfactant non-responders, felt to be at high risk of imminent death (Tables 1 and 2). Seven of 13 infants survived. At 36 weeks of age, 3 were on room air and 4 received oxygen by nasal cannula. Six of 13 infants died. Causes of death were: acute respiratory failure (3), intraventricular hemorrhage (2), and severe bronchopulmonary disease (1). In a phase 2 study of children with ARDS, 10 patients were enrolled. All were thought to be at greater than 40% risk

Table 1. Entry criteria – Premature neonates

24–34 weeks gestation
600–2000 g birth weight
Less than 5 days of age at enrollment
Diagnosis of ARDS
– failure to respond to at least one dose of surfactant
– high risk or mortality as assessed by referring physician

Table 2. Characteristics of enrolled premature infants

28.3 ± 0.7 weeks gestation
1057 ± 100 g birth weight
43.8 ± 11.5 h of life at enrollment
8/5 male/female
2.5 ± 0.2 doses of surfactant failed

Table 3. Physiologic responses to PLV in premature neonates

	baseline	1 h	24 h
FiO_2	1.0	0.95	0.60
paO_2	60	143	100
CL (dynamic)	0.18	0.29	0.4
mean Paw	17	12	—
Oxygenation index	49	17	9

Table 4. Demographics of children with ARDS treated by PLV

Age, yr	4.3 ± 1.6
Weight, kg	18 ± 6
A-aDO$_2$	457 ± 133
Oxygenation index	21.7 ± 15.7
pO$_2$/FiO$_2$	127 ± 71
PEEP	11.3 ± 2.8
PIP	37.6 ± 6.2
mean Paw	20.6 ± 5.5

of mortality (Table 4). Eight of 10 patients survived. There were no serious, unexpected adverse events deemed by the investigators to be related to the treatment. Five of the patients had episodes of desaturation which were treated by suctioning. Three patients had pneumothoraces, an incidence expected from the literature. Overall, PLV was well tolerated. In this group of children, A-aDO$_2$ fell from 450 to less than 300 in 24 h, and the benefit was sustained throughout the treatment period.

Conclusion

Pre-clinical and early clinical trials give cause for optimism as perflubron PLV proceeds into pivotal randomized, controlled trials. The technique and the perfluorocarbon required for its implementation (perflubron) offer a multifaceted approach to ALI and ARDS. The technique reduces pulmonary surface tension in surfactant dysfunction states, recruits atelectatic alveoli, and creates an oxygen reservoir in segments that would otherwise collapse in expiration. It represents an "open lung" approach to ventilation. In addition, PLV redistributes pulmonary blood flow toward non-dependent lung. It mobilizes secretions, quenches inflammation (both *in vitro* and *in vivo*), and stimulates surfactant production. To learn how PLV affects outcome in ARDS will require a large, multicenter, randomized, controlled trial.

References

1. Fuhrman BP, Paczan PR, DeFrancisis M (1991) Perfluorocarbon associated gas exchange. Crit Care Med 19:712–723
2. Hernan LJ, Penfil S, Fuhrman BP, et al (1996) Functional FiO$_2$ predicts alveolar pO$_2$ during perfluorocarbon associated gas exchange. Crit Care Med 24:A149 (Abst)
3. Hernan LJ, Fuhrman BP, Kaiser R, et al (1996) Perfluorocarbon associated gas exchange in normal and acid injured large sheep. Crit Care Med 24:475–481
4. Hernan LJ, Fuhrman BP, Papo MC, Steinhorn DM, Leach CL, Salman N, Paczan P, Kahn B (1995) Cardiopulmonary effects of perfluorocarbon associated gas exchange at reduced oxygen concentrations. Crit Care Med 23:553–559
5. Salman N, Fuhrman BP, Steinhorn DM, et al (1995) Prolonged studies of perfluorocarbon associated gas exchange and of resumption of conventional mechanical ventilation. Crit Care Med 23:919–924

6. DeLemos R, Winter D, Fields T, et al (1994) Prolonged partial liquid ventilation in the treatment of hyaline membrane disease (HMD) in the premature baboon. Pediatr Res 35:330A (Abst)
7. Tutuncu AS, Faithfull NS, Lachmann B (1993) Comparison of ventilatory support with intratracheal perfluorocarbon administration and conventional mechanical ventilation in animals with acute respiratory failure. Am Rev Respir Dis 148:785–792
8. Leach CL, Fuhrman BP, Morin FC III, Rath MG (1993) Perfluorocarbon associated gas exchange (PAGE) in respiratory distress syndrome. Crit Care Med 21:1270–1278
9. Leach CL, Holm B, Morin FCC III, et al (1995) Partial liquid ventilation in premature lambs with respiratory distress syndrome: Efficacy and compatibility with exogenous surfactant. J Pediatr 126:412–210
10. Wilcox DT, Glick PL, Karamanoukian HL, Morin FC, Fuhrman BP, Leach CL (1995) Perfluorocarbon associated gas exchange improves pulmonary mechanics, oxygenation, ventilation and allows nitric oxide delivery in the hypoplastic lung congenital diaphragmatic hernia lamb model. Crit Care Med 23:1858–1863
11. Thompson AE, Fuhrman BP, Allen J (1993) Perfluorocarbon associated gas exchange in experimental meconium aspiration. Pediatr Res 33:239A (Abst)
12. Papo MC, Paczan P, Fuhrman BP, et al (1996) Perfluorocarbon associated gas exchange improves oxygenation, lung compliance and survival in an animal model of adult respiratory distress syndrome. Crit Care Med 24:466–474
13. Nesti FD, Fuhrman BP, Steinhorn DM, et al (1994) Perfluorocarbon associated gas exchange (PAGE) in gastric aspiration. Crit Care Med 22:1445–1452
14. Hirschl RB, Tooley R, Parent AC, Johnson K, Bartlett RH (1995) Improvement of gas exchange, pulmonary function and lung injury with partial liquid ventilation. A study model in a setting of severe respiratory failure. Chest 108:500–508
15. Smith T, Dandona P, Fuhrman B, Marcucci K, Steinhorn D, Thusu K (1995) A liquid perfluorochemical decreases the in vitro production of reactive oxygen species by alveolar macrophages. Crit Care Med 23:1533–1539
16. Colton D, Bartlett R, Gill G, Hirschl R, Johnson K (1994) Neutrophil infiltration is reduced during partial perfluorocarbon liquid ventilation in the setting of lung injury. Surg Forum Proc XLV:668–670
17. Steinhorn DM, Fuhrman BP, Smith T (1995) Liquid perfluorocarbon affects phagocytosis by alveolar macrophages after in vitro exposure. Crit Care Med 23:A213 (Abst)
18. Steinhorn DM, Fuhrman BP, Smith T (1995) Perflubron decreases nitric oxide production by alveolar macrophages in vitro. Pediatr Res 27:55A (Abst)
19. Steinhorn DM, Sajan I (1996) Partial liquid ventilation reduces colonization of the lung during experimental nosocomial pneumonia. Pediatr Res 39:54A (Abst)
20. Steinhorn DM, Fuhrman BP, Holm B, Leach C (1996) Partial liquid ventilation enhances surfactant production. Am J Respir Crit Care Med 153:A640 (Abst)
21. Leach CL, Hernan LJ, Fuhrman BP, Holm B, Morin III F, Papo MC (1995) Partial liquid ventilation with LiquiVent increases endogenous surfactant production in premature lambs with respiratory distress syndrome. Pediatr Res 37 (4 Part 2):238A (Abst)
22. Leach CL, Greenspan JS, Rubenstein SD, et al (1996) Partial liquid ventilation with perflubron in fremature infants with severe respiratory distress syndrome. N Engl J Med 335:761–767
23. Toro-Figueroa L, Curtis S, Fackler J, et al (1996) Perflubron partial liquid ventilation (PLV) in children with ARDS. A safety and efficacy pilot study. Crit Care Med 24:A150 (Abst)

Experience in Liquid Ventilation

R. B. Hirschl

Introduction

Perfluorocarbons are structurally similar to hydrocarbons with the hydrogen replaced by fluorine. The carbon chains vary in length and an additional moiety often is attached to the molecule which, together, give unique properties to each perfluorocarbon. In general, perfluorocarbons have excellent oxygen and carbon dioxide carrying capacity (50 mL O_2/dL and 160–210 mL CO_2/dL, respectively) [1]. They are clear, odorless, inert fluids which are immiscible in aqueous and most other solutions. They are relatively dense (1.7–1.9 g/mL), have a low surface tension (15–19 dynes/cm), and are relatively volatile with vapor pressures which range from 11 to 85 torr at 37°C. The vapor pressure of the individual perfluorocarbon governs the rapidity with which it evaporates from the lungs after intra-

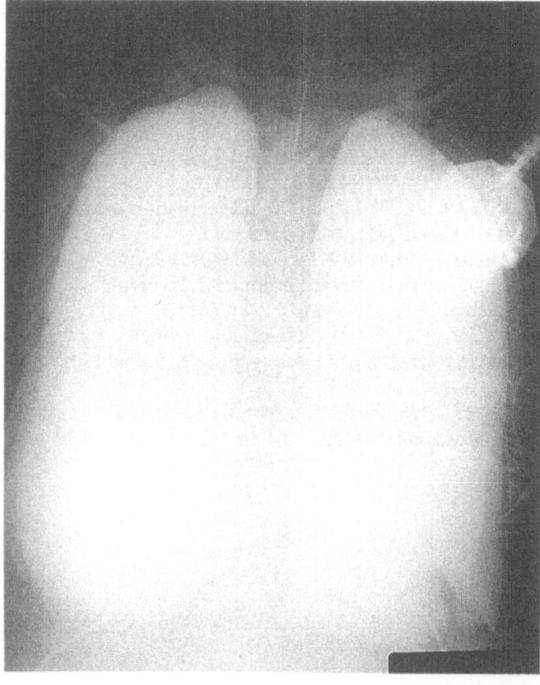

Fig. 1. Representative anteroposterior radiograph of a 51 year old adult with pneumonia on extracorporeal life support (ECLS) following administration of perflubron during PLV. The lungs are well-inflated and radiopaque. (From [27] with permission)

tracheal administration. As is demonstrated in Fig. 1, perflubron (LiquiVent®, Alliance Pharmaceutical Corp., San Diego, CA), which is currently the perfluoro-carbon most commonly used in clinical studies, is radiopaque, although this is not a characteristic of all of these fluids.

Total and Partial Liquid Ventilation

Clark and Gollan [2] first reported the ability to sustain gas exchange in the sub-merged, spontaneously perfluorocarbon-breathing mouse. The work of breath-ing, however, is markedly increased during spontaneous perfluorocarbon breath-ing because of the elevated resistance to flow of a fluid in the airways. For this rea-son, mechanical devices have been developed and tested in the laboratory to provide total liquid ventilation (TLV) in which the lungs are first filled to a vol-ume equivalent to the functional residual capacity (FRC), approximately 30 mL/kg), and then ventilated with perfluorocarbon. Shaffer and Moskowitz [3], in 1974, documented that such a device could provide demand-regulated total liq-uid ventilation. In 1989, the first reports of the use of total liquid ventilation in humans were published [4, 5]. Three moribund, preterm newborns who had failed surfactant therapy were managed with TLV. Pulmonary compliance in-creased during the period of TLV. The gas exchange response was variable. How-ever, this was the first demonstration of the ability to sustain gas exchange during TLV in humans. Although TLV is *not* being applied clinically at this time, research intending to further develop the technique of TLV is actively being performed [6].

In 1991, the first experience with *partial* liquid ventilation (PLV) in a normal rabbit model was reported [7]. With this technique, the lungs are filled with per-fluorocarbon, in general to a volume equivalent to FRC, and then gas ventilated with a standard gas mechanical ventilator. The adequacy of perfluorocarbon dose is assessed during PLV by visually identifying a meniscus of perfluorocar-bon within the endotracheal tube at end-expiration. There are many advantages to this technique over that of TLV: It does not require the use of a new device nor an understanding of the physics and physiology of fluid flows in the airways, en-dotracheal tube, and liquid ventilation device. Therefore, PLV can be relatively easily performed if one has an understanding of the ventilator management of critically ill patients with respiratory failure. A number of studies have demon-strated the efficacy of PLV in improving gas exchange in preterm neonatal; pedi-atric; and adult lung injury models which have included those induced by intra-venous oleic acid administration, gastric acid aspiration, and saline lavage [8–13].

Mechanisms of Liquid Ventilation

The mechanisms by which gas exchange and pulmonary function are increased in the setting of liquid ventilation have been explored over the last few years. We [14] previously demonstrated the ability of total liquid, in comparison to gas ventilation, to recruit collapsed lung regions in an *ex vivo* lung model of atelectasis. End-expiratory lung volume (EELV) increased 8-fold in otherwise normal, atelectatic lungs, and 14-fold in surfactant deficient, atelectatic lungs during total liquid when compared to gas ventilation. These data would suggest that perfluorocarbon might serve to enhance alveolar recruitment in the setting of atelectasis with or without surfactant deficiency, and, thereby, to improve pulmonary gas exchange. We [15] subsequently evaluated the ability of both TLV and PLV to resolve the lung atelectasis/consolidation which is prominent in the dependent regions of the lungs in patients with the acute respiratory distress syndrome (ARDS). Perfluorocarbon appears to effectively distribute into those dependent lung regions during either TLV or PLV with associated alveolar recruitment [16, 17]. Gauger et al. [18] evaluated FRC in an oleic acid model of lung injury during gas and PLV. FRC was measured by helium dilution as well as by null point plethysmography which is a technique similar in concept to body plethysmography. The gas FRC as measured by helium dilution decreased from 33.0 ± 3.3 to 22.1 ± 2.1 mL/kg ($p < 0.05$) following induction of lung injury, and further decreased to 11.8 ± 1.6 mL/kg following initiation of PLV ($p = 0.03$). However, when one added the gas FRC to the volume of perflubron administered, the mean total end-expiratory lung volume (gas plus perflubron) in the PLV animals was at least as great as that observed pre-injury (33.0 ± 3.3 pre-injury versus 41.8 ± 1.6 mL/kg during PLV, $p \leq 0.001$). Similar changes were observed in the end-expiratory lung volume as measured by body plethysmography. These data suggest that administration of perfluorocarbon during PLV results in the recruitment of otherwise atelectatic, consolidated lung regions which may enhance ventilation/perfusion matching and gas exchange. In addition, administration of perfluorocarbon tends to redistribute pulmonary blood flow away from the dependent and toward the non-dependent lung regions during TLV when compared to gas ventilation in normal lungs [19]. This pattern of redistribution of pulmonary blood flow toward the better aerated, non-dependent lung regions may also result in an improvement in ventilation/perfusion matching and gas exchange during PLV in the setting of lung injury.

One intriguing finding, which was initially observed in the oleic acid model, is a reduction in the degree of lung injury and inflammatory infiltrate observed during liquid when compared to gas ventilation [10, 20]. A decrease in neutrophil count, myeloperoxidase content, albumin leak, and intraalveolar hemorrhage has been documented during PLV when compared to gas ventilation in a model of cobra venom factor-induced lung injury [21, 22]. We have observed similar reductions in myeloperoxidase content and neutrophil count when positive end-expiratory pressure (PEEP) was applied in this model. This would suggest that alveolar recruitment may be an important component of the protective effects observed. Other studies have demonstrated that neutrophil and alveolar macrophage function are suppressed in the presence of perfluorocarbon, although experiments from our laboratories would indicate that neutrophil function is unchanged following exposure to perflubron [23–25]. Finally, it has been suggested that a lavage effect is associated with PLV which may result in the removal of inflammatory mediators and cellular elements from the peripheral airways and alveoli.

Pulmonary compliance is markedly increased during PLV in smaller animal models of respiratory failure, such as in the setting of congenital diaphragmatic hernia and preterm newborn respiratory distress syndrome [8, 26]. However, in mid-size and adult animal models of oleic acid lung injury, only a small increase or even a decrease in pulmonary compliance may be observed during PLV following administration of perfluorocarbon [9–11]. This may be related to the fact that alveolar surface tension is still not optimized during PLV in the setting of respiratory failure. In addition, fluoroscopy, chest radiography, and lung cross sectional imaging have been used to document that perflubron distributes in the lungs in an inhomogeneous fashion: The majority of the perflubron tends to pool in the dependent regions whether the patient is supine or upright [27]. The distribution of gas in the partially perfluorocarbon-filled lungs may be, therefore, inhomogeneous, and the volume available for distribution of the ventilating gas reduced as the dose of perfluorocarbon increases; a reduction in lung compliance is the result. The smaller the anteroposterior diameter of the patient, the less effect the dependent/non-dependent distribution of gas and perfluorocarbon in the lungs would be expected to have upon pulmonary compliance during PLV: This may contribute to the observation that the pulmonary compliance is frequently increased during PLV in newborns and infants, but not routinely in older patients.

Evaluation of PLV

Phase I/II studies evaluating the efficacy of PLV in premature newborn, pediatric, and adult patients with respiratory insufficiency have been completed and have demonstrated encouraging results. The multicenter study by Leach et al. [28], involving 13 premature newborns who had failed two doses of surfactant and had an a/A ratio <0.2 demonstrated a two-fold increase in mean pulmonary compliance from approximately 0.2 to 0.4 mL/cm H_2O/kg and a decrease in mean oxygen index (OI = mean airway pressure $\cdot FiO_2 \cdot 100/PaO_2$) from approximately 50 to 10 over the 24-h period following initiation of PLV with perflubron. In similar phase I/II studies, we [29] evaluated parameters of pulmonary function and gas exchange in adults, children, and newborns with respiratory failure on extracorporeal life support (ECLS). This series of patients included 10 adults with a variety of diagnoses (pneumonia = 7, charcoal aspiration = 1, ARDS = 1, and asthma = 1); 4 pediatric patients (pneumonia = 2, hydrocarbon aspiration = 1, ARDS = 1); and 5 neonates (congenital diaphragmatic hernia (CDH) = 4, primary pulmonary hypertension of the newborn = 1). As demonstrated in Fig. 2 and 3, a decrease in (A-a)DO_2 and an increase in static pulmonary compliance corrected for weight were observed in the 72-h following initiation of PLV in the adult patients [27]. Similar improvements were observed in the pediatric and neonatal populations [30, 31]. Half of the perflubron had evaporated from the lungs by a mean of 3.5 days after the last intratracheal dose (range 1–16 days) in the adult patients [32].

PLV has now been evaluated in 9 adult and 10 pediatric patients with respiratory insufficiency who were not on ECLS (Hirschl et al. unpublished results) [33]. PLV was performed for a total of 96 h with 28 day survival noted in 7 of 9 adults

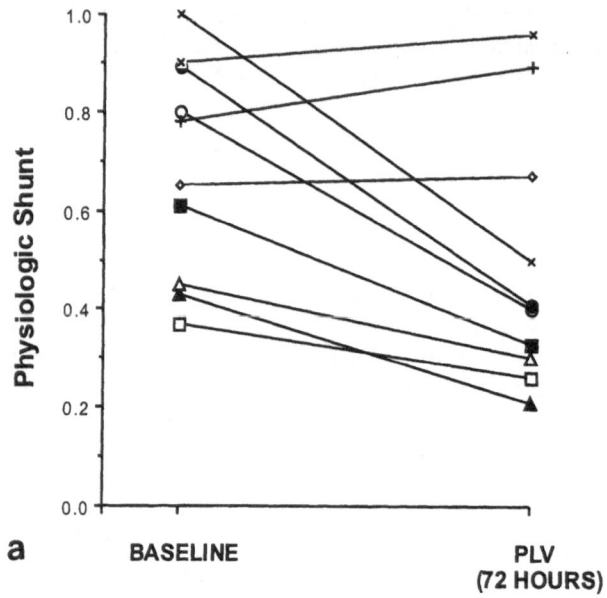

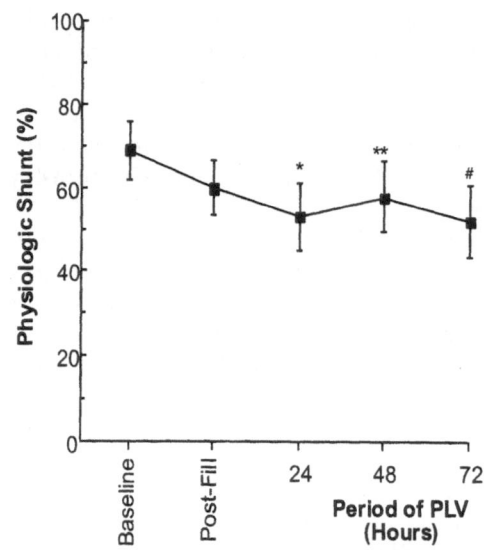

Fig. 2. a. Individual calculated pulmonary physiologic shunt at baseline and after 72 h of PLV. **b.** Calculated pulmonary physiologic shunt at baseline, after initial perfluorocarbon dose administration, and for the subsequent 3 days in patients with respiratory failure managed with extracorporeal life support and PLV. Data as mean ± SEM (p = 0.014 by one way repeated measures ANOVA, * p = 0.013, ** p = 0.022, # p = 0.031 by post-hoc paired t-test with Bonferroni corrected significant p < 0.013) (From (27] with permission)

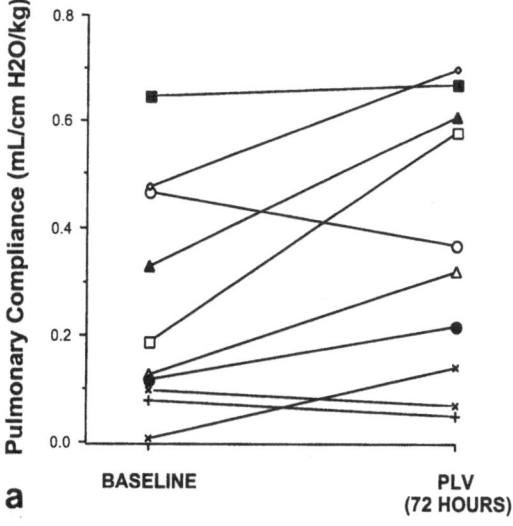

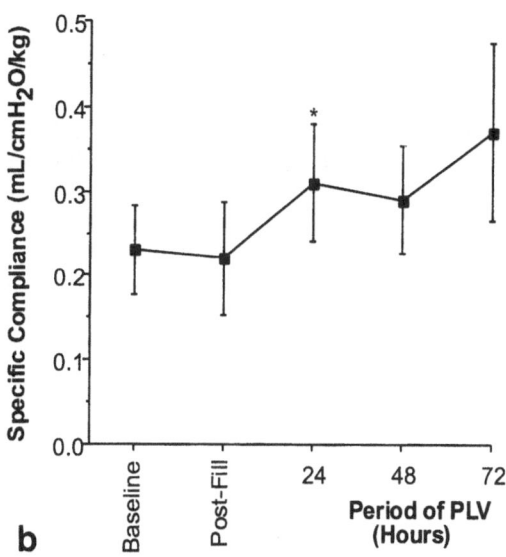

Fig. 3. a. Individual static pulmonary compliance at baseline and after 72 h of PLV. **b.** Static pulmonary compliance at baseline, after initial perfluorocarbon dose administration, and for the subsequent 3 days in patients with respiratory failure managed with extracorporeal life support and PLV. Data as mean ± SEM (From (27) with permission)

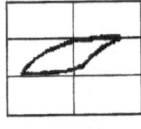   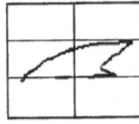   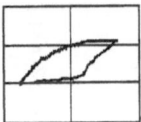

Baseline   **After 10 ml/kg fill**   **60 Minutes After Fill**

Fig. 4. Demonstration of the presence of the hydrostatic effect observed in the pressure/volume curve after filling with 10 mL/kg which has been termed the "beak". This phenomenon appears to be related to the presence of perfluorocarbon in the central airways at end-expiration and may be used to monitor the degree of perfluorocarbon filling during initial and subsequent dose administration. In this example, the beak is observed to resolve over the ensuing 60 min as the majority of the perfluorocarbon distributes into regions of the lungs that were likely atelectatic/consolidated. (From [35] with permission)

and 8 of 10 children. The (A-a)DO$_2$ decreased over the first 48 h in both groups from approximately 450 to 250 mmHg. Complications which were possibly related to administration of perflubron and performance of PLV included development of pneumothorax in 4 patients and transient episodes of oxygen desaturation in 5.

Protocols which are now active involve adults, children, fullterm newborns (non-CDH), CDH newborns, and preterm newborns who are not on ECLS. In these prospective, randomized, controlled trials, perflubron is being administered every 2–4 h to maintain lung perflubron volume equivalent to FRC as identified by the presence of a meniscus within the endotracheal tube at end-expiration during transient ventilator disconnect. In some patients, however, gas exchange, tidal volume, and hemodynamics will be optimal at a dose less than that necessary to fill to FRC. It is important to follow tidal volume during dosing: A significant decrease in tidal volume should indicate cessation of dose administration until subsequent peripheral distribution of the perfluorocarbon, along with alveolar recruitment, results in resolution of the decrease in pulmonary compliance. Examination of pressure/volume curves during liquid ventilation reveals a hydrostatic phenomenon early in the breath which is present when perfluorocarbon fills the central airways at end-expiration (Fig. 4) [34]. Referred to as "the beak" its presence can be used to indicate that the lungs are filled with perfluorocarbon to a volume approaching FRC during initial and subsequent dosing.

Conclusion

The technique of liquid ventilation is at an early stage in its evolution. There is much to be learned regarding optimal dosing, positioning, ventilator settings, and overall technique. However, liquid ventilation, with the associated ability to effectively recruit alveoli and to improve pulmonary function and gas exchange, represents a novel intervention with the promise of enhancing our ability to effectively manage patients with respiratory failure.

References

1. Shaffer TH, Wolfson MR, Clark L, Jr (1992) Liquid ventilation. Pediatr Pulmonol 14:102–109
2. Clark LC Jr, Gollan F (1966) Survival of mammals breathing organic liquids equilibrated with oxygen at atmospheric pressure. Science 152:1755–1756
3. Shaffer TH, Moskowitz GD (1974) Demand-controlled liquid ventilation of the lungs. J Appl Physiol 36:208–213
4. Greenspan JS, Wolfson MR, Rubenstein SD, Shaffer TH (1989) Liquid ventilation of preterm baby. Lancet 2:1095
5. Greenspan JS, Wolfson MR, Rubenstein SD, Shaffer TH (1990) Liquid ventilation of human preterm neonates. J Pediatr 117:106–111
6. Hirschl RB, Merz S, Montoya P, et al (1995) Development of a simplified liquid ventilator. Crit Care Med 23:157–163
7. Fuhrman BP, Paczan PR, DeFrancisis M (1991) Perfluorocarbon-associated gas exchange. Crit Care Med 19:712–722
8. Leach CL, Fuhrman BP, Morin Fd, Rath MG (1993) Perfluorocarbon-associated gas exchange (partial liquid ventilation) in respiratory distress syndrome: A prospective, randomized, controlled study. Crit Care Med 21:1270–1278
9. Overbeck MC, Pranikoff T, Yadao CM, Hirschl RB (1996) The efficacy of perfluorocarbon liquid ventilation in a large animal model of acute respiratory failure. Crit Care Med 24:1208–1214
10. Hirschl RB, Tooley R, Parent AC, et al (1995) Improvement of gas exchange, pulmonary function, and lung injury with partial liquid ventilation. A study model in a setting of severe respiratory failure. Chest 108:500–508
11. Hernan LJ, Fuhrman BP, Kaiser R, et al (1995) Perfluorocarbon associated gas exchange in normal and acid-injured-large sheep. Crit Care Med 23 (Suppl):A264 (Abst)
12. Nesti FD, Fuhrman BP, Papo MC, et al (1994) Perfluorocarbon-associated gas exchange in gastric aspiration. Crit Care Med 22:1445–1452
13. Tutuncu AS, Faithfull NS, Lachmann B (1993) Intratracheal perfluorocarbon administration combined with mechanical ventilation in experimental respiratory distress syndrome: Dose-dependent improvement of gas exchange. Crit Care Med 21:962–969
14. Tooley R, Hirschl RB, Parent A, Bartlett RH (1996) Total liquid ventilation with perfluorocarbons increases pulmonary end-expiratory volume and compliance in the setting of lung atelectasis. Crit Care Med 24:268–273
15. Gattinoni L, D'Andrea L, Pelosi P, et al (1993) Regional effects and mechanism of positive end-expiratory pressure in early adult respiratory distress syndrome. JAMA 269:2122–2127
16. Hirschl RB, Overbeck MC, Parent A, et al (1994) Liquid ventilation provides uniform distribution of perfluorocarbon in the setting of respiratory failure. Surgery 116:159–167
17. Quintel M, R.B. H, Roth H, et al (1995) Assessment of perfluorocarbon (PFC) distribution during partial liquid ventilation (PLV) in the setting of acute respiratory failure. Am J Respir Crit Care Med 151:A446 (Abst)
18. Gauger PG, Overbeck MC, Chamber SD, et al (1995) Perfluorocarbon partial liquid ventilation improves gas exchange while augmenting decreased functional residual capacity in an animal model of acute lung injury. Surgery Forum 46:669–671
19. Gauger PG, Overbeck MC, Koeppe RA, et al (1997) Distribution of pulmonary blood flow and total lung water during partial liquid ventilation in acute lung injury. Surgery (In press)
20. Quintel M, Heine M, Hirschl RB, et al (1997) Effects of partial liquid ventilation (PLV) on lung injury in a model of acute respiratory failure a histologic and morphometric analysis. Crit Care Med (In press)
21. Colton DM, Hirschl RB, Till GO, et al (1997) Neutrophil accumulation is reduced during partial liquid ventilation. Crit Care Med (In press)
22. Colton DM, Hirschl RB, Till GO, et al (1995) Lung vascular permeability is reduced during partial liquid ventilation (PLV) in the setting of respiratory failure. Am J Respir Crit Care Med 151:A446 (Abst)
23. mith T, Steinhorn D, Marcucci K, et al (1994) Perflubron (PFB) decreases free radical (FR) production by alveolar macrophages (A-) *in vitro*. Crit Care Med 22:A196 (Abst)

24. Virmani R, Fink LM, Gunter K, English D (1984) Effect of perfluorochemical blood substitutes on human neutrophil function. Tranfusion 24:343–347
25. Varani J, Hirschl RB, Dame M, Johnson K (1996) Perfluorocarbon protects lung epithelial cells from neutrophil-mediated injury in an *in vitro* model of liquid ventilation therapy. Shock 6:339–344
26. Wilcox DT, Glick PL, Karamanoukian HL, et al (1995) Perfluorocarbon-associated gas exchange improves pulmonary mechanics, oxygenation, ventilation, and allows nitric oxide delivery in the hypoplastic lung congenital diaphragmatic hernia lamb model. Crit Care Med 23:1858–1863
27. Hirschl RB, Pranikoff P, Wise C, et al (1996) Initial experience with partial liquid ventilation in adult patients with the acute respiratory distress syndrome. JAMA 275:383–389
28. Leach CL, Greenspan JS, Rubenstein SD, et al (1996) Partial liquid ventilation with perflubron in premature infants with severe respiratory distress syndrome. N Engl J Med 335:761–767
29. Hirschl RB, Pranikoff T, Gauger P, et al (1995) Liquid ventilation in adults, children, and full-term neonates: Preliminary report. Lancet 346:1201–1202
30. Pranikoff T, Gauger P, Hirschl RB (1996) Partial liquid ventilation in newborn patients with congenital diaphragmatic hernia. J Ped Surg 31:613–618
31. Gauger PG, Pranikoff T, Schreiner RJ, Hirschl RB (1996) Initial experience with partial liquid ventilation in pediatric patients with the acute respiratory distress syndrome. Crit Care Med 24:16–22
32. Kazerooni EA, Pranikoff T, Cascade PN, Hirschl RB (1996) Perfluorocarbon partial liquid ventilation during extracorporeal life support in adults: radiographic appearance. Radiology 198:137–142
33. Toro-Figueroa LO, Melinoes JN, Curtis SE, et al (1996) Perflubron partial liquid ventilation (PLV) in children with ARDS: A safety and efficacy pilot study. Crit Care Med 24:A150 (Abst)
34. Hirschl RB (1997) Pulmonary function during liquid ventilation. In: Donn S (ed) Neonatal and pediatric pulmonary graphic analysis: Principles and clinical applications. Futura, Mount Kisco, NY (In press)

Extra-Pulmonary Adjuncts
to Ventilatory Support

Extracorporeal Respiratory Support

A. Pesenti and R. Fumagalli

Introduction

In this brief review, we will discuss the use of extracorporeal respiratory support (ERS) in acute respiratory failure. Focus will be mainly on adult patient applications, but information and hints from the large experience collected in neonates and pediatric patients will also be brought to the attention of the reader. Many articles [1–3], reviews [4–6], editorials [7], and textbook chapters [8–9] have been written on this topic: We will therefore proceed by trying to answer a few crucial questions about the procedure and its clinical application.

What is Extracorporeal Respiratory Support?

ERS in its various forms is conceived as a life support procedure. The use of an extracorporeal artificial organ designed to oxygenate blood and remove carbon dioxide is intended to maintain viable blood gases, and life, while substituting for the gas exchange function of the failing natural lungs.

The appropriate artificial organ to substitute for pulmonary gas exchange is represented by the membrane lung: such devices have been available for clinical routine use for more than three decades [10–11]. ERS has been applied in various forms and technical modifications. Different acronyms are used in the literature to emphasize both technical aspects and differences in the physiological goals of life support. ECMO [14] (extracorporeal membrane oxygenation) stresses the importance of oxygenating the blood; it usually implies the use of a venoarterial bypass, providing therefore not only respiratory support but also some degree of cardio-circulatory support.

Extracorporeal CO_2 removal ($ECCO_2R$) [1] is a name coined by Kolobow and Gattinoni [4] to identify an approach that, by exploiting CO_2 removal rather than oxygenation, allows respiratory assistance to be performed at lower blood flows and through a simplified veno-venous bypass. Extracorporeal lung assist (ECLA) or extracorporeal life support (ELS) [9] are other descriptors of ERS. It should always be kept in mind, however, that ERS has been applied almost exclusively as a life support procedure. ERS is therefore intended to maintain life while the natural history of the disease progresses according to factors or determinants not necessarily linked to the ERS procedure. Disease evolution may eventually take the patient's lungs back to a normal gas exchange function, or otherwise lead to irreversible damage.

To avoid the complexity of pumping blood through an extracorporeal device, attempts have been made to apply the artificial gas exchanger inside the body (IVOX) [12, 13]. Though potentially very promising, this approach has had limited success, and did not change the general picture of the field.

Extracorporeal gas exchange normally requires the pumping of 15 to 75% of the cardiac output through an artificial lung. Systemic blood anticoagulation is needed to avoid clotting of the extracorporeal devices and circuitry. These requirements imply a degree of invasiveness and the potential for major side effects. Among these, bleeding due to anticoagulation is of paramount importance.

Is ERS an Effective Life Support Treatment?

There are no doubts that the available technology is good enough to provide viable gas exchange for weeks or months, even if natural lung function is totally lost and natural gas exchange approaches or reaches zero.

Forst et al. [15] reported on a successful extracorporeal perfusion in a patient with ARDS (acute respiratory distress syndrome) lasting 104 days. Total or almost total extracorporeal gas exchange for periods of several weeks is not exceptional, but rather is becoming the rule in the last decade [8]. These results were anticipated by the conclusion of the NIH ECMO study [16], which showed that the procedure was feasibile and capable of providing the intended supplemental respiratory support. The average ECMO patient lived longer than control, life being supported for days or weeks.

What do we need ERS for?

In the 70's, the incidence of ARDS was estimated at 150000 cases per year in the USA, with an average mortality of 40% [16]. This incidence appears substantially reduced in recent years: In Europe, it ranges between 1.5 to 4.5 cases/100000 inhabitants per year [17–19], while it is now reported to be 5.3 to 10.5 cases/100000 inhabitants in the USA [20–21]. In spite of the fact that the majority of published clinical investigations report mortality rates above 50%, a substantial amount of evidence has suggested that a trend toward improved survival in severe ARDS is indeed present [22]. More importantly, the role of gas exchange impairment as a predictor or a cause of mortality has been challenged.

In 1985, an important study [23] indicated that sepsis and multiple organ failure, rather than the impaired gas exchange, were the major causes of mortality in ARDS patients. In 1992, however, Suchita et al. [24] reported that a very substantial proportion of patients (40%) died because of progressive respiratory failure, and not because of sepsis or failure of other organ systems. Recently, Milberg et al. [25] reported a decrease in ARDS mortality rate which is in fact limited to the septic patient subpopulation. It might therefore be possible that in recent years we have gained better control over septic complications and improved the management of septic patients. This in turn has reestablished altered gas exchange and hypoxia as major causes of death in ARDS patients.

In spite of the wave of moderate optimism running through the intensive care community about ARDS survival, one should perhaps consider that [23]:

1) 40% of all ARDS deaths are associated with subvital gas exchange (PaO_2 < 40 mmHg at FiO_2 of 1.0), and

2) Any intervention which prevents sepsis would be beneficial. If improved respiratory support shortened the course or severity of ARDS, it also might be helpful in reducing the incidence of sepsis (and therefore death).

Vasilyev et al. [26] in 1995 reported survival rates of a large number of patients and concluded that 67% of patients requiring positive pressure ventilation (PaO_2 < 60 mmHg with FiO_2 ≥ 0.6) still die. If death is directly caused or strictly related to gas exchange impairment, or to invasive supportive treatments deemed necessary to overcome it, then the use of an artificial gas exchanger is justified, in analogy to the use of continuous hemofiltration in acute renal failure.

Which are the Goals of ERS in ARDS?

ERS has two main goals:

1) to maintain viable blood gases, hence avoiding respiratory death, while tiding the patient over the acute phase. As already stated, the capability of the system to substitute for gas exchange has been proven, and

2) to avoid the damage of mechanical ventilation (provide lung rest).

The major pathophysiological trait of ARDS is a reduction in functional residual capacity (FRC), a decrease in the number of ventilated alveoli, and severe impairment of gas exchange. To maintain life, the residual aerated lung ("baby lung") must be mechanically ventilated. In fact, a small number of alveoli have to provide for the entire gas exchange, and the residual healthy lung is hyperventilated at high volume and pressure. This leads to barotrauma and further lung damage [27]. Minute ventilation in the range of 20 L/min is not exceptional in severe ARDS. If the size of the "baby lung" is reduced to 1/5 of the normal, then the equivalent of the effects of a minute ventilation of 100 L/min in a normal lung might be expected. By substituting for the gas exchange function, ERS may relieve the residual healthy lung from the burden of ventilation.

No direct proof exists that extracorporeal respiratory support provides a better environment for lung healing: experimental evidence however shows that hyaline membrane disease may be prevented [28], acute respiratory failure reversed [29], and hemodynamics and renal function ameliorated [30].

Which are the Major Problems limiting the Clinical Application of ERS?

ERS is still a very invasive technique. Total respiratory support requires blood flows of the order of 1.5 to 1.8 L/min/m2. Large bore cannulas (7 to 10 mm internal diameter) must be appropriately inserted into central vessels.

The introduction of $ECCO_2R$ was a first step in reducing invasiveness [1]: Blood flows of the order of 10 to 15% of the cardiac output will suffice for to extracorporeal removal of the total CO_2 production. Since oxygenation must be achieved largely by the patient's own lung, venous admixture cannot be higher than 70 to 80%, if vital blood gases have to be maintained. The capability for total oxygenating support, and therefore for blood flows higher than 4 L/min has to be built into any ERS circuitry, even when $ECCO_2R$ is the intended technique.

Artificial lungs are far from ideal: their design allows sites for blood stagnation, and blood is exposed to very large foreign surfaces (up to 9 m²). Blood coagulation must be accurately managed, walking the tightrope between clotting of the circuitry and bleeding by the patient. Heparinized surfaces are now available. Even if laboratory studies show that ERS can be applied for days without heparin at normal clotting times without major side effects, systemic heparinization is usually maintained when heparinized surfaces are applied in patients. This is mostly to prevent clotting of the circuitry, and fatal embolism, were blood flow in the circuitry to stop for any reason. Baseline continuous heparinization is therefore maintained, except when it is electively stopped in cases of major bleeding or surgery. We [8] reported a substantial decrease in blood product requirement with the use of heparinized surfaces and percutaneous cannulation; packed red cells requirements decreased from an average of 976 ± 830 to 360 ± 363 mL/day.

Bleeding, however, is still the major complication of ERS, and intracranial hemorrage (ICH) is feared the most. In our own experience, out of 106 non-neonate patients, ICH was identified as the cause of death in 14. $PaCO_2$ higher than 75 mmHg before connection, disseminated intravascular coagulation and pathological brain CT scan were the major factors related to ICH during bypass.

Long-term extracorporeal support is a complex technique: it requires a well trained and well organized multidisciplinary team, and it has a major impact on other hospital services and departments. After a few days of bypass, human fatigue becomes an important source of error and misjudgment. Work shifts have to be short, and enough free time has to be provided.

Has the Introduction of New Therapies changed the Indications for ERS?

New modes of management are being proposed and tested for ARDS, and our last ditch, life saving indications for ERS must be continuously updated to the most advanced respiratory support and treatment. We are faced today with decisions about nitric oxide inhalation, or prone positioning. In a similar way, our pediatric colleagues are faced with high frequency oscillation (HFO). Permissive hypercapnia has changed our feelings about the need to aggressively improve CO_2 elimination efficiency in patients who are difficult or impossible to ventilate. Since we have become used to limiting ventilation to reasonable settings, we tolerate quite lightheartedly $PaCO_2$ levels often between 60 and 70 mmHg, even approaching 100 mmHg. When the disease gets really bad, we have no other choice than to accept high $PaCO_2$ values, in spite of high and very high minute volumes. We recently reported that $PaCO_2$, before connection to bypass, has increased from an average of 46.9 ± 13.5 mmHg in the decade 1980–1987 to 68.5 ± 19.4 in 1992–1995, and that was in spite of the fact that minute ventilation figures were not significantly different (Table 1).

New treatments are often successful in achieving some clinical improvement in patients that otherwise, years ago, would have been considered desperate ERS candidates. Since ERS is considered a last resort, all other options are exhausted before connection to bypass. This strategy not only impacts on the decision to cannulate, but most often delays the decision to transfer the patient to the referral ERS center.

These considerations bring up the problem of patient selection for ERS. An effort is made to identify the patient with a sufficiently high risk of death to undergo what generally is considered an experimental therapy. Experimental work has shown that the severity of the disease might be an important factor in determining whether extracorporeal support is advantageous or not. Using an animal model of acute respiratory failure in which the offending agent was mechanical ventilation at peak inspiratory pressure of 50 cmH_2O, Borelli et al. [29] evaluated ERS against conventional mechanical ventilation in a randomized, controlled animal study. Two levels of injury were evaluated: mild and severe. In the mild injury model, ERS achieved 100% survival versus 27% in the control group. At the opposite extreme, no difference in mortality between ERS and control could be found in the severe model, and all animals died of progressive multiple organ failure. The investigators concluded that, in the severe model, the damage had progressed to a stage in which neither conventional treatment nor extracorporeal support could succeed in reversing lung failure, and that there is a stage of disease beyond which ERS is no longer able to affect survival.

Mirroring these experimental results, Green et al. [31] report data on a pediatric non-neonatal population (2 weeks to 18 years). In a retrospective, multicenter cohort analysis on 331 patients from 32 hospitals, they concluded that the use of ECMO was associated with a reduction in mortality. Using matched pair analysis, a 26% mortality rate favorably compared with 49% in the non-ECMO patients. The ECMO beneficial effect was concentrated on the group of patients with a risk of death between 50 and 75%. No effect was detected in the other risk groups.

Table 1. Respiratory parameters before bypass (Milan-Monza – 1980 to 1995)

	1980–1987	1988–1991	1992–1995	ANOVA p value
Qs/Qt,%	49.0 ± 13.5	44.5 ± 9.3	50.5 ± 9.6	NS
PEEP, cmH_2O	11.8 ± 4.7	13.6 ± 5.3	13.4 ± 2.9	NS
$PaCO_2$, mmHg	46.9 ± 13.5	63.9 ± 25.1	68.5 ± 19.4	< 0.0001
VE/Kg, l/kg/min	0.25 ± 0.15	0.19 ± 0.05	0.21 ± 0.07	NS
Peak, cmH_2O	45.3 ± 10.4	46.7 ± 8.1	46.3 ± 7.3	NS

Qs/Qt: intrapulmonary shunt, VE/Kg: expired volume l/Kg/min, PEEP: positive end expiratory pressure, Peak: peak pressure

These data support the observation that ERS is associated with increased survival in patients with a high mortality risk. However, it is important to notice that there was no apparent benefit from ECMO in either the lowest or the highest risk quartile. Patients with mild disease do not warrant the risk and cost of ECMO: patients in the highest risk group may have passed the time point and pathophysiologic evolution of their disease when they may have benefitted from ECMO.

Does ERS Pass the Test of Randomized, Controlled Studies?

Three randomized studies have been published in neonates, and two in adults. To do a randomized study, the participant investigator must not be biased in favor of one or the other of the tested treatments. ERS is a complex and demanding technical procedure. A strong motivation is required to acquire the competence and experience needed to run an ERS program, certainly implying a bias in favor of ERS. An unbiased team will almost certainly be a team with minimal experience: a major obvious difficulty exists in finding a team of dedicated people, competent in ERS, and with no bias in favor of it.

Three prospective, randomized neonatal studies have been completed. The first one was performed by Bartlett et al. [33], undoubtely the most experienced group in the US and probably in the world. An unusual "play the winner" randomization strategy was planned to minimize the number of deaths necessary to reach a significant conclusion, while taking into account an intrinsic institutional bias toward ECMO. 100% survival was achieved in the ECMO group. The second randomized study came two years later from Boston [34]. In this study, all neonates meeting entry criteria were randomized either to ECMO or to maximal conventional treatment according to the standard of the attending neonatologist. An adaptive randomization design led the 29 patients in the ECMO group (28 survivors) to be compared to 10 patients in the conventional arm, with only 6 survivors. The third study was the UK randomized trial [35], in which 63 of 93 neonates allocated to ECMO survived compared with 38 of 92 allocated conventional care. In this trial, the patients were randomized either to referral to one of the specialized ECMO centers or to continued intensive conventional management at the original hospital. The results therefore show that allocation to ECMO decreased the risk of death or severe disability. This study proves that a standardized approach including ERS compares favorably to neonatal respiratory care as generally practiced in the United Kingdom.

Randomized studies in adults have been less successful: The first study was the NIH-sponsored ECMO study [14], which was performed as a collaborative effort by 9 US centers, starting in 1974. The NIH study was undertaken because ERS was felt as a costly procedure gaining ever wider use without clear evidence of its benefits. Initial enthusiasm had indeed been damped by Gille and Bagniewskis' scrutiny of published case reports [36], which yielded a bare 15% survival rate out of 233 patients treated by 90 different medical teams in 7 countries from 1966 to 1975. Unexpectedly, in the NIH ECMO study, survival was extremely low both in the treated and in the control group. The entry criteria, which were mainly based on gas exchange impairment (Table 2), had in fact defined a patient population with a mortality higher than 90%, and this result was somehow surprising, since the expert panel had expected a 65% mortality rate.

Another view of the results is provided by HL Anderson who stated: "Some of the nine study centers were inexperienced, coagulation control was crude, veno-arterial bypass was used, and many of the patients were maintained on high pressure, high oxygen mechanical ventilation. Looking back on this experience, it is somehow surprising that any patient survived" [37]. An additional data collection [16] on a less severely ill population of 750 patients intubated for more than 24 h and mechanically ventilated with $FiO_2 \pm 50\%$, revealed a 68% mortality rate, still astonishingly high.

The NIH ECMO study, though it caused a temporary moratorium on the US use of ECMO in adult patients, is a milestone since it proved among other things that:
1) ECMO was highly effective in providing temporary life support;
2) In both ECMO and control patients, the predominant cause of death was progressive pulmonary failure; and
3) ECMO allowed patients to be maintained at lower PEEP and tidal volume.

Following the publication of clinical series of ARDS patients treated by ERS with historical controls by European [1] and American [37] groups, Morris et al. [3] published in 1994 the result of a randomized, controlled study comparing EC-CO$_2$R to conventional treatment. Once again survival was not different in the ERS group as compared to control. The Salt Lake study found approximately 30 to 40% survival in both groups, which is much better than expected in the control group and somehow lower than expected in the ERS group. The study was designed to enroll 60 patients. At the first interim analysis (20 patients), more control patients were surviving (42%) than ERS patients (23%). The study was continued due to lack of statistical significance, but at the second interim analysis (40 patients), the difference in mortality had become so small, that even prolonging the study to include 60 or 100 patients would not have been sufficient for a significant difference. One might wonder whether, as suggested by these data, the survival of the ERS group would have kept increasing, and whether increasing the number of patients, and therefore experience, could have led to different results.

Table 2. The NIH ECMO entry criteria

Fast entry
- PaO$_2$ < 50 mmHg at FiO$_2$ 1.0
- PEEP ≥ 5 cmH$_2$O
- 3 determinations 1 h apart

Slow entry
- PaO$_2$ < 50 mmHg at FiO$_2$ 0.6
- PEEP ≥ 5 cmH$_2$O
- plus
- shunt fraction ≥ 30% at FiO$_2$ 1.0
- 3 determinations 6 h apart after 48 h of ICU

Of the 21 ERS patients, 7 are reported survivors. Of these, 1 never underwent ECMO because he improved with no need for it. Of the remaining 6 survivors, 5 had been disconnected from bypass because of excessive bleeding. To look at it from another perspective, out of the 19 bypassed patients, an astounding 7 were disconnected due to uncontrollable bleeding. What is really confusing is that 5 of the 6 ERS survivors came from this bleeding group of 7, and one cannot avoid the paradox of thinking that they survived because, luckily enough, they almost bled to death during bypass. The study concluded that there is no difference in survival between the mechanical ventilation group and the extracorporeal CO_2 removal group.

The authors recommended therefore that extracorporeal support for ARDS be restricted to controlled clinical trials. We think however that we need more research on the ERS field to understand why both adult randomized studies showed no advantage for extracorporeal support; we need to identify the reasons and the flaws that nullified the advantage of the very sound pathophysiological basis of ERS treatment. This information cannot be gathered from a randomized, controlled study. A randomized, controlled clinical study could only provide either the same result as the NIH and Morris' study, or negate it. What we need is not yet a dichotomous "yes or no" response, but rather well structured clinical research observations, and technical development.

The ethics of this are very straightforward, since randomized study has proven, at worst, no advantage, but no disadvantage to ERS either.

Cost is an important consideration: In the randomized UK study [35], the cost per survivor in the ECMO group was £ 24 123 versus £ 23 450 in the conventional group. Mean charges per ECMO infant amounted to £ 17 154 versus £ 9 901 for the conventional treatment.

Conclusion

The membrane lung is an extracorporeal device for exchanging blood gases. By preventing hypoxia and hypercapnia, the use of the membrane lung can maintain life while otherwise intolerable pulmonary damage heals. A membrane lung may avoid the side effects of mechanical ventilation, baro- and volu-trauma. ERS is a standard accepted therapy for neonates and probably for some pediatric age groups. In the adult patient population, the USA ELSO registry has collected a 47% survival rate, while in Europe more than 600 patients have been treated, with a survival rate higher than 50%. ERS has developed from the collective effort of many individuals of different backgrounds – pediatrics, neonatology, surgery, anesthesiology, intensive care and many others. Research is ongoing in various directions to expand the use of ERS. ERS is a highly rational approach to the supportive management of severe gas exchange impairment. Many problems still limit the clinical application of ERS technique: the target of research and technological development might be to make extracorporeal support as simple and as safe as renal support techniques.

References

1. Gattinoni L, Pesenti A, Mascheroni D, et al (1986) Low frequency positive pressure ventilation with extracorporeal CO_2 removal in severe acute respiratory failure. JAMA 256: 881–886
2. Brunet F, Belghith M, Mira JP, et al (1993) Extracorporeal carbon dioxide removal and low frequency positive pressure ventilation improvement in arterial oxygenation with reduction of risk of pulmonary barotrauma in patients with adult respiratory distress syndrome. Chest 104: 889–898
3. Morris AH; Wallace CJ; Menlove RL, et al (1994) Randomized clinical trial of pressure controlled inverse ratio ventilation and extracorporeal CO_2 removal for adult respiratory distress syndrome. Am J Respir Crit Care Med 149: 295–305
4. Pesenti A, Kolobow T, Gattinoni L (1988) Extracorporeal respiratory support in the adult. Trans Am Soc Artif Intern Organs 34: 1006–1008
5. Levy FH, O'Rourke PP, Crone RK (1992) Extracorporeal membrane oxygenation. Anesth Analg 75: 1053–1062
6. Pesenti A, Gattinoni L, Bombino M (1993) Long term extracorporeal respiratory support: 20 years of progress. Intensive and Critical Care Digest 12: 15–17
7. Zapol WM, Kitz RJ (1972) Buying time with artificial lungs. New Engl J Med 286: 657–658
8. Gattinoni L, Pelosi P, Brazzi L, Pesenti A (1995) Extracorporeal membrane oxygenation. In: Parrillo JE, Bone RC (eds) Critical care medicine: Principles of diagnosis and management. 1st Edition Mosby Year Book, St Louis, pp 881–892
9. Bartlett RH (1990) Extracorporeal life support for cardiopulmonary failure. Curr Probl Surg 27: 623–706
10. Clowes GHA, Hopkins AL, Neville WE (1956) An artificial lung dependent upon diffusion of oxygen and carbon dioxide through plastic membranes. J Thorac Cardiovasc Surg 32: 630–637
11. Kolobow T, Bowman RL (1963) Construction and evaluation of an alveolar membrane artificial heart-lung. Trans Am Soc Artif Intern Organs 9: 238–243
12. Mortensen JD (1992) Intravascular oxygenator: A new alternative method for augmenting blood gas transfer in patients with acute respiratory failure. Artif Organs 16: 75–82
13. High KM, Snider MT, Richard R, et al (1992) Clinical trials of an intravenous oxygenator in patients with adult respiratory distress syndrome. Anesthesiology 77: 856–863
14. Zapol W, Snider MT, Hill JD, et al (1979) Extracorporeal membrane oxygenation in severe acute respiratory failure. A randomized prospective study. JAMA 242: 2193–2196
15. Forst H, Manert W, Niedermeier A, et al (1994) Extracorporale Lungenersatz-therapie in Munchen. In: Peter K, Lawin P, Briegel J (eds) Schriftenreihe Intensivmedizin, Noftallmedizin , Anaesthesiologie, Intensivmedizin, Organdysfunktionen Vol 84, Georg Thieme Verlag, Stuttgart, pp 148–157
16. NHLBI Division of Lung Diseases (1979) Extracorporeal support for respiratory insufficiency. A collaborative study in response to RFP. NHLI: 73–20
17. Villar J, Slutsky AS (1989) The incidence of the adult respiratory distress syndrome. Am Rev Respir Dis 140: 814–816
18. Lewandowski K, Metz J, Deutschnann C, et al (1995) Incidence, severity, and mortality of acute respiratory failure in Berlin, Germany. Am J Respir Crit Care Med 151: 1121–1125
19. Webster Nr, Cohen AT, Nunn JF (1988) Adult respiratory distress syndrome – How many cases in the UK. Anaesthesia 43: 923–926
20. Thomsen GE, Morris AH (1995) Incidence of the adult respiratory distress syndrome in the State of Utah. Am J Respir Crit Care Med 152: 965–971
21. Earle LA, Grimm AM, Hopkins LE, Gottlieb JE (1993) Identifying patients with adult respiratory distress syndrome by utilizing a search strategy employing ICD 9 Codes. Am Rev Respir Dis 147 S: A348 (Abst)
22. Lemaire F (1996) The prognosis of ARDS: Appropriate optimism? Intensive Care Med 22: 371–373
23. Montgomery AB, Stager MA, Carrico CJ, Hudson LD (1985) Causes of mortality in patients with the adult respiratory distress syndrome. Am Rev Respir Dis 132: 485–489

24. Suchyta MR, Clemmer TP, Elliott CG, et al (1992) The adult respiratory distress syndrome. A report of survival and modifying factors. Chest 101:1074–1079
25. Milberg JA, Davis DR, Steinberg KP, Hudson LD (1995) Improved survival of patients with acute respiratory distress syndrome (ARDS) 1983–1993. JAMA 273:306–309
26. Vasilyev S, Schaap RN, Mortensen JD (1995) Hospital survival rates of patients with acute respiratory failure in modern respiratory intensive care units. An international multicenter prospective survey. Chest 107:1083–1088
27. Slutsky AS (1994) Mechanical ventilation. Intensive Care Med 20:64–79
28. Pesenti A, Kolobow T, Buckold DK, et al (1982) Prevention of hyaline membrane disease in premature lambs by apneic oxygenation and extracorporeal CO_2 removal. Intensive Care Med 8:11–17
29. Borelli M, Kolobow T, Spatola R, et al (1988) Severe acute respiratory failure managed with continuous positive airway pressure and partial extracorporeal carbon dioxide removal by an artificial membrane lung. A controlled randomized animal study. Am Rev Respir Dis 138:1480–1487
30. Gattinoni L, Agostoni A, Damia G, et al (1980) Hemodynamics and renal function during low frequency positive pressure ventilation with extracorporeal CO_2 removal. Intensive Care Med 6:155–161
31. Green TP, Timmons OD, Fackler JC, et al (1996) The impact of extracorporeal membrane oxygenation on survival in pediatric patients with acute respiratory failure. Crit Care Med 24:323–329.
32. O'Rourke PP (1995) Extracorporeal life support: How can it be studied? In: Zwischenberger JB, Bartlett RH (eds) ECMO extracorporeal cardiopulmonary support in critical Care. Extracorporeal Life Support Organization, Ann Arbor, USA, pp 511–520
33. Bartlett RH, Roloff DW, Cornell RG, et al (1985) Extracorporeal circulation in neonatal respiratory failure: A prospective randomized study. Pediatrics 76:479–487
34. O'Rourke PP, Crone RK, Vacanti JP, et al (1989) Extracorporeal membrane oxygenation and conventional medical therapy in neonates with persistent pulmonary hypertension of the newborn: A prospective randomized study. Pediatrics 84:957–963
35. UK collaborative ECMO trial group (1996) UK collaborative randomised trial of neonatal extracorporeal membrane oxygenation. Lancet 348:75–82
36. Gille JP, Bagniewski A (1976) Ten years of use of extracorporeal membrane oxygenation (ECMO) in the treatment of acute respiratory insufficiency. Trans Am Soc Artif Intern Organs 22:102–108
37. Anderson HL, Delius RE, Sinard JM, et al (1992) Early experience with adult extracorporeal membrane oxygenation in the modern era. Ann Thorac Surg 53:553–563

Permissive Hypercapnia or the Prone Position in ARDS?

R. K. Albert

Introduction

Permissive hypercapnia has been widely accepted in the ventilatory support of patients with the acute respiratory distress syndrome (ARDS) as a result of the rediscovery that the tidal volume (VT) and level of positive end-expiratory pressure (PEEP) used in the support of these patients might, and of themselves, cause further injury. The rationale for permissive hypercapnia is that the smaller tidal volumes resulting from lower peak and higher expiratory alveolar pressure would limit lung stretch, thereby reducing the risk of ventilation-induced lung injury [1].

Several studies [2, 3] have now confirmed older ones [4, 5] in showing that gas exchange can be improved in patients with ARDS when they are turned from supine to prone, and the mechanism by which this improvement occurs in animal models has been elucidated [6].

Interpreting studies investigating the pathophysiology of ventilation-induced lung injury in terms of the effect of the prone position on the gravitational pleural pressure (Ppl) gradient suggests that the rationale supporting permissive hypercapnia may be flawed, and that ventilating patients in the prone position may be a better way to minimize the possibility of ventilator-induced lung injury. The purpose of this chapter is to review the information supporting these conclusions.

Permissive Hypercapnia

Despite numerous reports in the 1970's and 1980's indicating that ventilating the lung with excessive volume was deleterious [7–11], the principle of limiting the degree of inflation was not widely accepted until Dreyfuss and colleagues [12] demonstrated the adverse effects of large volume ventilation delivered to laboratory animals for only 5 min and coined the term "volutrauma", correctly indicating that the injury resulted from excessive lung volume trans alveolar pressures, and Gattinoni and colleagues [13, 14] used the idea of a "baby lung" to explain the fact that the reduced compliance seen in ARDS results from overdistension of that fraction of the lung into which the tidal volume is being delivered, rather than from a generalized stiffening of the parenchyma from the inflammatory process.

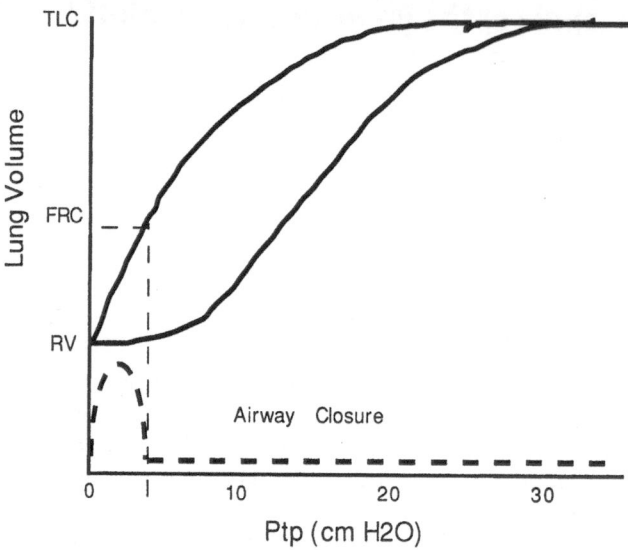

Fig. 1. Schematic representation of the pressure-volume characteristics of a normal lung, along with a depiction of the frequency distribution of airway closure

Consensus rapidly emerged that patients with ARDS should be ventilated with VT that were smaller than the customary 10 mL/kg, limiting the degree of lung expansion to that produced by a static inflation pressure of 35 cmH$_2$O, (in a patient with a normal chest wall this would approximate to the transalveolar pressure associated with total lung capacity). Further PEEP should be titrated on the basis of pressure-volume (P-V) curves for each patient, seeking a value that exceeded airway opening pressure [1].

A schematic P-V curve of a normal lung is shown in Fig. 1, along with a depiction of the hypothetical frequency distribution of airway closure (see chapter on Recruitment by Marini and Arrato). Most airways remain open as the lung deflates from total lung capacity (TLC) to functional residual volume (FRC), but closure intensifies as the lung drops below FRC, ending at residual volume (RV). Fig. 2 demonstrates the effect of ARDS. Several differences are indicated including reductions in lung volumes and increased airspace closure (i.e. alveolar collapse and/or airway closure) that begins at a lung volume exceeding FRC (as indicated by the reduction in shunt that results from adding PEEP) and occurs over a wider range of transpulmonary pressures.

The method by which VT and the level of PEEP are set when employing permissive hypercapnia in conjunction with PV curve definition is shown in Fig. 3. PEEP is titrated to exceed that point on the inflation P-V curve at which compliance improves (i.e. the P$_{flex}$). VT is limited to whatever is produced by the cycling of airway pressure between the set level of PEEP and a plateau pressure limited to 35 cmH$_2$O. As shown on Fig. 3, there can be a considerable difference between airway opening and closing pressures.

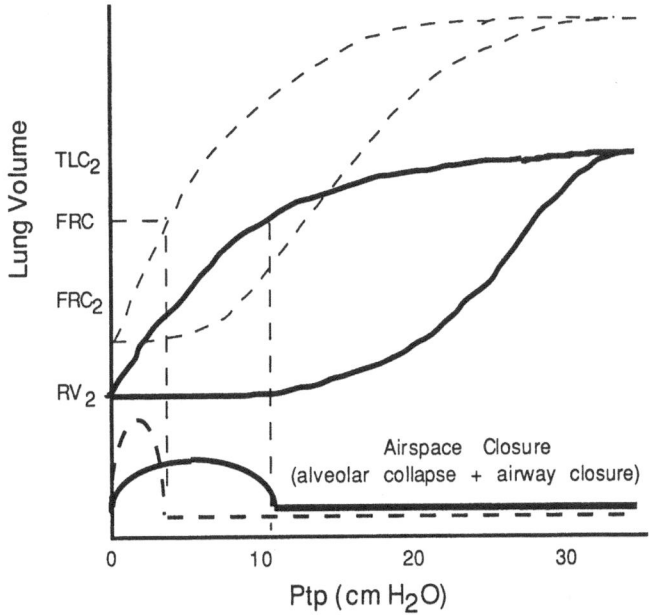

Fig. 2. Schematic representation of the pressure-volume characteristics of a normal lung (dotted lines) and a lung with ARDS (solid lines), along with a depiction of the frequency distribution of airway closure for the two conditions

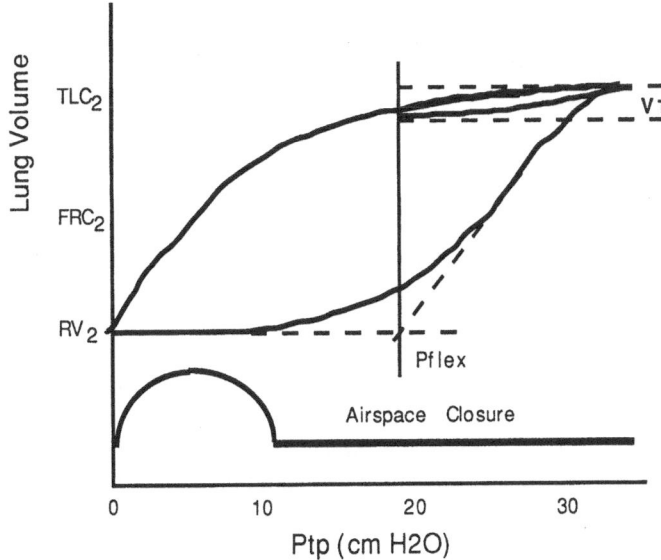

Fig. 3. Permissive hypercapnia. The level of PEEP is set using the inflection point of inflation curve and tidal volume is limited to that delivered as airway pressure cycles between the level of PEEP and 35 cmH$_2$O

Potential Problems with Permissive Hypercapnia

VT Limited by an Airway Pressure of 35 cmH$_2$O

It is quite reasonable to limit lung inflation to that present at a transpulmonary pressure (Ptp) of 35 cmH$_2$O as this pressure is certainly sufficient to inflate lungs of normal human subjects to TLC. The difficulty lies with the fact that a static airway or plateau pressure of 35 cmH$_2$O does not equate to a Ptp of 35 cmH$_2$O, particularly if chest wall compliance is decreased. Limiting VT to that produced by a plateau pressure of 35 cmH$_2$O could result in lungs being ventilated with smaller volumes than is necessary in some patients (15), and this practice has been shown to augment lung injury [16].

In some patients the fact that the plateau pressure does not equate with Ptp is clearly apparent (e.g. those with a large volume of ascites, a marked ileus, or large pleural effusion). In most patients, however, there is no convenient way of recognizing when chest wall compliance is abnormal, and, if so, how much it may be affecting lung mechanics.

Need for Paralysis

When VT is bracketed between PEEP and a plateau airway pressure of 35 cmH$_2$O there is frequently insufficient alveolar ventilation to accommodate removal of the CO$_2$ produced at normal PaCO$_2$, and the resulting respiratory acidemia frequently requires that patients be sedated and even paralyzed to suppress their ventilatory response and prevent agitation.

Many, if not most patients with ARDS, have marked regional heterogeneity in the degree of airspace collapse, with the dorsal lung regions preferentially affected when patients are supine. This is manifested by the fact that pleural pressure (Ppl) actually becomes positive in these dorsal regions when lungs are edematous [17]. This problem is particularly important with regard to permissive hypercapnia because of the frequent need for paralysis.

Twenty years ago, Froese and Bryan [18] found that the reduction in FRC that occurred when patients were paralyzed resulted from a cephalad shift of dependent (i.e. dorsal) portion of the diaphragm. Accordingly, when patients with ARDS are paralyzed, the airspace collapse that already occurs preferentially in the dorsal lung regions is likely to increase, worsening the shunt. Froese and Bryan also found that neither PEEP nor large VT ventilation were able to reverse the changes brought about by paralysis. They concluded that "the only way to ventilate those regions is to modify the effect of abdominal mass by manipulating posture. In this respect the optimal position would be prone with the abdomen unsupported" [18].

Lung Over-distension versus Airspace Opening and Closing

In one of the first studies indicating that high VT ventilation caused lung injury, Webb and Tierney [19] demonstrated that the injury was markedly reduced by adding PEEP. This observation has been confirmed by others [16]. This finding strongly suggests that the end-inspiratory lung volume (i.e. over-stretching) is not solely responsible for the lung injury that occurs from ventilation as the peak pressures (and presumably the end-inspiratory lung volumes) were the same in the animals that did or did not receive PEEP.

One hypothesis proposed to explain how PEEP might reduce ventilation-induced lung injury is that the increase in end-expiratory lung volume induced by PEEP reduces repeated airspace opening and closing which could generate shear forces sufficient to create the injury [19], especially if such opening occurs at high alveolar pressure. This idea is supported by the recent report by Gattinoni and colleagues [13], noting that the cysts or bullae developing in the lungs of patients with prolonged ARDS were preferentially located in dorsal lung regions. If volu-trauma were caused by lung overdistension, these cysts should have been preferentially located in ventral regions where lung distension is greatest. If the end-inspiratory lung volume were not a critical determinant of ventilation-induced lung injury, then limiting end-inspiratory pressure with the idea of limiting this volume makes little sense and our attention should be redirected to assuring that the end-expiratory lung volume exceeds that at which airspace collapse occurs. In fact both high tidal pressures and insufficient end-expiratory pressures are likely to contribute, with preservation of alveolar patency perhaps the most important.

The gravitational Ppl gradient that exists in supine patients produces regional differences in alveolar volume at FRC, and results in airspace closure occurring over a rather wide range of end-expiratory pressures. Accordingly, physiologic principles would indicate that it is not possible to generate VT and PEEP level that can keep dorsal airspaces open without overdistending the non-dependent lung in the supine position as, because of lung interdependence, there can only be a continuum between airspace opening and overdistension. Additionally, variations in regional lung compliance, abnormalities in chest wall compliance and the inability to measure Ptp conveniently make the problem of finding the "best PEEP" quite difficult.

Potential Alternatives for Adjusting VT and PEEP

PEEP Adjustment using the Deflation Portion of the Lung P-V Curve

The purpose of using the inflection point on the inflation portion of lung P-V curve to adjust the level of PEEP is to keep the end-expiratory airway pressure above that which opens the majority of lung units. To the extent that airspace opening and closing pressures differ, patency could be maintained at a lower level of PEEP if PEEP were titrated to prevent closure rather than to achieve opening

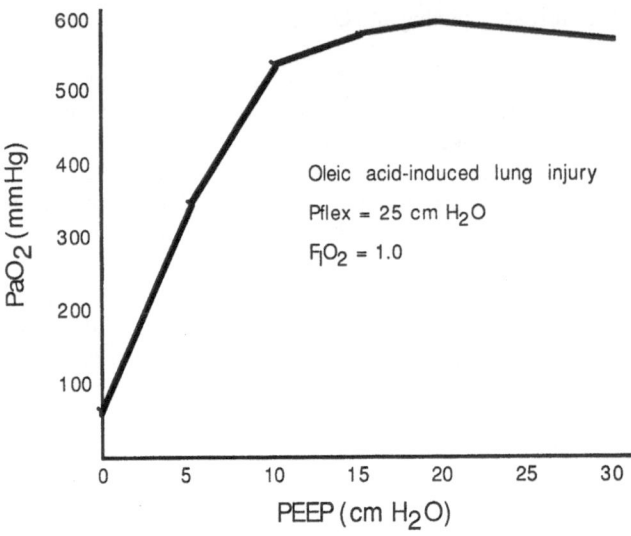

Fig. 4. Effects of increasing and decreasing PEEP on oxygenation in a single animal with oleic acid-induced lung injury. FiO_2 was constant at 1.0, respiratory rate was unchanged, and peak pressure was set at 35 cmH_2O. P_{flex} was located between 10 and 15 cmH_2O in this experiment

(i.e. titrating PEEP on the basis of the deflation, rather than the inflation portion of the curve). Doing so should allow the level of PEEP to be reduced below P_{flex} without extensive airway closure and, accordingly, without oxygenation falling. An example of such an effect is shown in Fig. 4 in which the level of PEEP was initially set by establishing the P_{flex} (i.e. 25 cmH_2O in this instance) and then lowered in a single animal with oleic acid-induced acute lung injury breathing 100% O_2. Peak inflation pressure was held constant at 35 cmH_2O and respiratory rate remained unchanged. In this instance, the pH was 7.10, the $PaCO_2$ was 70 mmHg and VT was 200 mL when PEEP was set just above P_{flex}. PEEP could be reduced to 5 or 10 cmH_2O, increasing VT to as much as 550 mL without affecting the PaO_2 to any clinically important extent and doing so decreased $PaCO_2$ to as low as 25 mmHg (despite reducing VT at the lower levels of PEEP so as to prevent pH from exceeding 7.5).

Although it would be nice if the pressure at which airway closure occurred could be discerned from the deflation portion of the P-V curve, akin to the way P_{flex} marks the point of airspace opening (in many, but not all patients), the gravitational gradient of Ppl that exists in supine patients mandates that there cannot be a single airway pressure at which closure (or opening) occurs in the majority of the lung.

Prone Position

Patients with ARDS have increases in radiographic lung density in the dorsal lung when they are supine [14, 20]. That these must result from airspace collapse rather than from non-uniform lung injury is apparent from the fact that the densities rapidly improve when patients are turned prone [21]. Although PEEP can reverse these densities to some extent, the effect is largely confined to more ventral areas (as was predicted by Froese and Bryan [18] in the article summarized above).

Numerous studies have indicated that the gravitational Ppl gradients seen in the upright, lateral decubitus, and supine positions are almost completely eliminated in the prone position [22], regardless of whether lungs are normal or edematous [23]. In the absence of a gravitational Ppl gradient, all lung units, regardless of whether they are located in the dependent or non-dependent regions, have a similar volume when the lung is at FRC. Accordingly, as demonstrated on Fig. 5, 1) airspace opening and closure should occur over a narrower range of Ptp; and 2) the Ptp required to generate TLC should be lower. If these suggestions are correct, it may be possible to select a "best PEEP" from the deflation portion of the lung P-V curve, *if the subjects are prone*, as an abrupt break in the curve should be more apparent as closure begins. If this reasoning is correct, PEEP might be reduced to a lower level, allowing a greater VT (Fig. 6) without exceeding product guidelines for maximum tidal alveolar pressure. Increased ventilation would avoid, respiratory acidosis and the need for paralysis and sedation. Additionally,

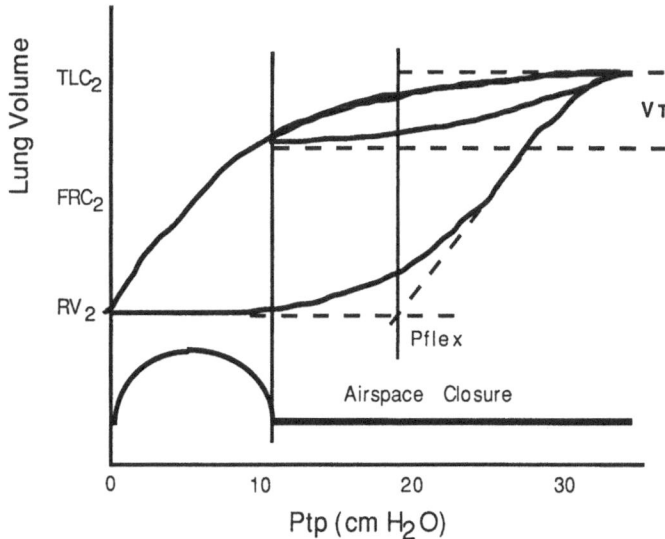

Fig. 5. Effects of using the deflation curve to set the level of PEEP. To the extent that airway opening and closing pressures differ the level of PEEP can be reduced, augmenting tidal volume and reducing the degree of respiratory acidemia that occurs as a result of titrating PEEP by the inflation curve

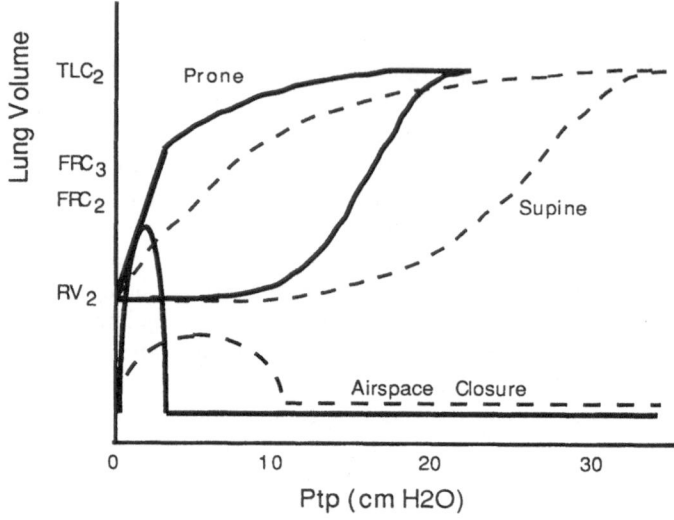

Fig. 6. Lung P-V curve in ARDS with patient in the prone position (solid line). Note sharper inflection and deflection zones when conpared to the supine curve (dashed)

if airspace opening and closing does indeed prove to be the cause for ventilation-induced lung injury, the prone position should narrow the range of Ptp over which opening and closing occurs and could reduce the injury considerably.

Conclusion

The pathophysiologic changes associated with ARDS, together with the concept that ventilation-induced lung injury results from airspace opening and closing leads to the reasonable hypothesis that ARDS may be a iatrogenic disease in many instances, resulting from the methods of ventilatory support employed in this setting. The fact that the gravitational Ppl gradient is eliminated in the prone position suggests that, in addition to improving gas exchange in the setting of ARDS, the prone position may also allow optimal PEEP adjustment to minimize ventilation-induced lung injury.

References

1. Slutsky AS (1993) Mechanical ventilation. American College of Chest Physicians' Consensus Conference. Chest 104: 1833–1859
2. Chattel G, Sab JM, Dubois JM, Sirodot M, Gaussorgues P, Robert D (1997) Prone position in mechanically ventilation patients with severe acute respiratory failure. Am J Respir Crit Care Med (In press)
3. Langer M, Mascheroni D, Marcolin R, Gattinoni L (1988) The prone position in ARDS patients. A clinical study. Chest 94: 103–107

4. Piehl MA, Brown RS (1976) Use of extreme position changes in respiratory failure. Crit Care Med 4:13–14.
5. Douglas WW, Rehder K, Beynen RM, Sessler AD, Marsh HM (1977) Improved oxygenation in patients with acute respiratory failure: The prone position. Am Rev Respir Dis 115:559–566
6. Lamm WJE, Graham MM, Albert RK (1994) Mechanism by which the prone position improves oxygenation in acute lung injury. Am J Respir Crit Care Med 150:184–193
7. Egan EA, Nelson RM, Olver RE (1976) Lung inflation and alveolar permeability to non-electrolytes in the adult sheep *in vivo*. J Physiol 260:409–424
8. Baile EM, Albert RK, Kirk W, Lakshminarayan S, Wiggs BJR, Pare PD (1984) Positive end-expiratory pressure decreases bronchial blood flow in the dog. J Appl Physiol (Respir Environ Exercise Physiol) 56:1289–1293
9. Lakshminarayan S, Jindal SK, Kirk W, Butler J (1990) Acute increases in anastomotic bronchial circulation to pulmonary blood flow die to generalized lung injury. J Appl Physiol 62:2358–2361
10. Coffey RL, Robertson HT, Albert RK (1983) Mechanisms of physiological dead space response to PEEP after oleic acid lung injury. J Appl Physiol (Resp Environ Exercise Physiol) 54:1550–1557
11. Parker JC, Townsley MI, Rippe B, Taylor AE, Thigpen J (1984) Increased microvascular permeability in dog lungs due to high peak airway pressures. J Appl Physiol 57:1809–1816
12. Dreyfus D, Basset G, Soler P, Saumon G (1985) Intermittent positive-pressure hyperventilation with high inflation pressures produces pulmonary microvascular injury in rats. Am Rev Respir Dis 132:880–884
13. Gattinoni L, Bombino M, Pelosi P, et al (1994) Lung structure and function in different stages of severe adult respiratory distress syndrome. JAMA 271:1772–1779
14. Gattinoni L, Mascheroni D, Torresin A, et al (1986) Morphological response to positive end-expiratory pressure in acute respiratory failure. Computerized tomography study. Intensive Care Med 12:137–142
15. Presenti A, Pilosi P, Rossi N, Virtuani A, Brazzi L, Rossi A (1991) The effect of positive end-expiratory pressure on respiratory resistance in patients with the adult respiratory distress syndrome and in normal anesthetized subjects. Am Rev Respir Dis 144:101–107
16. Muscedere JG, Mullen JMB, Gan K, Slutsky AS (1994) Tidal ventilation at low airway pressures can augment lung injury. Am J Respir Crit Care Med 149:1327–1334
17. Mutoh T, Guest RJ, Lamm WJE, Albert RK (1992) Prone position alters the effect of volume overload on regional pleural pressures and improves hypoxemia in pigs *in vivo*. Am Rev Respir Dis. 146:300–306
18. Froese AB, Bryan AC (1974) Effects of anesthesia and paralysis on diaphragmatic mechanics in man. Anesthesiology 41:242–255
19. Webb H, Tierney D (1974) Experimental pulmonary edema due to intermittent positive pressure ventilation with high inflation pressures: Protection by positive end-expiratory pressure. Am Rev Respir Dis 110:556–565
20. Maunder RJ, Shuman WP, McHugh JW, Marglin SI, Butler J (1986) Preservation of normal lung regions in the adult respiratory distress syndrome: Analysis by computed tomography. JAMA 255:2463–2465
21. Gattinoni L, Pelosi P, Vitale G, Pesenti A, D'Andrea L, Mascheroni D (1991) Body position changes redistribute computed-tomographic density in patients with acute respiratory failure. Anesthesiology 74:15–23
22. Lai-Fook S, Rodarte JR (1991) Pleural pressure distribution and its relationship to lung volume and interstitial pressure. J Appl Physiol 70:967–978
23. Mutoh T, Guest RJ, Lamm WJE, Albert RK (1992) Prone position alters the effect of volume overload on regional pleural pressures and improves hypoxemia in pigs *in vivo*. Am Rev Respir Dis 146:300–306

The Effects of Prone Position on Respiratory Function

L. Gattinoni, P. Pelosi, and L. Brazzi

Introduction

Acute respiratory failure (ARF) is characterized by radiographic diffuse bilateral infiltrates, decreased respiratory compliance, small lung volumes, and severe hypoxia [1, 2]. Correction of life-threatening hypoxia is one of the main goals of treatment, and different approaches have been suggested, including high airway pressures, jet ventilation, nitric oxide inhalation, and extracorporeal oxygenation. However, some of them may damage the lung, while others are extremely complex.

In 1974, Bryan [3] suggested that anesthetized and paralyzed patients, in the prone position, should exhibit a better expansion of the dorsal lung regions, than in the supine position where perfusion is believed to be prevalent, with a consequent improvement in oxygenation. Since then, several authors [4–7] showed, in small case series, that turning prone a mechanically ventilated patient with life-threatening hypoxia can produce a dramatic improvement in oxygenation. Thus, the prone position started to be considered as a simple and safe method to improve oxygenation in patients with ARF, and a "good turn" is now recommended early in the course of ARF [8]. However, the oxygenation improvement is not a consistent finding and the pathophysiological basis has not yet been completely elucidated.

In this chapter, we will discuss:
1) the effects of prone position on respiratory function in normal subjects;
2) the effects of prone position on respiratory function in patients with ARF; and
3) the different pathophysiological mechanisms involved in oxygenation response in the prone position.

Normal Subjects

Distribution of Alveolar Inflation in Supine Position

Awake: The distribution of alveolar inflation follows a gravitational gradient, with the non-dependent alveoli, located near the sternum, being more distended than the dependent ones, located near the vertebra (Fig. 1) [9–12]. This behavior is attributable to the elastic characteristics of the lung. In fact, in a normal lung, the alveolar dimensions depend on the transpulmonary pressure, i.e. the differ-

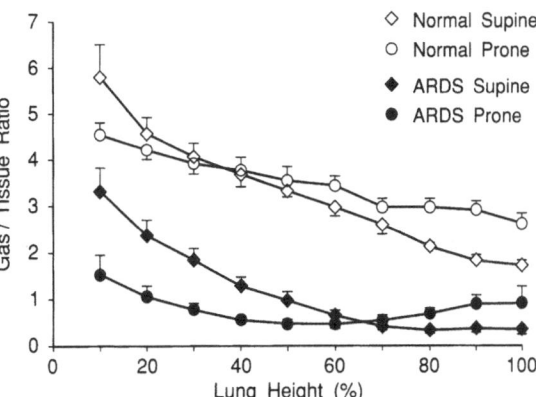

Fig. 1. The gas-tissue ratio, an index of alveolar inflation in the supine (rhombus) and prone (circles) positions. The white symbols refer to normal lung (n = 14) and the black symbols to lungs of ARF patients (n = 20). A height 0 refers to the ventral surface in supine position and to the dorsal surface in prone position. (From [20] with permission)

ence in pressure between alveolar pressure and pleural pressure. Since alveolar pressure is similar in the different alveoli, while pleural pressure is more negative in the non-dependent regions, transpulmonary pressure is greater in the non-dependent compared to the dependent part of the lung. The nature of this transpulmonary gradient is unclear and it is mainly attributed to the following factors: 1) lung weight; 2) shape and mechanical properties of the chest wall; and 3) shape and mechanical properties of the lung [13]. Lung weight is generally considered the most important contributor to the alveolar distension gradient, assuming that the lung behaves as a fluid and that a modified hydrostatic pressure is transmitted through the lung parenchyma as in a fluid [14–17]. In this way, the dimensions of the alveoli depend on the superimposed hydrostatic pressure: the more dependent the alveolus, the higher the superimposed pressure and the lower the alveolar dimension. However, other factors, alone or together with lung weight, may help determine transpulmonary pressure. Among them, lung and thoracic shape seem to play the major role.

Anesthesia-Paralysis: During mechanical ventilation, the inflation gradient probably follows the same pattern observed during spontaneous ventilation [9–12], although no data, to our knowledge, is available. Computerized tomography has shown induction of anesthesia causes a reduction in lung volume with atelectasis occuring in the most dependent part of the lung (Fig. 2) [18, 19]. The administration of a neuromuscular blocking agent does not cause any further change in lung morphology. The reduced muscular tone, produced by anesthesia, is likely involved in the generation of dependent atelectasis. Reduced muscular tone produces its effects on the rib cage, diaphragm and mediastinum. The rib cage becomes much more flat and reduces its ventral-dorsal height. The diaphragm, loosing its muscular tone, becomes a flaccid membrane cranially shifted in its dorsal part by the abdominal hydrostatic pressure. Finally the mediastinum, no longer suspended by the rib cage, weights on the most dependent lung regions. The combination of these three factors cause the formation of atelectasis in the most dependent lung regions.

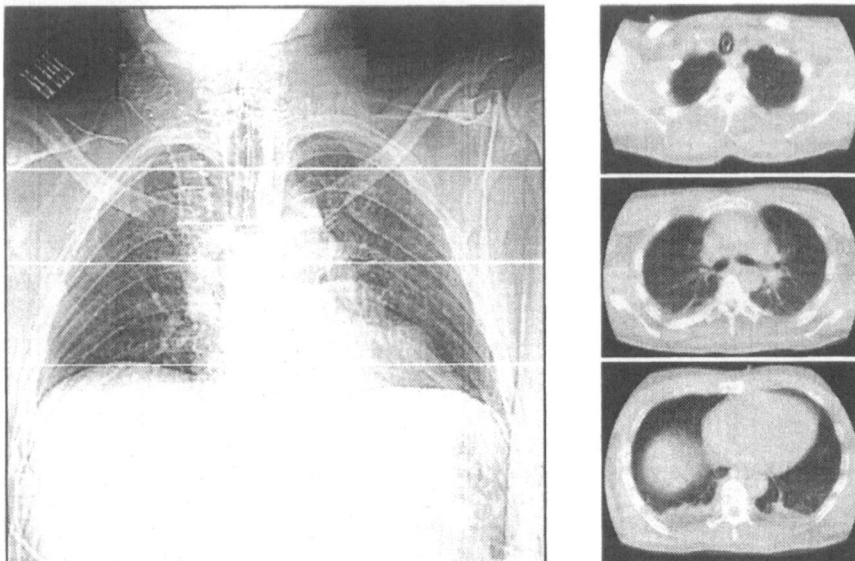

Fig. 2. Conventional radiography and CT scan of the lung (Apex, Hilum and Bases) of a normal anesthetized subject. CT scan shows the presence of atelectatic areas in the most dependent part of the lung

Distribution of Alveolar Inflation in Prone Position

Awake: When a normal subject is shifted from the supine to the prone position, the distribution of alveolar inflation changes, increasing in the dorsal regions and decreasing in the ventral ones (Fig. 1) [11]. Moreover, the alveolar inflation distribution is more homogeneous in the prone than in the supine position [12, 20], and therefore the prone position does not simply reverse the regional distribution of inflation.

Anesthesia-Paralysis: Again, few data are available regarding the distribution of regional inflation in the prone position. However, as for the supine position, it should follow the same behavior found in awake subjects [12, 20]. Really, the change of position during anesthesia and paralysis may cause a reversal of dependent density.

Distribution of Ventilation in Supine Position

Awake: Ventilation in the spontaneously breathing normal subject distributes predominantly to the dependent lung regions [21]. The major determinants of the distribution of ventilation are: 1) the regional inflation distribution; and 2) the pattern of diaphragm movements. As discussed above, the non-dependent alveoli are more distended than the dependent ones. Thus, the upper alveoli are closer to the flat (low-compliance) portion of their pressure-volume curve, while the lower ones are located on the steeper part of the curve [22, 23]. Since the amount of ventilation depends on the change in transpulmonary pressure, for a given applied transpulmonary pressure, ventilation is greater in the lower lung regions than in the upper ones. Moreover, in the supine position, a large portion of the lung is close to the diaphragm, which may vary its tension, shape, and position. During spontaneous breathing, there is a greater displacement of the dependent diaphragm, consequently with greater ventilation of the dependent lung [24–26].

Anesthesia-Paralysis: During anesthesia and paralysis, ventilation is always mainly distributed in the lower part of the lung, but this gradient is less evident than during awake spontaneous breathing. The diaphragm appears to play a major role in the distribution of ventilation [27–29]. In this case, in fact, the diaphragm behaves as a flaccid membrane that is faced with the vertical pressure gradient of the abdominal contents. The non-independent part of the diaphragm moves passively and faces a lower abdominal pressure; thus, in proportion, ventilation is greater in the non-dependent lung regions.

Distribution of Ventilation in Prone Position

Awake: Data are conflicting regarding the distribution of ventilation in the prone position. In fact, some authors found a uniform vertical distribution of ventilation [30], while others found a vertical gradient with greater ventilation either in the dependent or in the non-dependent lung regions [11, 31].

Anesthesia-Paralysis: During anesthesia and paralysis, Rheder et al. [31] found that ventilation was distributed predominantly to the dorsal part of the lung. However this pattern was not modified compared to spontaneous breathing.

Distribution of Perfusion in Supine Position

Awake and during Anesthesia-Paralysis: In awake subjects, a progressive increase in the perfusion distribution from non-dependent to the dependent regions has been demonstrated. However, the determinants of this gravitational perfusion gradient are not yet clear and different theories have been formulated. A gravitational theory initially proposed by West et al. [32] considers that the relationships between blood flow, pulmonary artery pressure, alveolar pressure and venous return can be modeled as a Starling resistor. The Starling resistor may be described as a collapsable tube (pulmonary vessels) across a closed chamber (alveoli) in which pressure may be varied: when the inflow pressure (pulmonary artery pressure) is lower than the chamber pressure (alveolar pressure), blood flow stops; when the inflow pressure is higher than the chamber pressure, flow is governed by either the difference between pulmonary artery pressure and alveolar pressure, or by the difference between pulmonary artery and venous pressures. Following this "gravitational" point of view, perfusion should increase steadily down the lung.

Other theories do not consider gravity as the main factor explaining the gravitational gradient of perfusion [33–37]. It is evident that, if these theories are correct and the gravitational effect does not play an important role in determining perfusion distribution, positioning should not seem to be really important in determining perfusion characteristics.

Distribution of Perfusion in Prone Position

Awake and during Anesthesia-Paralysis: According to the "gravitational" theory, a perfusion gradient should exist from dorsal to ventral regions. However, few data confirm this pattern in humans [11] and indeed in dogs, a dorsal to ventral gradient in perfusion has not been observed in the prone position [38].

Respiratory Mechanics and Lung Volumes in Prone Position

Awake: The modifications in respiratory mechanics and lung volume which occur in the prone position have not been thoroughly investigated [39]. Lumb and Nunn [40] found a moderate increase in end-expiratory lung volume from supine to prone position, while other authors found that subjects assuming the prone position failed to show a significant change [41]. Unfortunately, to our knowledge, little data are available regarding respiratory mechanics for the prone position. Nevertheless, forced vital capacity is reduced in prone position, without changes in obstructive respiratory indices [42]. On the other hand, the contribution of the diaphragm is increased in prone position indicating that diaphragmatic movement is probably enhanced in prone position [43].

Anesthesia-Paralysis: We recently investigated the effects of prone positioning on respiratory mechanics and lung volumes during general anesthesia in normal and obese subjects [39, 44]. In normal subjects, we found that the prone position does not alter total respiratory system compliance or either of its lung and chest wall components. Similar results have been obtained in obese subjects. However, in obese patients, prone positioning resulted in an increase in lung compliance and in a reduction in chest wall compliance, with the compliance of the total respiratory system remaining unmodified. It is possible that different effects of abdominal content, and consequently of the intraabdominal pressure on thoraco-abdominal mechanics may explain this behavior. These mechanical changes were paralleled by increases in lung volume and arterial oxygenation, both in normal and in obese subjects. However, no direct relationship was found between changes in lung volume and improvement in oxygenation. This indicates that in normal and obese subjects, under general anesthesia and paralysis, modifications in lung volume probably are not the main causes for improved oxygenation.

Patients with Acute Respiratory Failure (ARF)

Since data on respiratory mechanics, alveolar inflation, distribution of ventilation and perfusion reported in the literature for patients with ARF refer only to patients treated with anesthesia and paralysis, our discussion will be confined to those subjects.

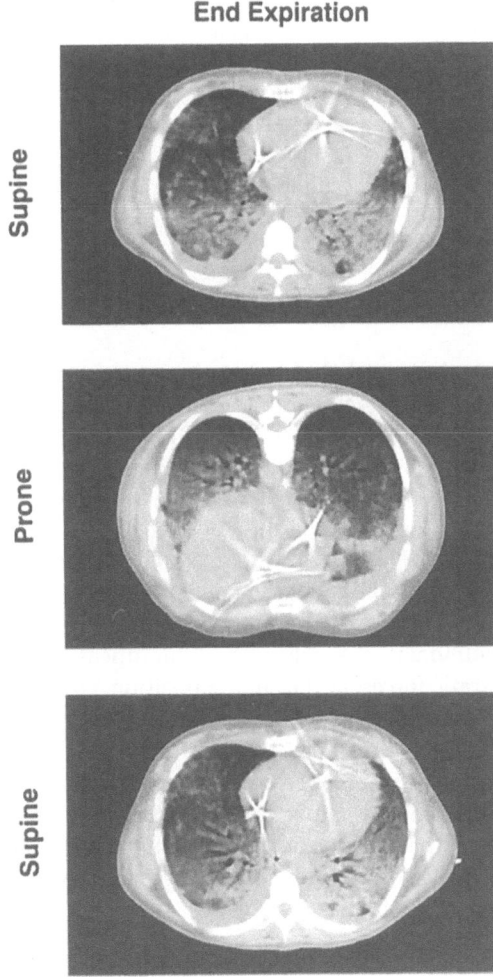

End Expiration

Fig. 3. A representative CT scan image in supine, prone and after return to supine position of an ARF patient. Note the typical redistribution of lung densities in prone position

Distribution of Alveolar Inflation in Supine Position

Anesthesia-Paralysis: Using computed tomography (CT), the lung image in ARF is characterized by radiographic densities, primarily located in the dependent regions, that are dorsal in the supine position (Fig. 3) [45]. Applying a regional CT analysis of the lung, it was found that alveolar inflation is markedly reduced both in the ventral regions (near the sternum in supine position) and in the dorsal ones (near the vertebra in supine position), following a gravitational gradient (Fig. 1) [46]. Thus, the non-dependent alveoli are more expanded than the dependent ones. In contrast, the distribution of edema is uniform throughout the lung parenchyma, suggesting that the disease process is uniformly distributed. As the total mass of the ARF lung is more than twice that of a normal lung [47, 48], the lung progressively collapses under its own weight, squeezing out the gas from the dependent regions with formation of compression atelectasis. This suggests that the lung weight hypothesis previously discussed may apply to patients with ARF. However, other factors, such as lung and chest wall shape, may be involved in determining this alveolar inflation gradient. It is possible to model the ARF lung as composed of three compartments: one affected by the disease but continuously open to gases (open diseased zone); one fully diseased without any possibility of recruitment (closed diseased zone); and one composed of collapsed alveoli potentially recruitable with increasing pressure (recruitable diseased zone) [46, 49].

Distribution of Alveolar Inflation in Prone Position

Anesthesia-Paralysis: In changing patient position from supine to prone, we observed a movement of the densities, i.e. lung inflation, from dorsal to ventral regions (Fig. 3) [12]. This movement from previously dependent to newly dependent regions of the lung is probably due to different gravitational forces acting on the lung parenchyma. In fact, the rapid redistribution we observed can hardly be explained by the sudden formation of edema in the newly dependent regions and a reabsorption of the earlier edema in the newly non-dependent regions. Moreover, the changes in densities are too great to be explained only by a shift of blood mass. Consequently, the most likely explanation is a redistribution of intrapulmonary gas, caused by a modification of hydrostatic pressures. The hydrostratic forces, in the supine position, collapse the dorsal lung, which is the most dependent one, whilst, in the prone position, the most dependent lung, with higher hydrostatic forces, is the ventral one which, hence, become collapsed. Prone position does not only cause a reversal of regional inflation gradient, but also a more homogeneous distribution of lung inflation [20]. As in normal subjects, the modifications of the lung and chest wall shape, in the prone position, also play a role in inducing changes in transpulmonary gradient and thus in alveolar inflation.

Distribution of Alveolar Ventilation in Supine Position

Anesthesia-Paralysis: Looking at CT scans taken at end-expiration and at end-inspiration, it is possible to quantitatively estimate regional ventilation [50]. In the early phase of ARF, ventilation distributes mainly to the non-dependent lung regions, probably because the dependent lung is usually collapsed and/or consolidated. This pattern is partly modified by the application of PEEP: when PEEP is increased, the dependent lung regions are recruited and ventilation becomes more uniformly distributed.

Distribution of Alveolar Ventilation in Prone Position

Anesthesia-Paralysis: Unfortunately, data regarding the distribution of ventilation in the prone position are not currently available. However, from regional inflation data, we may infer that ventilation should redistribute from the ventral regions (collapsed in prone position) to the dorsal ones (recruited in prone position) [12]. Moreover, as regional inflation is more uniform in the prone position, we expect that ventilation in this position is, probably, more homogeneous as well.

Distribution of Perfusion in Supine Position

Anesthesia-Paralysis: During ARF, several factors may alter the distribution of perfusion, including hypoxic vasoconstriction [51], vessel obliteration [52], and extrinsic vessel compression. However, it is not clear if, even during ARF, perfusion distribution follows a gravitational gradient or is dependent on anatomical factors. Some evidence supports the first hypothesis. In fact, using selective angiography in patients with ARF, defects in intravascular filling or diffuse vascular pruning have been observed [53]. Selective angiography was usually positive when the tip of the catheter was in CT dense regions, and usually negative when the catheter tip was located in inflated regions, suggesting the presence of external compression of the vessels [54]. Thus, it seems from these observations, that regional perfusion in ARF is abnormal and probably diverted towards innated and non-dependent regions.

Distribution of Perfusion in Prone Position

Anesthesia-Paralysis: To our knowledge no data are available regarding the distribution of pulmonary blood flow in ARF patients in the prone position. However, experimental evidence in dogs [38] suggests that perfusion to the dorsal region is greater than to the ventral one in the prone position, suggesting that mechanisms other than gravity may operate in this situation.

Respiratory Mechanics and Lung Volume in Prone Position

Anesthesia-Paralysis: We recently investigated modifications in respiratory mechanics and lung volumes that occur in the prone position in mechanically ventilated patients with ARF [55]. We found that the prone position decreased thoraco-abdominal compliance, but did not affect total respiratory system compliance or lung volumes. The reduction in the thoraco-abdominal compliance could be explained by a decrease in the thoracic wall and/or the diaphragmatic wall compliance. Assuming that overall compliance of the diaphragmatic wall remains unchanged in the prone position (since intraabdominal pressure did not change), the decrease in thoraco-abdominal compliance may best be explained by a greater stiffness of the posterior wall of the thorax free to move only in the prone position, compared to the anterior wall of the thorax free to move only in the supine position.

Mechanisms of Improvement in Oxygenation in Prone Position

From a pathophysiological view, hypoxemia in ARF is a consequence of a reduction in the ventilation/perfusion (VA/Q) ratios and of the presence of a true shunt due to alveolar units not ventilated but perfused, i.e. with a VA/Q = 0. The combination of these two phenomena is called "physiological shunt". Prone positioning can improve oxygenation due to different mechanisms which in general improve the VA/Q ratio, and consequently cause a reduction in physiological shunt.

Increase in Lung Volume

An increase in lung volume was first hypothesized by Douglas et al. [5] to explain the improvement in oxygenation in the prone position. The increase in lung volume should be due to an unloading of the diaphragmatic movement in the prone position compared to supine, owing to a reduction of the forces opposing the passive movement of dorsal regions. However, this hypothesis has not been confirmed in ARF patients, since lung volume does not appear to change in the prone position [55]. Moreover, modifications in oxygenation seem not to relate to changes in lung volume. As discussed above the lack of a relationship between changes in lung volume and oxygenation in the prone position has been also reported, both in normal [39] and obese [44] subjects during general anesthesia.

Redistribution of Perfusion

This attractive hypothesis is based on the fact that perfusion in the supine position is gravity-dependent, i.e. most prevalent in the most dependent part of the lung, and lung densities are also mainly located in the dependent lung regions. Thus, in the supine position, perfusion should predominate in the most diseased lung regions, with a consequent increase in "shunt" fraction (reduced VA/Q). If we were to turn a patient and densities remained in the dorsal part, while perfusion following a gravitational gradient increased in the ventral one, one should expect an improvement of VA/Q matching with an increased oxygenation. Unfortunately, this simple and attractive mechanism does not apply in patients with ARF. In fact, although the perfusion behavior is unstudied in human patients with ARF, prone positioning redistributes lung densities from dorsal to ventral lung regions [12].

Recruitment of Dorsal Spaces

This seems to be one of the most likely causes of increased oxygenation in the prone position. In fact, densities in the dorsal part of the lung decrease in prone position, while perfusion probably remains most prevalent in the dorsal lung regions aided in part by release of hypoxic vasconstriction. Thus VA/Q improves, with a consequent increase in oxygenation.

More Homogeneous Distribution of Ventilation

Application of a positive end-expiratory pressure (PEEP) generally improves oxygenation in ARF patients [47]. The mechanisms by which PEEP improves oxygenation are essentially two: recruitment of previously collapsed lung regions, and the recreation of a more homogeneous distribution of ventilation [50]. Prone positioning has also been found to reduce the transpulmonary gradient [56], thus producing a more homogeneous inflation gradient and, possibly, a more homogeneous distribution of ventilation. Modifications in the shape and mechanical properties of the thoraco-abdominal cage, which have been described to occur in the prone position [20, 55, 57], may attenuate the transpulmonary pressure gradient. Changes in the mechanical properties of the thoraco-abdominal cage may play an important role in determining the oxygenation response to prone positioning.

Conclusion

Prone positioning improves oxygenation in the majority but not in all patients with ARF. To completely elucidate the physiological mechanisms underlying oxygenation changes, knowledge of regional perfusion is required. Nevertheless, both a recruitment of previously collapsed alveolar spaces and a more homogeneous distribution of ventilation, probably due to modifications in the mechanical properties of the thoraco-abdominal cage, together with a relatively unchanging distribution of perfusion, probably play an important role in determining the oxygenation response to prone positioning.

References

1. Asbaugh DG, Bigelow DB, Petty TL, Levine BE (1967) Acute respiratory distress in adults. Lancet 2:319–323
2. Bernard GR, Artigas A, Brigham KL, et al (1994) The American-European conference on ARDS. Definitions, mechanisms, relevant in outcomes and clinical trial coordination. Am J Respir Crit Care Med 149:818–824
3. Bryan AC (1974) Comments of a devil's advocate. Am Rev Respir Dis 110:143
4. Piehl MA, Brown RS (1976) Use of extreme position changes in respiratory failure. Crit Care Med 4:13–14
5. Douglas WW, Rehder K, Beynen RM, Sessler AD, Marsh HM (1977) Improved oxygenation in patients with acute respiratory failure: The prone positon. Am Rev Respir Dis 115:559–566
6. Langer M, Mascheroni D, Marcolin R. Gattinoni L (1988) The prone position in ARDS patients. A clinical study. Chest 94:103–107
7. Pappert D, Rossaint R, Slama K, Gruning T, Falke KJ (1994) Influence of positioning on ventilation-perfusion relationships in severe adult respiratory distress syndrome. Chest 106:1511–1516
8. Albert RK (1994) One good turn... Intensive Care Med 20:247–248
9. Rehder K, Sessler AD, Rodarte JR (1977) Regional intrapulmonary gas distribution in awake and anesthetized-paralyzed man. J Appl Physiol 42:391–402
10. Bryan AC, Milic-Emili J, Pengelly D (1966) Effect of gravity on the distribution of pulmonary ventilation. J Appl Physiol 21:778–784
11. Kaneko K, Milic-Emili J, Dolovich MB, Dawson A, Bates DV (1966) Regional distribution of ventilation and perfusion as a function of body position. J Appl Physiol 21:766–777
12. Gattinoni L, Pelosi P, Vitale G, Pesenti A, D'Andrea L, Mascheroni D (1991) Body position changes redistribute lung computed tomographic density in patients with acute respiratory failure. Anesthesiology 74:15–23
13. Agostoni E (1986) Mechanics of the pleural space. In: Handbook of physiology: The respiratory system. Vol. 3; Chap 30. American Physiological Society, Bethesda, MD, pp 531–559
14. Milic-Emili J, Henderson JAM, Dolovich D, Trop D, Kaneko K (1966) Regional distribution of inspired gas in the lung. J Appl Physiol 21:749–759
15. Glaister DH (1970) Distribution of pulmonary blood flow and ventilation during forward (+ Gx) acceleration. J Appl Physiol 29:432–439
16. Michels DB, West JB (1978) Distribution of pulmonary ventilation and perfusion during short period of weightlessness. J Appl Physiol 45:987–998
17. Krugger JJ, Bain T, Patterson JL (1961) Elevation gradient of intrathoracic pressure. J Appl Physiol 16:465–468
18. Brismar B, Hedestierna G, Lundquis H, et al (1985) Pulmonary density during anesthesia with muscular relaxation. A proposal of atelectasis. Anesthesiology 62:422–428
19. Hedestierna G, Strandberg A, Brismar B, et al (1985) Functional residual capacity, thoraco-abdominal dimension and central blood volume, during general anesthesia with muscle paralysis and mechanical ventilation. Anesthesiology 62:247–254
20. Gattinoni L, Pelosi P, Valenza F, Mascheroni D (1994) Patient positioning in acute respiratory failure. In: Tobin MJ (ed) Principles and practice of mechanical ventilation. McGraw Hill, New York, pp 1067–1076
21. Engel LA, Utz G, Wood DH, Macklem PT (1974) Ventilation distribution in anatomical lung units. J Appl Physiol 37:194–200
22. Otis AB, Mckernow CB, Bartlett RA, et al (1995) Mechanical factors in distribution of pulmonary ventilation. J Appl Physiol 8:427–433
23. Pedley TJ, Sudlow MF, Milic-Emili J (1972) A non-linear theory of the distribution of pulmonary ventilation. Respir Physiol 15:1–38
24. Froese AB, Bryan AC (1974) Effects of anesthesia and paralysis on diaphragmatic mechanics in man. Anesthesiology 41:242–255
25. Chevrolet JC, Emrich J, Martin RR, Angel LA (1979) Voluntary changes in ventilation distribution in lateral posture. Respir Physiol 38:313–323

26. Chevrolet JC, Martin JG, Flood R, Martin RR, Engel LA (1978) Topographical ventilation and perfusion distribution during IPPB in the lateral posture. Am Rev Respir Dis 118:847–854
27. Potgieter SV (1959) Atelectasis: Its evolution during upper urinary tract surgery. Br J Anesth 31:472–483
28. Nunn JF (1961) The distribution of inspired gas during thoracic surgery. Ann R Col Surg Engl 28:223–237
29. Rheder K, Hatch DJ, Sessler AD, Fowler WS (1972) The function of each lung of anesthetized and paralyzed man during mechanical ventilation. Anesthesiology 37:16–26
30. Amis TC (1979) Regional lung function in man and in dog. PhD thesis. London. University of London
31. Rheder K, Knopp JJ, Sessler AD (1978) Regional intrapulmonary gas distribution in awake and anesthetized-paralyzed prone man. J Appl Physiol 45:528–535
32. West JB, Dolley CT, Naimark A (1964) Distribution of blood flow in isolated lungs: Relation to vascular and alveolar pressures. J Appl Physiol 19:713–724
33. Amis TC, Jones HA, Hughes JMB (1984) Effect of posture on intraregional distribution of pulmonary perfusion and Va/Q ratios in man. Respir Physiol 56:169–182
34. Orphanidou D, Hughes JMB, Myers MJ, Al-Suhali AR, Henderson B (1986) Tomography of regional ventilation and perfusion using Kripton 81m in normal subjects and asthmatic patients. Thorax 41:542–551
35. Reed JH, Wood EH (1970) Effect of body position on vertical distribution of pumonary blood flow. J Appl Physiol 28:303–311
36. Wiener CW, Kirk W, Albert RK (1990) Prone position reverses gravitational distribution of perfusion in dogs lungs with oleic acid-induced injury. J Appl Physiol 68:1386–1392
37. Glenny RW, Robertson HT (1990) Fractal properties of pulmonary blood flow: Characterization of spatial heterogeneity. J Appl Physiol 69:532–545
38. Glenny RW, Lamm WJE, Albert RK, Robertson HT (1991) Gravity is a minor determinant of pulmonary blood flow distribution. J Appl Physiol 71:620–629
39. Pelosi P, Croci M, Calappi E, et al (1995) Prone positioning during general anesthesia minimally affects respiratory mechanics while improving functional residual capacity and increasing oxygen tension. Anesth Analg 80:855–860
40. Lumb AB, Nunn JF (1991) Respiratory function and rib cage contribution to ventilation in body positions commonly used during anesthesia. Anesth Analg 73:422–426
41. Moreno F, Lyons HA (1961) Effect of body posture on lung volume. J Appl Physiol 16:27–29
42. Cortese DA, Rodarte JR, Rehder K, Hyatt RE (1976) Effect of posture on the single breath oxygen test in normal subjects. J Appl Physiol 41:474–479
43. Krayer S, Rehder K, Wetterman J, Didier EP, Ritman EL (1989) Position and motion of the diaphragm during anesthesia and paralysis. Anesthesiology 70:891–898
44. Pelosi P, Croci M, Calappi E, et al (1996) Prone positioning improves pulmonary function in obese patients during general anesthesia. Anesth Analg 83:578–583
45. Gattinoni L, Mascheroni D, Torresin A, et al (1986) Morphological response to positive end-expiratory pressure in acute respiratory failure. Computerized tomography study. Intensive Care Med 12:137–142
46. Pelosi P, D'Andrea L, Vitale G, Pesenti A, Gattinoni L (1994) Vertical gradient of regional lung inflation in adult respiratory distress syndrome. Am J Respir Crit Care Med 149:8–13
47. Gattinoni L, Pesenti A, Bombino M, et al (1988) Relationship between lung computed tomographic density, gas exchange and PEEP in acute respiratory failure. Anesthesiology 69:824–832
48. Teplitz C (1976) The core pathobiology and integrated medical science of acute respiratory insufficiency. Surg Clin N Am 56:1091–1130
49. Gattinoni L, Pesenti A, Avalli L, Rossi F, Bombino M (1987) Pressure-volume curve of total respiratory system in acute respiratory failure. Computed tomographic scan study. Am Rev Respir Dis 136:730–736
50. Gattinoni L, Pelosi P, Crotti S, Valenza F (1995) Effects of positive end-expiratory pressure on regional distribution of tidal volume and recruitment in acute respiratory distress syndrome. Am J Respir Crit Care Med 151:1807–1814
51. Arborelius M, Lunding G, Svanberg L, Defares JG (1960) Influence of unilateral hypoxia on blood flow through the lungs in man in lateral position. J Appl Physiol 15:595–597

52. Jones R, Reid LM, Zapol WM, Tomashefski JF, Kirton OC, Kobayashi K (1985) Pulmonary vascular pathology: Human and experimental study. In: Zapol WM, Falke KJ (eds) Acute respiratory failure. Vol. 24. Marcel Dekker New York, pp 23–160
53. Greene R, Zapol WM, Snider MT, et al (1981) Early bedside angiographic diagnosis of pulmonary vascular occlusion during acute respiratory failure. Am Rev Respir Dis 125:593–601
54. Vesconi S, Rossi GP, Pesenti A, Fumagalli R, Gattinoni L (1988) Pulmonary microthrombosis in severe adult respiratory distress syndrome. Crit Care Med 16:111–115
55. Tubiolo D, Vicardi P, Pelosi P, et al (1995) The effects of prone position on lung volume, respiratory compliance and gas exchange in ARDS patients. In: Anesthesia, Pain, Intensive Care and Emergency Medicine. APICE, Trieste, pp 78–79
56. Mutoh T, Guest RJ, Lamm WJE, Albert RK (1992) Prone position alters the effect of volume overload on regional pleural pressures and improves hypoxemia in pigs *in vivo*. Am Rev Respir Dis 146:300–306
57. Margulies SS, Rodarte JR (1990) Shape of the chest wall in the prone and supine anesthetized dog. J Appl Physiol 68:1970–1978

Pharmacological Manipulation of V/Q in ALI and ARDS

Inhaled Nitric Oxide: Clinical Experience

H. Gerlach, D. Keh, and J. Falke

Introduction

Since the classic study of Furchgott and Zawadzki [1] demonstrating the need of an intact endothelial cell layer for agents such as acetylcholine to have a relaxing effect on the blood vessel, an exploding body of literature has implicated the vascular endothelium as a source of relaxing factors. An important endothelial-derived relaxing factor (EDRF) is nitric oxide (NO), a short-lived gas molecule. NO is a highly reactive radical made from the amino acid L-arginine by the action of the enzyme nitric oxide synthase (NOS), releasing citrulline and NO [2]. A number of cofactors are required for this enzymatic reaction, as well as the availability of molecular oxygen. NO is formed throughout all vascular beds, and its basal release from endothelial cells may maintain normal blood vessel tone [3]. NO is also made by many different cell types in addition to endothelial cells, such as neutrophils, platelets, macrophages, and smooth muscle cells (SMC), as well as neurons [4, 5]. In fact, there is increasing evidence that NO may function as a neurotransmitter in the brain to mediate the glutamate receptor signal transduction, and as an inhibitory, non-adrenergic, non-cholinergic neurotransmitter in the gastrointestinal and genito-urinary tracts [6]. Inflammatory cells and SMC express NO only in response to activation by endotoxin, interleukin(IL)-1, tumor necrosis factor (TNF), or interferon. This multifaceted molecule can therefore regulate a number of different processes, from inflammation, to neuronal signal transduction, to regulation of vascular tone.

Several species of the enzyme NOS have been described, and several distinct NOS genes have been identified. There is the "immunetype" NOS (iNOS), expressed by most cells except platelets [7–9]; the neuronal subtype of NOS (nNOS), which mediates non-adrenergic, non-cholinergic nerve stimulation [10, 11]; and the eNOS, which is expressed by endothelial cells [12–14]. The eNOS regulates normoxic pulmonary vasodilation, whereas nNOS and iNOS are expressed by airway epithelial and muscle cells, and these enzymes are involved in bronchodilation. The nomenclature is confusing because one cell type may express more than one NOS, or each NOS isoform may be expressed by more than one cell type.

The development of drugs that inhibit NOS has been very useful to determine the physiological role of NO. Analogs of L-arginine act as false substrates for NOS and therefore block formation of NO. Administration of L-arginine, but not D-arginine, restores enzymatic activity. Examples of arginine analogs used in several studies include N^G-monomethyl-L-arginine (L-NMMA), N^G-nitro-L-arginine methyl ester (L-NAME), and N^{ω}-nitro-L-arginine (L-NNA). Selective inhibitors of iNOS are being developed, and they may be important therapeutic agents in inflammatory states.

NO activates soluble guanyl cyclase by binding to its heme moiety and by altering its configuration, resulting in production of the second messenger, cyclic guanosine monophosphate (cGMP) from guanosyl triphosphate (GTP). Via incompletely understood inhibition of locally derived mechanisms, cGMP results in SMC relaxation by decreasing intracellular calcium. In addition, NO directly stimulates calcium-dependent K^+ channels, leading to hyperpolarization and relaxation of vascular SMC via a cGMP-independent mechanism [15]. Nitrovasodilators, such as sodium nitroprusside and nitroglycerine, work via releasing NO either spontaneously or by intracellular conversion. NO can be bound by heme-containing molecules, such as guanyl cyclase and hemoglobin; the latter acts as a scavenger of NO, resulting in its inactivation. In addition, it has been suggested that NO may complex with thiols, (such as cysteine) forming S-nitrocysteine. Such complexes prolong the half-life of NO, with effects distal from its site of release [16]. In addition to SMC relaxation, NO inhibits platelet aggregation or adhesion to endothelium and may therefore prolong the bleeding time [17]. Regulation of NO production in the lung, both in the basal state and in models of pulmonary hypertension, is an active area of research.

Acute Lung Injury and the Need for Vasodilation

Acute lung injury (ALI) or its aggravated form, the acute respiratory distress syndrome (ARDS), is characterized by a sudden, generalized inflammation of the lung, which induces
1) non-cardiogenic pulmonary edema,
2) pulmonary arterial hypertension,
3) a reduction of total compliance of the lung, and
4) progressive systemic hypoxemia due to a pulmonary ventilation/perfusion-mismatch leading to an increased portion of intrapulmonary right-to-left shunt areas [18].

Pulmonary hypertension causes a rise of the microvascular filtration pressure in the lung and, hence, the development of an interstitial pulmonary edema as well as overstress and dysfunction of the right ventricle [19].

Current strategies for treatment of ARDS tend toward a less aggressive ventilation therapy based on the use of pressure-controlled ventilation (PCV) with positive end-expiratory pressure (PEEP), permissive hypercapnia, differential lung ventilation (DLV), prone positioning, dehydration, as well as extracorporeal lung assist (ELA) with heparin-coated systems [20]. The additional treatment with systemically applied vasodilators is limited by the simultaneous dilation of pulmonary and systemic vessels, which induces systemic hypotension. Furthermore, vasodilation in the whole lung by systemic vasodilators induces a relative increase of blood flow in shunt areas, followed by a deterioration of systemic oxygenation. Hence, a further rise of the inspired oxygen fraction (FiO_2) and/or ventilation pressure is necessary to guarantee the same oxygenation as without vasodilators [21].

When the biological relevance and the physiological pathways of NO began to be obvious, the question arose if gaseous NO could be used for controlled inhalation. Inhaled NO, similar to the endogenous, endothelium-derived NO, should be able to induce vasodilation. Based on the two bio-characteristics of NO – to vasodilate and to bind to hemoglobin within seconds after diffusion into the intravascular space – inhaled NO might be inactivated immediately without influencing the systemic circulation, resulting in a so-called "selective pulmonary vasodilation". Animal studies on toxicity of NO inhalation for up to six months revealed no evidence of side effects using NO doses of less than 40 parts per million (ppm) [22, 23]. Pilot-studies in humans by Higenbottam et al. [24, 25] in 1988 demonstrated that the inhalation of NO was, indeed, able to reduce pulmonary hypertension in adult patients without major effects on the systemic circulation. Animal experiments by Frostell and Pison [26, 27] revealed that inhaled NO was also able to reverse hypoxic pulmonary vasoconstriction without impairing pulmonary gas exchange. In parallel, two other groups found that the beneficial effect of inhaled NO might also be useful in the therapy of the persistent pulmonary hypertension of the newborn (PPHN) [28, 29]. In all these studies, NO was inhaled in doses between 5 and 80 ppm, and no critical side effects such as systemic hypotension or methemoglobinemia were registered.

Low Dose Inhalation of NO in ARDS

The first ARDS patients were treated with inhaled NO using doses of 18 and 36 ppm, and the registered effects on hemodynamics and pulmonary gas exchange were compared with the effects after treatment of the same patients by intravenous infusion of prostacyclin (PGI2), using a dose of 4 ng/kg/min (Fig. 1) [30]. The results of these studies revealed that both inhaled NO and infused prostacyclin are able to reduce the pulmonary resistance about 20% [31]. In contrast to prostacyclin, which simultaneously caused systemic hypotension and a decreased arterial oxygen saturation, inhaled NO did not induce any change of systemic hemodynamics, but improved arterial oxygenation in a significant way. By measuring the ventilation/perfusion ratio it was confirmed that the portion of intrapulmonary shunt areas was expanded by the infusion of prostacyclin, but, in contrast, reduced by inhalation of 18 and/or 36 ppm NO due to a redistribution of pulmonary blood flow towards areas with nearly normal ventilation/perfusion ratios. This beneficial effect of NO was also observed in long-term studies with doses of less than 20 ppm (Fig. 2) [31]. However, the first studies with NO inhalation in ARDS patients demonstrated no difference between the two doses of 18 or 36 ppm regarding pulmonary resistance and systemic oxygenation. On the other hand, the patients developed no tachyphylaxis, but, in contrast, seemed to become "dependent" on NO inhalation, even when the course of the disease was posi-

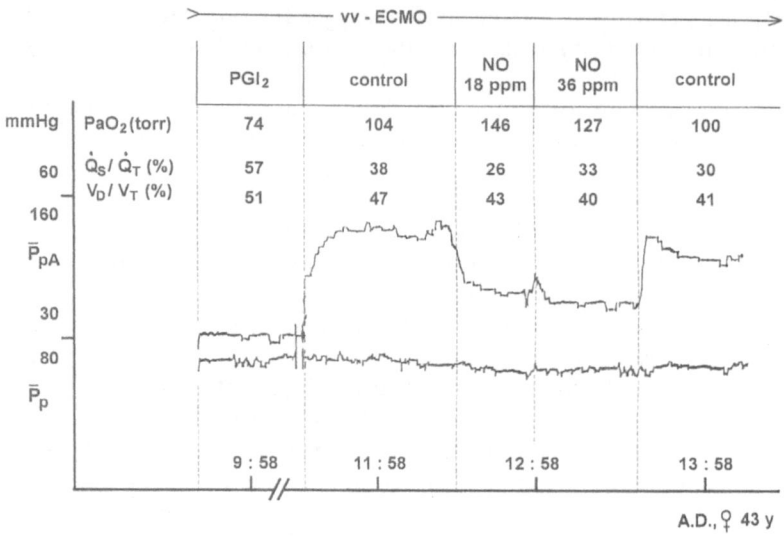

Fig. 1. Original recording from of the first patient with severe ARDS due to aspiration pneumonia receiving NO inhalation. On the y-axis, mean systemic and pulmonary arterial pressures are indicated (mmHg from 0–60 for PAP, from 0–160 for systemic pressure). On the x-axis, time course of the pressures is indicated (upper curve: PAP; lower curve: systemic pressure), subdivided for the following protocol: First, prostacyclin was infused systemically (PGI2), then, the infusion was stopped ("control"). This was then followed by the inhalation of 18 ppm NO and 36 ppm NO. Finally, inhalation was stopped for another control. The monitored data for oxygenation (PaO₂), intrapulmonary right-to-left shunt (QS/QT), and dead space ventilation (VD/VT) after reaching a steady-state for each treatment are inserted as a time-dependent table. As demonstrated, both systemic prostacyclin and inhaled NO are able to reduce PAP, whereas only inhaled NO improves the systemic oxygenation. In contrast, systemic prostacyclin decreases PaO₂ (compared to the control data) by increasing the intrapulmonary right-to-left shunt

tive. Finally, no severe side effects such as methemoglobinemia were observed, even during long-term inhalation.

After these first trials, we tested the dose-response of selective pulmonary vasodilation by NO in patients with severe ARDS. We used NO doses between 10 parts per billion (ppb) and 100 ppm. Surprisingly, it was found that an improvement of systemic oxygenation by NO can be achieved with much lower doses of NO than were used before (the ED50 for increasing oxygenation was approximately 0.1 ppm). In addition, the best dose for improved oxygenation is different from that for optimal reduction of pulmonary resistance (ED50 >2 ppm) [32]. The optimal improvement of systemic oxygenation is usually found with 10 ppm NO; higher doses of NO might reverse the beneficial effect. In some cases, however, ARDS patients had an impressive effect of NO, demonstrating the best systemic oxygenation with 1 ppm NO, whereas higher doses, e.g. 100 ppm, showed similar effects to systemic vasodilators, i.e. deteriorated systemic oxygenation due to increased intrapulmonary right-to-left shunt areas. The pulmonary resistance, in contrast, was continuously reduced by NO doses.

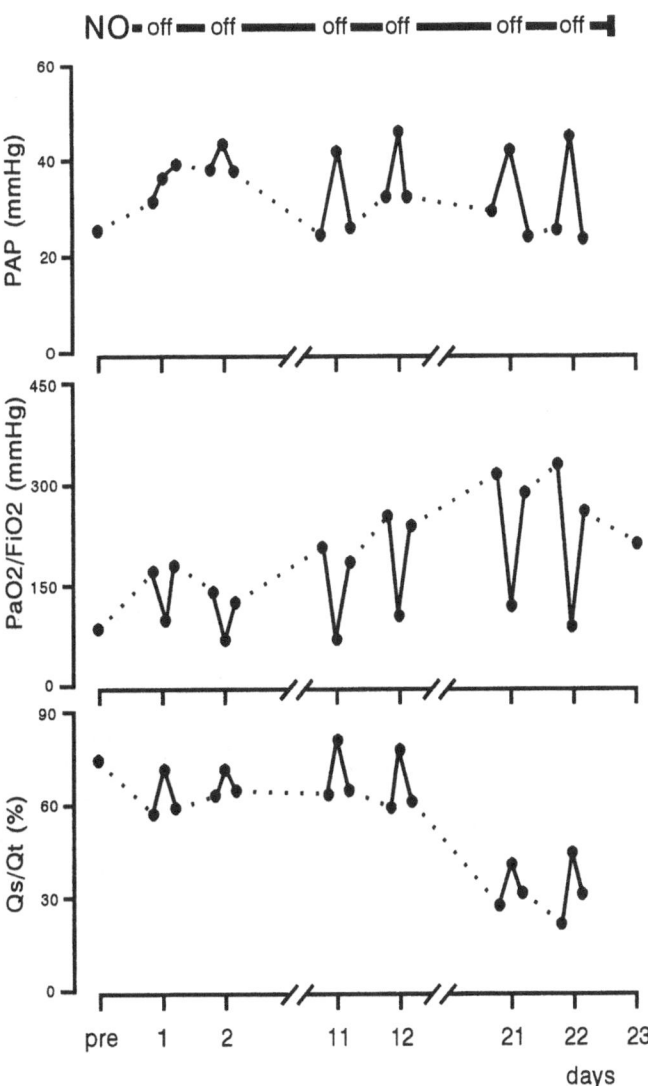

Fig. 2. Effect of long-term NO inhalation on pulmonary artery pressure (PAP), arterial oxygenation (PaO$_2$/FiO$_2$), and intrapulmonary right-to-left shunt (QVA/QT) of a patient with severe ARDS. Disruption of NO inhalation always leads to increased PAP and deteriorated oxygenation by enhanced intrapulmonary shunt. No tachyphylaxis could be registered. (Modified from [64])

The response to inhaled NO varied both inter-individually between the patients, and intra-individually during the treatment of the some individual. The optimal NO dose regarding systemic oxygenation was registered from 0.5 to 100 ppm; some patients showed no effect or only moderate effects after initiating NO inhalation ("non-responders"). In some cases, it was possible to improve systemic oxygenation for up to two weeks by inhaling 0.06 to 0.25 ppm NO [33]. These are similar NO concentrations as found in the exhaled air of animals and healthy human volunteers. NO is produced in the upper airways and auto-inhaled during normal ventilation [34, 35]. Thus, low dose NO inhalation might be considered as a replacement therapy, since mechanical ventilation disrupts the patient from inhaling his own NO!

Why is Less NO Better?

Results from our department [32] demonstrate that, in approximately 80% of patients with ARDS, a) lower doses of inhaled NO improve systemic oxygenation; b) higher doses, in contrast, may lower the arterial oxygen content; and c) improvement of systemic oxygenation and reduction of pulmonary artery pressure are not closely correlated during NO dose-response studies. This may be explained by two hypotheses:

1) The "diffusion theory" (Fig. 3): NO is a very lipophilic substance with a low molecular weight which quickly diffuses into tissue, reaching a balance between the rate of diffusion and the rate of NO oxidation or binding to target sites. Low doses of inhaled NO probably diffuse only into the vessels in their immediate proximity, i.e. capillaries of their "own", ventilated alveoli (Fig. 3, left side). Hence, with lower NO doses, there is a more or less "strictly selective" vasodilation in ventilated areas of the pulmonary vasculature, reducing intrapulmonary shunt and, thus, increasing systemic oxygenation. With higher NO doses, however, diffusion of the lipophilic NO through the lung tissue into non-ventilated areas, i.e. shunt areas, (Fig. 3, right side) still leads to a selective pulmonary vasodilation with further reduction of pulmonary resistance, but reversing the beneficial effect on oxygenation.

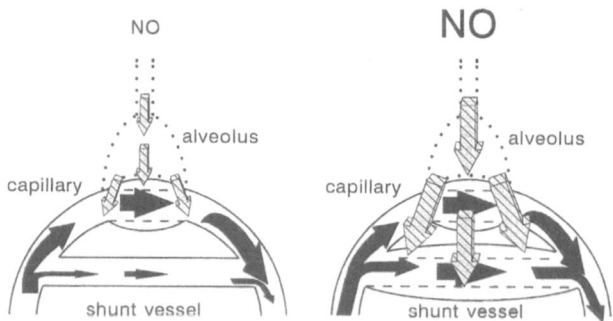

Fig. 3. Pathophysiologic model for the effect of low and high dose NO inhalation. The "diffusion theory": Low dose NO only diffuses in areas around the ventilated alveoli (left side), thus inducing relative reduction of shunt perfusion. High dose NO also diffuses to vessels of shunt areas (right side) and reduces the beneficial effect on systemic oxygenation. Both low and high dose NO reduce the total vascular resistance of the lung. (Modified from [65])

2) The "transport theory" (Fig. 4): This theory is based on the findings that NO binds to albumin and hemoglobin and, by this way, may be transported through the vessels before it affects other regions. The vascular system of the lung, in contrast to other organs like the liver, is strictly dichotomous. From the pulmonary artery to the end capillaries, each vessel divides in two smaller ones without transverse connections. Beyond the capillary bed, two vessels always re-join to a larger one, until the pulmonary veins are reached. This means that vessels of shunt (i.e. non-ventilated) areas and of areas with ideal ventilation/perfusion ratios are finally united in the pulmonary venous system. Hence, if NO is inhaled in low doses, it causes a low local concentration, and acts on the vascular smooth muscles of the vessel. Due to the low concentration, diffusion of NO into the intravascular space and binding to albumin and/or hemoglobin may not occur before the venous vessel re-joins with a shunt vessel, thus inducing vasodilation and an increase of the flow only in the ventilated area (Fig. 4, left side). If, however, high doses of NO are inhaled, intracapillary concentrations increase. Thus, NO may be transported to more distal regions, which might result in a decreased "after-load" for both ventilated and non-ventilated areas (Fig. 4, right side).

Although both theories currently remain speculative, the "diffusion theory" might be favored since NO is supposed to act on the vascular smooth muscle cell of the capillary before it is resorbed into the intravascular space. The marked reduction of pulmonary artery pressure by NO may also argue for the "diffusion theory", since the alveolar capillaries have few smooth muscle cells and the arteries and arterioles regulate pulmonary vascular resistance. How could NO get to the arteries if not by diffusion? If NO has to diffuse through the pulmonary tis-

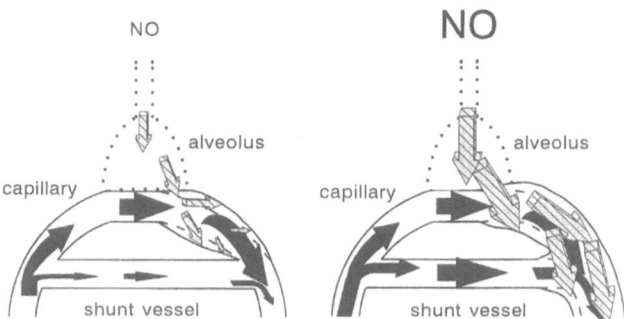

Fig. 4. Pathophysiologic model for the effect of low and high dose NO inhalation. The "transport theory": Low dose NO diffuses into the vascular smooth muscle cells before it is transported into the capillaries in higher concentrations. Therefore, NO is quickly inactivated in the venous system before shunt vessels are involved (left side), thus inducing relative reduction of shunt perfusion. High dose NO is also diffusing into the vessels. Here, it binds to albumin and/or hemoglobin. Transported by the blood stream NO remains active in venous vessels of shunt areas (right side). This reduces the beneficial effect of NO on systemic oxygenation. Both low and high dose NO reduce the total vascular resistance of the lung. (Modified from [65])

sue to achieve an effect, how is it possible to guarantee the selectivity for ventilated areas with low doses of NO? This might argue in favor of the "transport theory". Future studies must answer these questions; so far, the interesting dose-response characteristics of NO in patients with severe ARDS are an important feature which merit further attention to its clinical use.

NO Side Effect No 1: Bleeding Disorders

As demonstrated by several studies, inhalation of gaseous NO prolongs bleeding time in animals and healthy humans [17, 36], and inhibits platelet aggregation in patients with ARDS [37]. Additional case reports point out the possible danger of bleeding disorders during NO inhalation which might lead to a fatal outcome by intracerebral hemorrhage [38]. *In vitro*, NO released from endothelial cells inhibits platelet adhesion to endothelium [39], inhibits platelet aggregation [40], and has disaggregating properties [41]. Endogenous NO produced by a Ca^{2+} and NADPH-dependent cytosolic NOS via the L-arginine/NO-pathway down-regulates platelet aggregability. This was found to be an intra-platelet negative feedback mechanism which modulates platelet response after stimulation [5, 42]. Similar to its effect on smooth muscle cells, the inhibitory effect of NO on platelets is mediated through cGMP, which blocks phospho-inositide-pathway regulating phospholipase C, and indirectly increases cyclic adenosine monophosphate (cAMP) level by inhibiting cAMP-specific phosphodiesterase [43]. As a

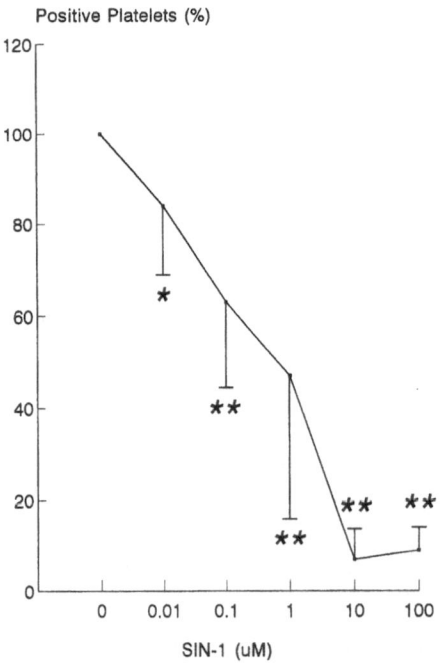

Fig. 5. Dose-dependent attenuation of GP IIb–IIIa activation by the NO donor SIN-1. Platelets were incubated with 0.01–100 μM SIN-1 and stimulated with 0.05 U/ml human α-thrombin. Positive platelets (PAC-FITC binding to activated GP IIb–IIIa) in percent from controls (* $p < 0.05$, ** $p < 0.01$, $n = 6$, mean ± SD). (Modified from [46])

result of the interaction of NO with intracellular signal transduction, platelet aggregation decreases by an inhibition of Ca^{2+} rise, release of granule contents, and phosphorylation of proteins [44]. Thus, NO plays an important role in regulation of vascular homeostasis by controlling vascular tone and platelet function.

Whereas NO-platelet interactions were intensively studied by numerous investigators using functional assays, measurement of secreted granule contents, ligand binding to receptors, and analysis of intra-platelet activation dependent metabolic pathways, few data exist about the effects of NO on platelet cell surface adhesion receptor expression during activation with α-thrombin, measured by flow cytometry [45]. We investigated the modulating effects of the NO releasing compound SIN-1 [46] on the availability of different functional platelet adhesion receptors by flow cytometry [47]. Using a specific antibody (PAC) against the acivated form of the fibrinogen receptor glycoprotein GP IIb–IIIa, it was demonstrated that SIN-1 inhibited on GP IIb–IIIa activation in a dose-dependent manner (Fig. 5). As an additional finding, the inhibition of α-thrombin induced platelet activation by SIN-1 was found up to 60 min after activation [47]. *In vivo*, NO inhalation may induce bleeding disorders by disaggregating platelets even when bleeding does not occur initially after surgical interventions. This is probably an important finding in terms of defining inclusion and exclusion criteria for future clinical studies with NO inhalation in ALI.

NO Side Effect No 2: Inhibition of Endogenous NOS

During several clinical trials, it was reported that patients need a special weaning procedure to terminate NO inhalation, especially after long-term treatment. In addition, rebound phenomena regarding both systemic oxygenation and pulmonary hypertension point to an increasing dependency of patients on inhaled NO [33]. These effects are probably due to a feedback inhibition of the endothelial NOS by the exogenously supplied NO. This was demonstrated *in vitro* using NO donors [48] as well as when using gaseous NO [49]. Thus, in ARDS patients vasoconstriction in the ventilated areas may occur after a sudden shut-off of NO, introducing the rebound phenomenon [49]. These findings, combined with other studies showing that the absolute level of pulmonary arterial pressure (PAP) is a marker for the severity of pulmonary microvascular injury in ARDS [50], and that pulmonary hypertension is associated with impaired NO production [51], confirm the hypothesis that even low doses of NO might reduce PAP in most severe cases of ALI [31–33]. In this condition endogenous NO production by the pulmonary vascular endothelium is considerably impaired. This was underlined by the observation that intravenous application of inhibitors of endogenous NOS was shown to increase systemic and pulmonary vascular resistance in septic patients with vasoplegia, but had little effect in ARDS patients who had been treated with NO inhalation for a longer time (unpublished data).

Effects versus Side Effects: Is NO Inhalation a Helpful Treatment?

Inhalation of NO appears to be an exciting advance in the treatment of ALI and pulmonary hypertension, and the rapidity with which this advance in basic science has gone from bench to bedside is truly breathtaking. Inhaled NO reduces PAP – a significant marker for severity and prognosis of ARDS – and increases arterial oxygenation. It selectively dilates vessels of ventilated lung areas and does not cause systemic vasodilation. Studies revealed that low dose NO inhalation might be considered as a replacement for the autoinhalation of endogenous gaseous NO, synthesized in the upper airways, which is interrupted in intubated patients. Other studies demonstrated that inhaled NO has an anti-inflammatory effect in ARDS patients – possibly another argument to use NO inhalation [52]. In conclusion, NO may be a cheap and safer alternative for more invasive strategies in the treatment of ARDS, e.g. veno-venous extracorporeal membrane oxygenation (vv-ECMO) [53, 54]!

The side effects of inhaled NO – increased bleeding disorders and inhibition of endogenous NOS causing rebound phenomena and weaning problems – cannot be neglected. So far, there is a general agreement that NO inhalation should be used at low doses in a range from 1–20 ppm, since higher doses confer no additional benefit [55, 56]. Furthermore, the improvement of systemic oxygenation and pulmonary hypertension by inhaled NO varies [57]. Interindividual variations have been interpreted in a contradictory manner: whereas two studies revealed that the NO effect on reduction of PAP was more prominent in patients with a higher baseline pulmonary vascular resistance [55, 56], another group claimed that the beneficial effect of NO was probably higher in patients with a better right ventricular output [58]. Some studies were performed to demonstrate additional or even synergistic effects of inhaled NO with other treatment strategies, e.g. surfactant therapy [54] or intravenous application of almitrine [59]. Finally, a direct comparison of inhaled NO and aerolized prostacyclin in ARDS patients revealed that individually titrated doses of NO and aerolized prostacyclin affect selective pulmonary vasodilation and redistribute blood flow from shunt areas to well-ventilated regions with nearly identical efficacy profiles [60].

So far, there are no studies published which are able to show that NO inhalation actually improves outcome. Most studies were performed with an uncontrolled protocol [53–58]. We first analyzed our own data retrospectively on the effect of NO inhalation [61]. 26 matched pairs were formed with respect to etiology and grade of ARDS, as well as to other organ failures, comparing patients with or without NO inhalation. The analysis revealed that there was a significant effect of NO inhalation on improvement of systemic oxygenation and pulmonary vascular resistance for all patients. However, only 60% of the NO-treated patients were really "responding" in terms of a PAP reduction (arbitrarily defined as a reduction of PAP of at least 3 mmHg). With respect to the clinical outcome, both the patients with or without NO inhalation had a survival rate of 69%, and no differences were found for the total time of ventilation or ICU stay [61]. Preliminary results of a first prospective, placebo-controlled, double-blinded multicenter clinical trial with 177 ARDS patients also supported the concept that low-dose inhaled NO can improve the hypoxemia associated with ARDS as well as lower the intensity of mechanical ventilation. The clinical outcome of the patients in both groups, however, was not significantly different [62].

We are currently performing a prospective, randomized, placebo-controlled monocenter clinical trial on the time-dependent dose-response, characteristics of long-term NO inhalation in patients with severe ARDS. The patients are evaluated according to a standard protocol. At the time of inclusion, no patient receives vv-ECMO. Patients are randomized after an initial dose-response analysis of NO, using inhalatory concentrations from 0.01 up to 100 ppm NO. The NO group receives a continuous inhalation of 10 ppm NO for at least 72 h, regardless of whether they were considered as "responders" or "non-responders" with respect to systemic oxygenation or pulmonary hypertension. Every day, the effect of the NO inhalation is controlled (on-off-on tests). After 72 h, a second dose-response curve is performed, as well as afterwards in a 72-h time course. In NO group dosing is continued until FiO_2 can be reduced to 0.4 while keeping PaO_2/FiO_2 higher than 60 mmHg under pressure-controlled ventilation with PEEP of ≤ 10 cmH$_2$O.

A first interim analysis after 20 patients (10 patients with, 10 patients without NO inhalation) revealed that the groups have no significant differences at time of inclusion with respect to the initial catastrophic event, hemodynamics, gas exchange, and other description parameters. The initial dose-response curves for the systemic oxygenation and reduction of pulmonary hypertension are more or less identical, demonstrating a peak effect for oxygenation at 10 ppm NO as described before [32]. In the following days, there was an overall tendency in terms of improving oxygenation and pulmonary hypertension. Interestingly, the data for PAP after 72 h demonstrate that a shut-off of NO results in a higher PAP baseline compared to the control group (Fig. 6), suggesting that the patients were sensitized by inhaled NO. Furthermore, the NO effect in the control group was no longer significant. This means that NO "treatment" is not really benefi-cial since PAP in the NO group during NO inhalation is not significantly differ-ent from the baseline PAP in the control group (Fig. 6). Hence, one might argue that, for reduction of PAP in ARDS patients, you can use NO inhalation or not!

Similar data were found for systemic oxygenation: compared to the control group, the initial reduction of FiO_2 in the NO group due to the positive effect of inhaled NO on systemic oxygenation is only significant on the day of inclusion (Fig. 7). Hence, the argument that NO inhalation makes it possible to reduce aggressive ventilation has to be doubted. Further studies are needed to clarify if this phenomenon is due to a feedback inhibition of endogenous NO synthesis by inhaled NO, or to a direct interaction of high oxygen concentrations with NO, possibly inducing toxic metabolites such as NO_2 or peroxynitrate. The outcome in terms of survival, ICU stay or ventilation days (regardless if for all or only for surviving patients) was identical in both groups. One interesting finding, however, was that patients in the NO group did not require any vv-ECMO, whereas 4 of the first 10 control patients fulfilled the inclusion criteria for vv-ECMO and required

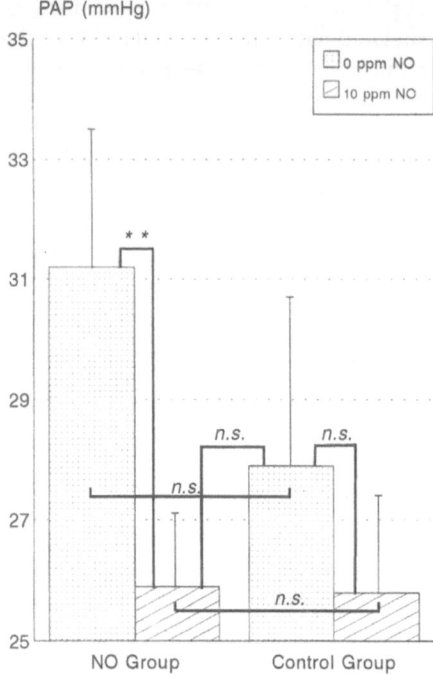

Fig. 6. Effect of a 10 ppm NO inhalation (20 min) on pulmonary arterial pressure (PAP) in ARDS patients (not treated with extracorporeal lung assist) who received a 3–day continuous NO inhalation with 10 ppm as an add-on therapy (NO Group) or were treated as usual (control Group; 3 patients who had to be connected to vv-ECMO within the first 72 h are excluded). In contrast to the data before randomization of the patients, NO inhalation did not have any significant effect within the control group, whereas the effect within the NO group was even more marked. Both groups had a similar PAP during NO inhalation, the "NO-off" value of the patients from the NO group was higher than from the control group (** $p < 0.01$, n.s. = not significant, two-sided paired (within the groups) and unpaired (between the groups) t-test, n = 10 (NO group), n = 7 (control group), mean ± SD

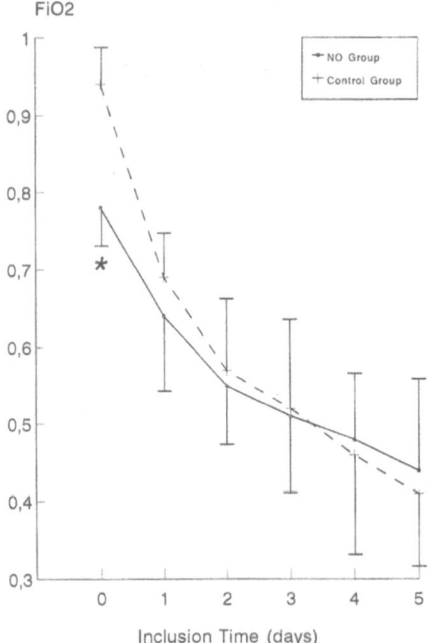

Fig. 7. Time course of FiO_2 in ARDS patients (not treated with extracorporeal lung assist) who received a continuous NO inhalation with 10 ppm as an add-on therapy (NO group) or were treated as usual (control group). The initial reduction of FiO_2 in patients from the NO group was no more significant after 24 h and during the following time

connection to an extracorporeal perfusion system ($p < 0.05$, Fisher's Exact Test). Although the total number of patients is very small, this indicates that NO inhalation might be considered as a useful bridging therapy to bypass more invasive and expensive strategies.

Conclusion

Inhalation of NO in patients with ALI or other forms of pulmonary hypertension seems to be a new, encouraging therapeutic concept, which, after performance of prospective randomized multicenter studies, might be able to lower mortality. However, the clinician has to bear in mind that, according to current results, NO does not necessarily have a beneficial effect for the patient. So far, there is no proof that NO inhalation improves the final outcome of ARDS patients. In addition, the reaction of the individual patient is not predictable. Trying different NO doses seems to be indicated; on the other hand, how can we guess if the best systemic oxygenation, or the most effective reduction of pulmonary resistance, or something in between is the optimal treatment for the patient? At the moment, definite statements about the physiological relevance of NO cannot be presented; however the rapid advance of NO science leads us to expect new developments every day. One important area for the future concerns the possible effects of NO inhalation on immunological and neurological functions, which must be investigated before NO inhalation can be accepted as a standard therapy for severe ARDS or other forms of pulmonary hypertension. Endogenous NO synthesis in the upper airways also merits further attention. Hence, NO inhalation in humans should only be performed following clear protocols and with caution [63].

Our recommendations for basic requirements of these protocols are the following:
1) Ethical requirements: So far, any form of NO inhalation is not a therapeutic trial but a clinical experiment. The Declaration of Helsinki, the rules for Good Clinical Practice, and the dictates of the hospitals ethical committee must be adhered to.
2) Evaluation of patients: Inclusion criteria depend on the individual protocol, i.e. whether patients with ALI, ARDS or pulmonary hypertension are studied. Repeated dose-response studies must be performed to identify "responders" and "non-responders". It has to be discussed before the study begins which NO dose should be used, e.g. a constant dose, or a variable dose based on the individual dose-response, and what is the "target" parameter, e.g. systemic oxygenation or pulmonary resistance.
3) NO/NO_2-measuring systems: For optimal patient safety, continuous measurement of NO and NO_2 must be guaranteed during inhalation. Electrochemical instruments with a sensitivity between 0.1 and 1 ppm are sufficient for long-term use. For dose-response studies, however, chemiluminescence instruments with a sensitivity up to 1 ppb are presupposed.

4) Storage of gases, environmental safety: NO gases must be stored according to the usual safety instructions which protect against tilting of the gas cylinders and control environmental NO concentrations in the patients' rooms by repeated measurements.

5) NO application systems: Self-made application systems without feedback controls and alarm systems have to be considered as dubious. Several systems are currently developed and offered commercially. These systems should be used in collaboration with the companies. If these systems are not available, NO inhalation should not be performed!

Acknowledgement. Supported by Deutsche Forschungsgesellschaft DFG, Grant No: Fa 139/4-1

References

1. Furchgott RF, Zawadzki JV (1980) The obligatory role of endothelial cells in the relaxation of arterial smooth muscle by acetylcholine. Nature 288:373–376
2. Palmer RM, Ashton DS, Moncada S (1988) Vascular endothelial cells synthesize nitric oxide from L-arginine. Nature 333:664–666
3. Vallance P, Collier J, Moncada S (1989) Effects of endothelium-derived nitric oxide on peripheral arteriolar tone in man. Lancet 2:997–1000
4. Marletta MA (1993) Nitric oxide synthase structure and mechanism. J Biol Chem 268: 12231–12234
5. Radomski MW, Palmer RM, Moncada S (1990) An L-arginine/nitric oxide pathway present in human platelets regulates aggregation. Proc Natl Acad Sci USA 87:5193–5197
6. Rand MJ (1992) Nitrergic transmission: Nitric oxide as a mediator of non-adrenergic, non-cholinergic neuro-effector transmission. Clin Exp Pharmacol Physiol 19:147–169
7. Geller DA, Nussler AK, Di SM, et al (1993) Cytokines, endotoxin, and glucocorticoids regulate the expression of inducible nitric oxide synthase in hepatocytes. Proc Natl Acad Sci USA 90:522–526
8. Xie QW, Cho HJ, Calaycay J, et al (1992) Cloning and characterization of inducible nitric oxide synthase from mouse macrophages. Science 256:225–228
9. Kobzik L, Bredt DS, Lowenstein CJ, et al (1993) Nitric oxide synthase in human and rat lung: Immunocytochenical and histochemical localization. Am J Respir Cell Mol Biol 9:371–377
10. Bredt DS, Hwang PM, Glatt CE, et al (1991) Cloned and expressed nitric oxide synthase structurally resembles cytochrome P-450 reductase. Nature 351:714–718
11. Nakane M, Schmidt HH, Pollock JS, et al (1993) Cloned human brain nitric oxide synthase is highly expressed in skeletal muscle. FEBS Lett 316:175–180
12. Janssens SP, Shimouchi A, Quertermous T, et al (1992) Cloning and expression of a cDNA encoding human endothelium-derived relaxing factor/nitric oxide synthase (published erratum appears in J Biol Chem 1992; 267:22694) J Biol Chem 267:14519–14522
13. Marsden PA, Schappert KT, Chen HS, et al (1992) Molecular cloning and characterization of human endothelial nitric oxide synthase. FEBS Lett 307:287–293
14. O'Dell TJ, Huang PL, Dawson TM, et al (1994) Endothelial NOS and the blockade of LTP by NOS inhibitors in mice lacking neuronal NOS. Science 265:542–546
15. Bolotina VM, Najibi S, Palacino JJ, et al (1994) Nitric oxide directly activates calcium-dependent potassium channels in vascular smooth muscle. Nature 368:850–853
16. Stamler JS, Jaraki O, Osborne J, et al (1992) Nitric oxide circulates in mammalian plasma primarily as an S-nitroso adduct of serum albumin. Proc Natl Acad Sci USA 89:7674–7677
17. Högman M, Frostell C, Arnberg H, Hedenstierna G (1993) Bleeding time prolongation and NO inhalation. Lancet 341:1664–1665

18. Zapol WJ, Snider MT (1977) Pulmonary hypertension in severe acute respiratory failure. N Engl J Med 296:476–480
19. Sibbald WJ, Driedger AA, Myers ML, Short AI, Wells GA (1983) Biventricular function in the adult respiratory distress syndrome. Chest 84:126–134
20. Suchyta MR, Clemmer TP, Orme JFJ, Morris AH, Elliott CG (1991) Increased survival of ARDS patients with severe hypoxemia (ECMO criteria). Chest 99:951–955
21. Radermacher P, Santak B, Becker H, Falke KJ (1989) Prostaglandin E1 and nitroglycerin reduce pulmonary capillary pressure but worsen ventilation-perfusion distributions in patients with adult respiratory distress syndrome. Anesthesiology 70:601–606
22. Oda H, Nogami H, Kusumoto S, Nakajima T, Kurata A, Imai K (1976) Long-term exposure to nitric oxide in mice. J Jpn Soc Air Pollut 11:150–160
23. Hugod C (1979) Effect of exposure to 43 ppm nitric oxide and 3.6 ppm nitrogen dioxide on rabbit lung. Int Arch Occup Environ Health 42:159–167
24. Higenbottam T, Pepke-Zaba J, Scott J, Woolman P, Coutts C, Wallwork J (1988) Inhaled "endothelium-derived relaxing factor" (EDRF) in primary hypertension. Am Rev Respir Dis 137:107 A (Abstr)
25. Pepke-Zaba J, Higenbottam TW, Dinh-Xuan AT, Stone D, Wallwork J (1991) Inhaled nitric oxide as a cause of selective pulmonary vasodilation in pulmonary hypertension. Lancet 338:1173–1174
26. Frostell C, Fratacci MD, Wain JC, Jones R, Zapol WM (1991) Inhaled nitric oxide. A selective pulmonary vasodilator reversing hypoxic pulmonary vasoconstriction. Circulation 83:2038–2047
27. Pison U, Lopez FA, Heidelmeyer CF, Rossaint R, Falke K (1993) Inhaled nitric oxide selectively reverses hypoxic pulmonary vasoconstriction without impairing pulmonary gas exchange. J Appl Physiol 74:7287–7292
28. Roberts JD, Polander DM, Lang P, Zapol WM (1992) Inhaled nitric oxide in persistent pulmonary hypertension of the newborn. Lancet 340:818–819
29. Kinsella JP, Neish SR, Shaffer E, Abman SH (1992) Low-dose inhalational nitric oxide in persistent pulmonary hypertension of the newborn. Lancet 340:819–820
30. Falke KJ, Rossaint R, Pison U, et al (1991) Inhaled nitric oxide selectively reduces pulmonary hypertension in severe ARDS and improves gas exchange as well as right heart ejection fraction: A case report. Am Rev Respir Dis 143 (Suppl):A248 (Abstr)
31. Rossaint R, Falke KJ, Lopez F, Slama K, Pison U, Zapol WM (1993) Inhaled nitric oxide in adult respiratory distress syndrome. N Engl J Med 328:399–405
32. Gerlach H, Rossaint R, Pappert D, Falke KJ (1993) Time-course and dose-response of nitric oxide inhalation for systemic oxygenation and pulmonary hypertension in patients with adult respiratory distress syndrome. Eur J Clin Invest 23:499–502
33. Gerlach H, Pappert D, Lewandowski K, Rossaint R, Falke KJ (1993) Long-term inhalation with evaluated low doses of nitric oxide for selective improvement of oxygenation in patients with adult respiratory distress syndrome. Intensive Care Med 19:443–449
34. Gustafsson LE, Leone AM, Persson MG (1991) Endogenous nitric oxide is present in the exhaled air of rabbits, guinea pigs and humans. Biochem Biophys Res Commun 181:852–857
35. Gerlach H, Rossaint R, Pappert D, Knorr M, Falke KJ (1994) Autoinhalation of nitric oxide after endogenous synthesis in nasopharynx. Lancet 343:518–519
36. Högman M, Frostell C, Arnberg H, Sandhagen B, Hedenstierna G (1994) Prolonged bleeding time during nitric oxide inhalation in the rabbit. Acta Physiol Scand 151:125–129
37. Samama CM, Diaby M, Fellahi JL, et al (1995) Inhibition of platelet aggregation by inhaled nitric oxide in patients with acute respiratory distress syndrome. Anesthesiology 83:56–65
38. Joannidis M, Buratti T, Pechlaner C, Wiedermann C (1996) Inhaled nitric oxide. Lancet 348:1448–1449
39. Radomski MW, Vallance P, Whitley G, Foxwell N, Moncada S (1993) Platelet adhesion to human vascular endothelium is modulated by constitutive and cytokine-induced nitric oxide. Cardiovasc Res 27:1380–1382
40. Furlong B, Henderson AH, Lewis MJ, Smith JA (1987) Endothelium-derived relaxing factor inhibits in vitro platelet aggregation. Br J Pharmacol 90:687–692

41. Radomski MW, Palmer RM, Moncada S (1987) The anti-aggregating properties of vascular endothelium: Interactions between prostacyclin and nitric oxide. Br J Pharmacol 92: 639–646

42. Radomski MW, Palmer RM, Moncada S (1990) Characterization of the L-arginine/nitric oxide pathway in human platelets. Br J Pharmacol 101:325–328

43. Maurice DH, Haslam RJ (1990) Molecular basis of the synergistic inhibition of platelet function by nitrovasodilators and activators of adenylate cyclase: Inhibition of cyclic AMP breakdown by cyclic GMP. Mol Pharmacol 37:671–681

44. Nguyen BL, Saitoh M, Ware AJ (1991) Interaction of nitric oxide and cGMP with signal transduction in activated platelets. Am J Physiol 261:H1043–H1052

45. Michelson AD, Benoit SE, Furman MI, et al (1996) Effects of nitric oxide/EDRF on platelet glycoproteins. Am J Physiol 270:H1640–H1648

46. Gerzer R, Karrenbrock B, Siess W, Heim JM (1988) Direct comparison of the effects of nitroprusside, SIN-1, and various nitrates on platelet aggregation and soluble guanylate cyclase activity. Thromb Res 52:11–21

47. Keh D, Gerlach M, K rer I, et al (1996) The effects of nitric oxide (NO) on platelet membrane receptor expression during activation with human α-thrombin. Blood Coag Fibrinol 7: 615–624

48. Assreuy J, Cunha FQ, Liew FY, Moncada S (1993) Feedback inhibition of nitric oxide synthase activity by nitric oxide. Br J Pharmacol 108:833–837

49. Kiff RJ, Moss DW, Moncada S (1994) Effect of nitric oxide gas on the generation of nitric oxide by isolated blood vessels: Implications for inhalation therapy. Br J Pharmacol 113:496–498

50. Villar J, Blazquez MA, Lubilio S, Quintana J, Manzano JL (1989) Pulmonary hypertension in acute respiratory failure. Crit Care Med 17:523–526

51. Dinh-Xuan AT, Higenbottam TW, Clelland CA, et al (1991) Impairment of endothelium-dependent pulmonary-artery relaxation in chronic obstructive lung disease. N Engl J Med 324:1539–1547

52. Chollet-Martin S, Gatecel C, Kermarrec N, Gougerot-Pocidalo MA, Payen DM (1996) Alveolar neutrophil functions and cytokine levels in patients with the adult respiratory distress syndrome during nitric oxide inhalation. Am J Respir Crit Care Med 153:985–990

53. Levy B, Bollaert PE, Bauer P, Nace L, Audibert G, Larcan A (1995) Therapeutic optimization including inhaled nitric oxide in adult respiratory distress syndrome in a polyvalent intensive care unit. J Trauma 38:370–374

54. Moller JC, Schaible TF, Reiss I, Artlich A, Gortner L (1995) Treatment of severe non-neonatal ARDS in children with surfactant and nitric oxide in a "pre-ECMO"-situation. Int J Artif Organs 18:598–602

55. Lowson SM, Rich GF, McArdle PA, Jaidev J, Morris GN (1996) The response to varying concentrations of inhaled nitric oxide in patients with acute respiratory distress syndrome. Anesth Analg 82:574–581

56. Bigatello LM, Hurford WE, Kacmarek RM, Roberts JD Jr, Zapol WM (1994) Prolonged inhalation of low concentrations of nitric oxide in patients with severe adult respiratory distress syndrome. Effects on pulmonary hemodynamics and oxygenation. Anesthesiology 80: 761–770

57. McIntyre RC Jr, Moore FA, Moore EE, Piedalue F, Haenel JS, Fullerton DA (1995) Inhaled nitric oxide variably improves oxygenation and pulmonary hypertension in patients with acute respiratory distress syndrome. J Trauma 39:418–425

58. Krafft P, Fridrich P, Fitzgerald RD, Koch D, Steltzer H (1996) Effectiveness of nitric oxide inhalation in septic ARDS. Chest 109:486–493

59. Wysocki M, Delclaux C, Roupie E, et al (1994) Additive effect on gas exchange of inhaled nitric oxide and intravenous almitrine bismesylate in the adult respiratory distress syndrome. Intensive Care Med 20:254–259

60. Walmrath D, Schneider T, Schermuly R, Olschewski H, Grimminger F, Seeger W (1996) Direct comparison of inhaled nitric oxide and aerolized prostacyclin in acute respiratory distress syndrome. Am J Respir Crit Care Med 153:991–996

61. Rossaint R, Gerlach H, Schmidt-Runke H, et al (1995) Efficacy of inhaled nitric oxide in patients with severe ARDS. Chest 107:1107–1115

62. Dellinger RP, Zimmerman JL, Hyers TM, et al (1996) Inhaled nitric oxide in ARDS: Preliminary results of a multicenter clinical trial. Crit Care Med 24:A7 (Abst)
63. Warren JB, Higenbottam T (1996) Caution with use of inhaled nitric oxide. Lancet 348:629
64. Gerlach H, Falke KJ (1995) The therapeutic role of nitric oxide in adult respiratory distress syndrome. Curr Anaesth Crit Care 6:10-16
65. Gerlach H, Falke KJ (1997) Low levels of inhaled nitric oxide in acute lung injury. In: Zapol WM, Bloch KD (eds.) Lung Biology in Health and Disease, Vol. 98. Nitric Oxide and the Lung. Marcel Dekker, New York, Basel, Hong Kong, pp 271-283

Pharmacological Modifications of the Pulmonary Circulation in ALI

D. Payen

Introduction

The clinical implications of pharmacologically modifying the pulmonary circulation concern both anesthesiology and intensive care. Anesthetic drugs frequently alter the pulmonary vasomotor tone directly via a direct action in vascular contraction but also indirectly by the central effect on neurogenic control. Critical illness, including acute lung injury (ALI) often leads to modifications of pulmonary vascular tone associated with alteration in vascular contractility [1–3]. In addition, therapeutic agents with vasoactive properties alter vascular tone and physiologic control mechanisms, such as hypoxic pulmonary vasoconstriction (HPV) [4]. In this chapter, we will review the effects of some drugs acting on pulmonary vascular tone which may affect gas exchange, especially PaO_2.

Physiological Background

For the clinician, the most popular parameter to assess the pulmonary vascular tone is the pulmonary vascular resistance (PVR), calculated as the direct ratio between pulmonary driving pressure and pulmonary blood flow (PBF), according to the Poiseuille law. However this approach has some limitations since it implies several assumptions which are not valid in human physiology. To be valid, the hydrodynamic equivalent of Ohm's law for electricity should be applied to rigid tubes with a fixed circular cross section, laminar flow, and a Newtonian fluid (i.e. a constant viscosity). Each of these conditions are violated by blood flowing through the pulmonary vascular bed, as evidenced by the non-linear relationship between pressure and flow. As a consequence, PVR (taken as the slope of the pressure-flow curve) varies in numerous conditions since: 1) the pulmonary vessels are viscoelastic and non-rigid, with a large compliance. This pliability accounts for the relatively large diameter variations which occur in response to changing intraluminal pressure, and 2) the pulmonary vessels are collapsible (and recruitable), defining a Starling resistor with a critical closure pressure. This later concept is of particular importance when an increase in the vessels' surrounding pressure is able to compress the vessel, as during positive pressure breathing.

Finally, it is difficult to accurately measure back pressure for PBF. This pressure can be estimated as the pulmonary artery occlusion pressure measured by a triple lumen catheter, but this pressure might be erroneous and/or difficult to measure during mechanical ventilation leading to a miscalculation of PVR.

The alternative is to use the pulmonary pressure-flow relationship which is characterized by a curvature to the pressure axis. Extrapolation of this curve allows a derivation of a mean critical pressure. In this concept, the curvature is due to the distensibility of vessels rather than a vascular recruitment. It is then useful to describe the more linear part of the curve by a slope and its intercept with the pressure ordinate [5–8].

Ventilation-Perfusion Ratio (VA/Q) and Hypoxic Pulmonary Vasoconstriction (HPV)

Since the predominant concern of respiratory intensive care is to simultaneously achieve adequate pulmonary gas exchange and stable hemodynamics, the pathophysiology and the pharmacology of the relationship between gas exchange and pulmonary blood flow is crucial [9].

The distribution of ventilation-perfusion (VA/Q) ratios has been characterized since the 1940s by the three-compartment model: venous admixture, dead space, and ideal VA/Q ratio. More recently, it has been improved by the use of a sophisticated 50-compartment mathematical model derived using 6 inert gases [10]. Such a concept is of particular importance to analyze the effects of vasoactive drugs and/or inhaled therapies on the flow component of this ratio.

Hypoxic pulmonary vasoconstriction (HPV) offers a defense against aveolar hypoxia. This phenomenon corresponds to the observed increase in pulmonary artery pressure during hypoxia resulting from pulmonary vasoconstriction. Although in the adult HPV might be only a vestigial memory of the fetal response, most investigators accept the explanation that HPV reduces the flow of desaturated blood through underventilated areas of lungs, improving VA/Q mismatching and then PaO_2. According to the mechanisms of HPV which are only partially understood, therapeutic interventions on the pulmonary vascular bed may have important positive or negative effects on gas exchange.

The basic mechanism of HPV is located in vascular smooth muscle and can be modulated by endogenous substances. Two different phases of HPV can be detected according to the time response: Phase 1 occurs early after hypoxia independently of endothelium, and phase 2 starts later, lasts longer and is endothelium-dependent. However, one has to recognize that the strength of HPV varies with age and species. The following 3 stimuli can activate HPV separately or in conjunction: alveolar hypoxia, mixed venous oxygen tension, and arterial oxygen tension [7, 11].

In addition to this, the reported variability in response also depends on the size of the effective hypoxic lung segment [12], and the influence of intravascular pressure [13]. The predominant reduction in blood flow when the atelectatic component is small becomes less apparent as more lung is involved. When the entire lung is involved as in severe ARDS, it becomes impossible to divert blood flow to another region, and the only available response is a rise in pulmonary artery pressure. In this case, despite a similar stimulus of HPV, the response in term of arterial oxygenation is different. Considering gas exchange, the diversion of blood flow from hypoxic to less hypoxic regions improves gas exchange. The size of hypoxic segment is therefore an important determinant of the overall response and effectiveness of HPV.

Since the pulmonary vessels are thin-walled, a narrowing by active constriction can be reexpanded to the limited diameter by appropriately increased transmural pressures. Then, the initial HPV is opposed by the increased pressure, causing normoxic and hypoxic curves to become closer. As a consequence, an increase in left atrial pressure impairs the HPV-induced partitioning of blood flow. One can understand that HPV limitation or inhibition by the therapy may have detrimental effects on gas exchange, since the very low VA/Q leads to a major worsening of PaO_2 unbuffered by HPV. The consequence of such HPV limitation may also have a different impact according to the homogeneity of the remaining lung. In acute pneumonia, HPV can effectively divert blood flow from poorly ventilated areas, improving VA/Q matching. However there is evidence that HPV is impaired in acute infection and/or inflammation, [1, 3] leading to disproportional increases in shunt in this condition. In addition, numerous mediators may alter pulmonary vascular tone. Therefore, according to the specific status of the remaining lung parenchyma (normal or abnormal), the impact of HPV might be quite different in terms of PaO_2 correction.

From HPV Mechanism to Pharmacology

To better understand the impacts of pharmalogic agents on the pulmonary circulation and their consequences for gas exchange, it might be useful to list the substances and or mediators involved in this mechanism and to try to clarify the cellular mechanism governing HPV. In this respect, serotonin, angiotensin, prostaglandins (PG) and leukotrienes have been proposed to mediate HPV, since they have been shown to be released by endothelial and mast cells during hypoxia. In fact, these substances are actually considered more as HPV-modulators than as direct mediators [5, 8]. Similarly, innervation and vasoactive susbstances also have important influences on the amplitude of HPV, but the basic response persists even when stimuli are removed.

Concerning the sensor for HPV, cytochrome P450 has been proposed as the trigger of HPV. However recent data indicate that cytochrome P450 inhibition does not alter the HPV response [14].

Endogenous NO is normally released by the pulmonary circulation, accounting for the resting low vascular tone of the pulmonary circulation. It has been proposed that HPV may result from an inhibition of nitric oxide (NO) synthesis during hypoxia. In isolated perfused lung models and in *in vivo* experimental situations [15], NO release is amplified during hypoxia, modulating HPV. NO synthase inhibitors are also able to reinforce HPV and to increase the regional conductance gradient associated with an improvement in VA/Q and PaO_2 [16]. Consequently, it is unlikely that HPV would be the result of an inhibition of NO synthesis or activity. However, based on this concept, inhibition of NO synthesis might be a way to enhance the conductance gradient in hypoxic situations with low VA/Q zones, as observed in patients with ARDS or ALI.

At the cellular level, the proposed mechanisms of HPV mainly concern Ca^{2+} and K^+ channels. Calcium enters the pulmonary vascular smooth muscle cell early in HPV through voltage-dependent calcium channels (VOC). The evidence for this statement is that calcium channel blockers inhibit [17], and calcium channel agonists enhance, HPV [18]. In addition, removal of calcium from the perfusate inhibits HPV in ferret or cat lungs. The calcium entry through VOC initiates the rise in smooth muscle cytosolic calcium caused by hypoxia. Then it may trigger the release of additional calcium from intracellular stores such as sarcoplasmic reticulum.

If we remember that VOC follows the depolarization of the membrane, what initiates such a depolarization? The role of K^+ channels are important in the control of smooth muscle membrane potential [8]. An outward potassium current promotes hyperpolarization and thus opposes calcium entry. Consequently, agents blocking such a K^+ channel will increase pulmonary constriction. Then, it is reasonable to propose that hypoxia inhibits such outward potassium channels, causing membrane depolarization, thus permitting the entry of calcium. A redox mechanism can influence potassium current in pulmonary vascular smooth muscle. Both hypoxia or glycolytic pathway inhibitors make the cytosol more reduced and induce a pulmonary vasoconstriction. One can then accept that hypoxia and the metabolic inhibitors may alter the gating of one or more potassium channels through changes in redox.

One can then expect an inhibition of HPV when calcium channel blockers are used for several reasons in ALI. The augmentation of venous admixture can occur, amplifying hypoxia. In a similar way, potassium channel blockers such as nicorandil can induce similar negative effects on gas exchange.

Pharmacologically Active Drugs on HPV

The use of drugs targeted to the pulmonary vascular bed might have different effects according to their route of administration [8]. The intravenous route allows the drug to reach the entire pulmonary circulatory bed, including the vessels of the poorly ventilated zones. Since the effect is non-selective, this might have positive or detrimental consequences in relation to the vascular tone modification [19]. For example, intravenously given prostacyclin (PGI_2) vasodilates the entire pulmonary vascular bed, resulting in a worsening of gas exchange in the presence of low VA/Q zones [20]. Conversely, the inhalation route appears suitable to restrict pulmonary vascular effects to well aerated zones, leading to the concept of selected vasodilation. The application of PGI_2 seems to be promising in this respect [20] since the intravenous dose of the drug might be reduced, avoiding and/or limiting the spillover into the systemic circulation.

Taking into account the pathophysiology of ALI and the more recent pharmacologic developments, this chapter will concentrate on the new aspects and new possibilities for therapeutic interventions concerning the pulmonary vascular bed. Three major systems have to be detailed with their proven or potential pharmacologic implications: endothelins, nitric oxide, and PGs.

Endothelins

Three similar but distinct endothelin 21 amino acid peptides (ET-1, ET-2, ET-3) are produced by endothelial cells after a cleavage of a prepropeptide via a propeptide. The conversion is mediated by an endothelin converting enzyme (ECE). ETs are not stored but synthesized *de novo* under various stimuli: shear stress, hypoxia, endotoxin, tumor necrosis factor (TNF)-α, epinephrine, angiotensin, thrombin, etc. ET induces smooth muscle contraction via several secondary messengers, the final pathway being an increase in intracellular calcium.

Two ET receptor subtypes have so far been cloned and expressed: ETA and ETB. ETA (not found on endothelial cells) mediates vasoconstriction, whereas ETB receptor stimulates the release of other substances. ET-1 is a potent vasconstrictor via direct ETA stimulation. There is now clear evidence that ET release stimulates NO release from the endothelial cells by ETB receptors, explaining the initial hypotension observed early after ET injection. This effect is blunted by NO synthase (NOS) inhibitors. ET-1 seems also to stimulate the release of PGI2 and thromboxane from endothelial cells. ET-1 is largely removed from the blood by the lung and its half life is close to 40 sec.

Normobaric hypoxia stimulates ET-1 gene expression, whilst hypoxia stimulates ET release in cultured bovine endothelial cells. ET-1 and ET-3 have both vasoconstricting and vasodilating properties in the rat lung [21] and can reverse the HPV response in isolated lungs, an effect unmodified by indomethacin or glibenclamide but attenuated by L-NMMA. More probably, ET-1 is not involved in the HPV response.

However, even if ET does not play any role in HPV, hypoxia not only stimulates ET release but alters its functional properties.

Prostaglandins

Arachidonic acid metabolites involve different biochemical pathways: cyclooxygenase (COX) produces prostaglandins (PG)s, lipoxygenase (LOX) forms leukotrienes. COX is known to exist in two isoforms: COX-1 is constitutive whereas COX-2 is induced by cytokines. Such a concept has direct implications in ALI, which concerns the acutely inflamed lung. It is thought that COX-2 predominates at the site of inflammation. The lung is the main generating site of prostanoids released during septic shock. Such a concept has led to the development of nonsteroidal anti-inflammatory drugs which specifically inhibit this isoform [22].

The relative importance of arachidonic acid derivatives in the vasomotor response to hypoxia appears to vary between species and vascular preparations.

Prostanoid inhibition by indomethacin augments HPV, whereas infusions of arachidonic acid decrease HPV and increase PGI_2 formation. In contrast, different non-steroidal anti-inflammatory drugs (NSAID) increase the contraction induced by hypoxia in human isolated arteries [23]. A recent study in an ovine ARDS model failed, however, to demonstrate any effect of $PGF_{2\alpha}$ to supplemental shift of pulmonary blood flow away from hypoxic zones. In this model $PGF_{2\alpha}$ essentially induced a global pulmonary vasoconstriction centered at the large pulmonary vessel level and reduced pulmonary blood flow [24].

Nitric Oxide and Pulmonary Vascular Tone

Since many chapters concern NO in ALI, only the most important aspects related to the pulmonary vasculature in ALI will be discussed. It is only recently that the role of endogenous release of NO in HPV has been demonstrated [15, 25]. In isolated perfused lungs, the administration of NOS inhibitors during ventilation with a hypoxic gas mixture augments the increase in pulmonary arterial pressure, suggesting that NO release may attenuate HPV. An impact of endogenous NOS on VA/Q matching has been well demonstrated in an anesthetized rabbit model by Sprague et al. [15]. The authors hypothesized that NO release by the lung would oppose regional HPV and support blood flow to hypoxic lung units, thereby decreasing PaO_2. Rabbit lungs were separately ventilated *in vivo* with unilateral alveolar hypoxia. The administration of a NOS inhibitor resulted in a dose-dependent reduction in the intrapulmonary distribution of the blood flow to hypoxic alveoli and in a concomitant increase in PaO_2. This effect was reversed by infusion of L-arginine, a NOS substrate. Moreover, this *in vivo* study demonstrated that significant intrapulmonary redistribution of blood flow away from hypoxic alveoli can occur in the absence of any change in pulmonary arterial pressure. These results strongly suggest that endogenous NOS present in the lung during alveolar hypoxia acts to oppose HPV.

The relatively frequent observation of an amplified pulmonary hypertension after NO inhibition by L-NMMA in septic patients confirms the importance of NO in the regulation of the pulmonary vascular tone in human beings during acute inflammation. Although little is known about the origin of NO (constitutive and/or inducible NOS), NO seems important to limit the pulmonary vasoconstriction observed in sepsis. However, if selective, blocking of NO might be effective. The reduction of flow in hypoxic zones will only improve the partition of flow and the VA/Q matching. Altough it is difficult to accomplish practically, it to combining intravenous NOS inhibitors and inhaled NO to limit the vasoconstriction to the non-ventilated area could be proposed. Improvement in VA/Q can then be expected if NO inhibition is able to constrict hypoxic vessels. Until now no data have been published confirming such as hypothesis.

A similar idea has been developed and tested in the past years with another compound called almitrine [26, 27]. Based on its pharmacological properties, almitrine has been used to reinforce HPV and/or to vasconstrict small pulmonary vessels. Although the mechanism by which hypoxia is sensed remains uncertain, it has been suggested that O_2 tension is detected in the vasculature through its effects on energy status, as reflected by the concentrations of high energy phosphates such as ATP [28, 29]. It has been shown in beef heart and in rat liver mitochondria [28, 29], that almitrine may influence energy metabolism such as oxidative phosphorylation. In aerobic organisms, this process is the major source of ATP formed, as electrons are transferred from NADH to O_2 through a series of electron carriers. It is carried out by respiratory assemblies that are located in the inner membrane of mitochondria. Almitrine inhibits ATP synthesis or impairs electron transport downstream from rotenone blocking site, localized in the NADH-cytochrome-Q reductase complex. These actions may correspond to the locus of hypoxic sensing [30] where the signal may be generated by ATP reduction in a distinct cellular compartment, as recently showed by Archer et al. [28] in the pulmonary vasculature.

In summary, almitrine is a large molecular weight lipophilic compound which stimulates the carotid body and improves ventilation-perfusion inequality by a direct action on the pulmonary vessels and the carotid body chemoreceptor. The observed strong similarities between the effects of almitrine and hypoxia suggest a similar mechanism of action, possibly through oxidative phosphorylation at the mitochondrial level. The observed benefit on PaO_2 has been related to the pulmonary vasoconstrictor effect of the drug. The dose range seems to be crucial since at low doses (< 10 mcg/kg/min), almitrine reinforces or restores HPV, whereas at higher doses the drug has no effect, or dilates pulmonary vessels. Interindividual differences in the magnitude of HPV response exist in humans, and minimal or no response has been recorded in selected patients. The effect of almitrine on HPV restoration is thus extremely attractive to improve VA/Q inequalities. Although the molecular mechanisms remain unknown, the use of such a drug as a continuous IV infusion seems to be effective. However, the benefit/ risk ratio has to be considered. In the acute situation in which we propose to use almitrine, short-term IV administration of low doses would probably limit the risk of sensory peripheral neuropathy.

Clinical Impact of Pharmacological Modifications of the Pulmonary Vascular Bed

The initial demonstration of the benefit of a combination of HPV reinforcement and NO inhalation in ARDS [31] has stimulated clinicians to test this in a larger population [32, 33]. The initial results demonstrated a larger increase in PaO_2 when NO inhalation and intravenous almitrine were associated. This strategy has been impressive in patients who are responding poorly to each drug separately [26]. Interestingly, the association of these two agents allows control of the pulmonary pressure elevation induced by almitrine, avoiding or limiting any resultant deterioration of right ventricular function.

Conclusion

The ability of NO to improve oxygenation should be enhanced when it is combined with infused vasoconstrictor judiciously selected. As Marshall et al. [7] concluded, "a clinical trial of such a combination is clearly warranted, which in fact may already have inadvertently been the basis for some reported successes with NO".

References

1. Graham L, Vasil A, Vasil M, Voelkel N, Stenmark K (1990) Decreased pulmonary vasoreactivity in an animal model of chronic *Pseudomonas* pneumonia. Am Rev Respir Dis 142: 221–229
2. Spaden H, Vincken W (1987) Pulmonary arterial hypertension in sepsis and the adult respiratory distress syndrome. Acta Clin Belg 47:30–40
3. Reeves J, Grover R (1974) Blockade of acute hypoxic pulmonary hypertension by endotoxin. J Appl Physiol 36:328–332
4. Light R (1996) Effect of sodium nitroprusside and diethylcarbamazine on hypoxic pulmonary vasoconstriction and regional distribution of pulmonary blood flow in experimental pneumonia. Am J Respir Crit Care Med 153:325–330
5. Voelkel N (1986) Mechanisms of hypoxic pulmonary vasoconstriction. Am Rev Respir Dis 133:1186–1195
6. Marshall B, Marshall C, Frasch F, Hanson C (1994) Role of hypoxic pulmonary vasoconstriction in pulmonary gas exchange and blood flow distribution. Intensive Care Med 20: 291–297
7. Marshall B, Hanson C, Frasch F, Marshall C (1994) Role of hypoxic pulmonary vasoconstriction in pulmonary gas exchange and blood flow distribution. Intensive Care Med 20:379–389
8. Weir E, Archer S (1995) The mechanism of acute hypoxic pulmonary vasoconstriction: The tale of two channels. FASEB J 9:183–189
9. West J (1977) Ventilation/blood flow and gas exchange. Blackwell Scientific Publications
10. Wagner P, Saltzman H, West J (1974) Measurement of continuous distribution of ventilation-perfusion ratios: Theory. J Appl Physiol 36:588–599
11. Payen D, Carli P, Brun-Buisson C, et al (1985) Lower body positive pressure versus dopamine during PEEP ventilation. J Appl Physiol 58:77–82
12. Marshall B, Marshall C (1980) Continuity of response to hypoxic pulmonary vasoconstriction. J Appl Physiol 49:189–196
13. Benumof J, Wahrenbrock E (1975) Blunted hypoxic pulmonary vasoconstriction by increased lung vascular pressures. J Appl Physiol 38:846–850
14. Chang S, Dutton D, Wang H, et al (1992) Intact lung cytochrome P-450 is not required for hypoxic pulmonary vasconstriction. Am J Physiol 263:L446–L453
15. Sprague R, Thiemermann C, Vane J (1992) Endogenous endothelium-derived relaxing factor opposes hypoxic pulmonary vasoconstriction and supports blood flow to hypoxic alveoli in anesthetized rabbits. Proc Natl Acad Sci USA 89:8711–8715
16. Mazmanian G, Baudet B, Brink C, et al (1989) Methylene blue potentiates vascular reactivity in isolated rat lungs. J Appl Physiol 66:1040–1045
17. McMurtry I, Davidson B, Reeves J, Grover R (1976) Inhibition of hypoxic pulmonary vasoconstriction by calcium antagonists in isolated perfused rat. Circ Res 38:99–104
18. McMurtry I (1985) Bay K 8644 potentiates and A 23 187 inhibits hypoxic vasoconstriction in rat lungs. Am J Physiol 249:H741–H746
19. Curzen N, Jourdan K, Mitchell J (1996) Endothelial modification of pulmonary vascular tone. Intensive Care Med 22:596–607

20. Scheeren T, Radermacher P (1997) Prostacyclin (PGI2): New aspects of an old substance in the treatment of critically ill patients. Intensive Care Med 23:146–158
21. Kourembanas S, Marsden P, McQuillan L, Faller D (1991) Hypoxia induces endothelin gene expression and secretion in cultured human endothelium. J Clin Invest 88:1054–1057
22. Masferrer JL, Zweifel BS, Manning PT, et al (1994) Selective inhibition of inducible cyclo-oxygenase 2 *in vivo* is anti-inflammatory and non-ulcerogenic. Proc Natl Acad Sci USA 91:3228–3232
23. Demiryurek A, Wadsworth R, Kane K, Peacock A (1993) The role of the endothelium in hypoxic constriction of human pulmonary artery rings. Am Rev Respir Dis 147:283–290
24. Kobayashi H, Tanaka N, Winkler M, Zapol W (1996) Combined effects of NO inhalation and intravenous PGF2α on pulmonary circulation and gas exchange in an ovine ARDS model. Intensive Care Med 22:656–663
25. Persson MG, Gustafsson LE, Wiklund NP, Hedqvist P, Moncada S (1990) Endogenous nitric oxide as a modulator of rabbit skeletal muscle microcirculation *in vivo*. Br J Pharmacol 100:463–466
26. Payen D, Gatecel C, Kermarrec N, Beloucif S (1997) Almitrine and inhaled nitric oxide in acute respiratory failure. In: Zapol W, Bloch K (eds) Nitric oxide and the lungs. Marcel Dekker, New York, Basel, Hong Kong, pp 313–332
27. Laubie M, Diot F (1972) A pharmacological study of the respiratory stimulant action of S 2620. J Pharmacol 3:363–374
28. Archer S, Huang J, Henry T, Peterson D, Weir E (1993) A redox-based O_2 sensor in rat pulmonary vasculature. Circ Res 73:1100–1112
29. Rounds S, Mc Murtry I (1981) Inhibitors of oxidative ATP production cause transient vasoconstriction and block subsequent pressor responses in rat lungs. Circ Res 48:393–400
30. Romaldini H, Rodriguez-Roisin R, Wagner P, West J (1983) Enhancement of hypoxic pulmonary vasoconstriction by almitrine in the dog. Am Rev Respir Dis 128:288–293
31. Payen D, Gatecel C, Plaisance P (1993) Almitrine effect on nitric oxide inhalation in adult respiratory distress syndrome. Lancet 341:1664
32. Wysocki M, Delclaux C, Roupie E, et al (1994) Additive effect on gas exchange of inhaled nitric oxide and intravenous almitrine bismesylate in the adult respiratory distress syndrome. Intensive Care Med 20:254–259
33. Lu Q, Mourgeon E, Law-Koune J, et al (1995) Dose-reponse curves of inhaled nitric oxide with and without intravenous almitrine in nitric oxide-responding patients with acute respiratory distress syndrome. Anesthesiology 83:929–943

Inhaled Nitric Oxide: Toxicity and Monitoring Issues

R. P. Dellinger

Introduction

Nitric oxide (NO) has a long environmental and industrial history. It is a major component of smog and cigarette smoke (as high as 1000 ppm in cigarette smoke). Commercially, it is produced by reacting sodium nitrite with sulfuric acid. Commercial uses include catalyst production, as an ozone scavenger in welding shield glasses, and in the semi-conductor industry. Over the last 10 years, NO has achieved major prominence as an important biomediator, with many characteristics of endothelium-derived relaxing factor (EDRF). Over the last 5 years, there has been an increasing interest and study of inhaled NO as a potentially useful pharmaceutical agent in patients with cardiopulmonary dysfunction characterized by some combination of pulmonary arterial hypertension and hypoxemia due to acute lung injury (ALI). This is somewhat remarkable since high concentrations of inhaled NO have long been known to be toxic and to have produced death in human accidents and in animal experiments. The difference between previously described toxicity and current thoughts of clinical benefit rests with the use of lower concentrations (1–100 ppm) for medical conditions as opposed to the higher concentrations (15000 ppm) that had been shown to produce death in humans and animals [1–3]. Initial concerns with the implementation of inhaled NO as a medical therapy were the production of 1) nitrogen dioxide (NO_2, a long known environmental pollutant) created as a breakdown product of NO reaction with oxygen, and 2) methemoglobin (metHb), created during the bloodstream phase of NO clearance from the body. The doses of inhaled NO currently used for medical purposes rarely produce clinically significant elevations in metHb or concentrations of NO_2 that have traditionally been of concern in the workplace. As use of inhaled NO continues to increase, attention is being directed toward more precise definition of threshold levels of concern for NO_2, and closer scrutiny of other byproducts of NO metabolism, including perioxynitrite and nitrosothiol compounds. It is also recognized that the different methods of inhaled NO delivery pose unique potential problems relative to NO delivery and NO_2 production. To follow is a presentation of the chemistry and clearance mechanisms of NO (as background for toxicity discussion), toxicity concerns, various methods of inhaled NO delivery to the mechanically ventilated patient (since toxicity issues may be different for different systems) and discussion of monitoring systems and issues (for assuring optimal medical therapy and minimizing chances of toxicity).

Chemistry and Clearance

The characteristic chemistry of the volatile gas NO, is largely due to the presence of a single unpaired electron in the $2 \cdot p\pi$ molecular orbit which defines the molecule as a free radical [4, 5]. The presence of this unpaired electron is sometimes annotated by writing the formula as $\cdot$NO. However, NO does not exhibit the high reactivity typical for most free radicals. In the presence of superoxide radicals, however, a reaction readily occurs, and this will be discussed later. In the presence of oxygen, auto-oxidation occurs forming NO_2. Currently NO_2 is the primary by-product for toxicity concerns. Although NO does not react with water, NO_2 does and this will be discussed later.

In normal humans, 80–95% of exogenously administered NO reaches the alveoli and is retained, whereas the remainder is expired [6–8]. NO clearance is facilitated by its remarkable capacity to diffuse through tissue and its avid binding to hemoglobin, forming metHb. Methemoglobin is reduced back to hemoglobin by metHb reductase, with nitrates as the byproduct. Approximately 70–80% of inhaled NO retained in the lung is excreted in the urine as nitrate [6] with the remainder being excreted as urea from a metabolic pathway which has not yet been clearly defined [9]. After a single inhalation of NO, the majority of nitrate and urea is excreted in the urine within the first 24 h after inhalation [6]. Some nitrite is also formed when NO dissolves in aqueous solutions, and very mild increases in plasma concentrations of nitrite may be noted. That the overwhelming majority of NO clearance is through the nitrate, as opposed to nitrite, pathway is important, since nitrite can nitrosate sulfhydryl groups and is of more concern for toxicity issues [9].

Oral ammonium nitrate has been used as a diuretic at doses of up to 10–15 g per day, with the only reported problem being transient methemoglobinemia [6]. Transient methemoglobinemia has also been reported in infants ingesting high levels of nitrates, both from drinking water and through direct absorption of nitrates used as topical therapy for burns [6]. Although no other consequences of increased blood nitrate concentrations have been noted in humans, some animal studies have shown reduced thyroid function, vitamin A deficiency, and increased frequency of spontaneous abortion [6]. The World Health Organization has recommended a maximum daily nitrate intake of 3.65 mg/kg. Assuming a typical minute ventilation, the use of up to 40 ppm inhaled NO in an adult with acute respiratory failure would produce no greater than two to three times this recommended value [10]. Impairment of renal function would be expected to increase serum nitrate and nitrite levels.

Toxicity Issues

Methemoglobin

Inhaled NO combines with hemoglobin in red blood cells to form metHb. Methemoglobin is reduced by metHb reductase back to hemoglobin with nitrate formation. Methemoglobin is not directly toxic but reduces the oxygen carrying capacity of the blood, thereby reducing oxygen delivery and producing a functional anemia. In addition, the oxyhemoglobin curve is shifted to the left, decreasing off-loading capability. Low amounts of metHb are normally produced each day through spontaneous auto-oxidation of hemoglobin. A wide variety of agents such as benzocaine, prilocaine, organic and inorganic nitrates and nitrites, metoclopramide, and dapsone may also produce methemoglobinemia. Methemoglobin levels are ascertained with a co-oximeter. Hyperlipemia and increased fetal hemoglobin falsely elevate metHb. Elevations in bilirubin also interfere with metHb measurement. With the typical range of inhaled NO utilized in clinical medicine (≤ 40 ppm), methemoglobinemia should not present significant clinical problems. Exceptions include neonates, who have diminished metHb reductase activity and adults with congenital or acquired metHb reductase deficiency. Partial and complete metHb reductase deficiency occurs more commonly in the native American Indian population. NO treatment may identify heterozygotes with partial reductase deficiency. Therefore, even in adults receiving low concentrations of inhaled NO, metHb measurements are needed initially to ensure that metHb reductase deficiency does not exist. Higher concentrations of inhaled NO (> 40 ppm) warrant periodic monitoring for methemoglobinemia, even in the absence of decreased metHb reduction activity.

Although significant metHb elevations (generally considered to be $> 5\%$) have rarely been encountered in adults with doses < 80 ppm, levels $> 5\%$ have been documented in children receiving doses of 20 ppm [11]. In a study by Young et al., [12] the decline in methemoglobin levels from a mean of 6.9 to 2% occurred within 100 min, with baseline being reached 175 min following discontinuation of inhaled NO. A published report described a faulty valve within a flow meter delivering high concentrations of inhaled NO in a neonate. This led to a metHb level of 14%, which dropped to 8% in 2 h and 2% at 4 h following discontinuation of inhaled NO [13]. Methemoglobinemia is not detected with ordinary pulse oximetry devices and requires co-oximetry measurement. Young and colleagues [12] studied metHb levels in 5 healthy adult volunteers receiving various concentrations of inhaled NO. Inhaled NO was delivered at 32, 64, 128, and 512 ppm in air. Administration continued for 3 h or until levels exceeded 5%. For the 32, 64, and 128 ppm concentrations, the average methemoglobin percentages at 3 h were 1.04, 1.75, and 3.75%, respectively. With the 512 ppm, all 5 volunteers had inhaled NO discontinued prior to 3 h with values averaging 6.93% and ranging from 5.70 to 8.16. Methemoglobin levels are initially a function of both the concentration of inhaled NO and the duration of exposure. Since the kinetics of metHb elimination are thought to be first order until 20% levels are reached [14, 4], it is likely that steady state metHb levels are likely to be attained in 3 to 5 h. A 5-h post-inhaled NO concentration change should therefore establish the maximal level for that inhaled NO dosage. Initial measurement should, however, be undertaken soon after a dosage change so as to identify early evidence of significant methemoglobinemia.

In patients with congenital methemoglobinemia, 10–20% methemoglobinemia is tolerated without ill effects [15]. The threshold for concern should be influenced significantly by other factors affecting O_2 delivery such as hemoglobin content and cardiovascular state. Critically ill patients who do not have lowered oxygen saturations in arterial and mixed venous blood are more likely to form metHb, since deoxyhemoglobin has greater avidity for NO than does oxyhemoglobin. Fetal hemoglobin may also be more prone to oxidation than adult hemoglobin. Methemoglobinemia may not be the most suitable marker of long-term red blood cell toxicity, since animals exposed to NO over long term show increased spleen weights, total bilirubin, and Heintz bodies, despite normal metHb levels [16, 17].

Nitrogen Dioxide

In the presence of oxygen, NO is auto-oxidized to NO_2. In contrast to NO itself, the potential toxicity of NO is of greater concern. NO_2 will react with water to form nitric and nitrous acids which may be responsible for pulmonary toxicity previously described with high concentrations of inhaled NO_2. The rate of formation of NO_2 from oxygen and NO depends upon the concentration of oxygen and the square of the NO concentration. Approximately 40% of inhaled NO_2 is retained in the lung [6]. Inhalation of 5000 ppm NO_2 has been demonstrated to produce pulmonary hemorrhage and death in animals. In 1988, the United States National Institute for Occupational Safety and Health recommended limiting the 8-h time weighted average NO concentration exposure to 25 ppm and the peak NO_2 concentration exposure to 5 ppm. Some animal studies, however, have shown that NO_2 concentrations less than 5 ppm can produce histopathologic abnormalities [18], lower resistance to infection [19], possibly induce mutagenicity [20], and produce loss of epithelial cilia [18]. NO_2 toxicity has been shown to be species and age specific [21]. The United Kingdom Health and Safety Executive standard is ≤ 3 ppm for NO_2.

There are differences that should be recognized when comparing workplace exposure to NO_2 with breathing NO_2 while being mechanically ventilated. NO inhaled from a mechanical ventilator is in association with higher oxygen concentrations than room air and could lead to greater NO_2 production during residence in the lung. Ascertaining the concentration of NO_2 in the deeper portions of the lung itself is also impossible. In addition, variations in concentration of measured NO_2 during nonconstant inspiratory flow may lead to sampling error during measurement. The time to reach a concentration of 5 ppm NO_2 can be calculated with the formula

$$1/(NO)_t - 1/(NO)_i = 2k(O_2)_t$$

where $(NO)_i$ is the NO concentration initially, $(NO)_t$ is that at time t, and k (rate constant) is 1.93×10^{-38} cm^6 mol^{-2} S^{-1} at 300°K. Based on this formula, Foubert and colleagues [22] calculated various times to reach 5 ppm at different oxygen concentrations and varying concentrations of NO. Table 1 reflects those calculations. It should be noted that it takes 60 min for room air and 20 ppm in-

Table 1. Time (min) to yield 5 ppm NO_2 with different mixtures of NO and O_2 (From [22] with permission)

O_2, %	NO (ppm)			
	20	40	80	120
20	60.08	12.86	3.00	1.32
30	40.05	1.56	2.00	0.088
40	30.03	6.43	1.75	0.66
50	24.03	5.15	1.20	0.52
60	20.01	4.28	1.00	0.44
70	17.16	3.66	0.85	0.37
80	15.01	3.20	0.75	0.33
90	13.35	2.85	0.66	0.29
100	12.01	2.56	0.60	0.26

haled NO, whereas at 100% oxygen and 120 ppm, it takes less than 30 sec. This calculation is based on the rate constant of 1.93×10^{-38} cm^6 mol^{-2} S^{-1}. Bouchet and colleagues [23] performed actual experimentation to confirm this rate constant. In their study, time to yield 5 ppm NO_2 (measured by chemolumines-cence) was on the average 2.5 times faster than those given by Foubert, implying in their experiment a higher rate constant. Rate of NO_2 formation is independent of humidity and faster at 25 than at 37°C [24]. Although the understanding of rate constants is of some practical value, it must be remembered that the application of these rate constants to mechanical ventilation systems with intermittent or constant gas movement and inhomogeneity of gases may be misleading.

Perioxynitrite

Since NO is a radical species it will readily react with other radicals. The one electron reduction product of O_2, superoxide (O_2), is a ubiquitous biological radical. It has one unpaired electron. NO and O_2 will therefore readily react with each other. This reaction produces perioxynitrite. Protonation of perioxynitrite ($-OONO$) gives perioxynitrous acid (HOONO) [25]. This unstable substance decomposes to nitrate (NO_3). This decompensation was originally thought to involve the generation of two potent oxidants, NO_2 and ·OH (the hydroxy radical), both with toxic potential [26]. Recently it has been demonstrated that HOONO itself is a potent oxidizing agent with ·OH-like activity and is unlikely to be a precursor for ·OH formation [27]. Perioxynitrite has been implicated as a potentially injurious agent in stroke, myocardial ischemia, and pulmonary edema [28]. However, it is not clear whether nitration in various pathological conditions is a marker of a primary pathology, is fundamentally related to that primary pathology, or could be protective (see discussion to follow). Nitration of tyrosine is a reaction pathway of potential high yield for perioxynitrite. In addition, perioxynitrite reacts quite rapidly with zinc-thiolate centers present in numerous transcription factors [29]. Therefore oxidation of such centers could alter the ability to recognize and bind DNA, exerting significant effects on gene regulation. Perioxynitrite is much more capable than H_2O_2 of oxidizing thiols and in addition readily catalyzes membrane lipid peroxidation, the latter in an iron independent manner unlike hydroxyl radical and hydrogen peroxide which require iron [30]. It has also been reported *in vitro* to damage surfactant protein A. Perioxynitrite reacts with metals or metalloproteins to form potent and toxic nitrosilating species such as nitronium ion [30]. Perioxynitrite is also bactericidal.

Surprisingly, in cell culture experiments, including Chinese hamster V79 cells, mesencephalic neuron cells, and H4 rat hepatoma cells, NO has been shown to protect against the cytotoxic effects of reactive oxygen species [31]. This protective effect in cell culture may be based on its proposed ability to scavenge more reactive oxygen intermediates, serving as an antioxidant itself. It is well established that hydrogen peroxide reacts with metals to yield powerful oxidants such as metallo-oxo species and hydroxyl radical. These reactants can rapidly interact with a variety of bi-organic molecules. It is proposed that these powerful oxidants mediate the cytotoxic action of hydrogen peroxide. NO can react directly with the hydroxyl radical to form perioxynitrite anion which can rapidly decompose to nitrate. Furthermore, the presence of NO prevents the oxidation of substrate mediated by the ferrous/peroxide mixture. NO can also scavenge Fe(IV)O pi cation radical hemeprotein, blocking a cascade of reactions which may lead to cytotoxicity. It has been suggested that protection from reperfusion associated, hydrogen peroxide-mediated cellular damage may be offered by NO reaction with reactive oxygen species [31]. Therefore, cells capable of generating NO may protect themselves from the insult of reactive oxygen species.

It is easy to ascertain from the above that the current status of potential perioxynitrite toxicity with inhaled NO is very controversial, with conflicting nonclinical studies and opinions on the toxicity of NO as it relates to reactive oxygen species. In the interim, it is important to continue to look for methods of experimentation to further elucidate any potential benefit or harm.

S-Nitrosylation

NO can react with sulfur in protein causing S-nitrosylation and forming S-nitrosothiol groups (RSNO) [32]. Most proteins would be possible targets for thiol formation when exposed to NO. Potential adverse reactions include inactivation of surfactant protein. Interestingly, inconsistencies between EDRF and NO in several biological actions might be explained by formation of RSNOs. One example includes the observed difference in *in vivo* half life of NO (approximately 0.1 sec) and *ex vivo* half life of EDRF (6–30 sec). This reported inconsistency may be explained by NO stabilization through reaction with intermediate molecular species that preserve biological activity and prolong physiologic half life [33]. Biomolecules bearing thiol functions appear likely candidates. RSNOs have potent platelet-inhibitory and vasorelaxant properties *in vivo* that resemble those of EDRF. RSNOs are produced as part of normal body homeostatic function such as the erection process.

Platelet Dysfunction

NO/EDRF inhibits platelet aggregation via a cyclic GMP-dependent mechanism. NO inhibits platelet adhesion to collagen, cell matrix, and endothelium [34, 35]. *In vivo*, it is likely that platelet aggregation is regulated by both intraplatelet and endothelial NO. Högman [36, 32] demonstrated prolongation of bleeding time in 6 volunteers breathing 30 ppm NO for 15 min, but not when re-tested with 10 ppm NO. Albert et al. [37] in a larger study of healthy volunteers breathing 30 to 80 ppm NO for up to 50 min failed to show any significant elevation of bleeding time or inhibition of platelet aggregation. Bleeding time has been shown to increase in rabbits exposed to 30 to 300 ppm NO over 15 min [36, 38]. Although bleeding time was not elevated in a human study by Samama, more subtle measurements of platelet function such as platelet aggregation studies with adenosine and ristocetin did show inhibition of platelet aggregation [39]. Interestingly, there was no dose dependency despite a dose range of inhaled NO between 1 and 100 ppm. Any systemic effect of platelet aggregation is likely to be insignificant is therms of the risk for bleeding complications at the concentrations of inhaled NO used clinically. It is conceivable that a local antiplatelet effect of inhaled NO might be beneficial in disease states such as ARDS, where pathology could be related at least in part to platelet activation.

Mutagenicity

NO has been demonstrated to produce mutageneses in *Salmonella typhimurium* cells in cell culture [40].

Gas Mixture

A patient being mechanically ventilated with 1–100 ppm inhaled NO and a minute ventilation of 10 L/min would require 0.01 to 1.0 mL/min of pure NO [41]. Such low flow rates would be difficult to monitor and control, with small errors producing large effects on the concentration of inhaled NO. Dilutant mixtures of NO in an inert carrier (nitrogen) are therefore used. The carrier cannot contain oxygen since NO rapidly oxidizes to NO_2, which is much more toxic than NO. Factors which should be considered when choosing a stock cylinder concentration of NO include 1) the need to have the flow rate in a manageable range since low flow rates are difficult to accurately maintain and high flow rates will result in unacceptable reduction in inspired oxygen concentration; and 2) the more dilute the mixture the faster the cylinders are exhausted. The cost of the NO mixture is primarily related to preparation and distribution and not to NO content. Therefore, differences in concentration make little difference to price. High concentrations of NO however are more hazardous if the delivery system leaks. The flow of NO mixture (V_{mix}) necessary to produce the desired final inspired nitric oxygen concentration can be expressed by the following formula [41]:

$$V_{mix} = \frac{V \cdot \cdot FINO}{(F_{mix}NO - FINO) - 1}$$

where V is the flow rate of the gas to which the NO will be added (gas flow around the continuous flow pediatric ventilator circuit or the minute ventilation of an adult ventilator), F_{mix}NO is the concentration of NO in the NO/nitrogen gas mixture, and FINO is the desired final inspired nitric oxygen concentration. The subsequent reduction in FiO_2 which will occur from the dilution due to addition of the NO mixture can be calculated as [41]:

$$\text{Final } FiO_2 = \frac{\text{Initial } FiO_2 \times V}{V + V_{mix}}$$

The majority of NO mixtures used in the United States and Europe are 400–1000 ppm. The prototype nitric oxygen delivery on the Siemens Servo 300 ventilator uses 2500 ppm. The EEC have raised concerns about tank concentrations greater than 1000 ppm. A downside to lowering the stock cylinder concentration is, however, the drop in maximal inspired oxygen fraction obtainable. For example, with 2000 ppm NO cylinders the maximal decrease in inspired oxygen fraction is only 1% when administering 20 ppm NO. In addition, one can estimate out the required stock NO flow, i.e. 1/1000th of the total flow passing through the inspiratory limb. An infant ordinarily on 10 L/min would therefore be started on 100 mL/min NO. This may add convenience in a hurried situation.

Cylinder contents are analyzed after mixing, and the actual concentration is displayed on the cylinder. In addition, the certificate gives the level of contamination by nitric dioxide in the cylinder. Small degreess of NO_2 contamination are acceptable (typically < 10 ppm NO_2 for tanks ≤ 1000 ppm NO). Higher thresholds for tanks of higher NO concentration are appropriate. The typical tank is scrubbed free of oxygen and should not result in NO conversion to NO_2 for at least 18 months. All NO used on patients should be of medical or pharmaceutical, (not industrial) grade.

Delivery Systems for NO Administration

Pediatric Constant Flow Ventilators

With constant flow ventilation systems, as frequently used for pediatric patients, an NO/NO_2 mixture is added to the inspiratory limb of the ventilator circuit as a fixed continuous gas injection. This delivery system results in a steady inspired concentration independent of an infant's minute ventilation. The NO flow will need to be reset only if the dose is changed or the continuous flow of gas within the circuit is altered. Since the NO will either be inspired or vented within seconds, oxidation to NO_2 is minimal. The gas is typically added after the humidifier to avoid any potential delay in passage of gas through the circuit. The injected gas mixture is a blend of NO source tank gas and N_2 from a second tank. Since a wide range of flow rates for NO mixtures may be required, a rotameter is selected that satisfies the flow requirements (0–250 mL/min versus 0–1 L/min).

Adult Ventilators

A continuous flow of NO can be applied to the inspiratory limb of an adult ventilator circuit in a manner similar to the continuous flow pediatric ventilator. This results in accumulation of NO in the inspiratory limb during expiration with delivery to the patient with each inspiration. NO transit time with this system is less than when applied prior to mechanical ventilation, and a soda lime absorber is not needed. This system allows delively of an average NO concentration over inspiration, although different sectors of that inspiratory breath will have different levels of NO. Delivering the NO gas mixture near the endotracheal tube prevents adequate downstream sampling for NO_2 and NO.

It is also possible to use timed-gas injection so that NO is only delivered during inspiration. Roissant and colleagues [42] used the nebulizer attachment on a Siemens 900C ventilator as a pneumatic valve for delivery of NO mixture with the flow adjusted by varying the driving pressure of the NO mixture delivered to the nebulizer. Since the nebulizer on this ventilator is only activated during inspiration, NO is only delivered during inspiration. Similar techniques have since been used on other ventilators. This system requires an electromechanical gas valve and an inspiratory signal derived from the ventilator. In order to avoid build up of pressure during the no-flow state, NO/N_2 mixture is wasted during expiration.

The addition of NO to the inspiratory limb in adult ventilation may, however, be problematic. Flow through the circuit is tidaled, transit time is longer, and minute ventilation may vary. With continuous injection into the inspiratory limb, tidal flow leads to different concentrations of NO in different areas of the delivered breath (despite a constant "average per breath" concentration). Variation in minute ventilation however will lead to different average concentrations of inhaled NO. The flow rate of NO, therefore, has to be adjusted when the minute ventilation changes to avoid changing concentrations of NO. It may also be more difficult to precisely measure NO and NO_2 delivered with this system since adequate mixing may not occur prior to entrance into the endotracheal tube. Blending NO into the ventilator breath prior to the mechanical ventilator should alleviate the potential problems described above. Even when NO is injected only during inspiration, NO concentration will vary widely throughout the breath unless a constant flow pattern (square wave flow pattern) is present. Furthermore, the users of slow response analyzers will fail to detect the variability whether or not the variation in concentration of NO is associated with continuous NO delivery into the inspiratory limb or with delivery only during inspiration. The use of slow response analyzers will fail to detect the high variability.

Many methods for pre-ventilation mixing of NO have been successfully used. One method suitable for mechanical ventilators with external oxygen blenders, such as the Siemens Servo 900C, is to use either the high or low pressure inlet (disconnecting the high pressure input for the latter) to receive gas that has been blended to achieve the desired NO concentration. A two blender system may be used with the first blender mixing NO/N_2 with N_2 and the second blender adding oxygen to this mixture. The blended gas input is into the internal reservoir bellows of the ventilator, which will then contain the desired NO concentration. Since all ventilator breaths are drawn from this reservoir, they will contain a constant inspired NO concentration. When the two blender system ("nitric blender" and "oxygen blender") are used for delivering a NO mixture prior to the ventilator, the relative contribution of each blender to the total gas flow varies with total flow and is not sufficiently precise at low flow rates of NO gas mixture. When delivering lower range NO concentrations in the presence of lower FiO_2s, small changes in the nitric blender mix produce greater changes in NO concentration. Nomograms have been constructed to provide a useful starting value for gas blending, however, fine tuning of the blenders while FiO_2 and NO is measured downstream is required before administering the gas to the patient. An oxygen analyzer is placed either just before or after the ventilator. It is also necessary to match the flow demands of the patient in order to ensure an adequate supply. A total flow into the reservoir that exceeds the minute ventilation will result in gas venting. This gas is then scavenged. Inadequate flows may occur with the low pressure system and result in inability to satisfy patient flow demands. A flow meter is placed distal to the two blenders prior to gas entrance into the ventilator when the low pressure system is used. The flow meter is adjusted to match patient demands. The primary disadvantage of pre-ventilation NO mixing is that the generation of NO_2 in the ventilator could be problematic, especially at high inspired oxygen fractions, high inhaled NO concentrations, and low minute ventilation. This can usually be countered by inserting a soda lime canister in the inspired limb of the ventilation circuit to absorb NO_2.

Another technique currently utilized is a single blender setup which delivers a nitrogen/NO mixture into the high pressure port of a ventilator with FiO_2 set directly on the ventilator (e.g. Puritan-Bennett 7200). The advantage of this delivery system is that there is no internal bellows and therefore less dwell time for production of NO_2.

Systems now exist that automatically detect changes in minute ventilation and adjust the flow of NO mixture into the circuit accordingly, either into the inspiratory limb or in the mechanical ventilator microprocessor system itself. These systems are available both for inspiratory limb delivery (Ohmeda I-NOvent) as well as with a prototype Siemens Servo 300 ventilator. Injection of NO varies as flow varies with pressure support, pressure control, and volume ventilation with other than square inspiratory flow wave form. A mass-flow controller is used to adjust the flow of NO with pneumatic sensing of inspiratory flow. This method avoids the bolusing of NO into the system during expiration, shortens exposure time for generation of NO_2, and injects NO only during inspiration. It is intended to ensure constant inspired NO concentration while matching the precise flow of the blended gas to flow during inspiration and to inject proportional amounts of NO. This system is similar to a theoretical unit shown to work with CO_2 delivery into the inspiratory limb [43]. CO_2 was used as a surrogate for NO in this study since rapid response NO sensors were not available at the time. The CO_2 sensor was needed to judge the mixing effectiveness of the delivery system. The Siemens Servo 300 has now been modified to use a mass controller and a single microprocessor chip to internally blend O_2 with air and then with NO, without using a mixing bag. A third port on the ventilator is used for adding the NO. This method of NO delivery, currently only available in Europe, also delivers a constant NO concentration only during inspiration and independent of minute ventilation. Finally, it should be remembered that there are no NO/N_2 blenders and when these gases are blended with an oxygen blender, the oxygen percentage selected will not be precise for the NO/N_2 flow. Final flow adjustments are therefore necessary with measurement of downstream NO concentration.

Soda Lime Absorbers and Humidifiers

When higher FiO_2s and higher NO concentrations are delivered pre-ventilator, a soda lime absorber may be placed in the inspiratory limb near the ventilator to remove NO_2. NO and NO_2 removal may vary among soda lime compositions. Soda lime is characterized by its indicator. Ishibe and colleagues [44] demonstrated that soda lime 1) completely absorbs NO_2 regardless of the presence of NO, 2) does not absorb NO when NO_2 is not present, and 3) when NO and NO_2 are both present absorbs both gases in nearly equimolecular amounts. Since the molecular amounts of NO will be considerably greater than NO_2, soda lime therefore becomes an effective remover of NO_2 in patients receiving inhaled NO therapy. Ethyl violet indicator soda lime has been demonstrated to remove 65–70% of NO_2 but only 7% of NO. It is recommended that the absorber be changed every third day. Placing the soda lime absorber closer to the Y piece in the inspiratory limb does not further reduce NO levels. The use of a charcoal absorber as opposed to soda lime significantly increases NO_2 scavenging but also increases NO scavenging, offering no advantage compared to soda lime.

Nitric acid is formed when NO_2 comes in contact with water. With excess NO, nitrous acid (a weaker acid) is formed. When heat and moisture exchangers (HMEs) were tested for pH changes after use during delivery of inhaled NO, no decrease in pH was noted in water used to rinse HMEs [45]. Therefore, the increase in dead space with HMEs does not appear to impact on generation of acid compounds in this saturated environment. Accumulations of nitric and nitrous acids (HNO_x) (below OSHA threshold for the workplace) have been demonstrated with 80 ppm NO, 90% oxygen, and 37°C maximally water vapor saturated gas [46]. Connecting two soda lime absorbers in series does not improve removal of NO_2 [45].

Scavenging

Scavenging systems may be employed to decrease atmospheric contamination with NO and NO_2. The general need for scavenging remains questionable and controversial [41]. For continuous flow systems at high NO concentrations, however, scavenging is appropriate, since during expiration the gas exiting the system will contain significant quantities of NO. The same is true where venting from bellows occurs. In non-continuous flow systems only expired gas is of primary concern. In normals only 10–20% of delivered NO is exhaled; however, this may be increased in diseases in which physiologic dead space is high. Scavenging is accomplished by venting into the hospital suction system or by using charcoal filters in line with the vented gas. The accepted upper limit for NO exposure in the workplace is 25 ppm over an 8-h period. In a non-continuous flow system or in any delivery system with low inspried concentrations of NO with any delivery system, the ambient air level of NO will be very low. Levels will tend to be higher in poorly ventilated rooms. Measurement of NO in the ambient air in the vicinity of the patient receiving inhaled NO has failed to reveal levels of 1 ppm or greater, the lower threshold for measurement on the electrochemical measuring device used [47]. With more sensitive chemoluminescent measurement devices, levels of 100 ppb NO and 30 ppb NO_2 have been measured around the bedside with charcoal filter scavenging in place [48]. It is nevertheless reasonable to take steps to minimize loss of NO enriched gas into the ICU during suctioning, bagging, ventilator disconnects, etc., especially when delivering high concentrations of NO. Even when inhaled NO is delivered by nasal cannula, NO concentrations in the room are very low [49]. Environmental measurements taken in London in 1994 showed a high of 996 ppb and a mean of 41 ppb for NO with 286 ppb and 36 ppb, respectively, for NO_2 [48]. It has been recommended that ambient levels of NO_2 in the workplace be kept less than 5 ppm. However, as previously mentioned there have been reports of subtle abnormalities occuring in animals exposed to 2 ppm NO_2. I recommend, therefore, to keep NO_2 concentrations delivered to the patient and in the ambient air as low as possible. Since the patient's inspired NO_2 concentration is targeted to stay below 5 ppm, the ambient NO_2 levels are unlikely to exceed 1 ppm. The World Health Organization and European Community recommend achieving a much more stringent NO_2 upper limit in ambient air in the workplace of 0.08 to 0.105 ppm.

NO and NO_2 Analyzers

The ideal analyzer is small, quiet, and provides precise continuous real-time analyses with small gas samples. It would be unaffected by water vapor, oxygen, or CO_2 concentrations. It would function reliably, require minimal maintenance, calibrate easily, and be inexpensive. The capability to monitor both NO and NO_2 with visual readout and adjustable alarms is desirable. Methods capable of monitoring NO include chemoluminescence, electrochemical, mass-spectrograph, and infrared devices [41, 50]. Devices currently used include the chemiluminescence and electrochemical detectors. The chemiluminescence device is extremely precise for measurement of NO and is capable of measuring concentrations 1000 times lower than those typically delivered to patients. Disadvantages include a large aspirating volume (0.7 L/min) which is associated with noisy aspirating pumps and the capability to decrease PEEP. Water vapor filters are also required to be inserted in the aspirating line and to be replaced frequently. Intermittent as opposed to continuous sampling decreases the need for frequent replacement of water vapor filters. These devices are also expensive. When chemiluminescence analyzing techniques are used "quenching" produces an underestimate of the concentration of NO_2 [51]. Quenching occurs when not all NO_2 molecules present yield a chemiluminescence signal [52]. This occurs because some NO_2 molecules collide with other molecules in the sample and are converted to NO. This process is called collisional deactivation. It is most likely to occur at higher concentrations of oxygen, when a stainless steel conversion chamber is being used, and when the specimen is heated. Molybdenum conversion chambers can reduce this effect but not eliminate it.

Smaller, less expensive electrochemical analyzers are enjoying increasing utilization. Separate devices are needed for NO_2 and NO [53]. The reliability, reproducibility, and accuracy of these devices are not as well established as chemiluminescence devices. Calibration is subject to drift, and accuracy should be assured with calibration gases prior to patient use. Recently developed monitors are becoming less expensive, alarm ready, and less affected by humidification of inspired gas.

Most currently used chemiluminescent and electrochemical devices compare favorably for measuring NO across currently utilized NO ranges. Electrochemical devices, however, tend to overread and chemoluminescent devices tend to underread actual NO_2 [54]. Variability for measuring NO_2 at higher concentrations of oxygen do exist [55, 56]. Differences may be because of sampling technique or because of a tendency for chemiluminescent devices to produce falsely low NO_2 measurements. Measurement of NO and NO_2 using analyzers that have been appropriately tested and calibrated with known concentrations of NO and NO_2 is essential prior to their clinical application. NO_2 calibration should be performed in an O_2 rich environment.

Monitoring

When assessing monitoring needs during NO therapy, it is important to recognize certain salient principles of monitoring. First, most analyzers currently being utilized have long response times, on the order of tens of seconds. Although the long response time is not a problem in constant flow systems, it is problematic in situations where gas flow is not constant (adult ventilators) and NO is added to the inspiratory limb. In this circumstance, the analyzer will tend to measure the average concentration over time at the point of measurement and not the true average or peak inspired concentration. This will usually lead to inaccurate measurement of the true mean inspired concentration.

Since a variable, but major amount of inspired NO and NO_2 is removed by the lungs, systems which sample in the expiratory limb will be of no use in determining inhaled levels. Likewise, sampling is also inappropriate at sites where up to two-thirds of the time expired gas will be sampled [29] (endotracheal tube or within the trachea).

In addition, the total dose of inhaled NO (and NO_2) may also be important to consider since higher minute ventilations at the same concentration will mean greater total exposures. Dwell times, reflected by I/E ratio, may also be an important consideration for NO_2.

Wessel and colleagues [57] reported regarding the use of inhaled NO in 123 patients, the majority of whom were neonatal and pediatric, with a wide variety of ventilatory support techniques. These included volume control in 53, pressure control in 5, and pressure-limited time-cycled infant ventilation in 25. They used the standard two blender mixing system previously described to successfully deliver inhaled NO to both constant flow (infant) and non-constant flow (adult) ventilator circuits. For adult ventilation, a flow meter was placed distal to these two blenders prior to entrance into either the low-pressure inlet or high-pressure inlet of a Siemens Servo 900C ventilator. An O_2 analyzer was placed in the inspiratory limb shortly after emergence from the ventilator with a humidifier in the inspiratory limb. The same blending system was utilized to accomplish infant ventilation. In this arrangement flow from the basic system provided all the ventilator gas. The final NO/nitrogen mixture derived from the flow meter distal to the second blender flowed into a humidifier, then to an oxygen analyzer, and on to the inspiratory gas line. The pressure-limited, time-cycled constant flow infant ventilator was used for alarm capability. Expiratory gas was scavenged. In both constant flow and non-constant flow systems, a chemoluminescence NO/NO_2 analyzer was inserted in the inspiratory portion of the Y connector just prior to the endotracheal tube. All patients received 80 ppm NO as the initial dose. In the majority of patients 80 ppm was the only dose. One-fifth of patients had NO weaned to ≤ 40 ppm before it was discontinued. In the overwhelming majority of patients, the NO_2 concentration was ≤ 1 ppm. In two infants with low minute ventilation, it increased transiently to 3 ppm. In 25 patients the NO and NO_2 concentrations in the immediate patient environment were less than 0.04 ppm and less than 0.01 ppm, respectively, even when the leak around the endotracheal tube was as much as 25% of tidal volume. The mean metHb concentration in these patients was $2.5 \pm 4\%$. In 4 patients, the metHb was $>4.6\%$. NO levels remained stable independent of minute ventilation.

Skimming and colleagues [58] investigated problems created by laminar gas flow at the injection point of NO into the inspiratory limb of a constant flow infant breathing circuit. They measured NO concentrations by chemoluminescence at varying locations from the injection point and at different positions inside the tubing beginning from the ipsilateral tubing wall relative to the NO injection point and continuing to the contralateral tubing wall. They also analyzed for mixing differences between corrugated and smooth tubing. Increasing NO source flow at the injection point was used to produce higher NO concentrations. For each NO flow rate and location testing there was significant variability in NO measurement across the inside diameter of the tube, with the highest NO concentration close to the ipsilateral tubing wall. Variations in NO concentrations measured across the injection of the tube decreased as the sampling moved more distant from the injection port. Corrugated tubing augmented mixing. A diaphragm device (Fig. 1) improved mixing of the NO source gas. The diaphragm was created by in-line insertion of a 4.0 mm endotracheal tube hub inserted into a 15 mm inside/22 mm outside diameter adapter, which was then placed in-line with the inspiratory limb tubing. This device did create increased resistance in the system but provided thorough gas mixing at flow rates as low as 2 L/min and only exceeded 12 cmH_2O resistance at gas flow rates >30 L/min. Exceeding the 12 cmH_2O threshold interfered with the performance characteristics of the pediatric ventilator utilized. Longer distances from infusion port are required to assure adequate mixing as 1) flow decreases, 2) internal tubing diameter increases, or 3) smooth tubing as opposed to corrugated tubing is used. Tubing with deep corrugation could be counterproductive if gas stagnation results in elevated inspired NO_2 concentration. Preliminary data would indicate that this does not occur with less pronounced corrugation. A flow transducer cartridge inserted in-line in the inspiratory port also provides improved mixing of gas, although it is not as proficient as the diaphragm device. It is also larger, more expensive, and cannot be inserted as close to the Y piece.

Westfelt and colleagues [45] measured test lung NO and NO_2 levels using the two basic types of NO source gas delivery, i.e. pre-ventilator and inspiratory limb. A NO_2 absorber (inserted in the inspiratory limb just as the gas exited the venti-

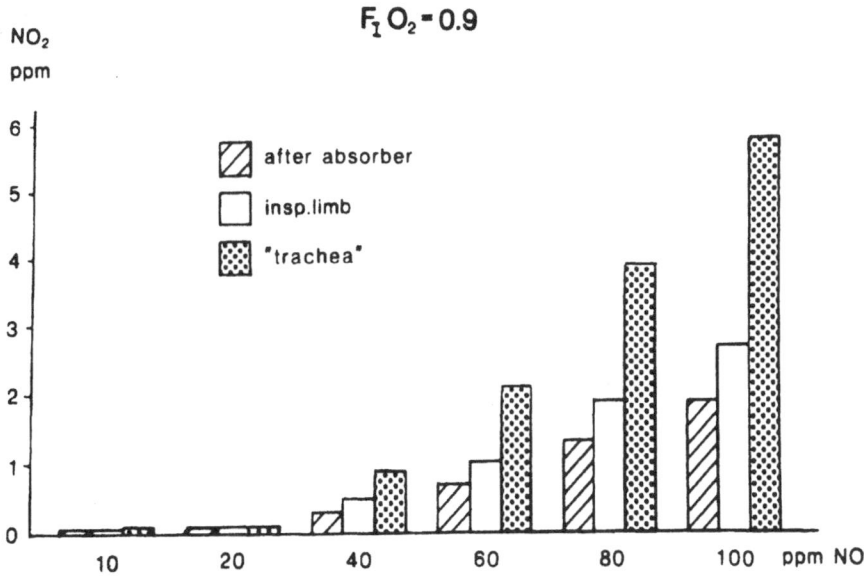

Fig. 1. Levels of nitrogen dioxide (NO_2) at three measuring points (2, 3 and 4) of the system at FiO_2 0.9, when delivering NO doses of 10, 20, 40, 60, 80 and 100 parts per million (ppm)

lator) was used when NO source gas was blended prior to the ventilator, and NO and NO_2 were measured 1) distal to the NO_2 absorber and prior to the humidifier, 2) just after gas exited from the humidifier, and 3) in the inspiratory limb close to the Y piece, and 4) in the trachea of the lung model. The low-pressure inlet of the Siemens Servo 900C ventilator was used for pre-ventilator administration. NO and NO_2 were measured using electrochemical technique and analyzers

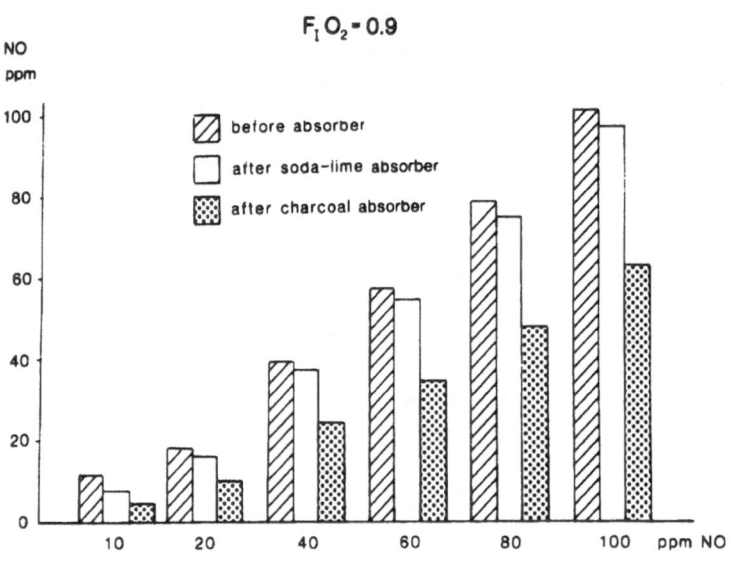

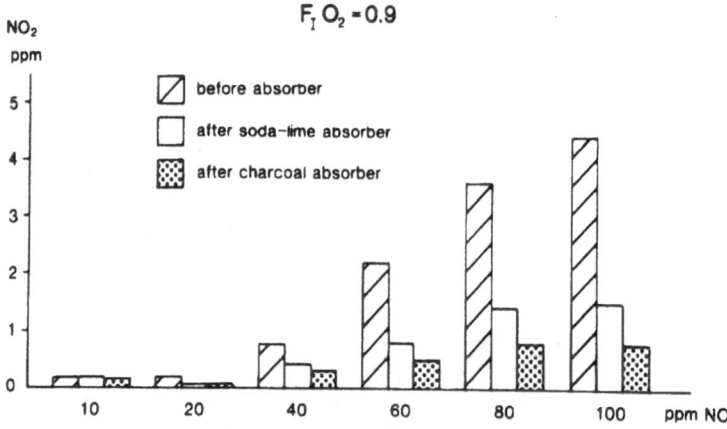

Fig. 2. Levels of nitric oxide (NO) (upper panel) and nitrogen dioxide (NO_2) (lower panel) measured before and after soda-lime and charcoal absorbers, at FiO_2 0.9 and NO-doses of 10, 20, 40, 60, 80 and 100 parts per million (ppm) (From [45] with permission)

calibrated twice daily. Response time was more than 10 sec. An ethyl violet color indicator soda lime absorber was used with measurement immediately after the absorber had been in place and at 72 h. Fig. 2 shows levels of NO_2 at three measuring points with varying concentrations of NO and FiO_2 of 0.9. Note that tracheal concentrations of NO_2 in test lung remained very low with 10, 20, and 40 ppm, rising to 2 ppm concentration in the trachea with 60 ppm NO, 4 ppm with 80 NO, and greater than 5 ppm with 100 ppm NO. When apnea was simulated in this study with temporary power supply interruption, there was a significant increase in NO_2 production in the lung, especially when the NO was being infused into the inspiratory limb. This problem would be circumvented if inspiratory limb infusion was synchronized with inspiration as is currently being done with some systems and as previously described in this manuscript.

Table 2. Inspiratory limb NO_2 concentrations over time with pre-ventilation delivery of inhaled NO in adults with ARDS

	NO₂ level					
	0 ppm	1.25 ppm	5 ppm	20 ppm	40 ppm	80 ppm
Day 1						
Mean	0.10	0.03	0.12	0.20	0.34	1.47
No of patients	54	21	34	28	27	7
Maximum value	1.00	0.05	1.00	2.00	0.90	2.25
Day 2						
Mean	0.10	0.09	0.10	0.16	0.31	1.42
No of patients	52	20	34	29	27	5
Maximum value	1.00	0.60	1.00	1.05	0.82	1.87
Day 3						
Mean	0.13	0.07	0.08	0.17	0.26	1.40
No of patients	48	20	28	28	25	5
Maximum value	0.58	0.72	0.55	0.70	0.92	1.88
Day 7						
Mean	0.09	0.12	0.09	0.16	0.30	1.92
No of patients	31	13	19	16	18	3
Maximum value	0.40	0.32	0.30	1.08	0.95	3.57
Day 14						
Mean	0.03	0.09	0.10	0.06	0.30	—
No of patients	11	3	5	10	11	0
Maximum value	0.25	0.17	0.40	1.00	1.03	—
Day 21						
Mean	0.07	0.12	0.15	0.16	0.45	—
No of patients	4	1	2	6	5	0
Maximum value	0.18	0.12	0.27	0.42	1.03	—
Day 28						
Mean	0.20	—	0.20	0.08	0.54	—
No of patients	1	0	1	5	3	0
Maximum value	0.20	—	0.20	0.14	1.12	—

Dellinger and colleagues [59] reported the use of inhaled NO in patients with ARDS. The study included 177 patients and was placebo controlled and blinded. The low pressure inlet of the Siemens Servo 900C was used after pre-ventilator blending of NO, N_2 and O_2. Nitrogen was used as placebo gas with treatment group patients receiving 1.25, 5, 20, 40, and 80 ppm inhaled NO. In this phase 2 study there was no difference in mortality between placebo and inhaled NO groups. There was also no difference in investigator–reported adverse events among treatment groups. Tables 2 and 3 show previously unpublished summaries of NO_2 (measured by electrochemical analyzer) and metHb monitoring data. This study demonstrated that there was no significant elevation in NO_2 measurements with pre-ventilator mixing of NO and a soda lime scrubber in the inspiratory limb. Methemoglobin levels of 5% or greater were reported in 4 patients, 2 of these patients receiving 80 ppm NO, one 40 ppm NO, and one placebo.

Table 3. Methemoglobin concentrations over time with pre-ventilation delivery of inhaled NO in adults with ARDS

	Mean Methemoglobin					
	0 ppm	1.25 ppm	5 ppm	20 ppm	40 ppm	80 ppm
Day 1						
Mean	0.83	0.84	0.93	1.01	1.39	2.45
No of patients	48	19	32	25	24	5
Maximum value	2.95	1.80	1.80	1.80	2.85	7.00
Day 2						
Mean	0.88	0.80	0.81	1.05	1.50	2.68
No of patients	51	20	31	28	24	4
Maximum value	3.40	1.95	1.75	1.85	2.75	3.80
Day 3						
Mean	0.88	0.80	0.86	0.18	1.54	2.47
No of patients	47	19	25	26	25	5
Maximum value	7.90	2.00	1.60	2.15	3.30	3.50
Day 7						
Mean	0.85	0.80	0.89	1.01	1.47	1.85
No of patients	28	12	18	15	18	3
Maximum value	1.60	1.30	2.55	1.65	5.10[a]	2.60[b]
Day 14						
Mean	0.79	0.83	1.33	1.10	1.55	0.75
No of patients	11	2	5	10	11	0
Maximum value	1.55	0.90	2.75	2.55	2.30	0.75
Day 21						
Mean	0.63	0.85	0.93	0.93	1.60	0.75
No of patients	3	1	2	6	5	0
Maximum value	1.15	0.85	1.05	1.60	2.05	0.75₄
Day 28						
Mean	1.05	0.75	0.90	0.85	1.27	0.75
No of patients	1	0	1	4	3	0
Maximum value	1.05	0.75	0.90	1.25	1.85	0.75

[a] 5.60 on Day 8 – [b] 6.50 on Day 9

Conclusion

When delivering inhaled NO it is important to consider potential toxicities of inhaled NO therapy to both patients and medical personnel and to counteract that possibility with sound delivery and monitoring practices. I recommend precise and accurate measurement of NO and NO_2 in the inspiratory limb, as close to the patient as feasable. NO_2 should be kept as low as efficacious and practical – optimally less than 5 ppm and ideally less than 2 ppm. Since potential toxicities of NO are still being investigated, it is important to minimize NO gas concentration and exposure. The length of time the gas remains in the.delivery circuit should also be minimized. I recommend precise control of the NO dose, on-line analysis of NO, NO_2, and O_2, and scavenging systems for the treatment of exhaust gases, as appropriate. Calibrated commercially purchased stock tanks of medical grade NO mixed with nitrogen should be used. I find soda lime useful in removing NO_2 from the breathing circuit in circumstances where it might be expected to reach significant levels in the inspiratory limb. Blood methemoglobin levels are measured as appropriate, based on the concentration of inhaled NO being delivered. MetHb levels should be measured initially in all patients until a steady state is reached to assure that there is no metHb reductase deficiency present.

References

1. Greenbaum R, Bay J. Hargreaves MD, et al (1967) Effects of higher oxides of nitrogen on the anaesthetized dog. Br J Anaesth 39:393–404
2. Shiel FO (1967) Morbid anatomical changes in the lungs of dogs after inhalation of higher oxide of nitrogen during anaesthesia. Br J Anaesth 39:413–424
3. Clutton-Brock J (1967) Two cases of poisoning by contamination of nitrous oxide with higher oxide of nitrogen during anesthesia. Br J Anaesth 39:388–392
4. Young JD, Sear JW, Valvini EM (1996) Kinetics of methaemoglobin and serum nitrogen oxide production during inhalation of nitric oxide in volunteers. Br J Anaesth 76:652–656
5. Stamler JS, Singel DJ, Loscalzo (1992) Biochemistry of nitric oxide and its redox-activated forms. Science 258:1898–1902
6. Westfelt UN, Benthin G, Lundin S, et al (1995) Conversion of inhaled nitric oxide to nitrate in man. Br J Pharmacol 114:1621–1624
7. Borland CDR, Higenbottom TW (1989) A simultaneous single breath measurement of pulmonary diffusing capacity with nitric oxide and carbon monoxide. Eur Respir J 2:56–63
8. Guenard H, Varene N, Vaida P (1987) Determination of lung capillary blood volume and membrane diffusing capacity in man by the measurements of NO an CO transfer. Respir Physiol 70:113–120
9. Edwards AD (1995) The pharmacology of inhaled nitric oxide. Arch Dis Child Fetal Neonatal Ed 72:F127–F130
10. Valvini EM, Young JD (1995) Serum nitrogen oxides during nitric oxide inhalation. Br J Anaesth 74:338–339
11. Frostell CG, Lönnqvist PA, Sonesson SE, et al (1993) Near fatal pulmonary hypertension after surgical repair of congenital diaphragmatic hernia: Successful use of inhaled nitric oxide. Anaesthesia 48:679–683
12. Young JD, Dyar O, Xiong L, Howell (1994) Methemoglobin production in normal adults inhaling low concentrations of nitric oxide. Intensive Care Med 20:581–584
13. Heal CA, Spencer SA (1995) Methaemoglobinaemia with high-dose nitric oxide administration. Acta Paediatr 84:1318–1319

14. Marrs TC, Bright JE (1996) Kinetics of methaemoglobin production (1). Kinetics of methae-moglobinaemia induced by cyanide antidotes, p-aminopropiophenone, p-hydroxyamino-propiophenone or p-dimethylaminophenol after intravenous administration. Hum Toxicol 5:295–301

15. Borgese N, Pietrini G, Gaetani S (1987) Concentration of NADH-cytochrome b 5 reductase in erythrocytes of normal and methemoglobinemic individuals measured with a quantitative radioimmunoblotting assay. J Clin Invest 80:1296–1302

16. Oda H, Nogami H, Kusumoto S, et al (1980) Lifetime exposure to 2.4 ppm nitric oxide in mice. Environ Res 22:254–263

17. Oda H, Nogami H, Kusumoto S, et al (1976) Long-term exposure to nitric oxide in mice. J Jpn Soc Air Pollut 11:150–160

18. Freeman G, Stephens RJ, Crane SC, et al (1968) Lesion of the lung in rats continuously exposed to two parts per million of nitrogen dioxide. Arch Environ Health 17:181–192

19. Goldstein E, Eagle MC, Hoeprich PD (1973) Effect of nitrogen dioxide on pulmonary bacterial defense mechanisms. Arch Environ Health 26:202–204

20. Von Nieding G (1978) Possible mutagenic properties and carcinogenic action of the irritant gaseous pollutants NO_2, O_3, and SO_3. Environ Health Perspect 22:91–92

21. Azoulay-Dupuis E, Torres M, Soler P, et al (1983) Pulmonary NO_2 toxicity in neonate and adult guinea pigs and rats. Environ Res 30:322–339

22. Foubert L, Fleming B, Latimer R, et al (1992) Safety guidelines for use of nitric oxide. Lancet 339:1615–1616

23. Bouchet M, Renaudin MH, Raveau C, et al (1993) Safety requirement for use of inhaled nitric oxide in neonates. Lancet 341:968–969

24. Miyamoto K, Aida A. Nishimura M, et al (1994) Effects of humidity and temperature on nitrogen dioxide formation from nitric oxide. Lancet 343:1099–1100

25. Fukuto JM (1995) Chemistry of nitric oxide: Biologically relevant aspects. Adv Pharmacol 34:1–15

26. Mahoney LR (1970) Evidence for the formation of hydroxyl radicals in the isomerization of pernitrous acid to nitric oxide in aqueous solution. J Am Chem 92:5262–5263

27. Koppenol WH, Moreno JJ, Pryor WA, et al (1992) Peroxynitrite, a cloaked oxidant formed by nitric oxide and superoxide. Chem Res Toxicol 5:834–842

28. Crow JP, Spruell C, Chen J, et al (1994) On the pH dependent yield of hydroxyl radical products from peroxynitrite. Free Rad Biol Med 16:331–338

29. Crow JP, Beckman JS (1995) Reactions between nitric oxide, superoxide, and peroxynitrite: Footprints of peroxynitrite *in vivo*. Adv Pharmacol 34:17–43

30. Freeman B (1994) Free radical chemistry of nitric oxide. Looking at the dark side. Chest 105 (Suppl):79S-84S

31. Wink DA, Hanbauer I, Laval F, et al (1994) Nitric oxide protects against the cytotoxic effects of reactive oxygen species. Ann NY Acad Sci 738:265–278

32. Frostell CG, Zapol WM (1995) Inhaled nitric oxide, clinical rationale and applications. Adv Pharmacol 34:439–456

33. Upchurch GR, Welch GN, Loscalzo J (1995) S-nitrosothiols: Chemistry, biochemistry, and biological actions. Adv Pharmacol 34:343–348

34. Merritt WT (1993) Nitric oxide: An important bioregulator. Transpl Proc 25:2014–2016

35. Radomski MW, Moncada S (1993) The biological and pharmacological role of nitric oxide in platelet function. In: Authi KS et al (eds) Mechanisms of Platelet Activation and Control. Plenum Press, New York pp 251–264

36. Högman M, Frostell C, Arnberg H, Hedenstierna G (1993) Bleeding time prolongation and NO inhalation. Lancet 341:1664–1665

37. Albert J, Wallen H, Bröjiersen A, et al (1995) Effects of inhaled NO on platelet function *in vivo* in healthy volunteers. FASEB J 9:A30 (Abst)

38. Högman M, Frostell C, Arnberg H, et al (1994) Prolonged bleeding time during nitric oxide inhalation in the rabbit. Acta Physiol Scand 151:125–129

39. Samama CM, Diaby M, Fellahi JL, et al (1995) Inhibition of platelet aggregation by inhaled nitric oxide in patients with acute respiratory distress syndrome. Anesthesiology 83:56–65

40. Tamir S, Lewis RS, Walker T, et al (1993) The influence of delivery rate on the chemistry and biological effects of nitric oxide. Chem Res Toxicol 6:895–899
41. Young JD, Dyar OJ (1996) Delivery and monitoring of inhaled nitric oxide. Intensive Care Med 22:77–86
42. Rossaint R, Falke KJ, Lopez F, et al (1993) Inhaled nitric oxide in adult respiratory distress syndrome. N Engl J Med 328:399–405
43. Young JD (1994) A universal nitric oxide delivery system. Br J Anaesth 73:700–702
44. Ishibe T, Sato T, Hayashi T, et al (1996) Absorption of nitrogen dioxide and nitric oxide by soda lime. Br J Anaesth 75:330–333
45. Westfelt UN, Lundin S, Stenqvist O (1994) Safety aspects of delivery and monitoring of nitric oxide during mechanical ventilation. Acta Anaesthesiol Scand 40:302–310
46. Putensen C, Räsänen J, Thomson MS, Braman RS (1995) Method for delivering constant nitric oxide concentrations during full and partial ventilatory support. J Clin Monitor 11:23–31
47. Gerlach H, Rossaint R, Pappert D, Falke KJ (1993) Time-course and dose-response of nitric oxide inhalation for systemic oxygenation and pulmonary hypertension in patients with the adult respiratory distress syndrome. Eur J Clin Invest 23:499–502
48. Goldman AP, Cook PD, Macrea DJ (1995) Exposure of intensive-care staff to nitric oxide and nitrogen dioxide. Lancet 345:923–924
49. Hess D, Kacmarek RM, Imanaka H, et al (1995) Administration of inhaled nitric oxide by nasal cannula. Am Rev Respir Crit Care Med 151:A44 (Abst)
50. Etches PC, Harris MD, McKinley R, Finer NN (1995) Clinical monitoring of inhaled nitric oxide: Comparison of chemiluminescent and electrochemical sensors. Biomed Instrum Technol 29:134–140
51. Miller CC (1994) Chemiluminescence analysis and nitrogen dioxide measurement. Lancet 343:300–301
52. Etches PC, Ehrenkranz RA, Wright LL (1995) Clinical monitoring of inhaled nitric oxide. Pediatrics 95:620–621
53. Mercier J-C, Zupan V, Dehan M, et al (1993) Device to monitor concentration of inhaled nitric oxide. Lancet 342:431–432
54. Sokol GM, Van Meurs KP, Thorn WI, et al (1996) Limitations in nitrogen dioxide measurement with commercially available analyzers. Pediatric Research 39:353A (Abst)
55. Goldman AP, Macrae DJ (1994) Nitrogen dioxide measurement in breathing systems. Lancet 343:850
56. Betit P, Grenier B, Thompson JE, Wessel DL (1996) Evaluation of four analyzers used to monitor nitric oxide and nitrogen dioxide concentrations during inhaled nitric oxide administration. Respir Care 41:817–825
57. Wessel DL, Adatia I, Thompson JE, Hickey PR (1994) Delivery and monitoring of inhaled nitric oxide in patients with pulmonary hypertension. Crit Care Med 22:930–938
58. Skimming JW, Cassin S, Blanch PB (1995) Nitric oxide administration using constant-flow ventilation. Chest 108:1065–1072
59. Dellinger RP, Zimmerman JL, Hyers TM, et al (1996) Inhaled nitric oxide in ARDS: Preliminary results of a multicenter clinical trial. Crit Care Med 24 (Suppl):A29 (Abst)

Clinical Trials in ARDS

Co-intervention Control:
A Critical Need in ICU Clinical Research

A. H. Morris

Introduction

Many Critical Care Problems have resisted Resolution

Modern medicine has fostered the development of unquestionable advances. Drug treatment of many illnesses, including hypertension and diabetes mellitus has brought renewed control and increased health to many patients. Pain treatment has provided relief from suffering and surgical techniques have provided previously undreamed of opportunities for recovery. The management of trauma, including immediate therapy, and both ground and air transportation has advanced strikingly since World War II. The treatment of severe burns has led to markedly increased survival.

Some important problems in critical care have, in contrast, resisted resolution. While our understanding of underlying mechanisms of injury and inflammation in sepsis and adult respiratory distress syndrome (ARDS) has blossomed, our understanding of clinical management of sepsis and ARDS has not. Several clinical trials of promising therapeutic agents have consistently failed to identify the promised advances in therapy [1-6]. The agents that have or are being tested include cyclooxygenase inhibitors (corticosteroids and ibuprofen), a platelet activating factor antagonist (BN 52021), an antioxidant (N-acetylcysteine), an opiate antagonist (naloxone), a bradykinin antagonist (CP-0127), a cyclic-guanidine monophosphate (GMP) stimulant (inhaled NO), anti endotoxins (E5 and HA1A), anti cytokines (interleukin (IL)-1 receptor antagonist and anti-TNF), and extracorporeal gas exchange (low frequency positive pressure ventilation-extracorporeal CO_2 removal). The absence of a clear benefit from this broad spectrum of tested interventions suggests either that the clinical problems are insoluble, that the needed interventions have not yet been tested, or that out clinical investigative strategy is not sound.

Inaccurate Human Perception

Although the survival of patients with ARDS appears to have increased, we do not understand why and cannot identify the responsible therapeutic elements that might underlie the putative improvement [7]. A recently reported single center clinical trial has provided the most encouraging evidence to date of the importance of both end-inspiratory and end-expiratory lung volumes in ARDS patients supported with mechanical ventilation [8]. This suggests that a lung protective strategy that avoids both low and high lung volumes is advantageous. Nevertheless, the general lack of success in clinical care improvement is disappointing.

Inaccurate human perception probably contributes to this lack of success. Human decision making limitations [9] likely contribute to inaccurate perceptions and thereby to the uncertainty in health care delivery. Humans are limited in their ability to estimate the degree of relatedness (covariation) between only two variables ("The theories we hold apparently lead us to expect and predict stronger empirical relationships than actually exist." [10]). Preconceived notions or hypotheses influence our estimates of relatedness of variables, and influence what we remember and how we recall items in memory [11, 12]. These limitations likely contributes strongly to the tendency of people, including clinicians, to perceive their behavior in terms incompatible with their actual performance. Data from a study of two rheumatologists indicate the disparity between their perceptions of the variables they used in clinical decision making and the variables that actually contributed to their decisions (inferred from systematic observation of their behaviors) [13].

Input information overload, a biospheric phenomenon [14], is a common problem in the complex ICU environment [15]. The number of variables (objects) humans are capable of managing simultaneously (the input) before decisions (the output) become degraded was reported to be 7 in a landmark psychological publication [16]. This may be an overestimate for ICU decisions. Faced with the challenge of adjusting four simple variables (I/E ratio, ventilatory rate, peak ventilator pressure, and positive end-expiratory pressure setting (PEEP)) for pressure controlled inverse ratio ventilation (PCIRV), experienced ICU physicians were not able to develop as systematic a response to ventilator management as was a computerized PCIRV protocol [17]. Within the more than 236 different variable categories noted in one of our ARDS patients one morning on rounds [15], many clinically important problems involved consideration of many more than four variables.

Lack of Clinical Standardization

Perhaps as a result of perceptual difficulties stemming from covariation misestimation and from input information overload, much fundamental medical terminology lacks specificity and standardization [18]. The common practice of ascribing different meanings to the same term fosters miscommunication and predisposes all of us to confounding interpretations of published information. These confounding interpretations likely increases unnecessary variation in clinical practice. Three examples
1) interpretation of different ARDS studies;
2) conflicting use of physiologic hemodynamic variables and recommendations for their use; and
3) inconsistent use of terms in fluid and electrolyte assessment, will illustrate the widespread nature of this pernicious contributor to clinical confusion.

1) The definition of ARDS has not been standardized. Comparison of two recent clinical trials [19, 20] of withdrawal of mechanical ventilation (weaning) techniques for ARDS patients is difficult because of differences in design and because of undefined rules for identifying the moment at which the intervention is begun. This latter decision is left to clinical judgment. Both the definition (selection) of ARDS patients and their management (care) are not standardized. The difficulties of interpretation and of comparison of results from different studies of ARDS patients are widely recognized [21, 22].

2) Inconsistencies were observed between the perceptions of physicians regarding their use of physiologic data and the actual use of such data in decision making for cardiac problems in the ICU [23]. This is in part due to the use of ill defined terms or statements, such as "..caution should be exercised when PAOP (pulmonary artery occlusion pressure) becomes increased to the extent that pulmonary edema is a risk" [24]. In fact, this example appeared in a journal issue containing three articles that presented mutually contradictory sets of recommendations about hemodynamic monitoring [25].

3) Variation in fluid and electrolyte practice patterns may be an important and uncontrolled cointervention that can influence patient outcome and obscure the effects of therapeutic interventions in clinical trials.

An analytical scheme addressing three major factors in fluid and electrolyte evaluation
1) effectiveness of the arterial circulation,
2) extracellular fluid volume (ECF)], and
3) state of hydration (osmolality)) is compatible with widely taught precepts [26–29].

Evaluating these three concepts separately is important for clarification of clinical fluid and electrolyte problems and thereby for reducing unnecessary variation in clinical practice. Several recent publications illustrate the confusion that follows the use of fluid and electrolyte terms in an unstandardized manner. An American Medical Association Council report identifies isotonic, hypertonic, and hypotonic dehydration, thereby confusing the evaluation of the state of the ECF and the state of hydration [30]. This publication also includes cardiovascular evaluation in the evaluation of hydration, thereby confusing the evaluation of the effectiveness of the arterial circulation with the evaluation of the state of hydration. A pediatric publication used the term hypernatremic dehydration (a tautology if standard definitions are used) to describe dehydration (hypernatremia) and ECF contraction [31]. A discussion of fluid management in traumatic brain injury used dehydration to refer to ECF contraction due to fluid restriction (negative fluid balance) and recommended avoiding attempts to control intracranial pressure (ICP) through dehydration, although they, earlier in the paper, clearly established the efficacy of ICP reduction via increased osmolality induced with mannitol (dehydration or underhydration according to the standard terminology) [32]. The use of terms in such contradictory ways must contribute to the current uncertainty concerning fluid and electrolyte therapy for important clinical problems such as sepsis [33], shock [34], and ARDS [35]. Fluid and electrolyte therapy may be an important non-experimental cointervention in ARDS care.

Variability in interpretation of commonly used terms, within and between clinicians and institutions, seems closely related to the lack of standardization of common terminology in many clinical areas. It is appropriate to ask how well we can expect clinicians to relate multiple clinical variables to each other. Given these limitations of human decision making, our perceptual inaccuracies, and the variation in use and in interpretation of important clinical variables, it seems unlikely that ordinary clinicians, in the complex ICU environment, can be expected to systematically generate therapeutic decisions that are coherent and that include consideration of all appropriate options.

People Do Not Do What They Claim

Proposals to employ decision support tools in clinical decision making frequently elicit objections from clinicians. The objections are often based on perceived uniqueness of their clinical environment. Common objections include claims of uniqueness of patients, institutions, and clinicians. Patients are frequently perceived to be more severely ill, institutional attributes are commonly perceived to be different from others, patient survival is perceived to be superior, and clinician background and current practice styles (with any operational protocols or guidelines) perceived to be special. It is wise to remember, when faced with objections to decision support based on the uniqueness of the objecting clinician or his environment, that humans commonly perceive their performance in terms incompatible with objective observation [9–13]. Opinion, unsupported by objective data, is often an unreliable foundation for decision making in complex circumstances.

It is of interest to note here that non-specific effects (placebo effect, Hawthorne effect, regression to the mean) can be important [36–39]. The placebo effect can be associated with a 43 to 75% positive clinical response in control patients [38, 39]. The placebo effect can, therefore, produce changes in patient outcome larger than those expected to be associated with many study interventions.

Signal-to-Noise Ratio

The clinical environment lacks a desirable level of control. Uncontrolled non-experimental clinical care elements, including cointerventions that influence patient outcome, likely contribute to our failure to define the impact of ICU therapies on patient outcome. The complexity of ARDS, sepsis, and other clinical problems is a major factor [1, 15, 40, 41]. The significant variation in clinical decision making and in clinical care produces a large amount of background noise that can obscure the changes in patient outcome due to interventions of interest. When coupled with the relatively small impact expected from many clinical interventions in complicated settings [42], this produces a low signal-to-noise ratio and disadvantages those trying to draw inferences about efficacy of clinical interventions [15, 41, 43].

The detection of an association between an input signal of interest and an outcome measure requires that the signal of interest be capable of separation from other, unwanted, signals with which it may be confused or by which it may be obscured. A common measure of this capability is the signal-to-noise ratio [44]. Unless the signal-to-noise ratio exceeds 1, the signal will be undetectable. Two major elements, the patient and the clinical caregiver, determine the intensity of patient care and the patient outcome (Fig. 1). Both the patient and the clinical caregiver are sources of random noise and of systematic noise (bias). The patient contributes noise because of uncontrollable host factors and because of variation in disease etiology, severity, extent, and duration. Local factors influence the patient's disease and spectrum of clinical problems. The patient identification and selection process is quite imperfect and may incorporate much local bias due to the prejudices of individual clinicians and clinical investigators. This bias is the result of many factors, among which are characteristics of local clinical environments and failure of the medical community to establish broadly accepted specific (executable) definitions of many diseases, including ARDS [21, 22]. The other major element, the clinical caregiver response to the patient, introduces both random noise and bias. Strong bias is injected into the response of clinical caregivers because of strongly held opinions based on many factors that influence behavior, including general and local cultural factors, local technical abilities, background, training, and experience. These biases, and other elements in the clinical environment, can be important non-experimental cointerventions and can influence pa-

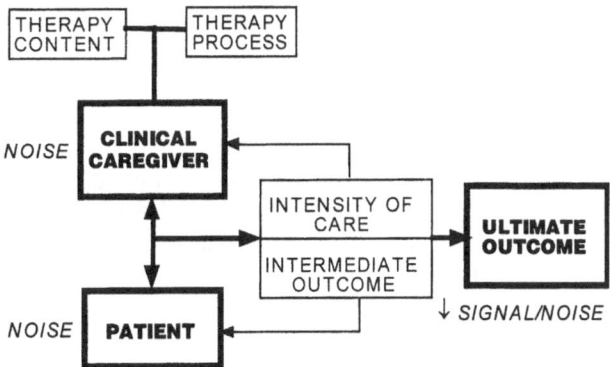

Fig. 1. The major elements (patient and clinical caregiver) that interact in an iterative feedback manner to determine the intensity of care, the level of intermediate outcomes (e.g. PaO_2, thoracic compliance Cth, etc.), and the ultimate outcome (e.g. survival). The intermediate outcomes and the intensity of care influence both the patient and the clinical caregiver during the iterative cycling of patient care. The patient finally exits form the iterative care process with some ultimate outcome. Both the patient and the clinical caregiver introduce random noise and non-random (systematic) noise (bias) that decrease the signal-to-noise ratio for important outcome events

tient outcome. The impact of random noise can be reduced by increasing the number (N) of observations (S/N varies inversely with N1/2). In contrast, the effect of systematic noise (bias) cannot be reduced by increasing N.

Non-experimental Co-interventions

Many interventional critical care studies, including those that incorporate mechanical ventilation techniques, cannot be double-blinded. Yet equal treatment of groups in randomized trials is important [45, 46]. Non-double-blinded studies must be scrutinized and the clinical care carefully assessed for comparability of the non-investigative cointerventions in the experimental treatment arms to assure internal validity of an experiment (Fig. 2) [37, 46]. While the determinants of patient outcome may include the intervention under study, these determinants are multiple and complex. Among the multiple variables that may determine outcome (e.g. survival) are variables, called non-experimental cointerventions, that are not part of the study. These variables or non-experimental cointerventions are frequently neither controlled nor measured.

Bias in experiments exerts its most pernicious effect when it is not equally expressed in the results of the different experimental groups. Non-experimental cointerventions that influence the different experimental groups unequally may produce a differential (between group) bias (Fig. 2). Differential bias threatens, and may invalidate, the assumptions of experimental group equation [46] necessary for the internal validity of a clinical trial (Fig. 2) [37]. Differential bias will be reduced in double blinded trials, but even with double blinding differential bias may not be eliminated. If the experimental treatment has an effect that, on the average, changes the clinical expression of the disease between the experimental groups, non-experimental treatment cointerventions may be applied differently to the treatment groups. For example fluid and electrolyte therapy (see below) in ARDS is variable and may lead to differential bias if the intervention being tested produces an effect that alters the frequency of pittiing edema in the treatment group. One experimental solution to this problem involves controlling as many of the non-experimental cointerventions as possible. The effect of many interventions on the outcome in complex clinical environments is likely to be small. It will, therefore, likely be obscured by the many non-experimental cointerventions involved in the clinical care of complex problems. Uncontrolled non-experimental clinical care process, with its cointerventions, may explain much of our failure to define the impact of ICU therapies on patient outcome.

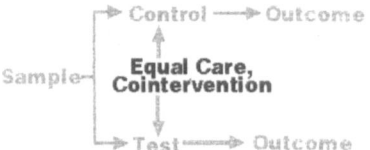

Fig. 2. Basic structure of patient allocation groups in a randomized clinical trial. Non-experimental cointervention (Cointervention) control is mandatory if the test and control groups are to be treated equally in all regards save for the intervention being investigated

Computerized Protocols: An Experimentally Attractive Decision Support Tool

The use of guidelines [47] and algorithms in clinical decision making is well established and appears to favorably influence patient outcome [48]. The most rigorous application of algorithms in clinical decision making is effected using rule-based computer systems [49]. Bedside (point-of-care) computerized protocols to standardize clinical decisions for mechanical ventilation for patients with ARDS have been used at the LDS Hospital for over 150 000 h in more than 150 ARDS patients [17, 50]. These computerized ARDS mechanical ventilation protocols have been exported to 11 other hospitals, uninvolved in their development, and have been used to support more than 60 ARDS patients through 1996, in a randomized clinical trial currently in progress [51].

The use of algorithms in clinical decision making generates tensions within the clinical community because of a perceived conflict between two paradigms of clinical decision making, to wit: the expert or authoritarian paradigm and the actuarial or numerical paradigm. Medicine has, since ancient times, traditionally employed the expert or authoritarian paradigm of decision making; this paradigm relies on expert clinical judgment. The clinician, empowered both by peers and the community, and licensed by the state, is the expert who provides the patient with the "best decision" based upon the expertís assessment of the particular problem for the individual patient at a specific time. This paradigm has traditionally ascribed special decision making power to the expert. This special power is derived from the background, experience, and training of the expert and has been described as intuitive, and therefore difficult to articulate and describe to others. This is one of the meanings of the "art" of medicine [52, 53].

The use of decision support tools, like computerized rule based algorithms, incorporates an actuarial paradigm, one based on numerical analysis and outcome data [54]. The tension between these two paradigms [15, 41] in the clinical community is not new. Arguments between proponents of each of these approaches raged before the French Academy in the early 19th century and involved important thinkers like Pascal, Poisson, Pinel and others [52, 53]. The conflict between these two approaches to clinical decision making is, in one sense, spurious since they are complementary rather that mutually exclusive approaches. The use of computerized protocols to standardize clinical decision making in complex clinical settings has, I believe, a sound ethical foundation [55].

Protocols Standardize Clinical Decision Making, They Do Not Standardize Clinical Care

Computerized protocols standardize clinical decision making [17, 50, 51, 56]. Since clinical decisions involve choices about therapy content (what we do) and therapy process (how we do it), standardization of clinical decision making involves standardization of content and process of therapy (Fig. 3). Executing computerized protocol instructions, different clinical caregivers (clinicians) provide the identical (standardized) response for a given set of patient data. Patient data are, however, not controlled by the clinician. Patient data are determined, in large

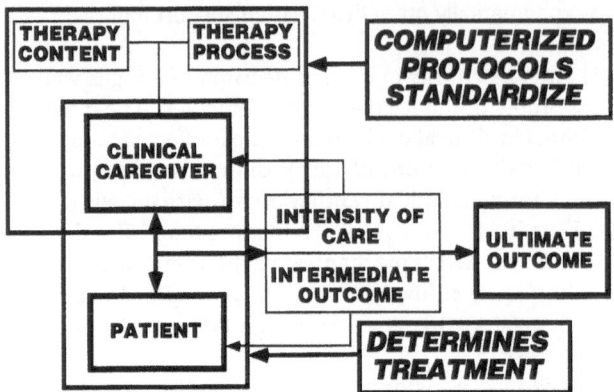

Fig. 3. Computerized protocols standardize clinical decisions but not clinical care. Computerized protocols standardize clinical decisions by leading clinicians to the same decision for a given patient expression of the disease. This does not standardize treatment. The two major elements in the health care encounter are the patient and the clinical caregiver. Treatment is determined by the interactions between these two elements, by both the standardized clinical decisions of the clinical caregiver and by the individualized patient expression of the disease. Since the response of patients to both the disease and to therapy are so variable and individualized, the treatment the patient receives is individualized and different for each patient. The standardization of clinical caregiver response does not produce a "cookbook" or patient-invariant treatment. (See Fig. 1)

part, by the patientís individualized expression of the disease and by the patientís individualized response to therapy. Clinical care (the treatment the patient receives) is, therefore, not standardized because it is determined not only by clinical decisions made by the clinical caregiver but also, and importantly, by the patientís individualized expression of the illness (Fig. 3). Without this crucial distinction one can easily, and erroneously, conclude that computerized protocol standardization of clinical decision making produces a "cookbook" or patient invariant clinical care or treatment. On the contrary, the clinical care delivered is patient specific and individualized, even though the clinical caregiver decision making is standardized by the computerized protocol.

Computerized Protocols Complement Meta-Analyses

Using meta-analysis to evaluate therapeutic efficacy addresses, in part, the problem of under powered randomized clinical trials due to low patient enrollment. Meta-analysis is the systematic assembly, critical appraisal, and synthesis of studies designed to address a single question. Meta-analysis provides valuable information about the credibility of clinical studies by subjecting the studies to a formal and rigorous review using explicit critical methods. From those studies that satisfy the rigorous review criteria, meta-analysis provides estimates of therapeutic efficacy. Meta-analysis is a powerful evidence-based medicine tool that allows credible inferences to be drawn from the combined analysis of small, independently non-definitive, but rigorously performed randomized clinical trials [3, 5, 42, 45]. Meta-analysis increases our ability both to detect real differences, and to conclude that no real differences exist (through increased power). By pooling results from rigorous individual studies, the number of observations is increased and more robust conclusions are thereby obtained from study results that cannot, independently, be convincing.

Meta-analyses cannot eliminate the non-random noise (bias) inherent in any single study or combination of studies. When the outcome effects (direction and magnitude) of these individual study differential biases are randomly distributed, meta-analysis has the maximum chance of providing an accurate estimate of treatment efficacy. If the differential biases are not randomly distributed among the studies included in the meta-analysis, the differential bias will appear in the meta-analysis result and reduce the accuracy of its estimate of treatment efficacy. Such non-random distributions of differential bias could occur if practice patterns produce differential bias in multiple single studies in a systematic manner through community-wide application of non-experimental cointerventions unequally between the treatment groups. For example, fluid and electrolyte therapy might play such a role. Such effects may be exposed by a rigorous clinical experimental approach in which cointerventions are explicitly controlled. Nevertheless, meta-analysis is a promising technique for advancing our understanding of therapeutic efficacy.

Protocols Have the Potential to Resolve Clinical Uncertainty if They are Used to Standardize Clinical Decision Making Between Institutions

The requirement for hundreds of patients in many clinical trials of critical care issues frequently necessitates multicenter trials lasting several years. The multiple year duration of many clinical trials introduces two serious limiting logistic problems: 1) unavoidable "secular" changes (changing non-experimental cointerventions that occur as a result of the passage of time); 2) faltering enthusiasm and interest among participating clinicians (MD, RN, RRT, etc.). The use of bedside (point-of-care) computerized protocols to standardize clinical decision making between institutions, makes possible the conduct of clinical trials with explicit methodology in large numbers of institutions. The acquisition of the required number of patients could then be realized in a short period of time, perhaps a few months. For example, a consortium of 100 hospitals configured to conduct clinical studies with computerized protocol standardization of clinical decision making, could likely enroll 800 ARDS patients within 6 months.

Widespread efforts to introduce separate, institution specific, guideline or protocol decision support are underway in many institutions. While this may further standardization within each institution, the development of separate and institution specific decision support tools will have little impact on the interinstitutional variation in health care delivery. The potential of computerized protocols to effectively address the problems of secular trends and faltering enthusiasm of participating clinicians, through the conduct of large multicenter trials, will not be realized by such institution specific protocols. The benefits of standardized explicit methodology in clinical trials, and the experimental rigor that they will convey on clinical trials, will only be realized by standardization of clinical decision making between large numbers of institutions. The development of separate, institution specific, decision support tools is, in this regard, counterproductive.

Protocols are Interventions

Protocols or algorithms, like all interventions, must be subjected to systematic evaluation, preferable in randomized clinical trials, in order to evaluate the benefits and risks that follow clinical protocol use. Evaluations should consider both internal and external validity issues [37, 38, 57–59]. Computerized protocols appear to produce favorable changes in clinically important outcomes [49]. Nevertheless the widespread distribution of most clinical decision support tools (Table 1) has not been matched by widespread systematic evaluation. The absence of systematic evaluation, including the absence of mechanisms for monitoring clinical performance, extends even to the extensive and scholarly output of several Agency for Heath Care and Policy Research activities.

Rationale

Patient Outcome: Good versus Harm

Improvement in the quality of medical care delivered to patients is widely desired and better therapies are actively sought. Because potential therapies have the power to do both good and harm, the evaluation of the balance between the good and the harm done to patients is a critical part of the assessment of clinical interventions The ethical principles of beneficence and non-maleficence should, therefore, play an important role in the decision to introduce new medical interventions into practice [60–62]. Unfortunately, most medical interventions are not supported by data that indicate the interventions produce more good than harm [63]. Equally disturbing is the observation that treatments based on uncontrolled clinical experience have a significant potential to be widely applied, even when useless or harmful [37, 42, 59, 64]. Uncontrolled and unblinded observational studies of patients, whose outcomes are compared with those of concurrent or historical series of patients, are often misleading. Treatments are much less likely to be judged efficacious when evaluated in randomized, double blinded clinical trials.

In 1917, Dr. Codman first proposed the use of patient outcome data for the monitoring and improvement of medical practice. Outcomes research has become an active investigative arena but it encompasses disparate approaches and goals, and is driven by different agendas, not all of which are primarily focused on improvement in quality of care (Table 1). In fact, the current widely voiced managed care imperative to "reduce cost and improve quality" implies a link between the two that, to my knowledge, does not exist. Among the approaches taken to increase the quality of care are those that focus on indications for, and general steps of, medical care. Proponents of outcomes measurement advocate the use of large data bases to evaluate specific treatment methodologies, medical technologies and the performance of medical care providers. Some promote the use of existing large data sets, such as the HCFA Medicare data base or large collections of patient data maintained by insurers [65]. Such databases are frequently acquired for financial or administrative reasons and are therefore not suitable for many investigations intended to lead to inferences about quality of care or about effectiveness or efficacy of interventions or clinical strategies. Others have proposed to create new collaborative data systems [66].

The approaches that rely only on medical outcomes inferred from large databases, suffer from the non-uniformity of patient care, from the frequent absence of explicit clinical methods, and from the observational (non-experimental) nature of the studies. Unfortunately, cointerventions [37, 59, 67, 68] and non-specific effects [36, 39] are expected to significantly influence many of the outcomes used to draw inferences about the effectiveness of clinical care from large databases such as the HCFA Medicare data. If cointerventions are institution specific, those data bases that incorporate information from many institutions may yield less biased results. If the cointerventions operate community-wide, multi-institutional, as well as single institutional results from such large data bases will be significantly biased and results drawn from studies of such databases could be misleading. The potential for error in conclusions drawn from observational epidemiologic studies is illustrated by the conflicting results from studies of the use of agents that block calcium channels in patients with acute myocardial infarction [69, 70]. The difference between the experimental results from randomized controlled trials and those from *post hoc* epidemiologic observational studies is dramatic.

Standardization of Clinical Care Process

There is community-wide interest in standardization of clinical care process as a means of either increasing the efficiency of care (reducing cost) or of increasing the quality of care (Table 1). Increasing efficiency is the primary goal of many recent observational studies in the managed care environment. Increasing efficiency involves reducing the consumption of resources associated with the delivery of care as currently practiced, generally without questioning the efficacy of the care delivered. The reduced consumption of resources is expected to reduce the costs of clinical care. Observational studies intended to increase efficiency might also identify some clinical interventions that result in improved quality of care, but they are only likely to do so for interventions that have a large, easily observed, effect on clinical outcome. Unfortunately, the clinical outcomes of interest for many complex clinical problems, including ICU problems, are influenced by multiple variables or cointerventions (large background noise). Changes in these outcomes due to a specific clinical intervention are frequently small (low signal) and assignment of these changes to interventions of interest is difficult because of the low signal-to-noise (S/N) ratio [15, 44].

Explicit Methodology

Standardization of elements of clinical care with protocols makes the clinical care method explicit. Explicit methods are exportable to other clinical care or clinical investigative sites (Table 1) [41]. Explicit methods are required for rigorous evaluation of clinical care process steps [37, 59]. Thousands of decision support products with different names, focus, and output are currently available to aid clinical practitioners (Table 2). Unfortunately most are useful only in a conceptual sense.

Table 1. Types of outcomes research studies. S/N = Signal-to-Noise Ratio Primary Driver = The major source of pressure for change (Reducing cost or increasing quality) Primary Goal = The major purpose of the activity (Increasing efficiency of currently practiced clinical intervention (accepting its clinical use) or defining whether or not the intervention works (questioning its clinical use) Observational = Observe and record only – no experiment involved Experimental = an intervention is intentionally manipulated to test its effect on an outcome Cointervention Control = non-experimental factors that might influence outcome are controlled to affect all experimental groups equally Exportable Method = the experimental or clinical method is explicitly documented so that it can be sent to another institution and used to duplicate the study or clinical intervention

Study Type (S/N level at which useful results are expected)	Primary Driver	Primary Goal	Study attributes			
			Observational	Experimental	Cointervention control (explicit method; standard decisions)	Exportable method
Database evaluation	↓ Cost	↑ Efficiency	×			
Continuous quality improvement	↓ Cost	↑ Efficiency	×			
Guidelines/ critical paths	↓ Cost	↑ Efficiency	×			
Case series/ historical controls (high S/N)	↑ Quality	Does it work?		×		
RCT (low S/N)	↑ Quality	Does it work?		×		
Meta-analysis (low S/N)	↑ Quality	Does it work?		×		
Computerized protocol (low S/N)	↑ Quality	Does it work?		×	×	×

Table 2. Common decision support products, their focus and outputs

Decision support product	Focus	Output
Guideline	Conceptual	Suggestions for clinical consideration
Critical path	Intermediate outcome steps	Timetable, reminders
Paper protocol	Clinical care process	Suggestions, instructions, general and specific
Computerized protocol	Clinical care process	Specific instructions, dynamic standing orders

They are usually incomplete, accounting for only some of the large number of combinations of clinical observations or intermediate patient outcomes encountered by clinicians. Because of this incompleteness, they are not robust clinical products and they lack specific instructions for at least some and often for many clinical circumstances. They cannot, therefore, standardize clinical decisions. Most of the decision support products fail to provide the support clinicians need when making difficult decisions with limited information in complex clinical environments. Since they cannot produce an explicit method, they are unlikely to contribute to the understanding and standardization of specific clinical care process steps in complex clinical settings.

As an example of the variable levels of detail and explicitness in decision support products, 4 different current clinical decision support tools for the withdrawal of post-operative mechanical ventilation are contrasted in Table 3. The variation in explicitness among these four decision support tools is obvious. The difference between the critical path recommendation that extubation should be achieved within 24 h and the specific rules of the computerized protocol is striking. For the clinical practitioner, only the computerized protocol rules provide an understanding of exactly what should constitute clinical management.

Before one can evaluate the outcome of a particular medical intervention, the intervention must be applied in a uniform manner to comparable patients [59]. This is a reflection of the widely recognized importance of experimental testing and replicability as a fundamental requirement of credible research in the physical [71] and in the social [46, 72] sciences. Existing large national data bases contain mixed groups of different treatments, even though they may be labeled with the same procedure or treatment code. Extending the analysis of practice pattern variation, James et al. studied detailed practice patterns within several well-defined procedures, including transurethral resection of the prostate (TURP) for symptomatic benign prostatic hypertrophy (BPH), cholecystectomy, total hip arthroplasty (non-fracture), cardiac pacemaker implantation, coronary artery bypass grafts (CABG), and treatment for pneumonia. Variations of 60 to more than 400% for common process of care steps for patients with comparable presentation and outcomes were observed [73–76]. Among 16 surgeons whose TURP practice patterns were tracked, median procedure times (by surgeon) ranged from 40 to 95 min, while average grams of prostatic tissue removed (by surgeon)

Table 3. Four different decision support tools for withdrawal of mechanical ventilation from patients after cardiac bypass surgery

Clinical practice guideline	Clinical or critical path	Nursing care plan	Computerized protocol
		Expected: Respiratory rate remains ±5/min of baseline, coughs effectively	
If the patient has a stable rhythm and stable hemodynamic status (PaO_2 >60 mmHg, FiO_2 <0.5, PEEP 5 cm H_2O)		Assess pulmonary status and record according to established policies. Do more frequently than required if client's condition is unstable	Assess weaning 8 h after surgery. Measure tidal volume (V_T), ventilatory rate (VR), maximum inspiratory pressure (MIP), and pHa
Follow the weaning technique ordered by the physician			Change to T-piece if: pHa >7.3, and spontaneous VR <30/min, and V_T >4 ml/kg mean body weight, and MIP ≤ 30 cm H_2O
			Check arterial blood gases 15 min after initiating T-piece
Extubate if: – 4 < tidal volume < 6 mL/kg, – 10 < vital capacity < 15 mL/kg, – 8 < ventilatory rate < 35/min, – maximum inspiratory pressure ≤ 20 cm H_2O, minute – ventilation < 10 L/min	Extubate within 24 h		

ranged from 11 to 42 g per case. These variations in TURP procedure had a strong statistical association with the occurrence of urethral strictures within one year of operation (the primary complication). The outcomes reported for treatments labeled "TURP" using insurance data, therefore leave much uncertainty about the actual procedures employed [59, 66, 77, 78]. A widely employed explicit methodology would significantly reduce this uncertainty.

Human Error

Finally, human errors are unavoidable [79, 80]. Even though they represent only 1% of clinical decisions and therefore indicate little room for improvement (decisions are error free 99% of the time), clinical ICU errors that threaten patient safety occur at a distressing frequency [81]. The clinical decision error rate can be reduced by simple computerized algorithms that generate reminders, alerts, or other information [54]. In addition to reducing error rates, such algorithms can reduce the clinical consequences of errors that take place. For example, an error of oversight in the ordering of a diuretic, without KCl, for a hypokalemic heart failure patient receiving Digoxin would have little impact if a computer reminder to order KCl supplementation were automatically generated.

Conclusion

Medicine, like social science, likely enjoys an "ecology of science ... in which there are available many more wrong responses than correct ones ...". There are probably many more bad choices than there are good choices among the possibilities faced by clinical decision makers. Individualized decision making unsupported by outcome data is therefore likely to be both variable and incorrect in complex clinical circumstances. The ability of experts to come to the "right therapeutic decision" when dealing with multivariate problems like ARDS should be questioned. This conclusion challenges the expert (authoritarian) paradigm that forms the foundation for much clinical decision making. This challenge leads to consideration of a complementary clinical decision making paradigm, one based on well defined rules constructed from the most scientifically credible information available with a preference for group data obtained under well controlled circumstances. Evidence-base medicine and meta-analyses provide one means for establishing such rules. Computerized protocols incorporating such rules, and used for decision support in the ICU, thus function as a tool for effecting this complementary clinical decision making paradigm. They possess a unique potential for increasing the rigor of experimental clinical research by providing explicit methodology. Clinical use of computerized protocols is compatible with ethical principles and imperatives.

Acknowledgement: Supported by the NIH (HL 36787), the AHCPR (HS 06594) the Deseret Foundation, the Respiratory Distress Syndrome Foundation, the LDS Hospital and IHC, Inc.

References

1. Lamy M, Deby-Dupont G, Deby C, Faymonville M, Damas P (1992) Why is our present therapy for Adult Respiratory Distress Syndrome so ineffective? Intens Crit Care Digest 11:6–12
2. Bone R (1995) Sepsis and controlled clinical trials: The odyssey continues. Crit Care Med 23:1313–1315
3. Cronin L, Cook D, Carlet J, et al (1995). Corticosteroid treatment for sepsis: A critical appraisal and meta-analysis of the literature. Crit Care Med 23:1430–1439
4. Eidelman L, Sprung C (1994) Why have new effective therapies for sepsis not been developed? Crit Care Med 22:1330–1334
5. Lefering R, Neugebauer E (1995). Steroid controversy in sepsis and septic shock: A meta-analysis. Crit Care Med 23:1294–1303

6. Morris A, Wallace C, Menlove R, et al (1994) Randomized clinical trial of pressure-controlled inverse ratio ventilation and extracorporeal CO_2 removal for ARDS (published erratum appears in Am J Respir Crit Care Med 1994, 149:838]. Am J Respir Crit Care Med 149:295–305

7. Milberg J, Davis D, Steinberg K, Hudson L (1995) Improved survival of patients with acute respiratory distress syndrome (ARDS): 1983–1993. JAMA 273:306–309

8. Amato MB, Barbas CS, Medeiros DM, et al (1995) Beneficial effects of the open lung approach with low distending pressures in acute respiratory distress syndrome. A prospective randomized study on mechanical ventilation. Am J Respir Crit Care Med 152:1835–1846

9. Arkes H (1986) Impediments to accurate clinical judgment and plossible ways to minimized their impact. In: Arkes H, Hammond K (eds) Judgment and decision making: An interdisciplinary reader. Cambridge University Press, pp 582–592

10. Jennings D, Amabile T, Ross L (1982) Informal covariation assessment: Data-based versus theory-based judgments. In: Kahneman D, Slovic P, Tversky A (eds) Judgment under uncertainty: Heuristics and biases. Cambridge University Press, pp 211–230

11. Beyth-Marom R, Dekel S (1985). An elementary approach to thinking under uncertainty.Hillsdale, New Jersey, Lawrence Erlbaum Associates, p 154

12. Tversky A, Kahneman D (1982) Availability: A heuristic for judging frequency and probability. In: Kahneman D, Slovic P, Tversky A (eds) Judgment under uncertainty: Heuristics and biases. Cambridge University Press, pp 163–178

13. Kirwan J, Chaput de Saintonge D, Joyce C, Currey H (1986) Clinical judgment in rheumaoid arthritis: II. Judging "current disease activity" in clinical practice. In: Arkes H, Hammond K (eds) Judgment and decision making: An interdisciplinary reader. Cambridge University Press, pp 364–368

14. Miller J (1978). Living systems. McGraw Hill, New York

15. Morris A (1993) Paradigms in management In: Pinsky M, Dhainaut JF (eds) Pathophysiologic foundations of critical care medicine. Williams and Wilkens, Baltimore, pp 193–206

16. Miller G (1956) The magical number seven, plus or minus two: Some limits on our capacity for processing information. Psychol Rev 63:81–97

17. East TD, Böhm SH, Wallace CJ, et al (1992) A successsful computerized protocol for clinical management of pressure control inverse ratio ventilation in ARDS patients. Chest 101:697–710

18. Shortliffe E, Barnett G (1990) Medical data: Their acquisition, storage, and use. In: Shortliffe E, Perreault L (eds) Medical informatics: Computer applications in health care. Addison-Wesley, Reading MA, pp 37–69

19. Brochard L, Rauss A, Benito S, et al (1994) Comparison of three methods of gradual withdrawal from ventilatory support during weaning from mechanical ventilation. Am J Respir Crit Care Med 150:896–903

20. Esteban A, Frutos F, Tobin MJ, et al (1995) A comparison of four methods of weaning patients from mechanical ventilation. N Engl J Med 332:345–350

21. Petty T, Bone R, Gee M, Hudson L, Hyers T (1992) Contemporary clinical trials in acute respiratory distress syndrome. Chest 101:550–552

22. Bernard G, Artigas A, Brigham K, et al (1994) The American-European consensus conference on ARDS: Definitions, mechanisms, relevant outcomes and clinical trial coordination. Am J Respir Crit Care Med 149:818–824

23. Ontario Intensive Care Study Group (1992) Evaluation of right heart catheterization in critically ill patients. Crit Care Med 20:928–933

24. Guidelines Committee Society of Critical Care Medicine (1992) Guidelines for the care of patients with hemodynamic instability associated with sepsis. Crit Care Med 20:1057–1059

25. Morris A (1993) Hemodynamic guidelines. Crit Care Med 21:1096

26. Windus D (1986) Fluids and electrolyte management. In: Orland M, Saltman R (eds) Manual of medical therapeutics. 25 ed. Little, Brown Co, Boston, pp 40–56

27. Levinsky N (1991) Fluids and electrolytes. In: Wilson J, Braunwald E, Isselbacher K (eds) Harrison's principles of internal medicine. 12 ed. McGraw Hill, New York, pp 278–283

28. DeVita M, Michelis M (1993) Perturbations in sodium balance. Clin Lab Med 13:135–148

29. Rose B (1994) Clinical physiology of acid-base and electrolyte disorders. (4 ed.) McGraw Hill, New York, pp 916-920

30. Weinberg A, Minaker K (1995) Dehydration. Evaluation and management in older adults. JAMA 274:1552-1556
31. Chilton L (1995) Prevention and management of hypernatremic dehydration in breast-fed infants. West J Med 163:74-76
32. Zornow M, Prough D (1995) Fluid management in patients with traumatic brain injury. New Horizons 3:488-498
33. Thijs L (1995) Fluid therapy in septic shock. In: Sibbald W, Vincent JL (eds) Clinical trials for the treatment of sepsis. Springer Verlag, Berlin, pp 167-190
34. Shoemaker W, Appel P, Kram H, Bishop M, Abraham E (1993) Temporal hemodynamic and oxygen transport patterns in medical patients: Septic shock. Chest 104:1529-1536
35. Mitchell J, Schuller D, Calandrino F, Schuster D (1992) Improved outcome based on fluid management in critically ill patients requiring pulmonary artery catheterization. Am Rev Resp Dis 145:990-998
36. Whitney C, Von Korff M (1992) Regression to the mean in treated versus untreated chronic pain. Pain 50:281-285
37. Hulley S, Cummings S (1988) Designing Clinical Research. Williams and Wilkins, Baltimore
38. Guyatt G, Drummond M, Feeny D, et al (1986) Guidelines for the clinical and economic evaluation of health care technologies. Soc Sci Med 22:393-408
39. Turner J, Deyo R, Loeser J, Von Korff M, Fordyce W (1994) The importance of placebo effects in pain treatment and research. JAMA 271:1609-1614
40. Bernard G, Plitman J (1995) The pharmacology of the acute respiratory distress syndrome: An update In: Parker M, Shapiro M, Porembka D (eds) Critical Care-state of the art. Soc Crit Care Med, Anaheim, pp 29-54
41. Morris A, Cook D 1997) Mechanical ventilation clinical trial issues. In: Marini J, Slutsky A (eds) Physiologic basis of ventilatory suport. Marcel Dekker, New York (In press)
42. Cook D (1994) Small trials in critical care medicine: What can intensivists learn from them? In: Vincent JL (ed.) Yearbook of intensive and emergency medicine. Springer-Verlag, Berlin, pp 779-785
43. Morris A (1996) ARDS clinical trial issues In: Haslett C, Evans T (eds) Adult respiratory distress syndrome. Chapman & Hall, London, pp 451-477
44. Tyson NdG (1996). Signal versus noise. Natural History 105:72-76
45. Guyatt G, Sackett D, Cook D (1993) User's guide to the medical literature: II. How to use an article about therapy or prevention A. Are the results of the study valid? JAMA 270:2598-2601
46. Campbell D, Stanley J (1966) Experimental and quasi-experimental designs for research (reprinted from Handbook of Research on Teaching, 1963) Houghton Mifflin Co, Boston, p 84
47. Grimshaw J, Russell I (1993) Effect of clinical guidelines on medical practice: A systematic review of rigorous evaluations. Lancet 342:1317-1322
48. Safran C, Rind D, Davis R, et al (1996) Effects of a knowledge-based electronic patient record on adherence to practice guidelines. MD Comput 13:55-63
49. Johnston M, Langton K, Haynes B, Mathieu A (1994) Effects of computer-based clinical decision support systems on clinician performance and patient outcome. Ann Intern Med 120:135-142
50. East T, Morris A, Gardner R (1995) Computerized management of mechanical ventilation. In: Grenvik A, Ayres S (eds) Textbook of critical care. 3 ed. WB Saunders, Philadelphia, pp 895-911
51. Kinder A, East T, Littman W, et al (1993) A computerized decision support system for management of mechanical ventilation in patients with ARDS: An example of exportation of a knowledge base. McGraw Hill, Washington, pp 888
52. Gigerenza G, Swijtink Z, Porter T, Daston L, Beatty J, Krüger L (1989) The empire of chance.Cambridge University Press
53. Matthews J (1995) Quantification and the quest for medical certainty. Princeton University Press
54. McDonald CJ (1996) Medical heuristics: The silent adjudicators of clinical practice. Ann Intern Med 124:56-62

55. Morris A, East T, Wallace C, et al (1994) Ethical implications of standardization of ICU care with computerized protocols. In: Ozbolt J (ed.) Proceedings of the 18th Annual Symposium on Computer Applications in Medical Care. Hanley & Belfus, Philadelphia, pp 501–505
56. Morris A (1994) Protocol control of mechanical ventilation in ARDS. In: Vincent JL (ed) Yearbook of Intensive and Emergency Care 1994. Springer-Verlag, Heidelberg, pp 495–510
57. Levine M (1992) Reader's guide for causation: Was a comparison group for those at risk clearly identified? ACP J : A12–A13
58. Rabeneck L, Viscoli C, Horwitz R (1992) Problems in the conduct and analysis of randomized clinical trials. Arch Intern Med 152 : 507–512
59. Pocock SJ (1983). Clinical Trials: A Practical Approach. Wiley & Sons, New York, p 266
60. Chalmers I (1986) Minimizing harm and maximizing benefit during innovation in health care: Controlled or uncontrolled experimentation? BIRTH 13 : 155–164
61. Warren K, Mosteller F (eds) (1993) Doing more good than harm: The evaluation of health care interventions. Ann NY Acad Sci 703 : 341
62. Jonsen A, Siegler M, Winslade W (1992). Clinical ethics. (3 ed.) McGraw Hill, New York
63. Williamson J, Goldschmidt P, Jillson I (1979) Medical Practice Information Demonstration Project-Final Report (Contract # 282–77–0068GS). Baltimore Office of the Asst. Secretary of Health, DHEW
64. Sackett D, Haynes R, Guyatt G, Tugwell P (1991) Clinical epidemiology: A basic science for clinical medicine. Little Brown, Boston, pp 187–248.
65. Wennberg JE (1988) Improving the medical decision making process. Health Affairs 7 : 99–106
66. Elwood PM (1988). Shattuck Lecture – Outcomes management: A technology of patient experience. NEJM 318 : 1549–1556
67. Schulz K, Chalmers I, Hayes R, Altman D (1995) Empirical evidence of bias: Dimensions of methodological quality associated with estimates of treatment effects in controlled trials. JAMA 273 : 408–412
68. Silverman W (1985). Human experimentation: A guided step into the unknown. Oxford University Press
69. Furberg C, Psaty B, Meyer J (1995) Nifedipine: Dose-related increase in mortality in patients with coronary heart disease. Circulation 92 : 1326–1330
70. Psaty B, Heckbert S, Koepsell T, et al (1995) The risk of myocardial infarction associated with antihypertensive drug therapies. JAMA 274 : 620–625
71. Giancoli D (1995). Physics. (3 ed.) Prentice Hall, Englewood Cliffs, p 3
72. Babbie E (1990) Survey research methods. Wadsworth Publishing Co, Belmont
73. Baird M (1988). Final analysis of the IHC coronary artery bypass graft quality utilization and efficiency (Q) study.Salt Lake City: Intermountain Health Care, Dept of Medical Affairs
74. Baird ML, Busboom SW, French TK, et al (1989) Final analysis of the IHC 1987 permanent pacemaker implant quality, utilization and efficiency (QUE) Study. Salt Lake City: Intermountain Health Care
75. James BC, Weed M, Lewis SW, Busboom S, Darricades G, Ingram B (1987) Final analysis of the IHC transurethral prostatectomy utilization study. Intermountain Health Care Department of Medical Affairs Technical Report No.1.Salt Lake City: Intermountain Health Care
76. Baird ML, Busboom SW, Ingram B, et al (1988) Final analysis of the IHC uncomplicated total hip arthroplasty quality, utilization, and efficiency (QUE) study. Salt Lake City: Intermountain Health Care
77. Wennberg JE (1987) Are hospital services rationed in New Haven or over-utilized in Boston? Lancet 1 : 1185–1189
78. Roos NP, Wennberg JE, Malenka DJ, et al (1989) Mortality and reoperation after open and transurethral resection of the prostate for benign prostatic hyperplasia. N Engl J Med 320 : 1120–1124
79. Abramson NS, Wald KS, Grenvik ANA, Robinson D, Snyder JV (1980) Adverse occurrences in intensive care units. JAMA 244 : 1582–1584
80. Wu A, Folkman S, McPhee S, Lo B (1991) Do house officers learn from their mistakes? JAMA 265 : 2089–2094
81. Leape L (1994) Error in medicine. JAMA 272 : 1851–1857

Designing the Perfect Trial in ARDS and ALI

R. J. Mangialardi and G. R. Bernard

Introduction

Since the adult respiratory distress syndrome (ARDS) was first described nearly 30 years ago, the definition used in clinical trials has varied considerably making comparison of their results difficult because of differences in underlying patient populations. A recent American-European consensus conference proposed a standardized definition that includes a PaO_2/FiO_2 ratio less than 200, bilateral lung infiltrates, and no clinical evidence of heart failure [1]. Even with this consensus definition, there is still subjectivity in the interpretation of chest radiographs used to discern bilateral lung infiltrates, and great variability in the underlying diseases ranging from aspiration to sepsis to multiple trauma. The reported survival rate has increased from approximately 10% in the extracorporeal membrane oxygenation (ECMO) trials in the early 1970s to approximately 50% today. Ongoing pathophysiologic research suggests that ARDS is a disease of lung inflammation resulting in increased capillary permeability, pulmonary edema, poor oxygenation, and deranged respiratory mechanics. Many clinical trials have evaluated agents designed to interrupt this inflammatory cascade in both ARDS and sepsis, but to date, no intervention has proven better than placebo under the scrutiny of randomized blinded clinical trials. Surprisingly, there have been no randomized clinical trials to evaluate the role of diuretic medications or to determine the optimal intravenous fluid solutions (colloid versus crystalloid) in ARDS, despite the fact that its major manifestation is pulmonary edema, and despite the fact that there is considerable clinical controversy over these issues. In this chapter, we will describel the rationale for conducting such a study and discuss the "ideal" versus the "practical" study design which could answer these important and basic clinical questions.

Rationale for Studying Albumin Supplementation in ARDS

Frank Starling discovered the physiologic relationship that governs fluid flux across semipermeable membranes nearly a century ago [2]. The Starling relationship provides four mechanisms for edema formation:
1) Elevation in hydrostatic pressures within the capillary;
2) Decrease in the oncotic pressure gradient between the capillary lumen and the interstitial space;

3) Increase in basement membrane permeability to proteins and other solutes; and
4) Decrease (or relative insufficiency) in lymphatic clearance of edema fluid from the interstitium back to the systemic circulation.

When clinicians apply the term "ARDS," they frequently imply that the patient has pulmonary edema secondary to increased lung capillary permeability (mechanism 3) [3]. However, the current clinical definition of ARDS (PaO_2/FiO_2 < 200, bilateral lung infiltrates, no evidence of heart failure) excludes the mechanism of increased hydrostatic pressure but does not exclude the possibility of any of the other three mechanisms. To evaluate the potential role of decreased oncotic pressure, we recently reviewed our experience in a clinical trial of ibuprofen in sepsis syndrome (unpublished material). That trial enrolled 455 patients with sepsis syndrome of which 178 patients developed ARDS. Patients with serum protein levels at study entry ≤ 5 g/dL were twice as likely to develop ARDS, and nearly three times as likely to die with ARDS as patients with serum protein levels at study entry ≥ 6 g/dL. The hypoproteinemic patients experienced significantly more weight gain over the first 5 days of the study and required significantly more ventilator support during the first 30 days of the study. These findings held true even after controlling for 16 possible confounding variables including Apache II scores.

No clinical study has ever examined the effects of altering serum protein levels in patients with ARDS by any intervention. The greatest number of clinical studies involving albumin administration have compared the use of colloid to crystalloid for the acute resuscitation of hypotensive patients, typically those with hemorrhagic shock [4–6]. These studies have generally been small and underpowered to detect mortality differences between crystalloid and colloid treated patients. The most consistent finding of these studies has been that use of albumin results in maintenance of serum albumin and protein levels while crystalloid resuscitation results in decreases in albumin and total protein levels. The second most consistent finding is that patients resuscitated with crystalloid generally require much larger volume infusions to achieve the same resuscitation endpoints (adequate hemodynamics) than patients receiving colloid. Some studies have found a trend toward better respiratory outcomes in the colloid-treated patients, but most have concluded that there was no difference. None of these studies has targeted patients with pre-existing ARDS or patients with pre-existing hypoproteinemia or hypoalbuminemia. If colloid therapy is useful in edematous, hypoproteinemic patients with ARDS but not in volume depleted normoproteinemic patients without ARDS, these studies have all been incapable of detecting such a finding.

A few studies have examined the impact of albumin supplementation in critically ill hypoalbuminemic patients and reached different conclusions [7–11]. Foley et al. [10] prospectively randomized critically ill patients with albumin levels ≤ 2.5 g/dL to receive either albumin or placebo in addition to standard nutritional support (enteral nutrition, EN, or parenteral, TPN). They randomized 18 patients to the treatment group and 22 patients to the control group and found no statistically significant differences in complication rate, length of hospital stay, or length of ICU stay between the groups. The patients were not selected on the basis of having pulmonary or systemic edema, and the respiratory complication event rate was low in both treatment and control groups. Furthermore, most of the complications that they measured could not be affected by the osmotic properties of albumin. These included complications such as myocardial infarction, arrhythmias, stroke, pneumothorax, gastrointestinal bleeding, and infection. Finally, the investigators based their intervention on albumin levels rather than total protein levels or measured plasma oncotic pressure, and their treatment endpoint (albumin ≥ 2.5 g/dL) was quite low compared to normal serum albumin levels.

Brown et al [9] prospectively randomized hypoalbuminemic patients requiring TPN to receive either albumin (31 patients) or placebo (30 patients) with a goal of achieving serum albumin levels ≥ 3 g/dL. They found a statistically significant decrease in pulmonary morbidity (18 controls versus 9 treated patients with "pneumonia") and in the incidence of sepsis (11 controls versus 2 treated patients) in treated patients. Their study did not target ARDS patients or patients with evidence of fluid overload, and the intervention was based on serum albumin level rather than total protein level.

Rationale for Studying Diuretics in ARDS

There has never been a prospective randomized clinical trial of diuretics versus placebo in ARDS [12], and this remains a controversial issue. Many clinicians advocate the cautious use of diuretics in the otherwise stable patient regardless of intravascular filling pressures because of animal data suggesting that edema formation is minimized by minimizing vascular pressures. [13, 14]. Others argue against the use of diuretics in these patients for several theoretical reasons. First, diuretic medications may decrease circulating volume and thus reduce cardiac output and tissue oxygen delivery [15]. Second, lower cardiac output caused by diuresis may impair renal function, and poor renal function is a known independent predictor of poor outcome in ARDS [16]. Third, many of these patients have shock, require pressor medications, or require ongoing fluid boluses for episodic hypotension, and diuretics may worsen shock or lead to increased pressor support to maintain an adequate blood pressure [15].

The largest clinical trial of volume management was reported by Mitchell et al [17]. The investigators used an extravascular lung water measurement technique to guide the use of diuretics in all patients with pulmonary edema including patients with both ARDS and congestive heart failure. Overall, patients who were randomized to the more aggressive diuretic regimen experienced more rapid improvement in lung function and had shorter duration of mechanical ventilation and ICU stay. Among the 50 patients with ARDS, the investigators found the same trends in net fluid balance and number of ventilator days as in the overall population, but the results did not quite reach statistical significance possibly because of the small sample size.

Simmons et al [18] retrospectively reviewed the records of 213 ARDS patients who were prospectively enrolled in a database. They examined weight change over the first 14 days of the study and found that patients who lost 3 or more kg had significantly better survival than those who gained 3 or more kg (67 versus 0%, p < 0.0001). Humphrey et al [19] retrospectively compared survival in ARDS patients based on change in pulmonary artery occlusion pressure. Patients with a 25% reduction in pulmonary capillary wedge pressure (PCWP) over the first 24 h after pulmonary artery catheter placement had a 75% survival compared to a 30% survival in patients who did not experience such a reduction. The difference remained statistically significant after adjusting for differences in age and initial Apache II scores.

We have had some success treating patients who have ARDS and low serum protein levels with a combination of diuretics and albumin (unpublished observation). We have generally found that this approach is associated with large volume diuresis without hemodynamic compromise and with improving oxygenation and improving respiratory mechanics. The combination may be especially effective at minimizing the potential problems of either therapy alone. For instance, albumin infusion may support intravascular volume and offset any tendency for diuretics to lower cardiac output, worsen tissue oxygen delivery, or impair renal function. Conversely, animal studies have shown that lung water is highly correlated with microvascular hydrostatic pressure in experimental lung injury. The diuretics may offset any tendency of albumin infusion to raise hydrostatic pressures and worsen pulmonary edema. Furthermore, diuretics may hasten the goal of raising serum protein level by concentration of the extracellular fluid compartment.

The Ideal Clinical Trial of Diuretics and Albumin in ARDS

Factorial Design

We now turn to the question of how best to design a randomized clinical trial to assess the role of albumin supplementation and diuretics in hypoproteinemic ARDS patients. Because we wish to test two interventions and we are especially interested in the possible synergy in the two treatments, we can obtain the most information from a factorial designed experiment as illustrated in Table 1. To examine the effect of albumin in ARDS, we could compare Group 1 + 2 to Group 3 + 4. To examine the effect of diuretics, we could compare Group 1 + 3 to Group 2 + 4. This design also makes it possible to examine the synergy between the two treatments, diuretics and albumin, by comparing Group 1 to all other groups. The

Table 1. Factorial design of albumin plus diuretics in ARDS clinical trial

Group 1	Albumin	Diuretics
Group 2	Albumin	Placebo for Diuretic
Group 3	Placebo for Albumin	Diuretics
Group 4	Placebo for Albumin	Placebo for Diuretics

factorial design is the most efficient way to answer the questions we have raised because it makes the best use of the placebo group. To evaluate albumin and diuretics in separate studies would require more patients to achieve the same power because each study would need a placebo group for comparison. The principle disadvantage of the factorial design is that it requires twice as many patients as a simple two-arm study such as one comparing only Group 1 to Group 4. However, if such a two-arm study produced positive results (i.e. treatment was better than placebo), it would be unclear whether the benefit arose as a result of albumin, diuretics, or the combination. If such a study produces a negative result (i.e. no difference between treatment and placebo), the possibility will remain that one of the treatments may be efficacious but that the efficacy is lost when the second drug is added.

Increasing Power by Decreasing Variability in Outcome Variables

A second consideration when designing a clinical trial of this type is minimizing the inherent variability in the underlying endpoints (the standard deviation in each of the continuous outcome variables). For a given number of patients in each group under comparison, the detectable effect size is directly proportional to the standard deviation in the variable of interest. For instance, a study of a given size might have an 80% power to detect (at a statistically significant level) a change in weight over 5 days equal to one half the standard deviation for weight change. If one of the outcome variables of interest is weight change over the first 5 days, and the study population includes both hemodynamically stable and unstable patients, ventilated and spontaneously breathing patients, early and late ARDS patients, and patients with various underlying diseases (sepsis, trauma, aspiration, etc.) there is likely to be great variability in fluid requirements, diuretic responsiveness, and hence weight change over 5 days. Alternatively, if the study targets only hemodynamically stable, mechanically ventilated patients who have been ventilated for at least 3 days, who have ARDS because of sepsis, and who are not deemed to be "weanable" at study entry, the population will be more homogeneous, the standard deviation for weight change will be much smaller, the standard deviation for weight change will be much smaller, and hence, the necessary difference in the measured weight change between groups necessary to reach statistical significance will be smaller and potentially more attainable. Furthermore, most ARDS patients who neither die nor recover rapidly are likely to meet the more restricted target criteria at some point in their clinical course. Another benefit of choosing such a stable population is that the dropout rate due to patient death during the study interval is likely to be smaller, thus making results for physiologic outcome variables easier to interpret. There are two disadvantages to narrowly targeting the study entry criteria. First, the result of the study may not be as broadly applicable as the investigator would like. For example, the results of a study targeted to hemodynamically stable, ventilator-dependent sepsis patients may not be applicable to hemodynamically compromised, non ventilator-dependent trauma patients, even though both groups have ARDS. Second, narrowly targeted inclusion criteria will reduce the number of patients who are eligible to participate in the study, thus increasing the cost, complexity, and duration of recruiting the desired number of patients. If the entry criteria are too narrowly defined, the study may not be practical.

Death as a Confounder of Physiologic Endpoints

A third consideration in clinical trial of ARDS is how to deal with patient dropout due to death [20]. One approach is to censor for patient death, i.e. simply leaving the patients who do not survive for the desired measurement interval (i.e. 5 days) out of the final analysis. This approach may miss significant differences between the groups. For instance, in our proposed study, it will be difficult to evaluate weight change over 14 days if 20–50% of the patients in each group die before day 14. The problem will be compounded if there is significantly greater mortality in one group than another. If one treatment arm is superior, we might expect to find that patients in that arm gain less weight over time. But, if patients receiving the inferior treatment die at a faster rate such that the patients with the worst outcomes are not alive to be weighed on day 14, we may not be able to detect a real difference in weight change between the two treatment arms. And, if the study is small, the difference in survival may not reach statistical significance. The opposite problem may occur if the follow-up interval is too short. If we establish the study endpoint as weight change after 1 day rather than 14 days, patient dropout will not be the problem. Instead, the follow-up interval may be too short to achieve meaningful differences between two treatments, and we may falsely conclude that there is no difference in therapies when a real difference exists. Thus, there is a precarious balance between allowing an adequate time interval for the effect of therapy to become apparent, and not allowing so long a time interval that patient demise makes the results uninterpretable.

The problem of assessing ventilator dependence is even more complex One could compare groups based on time to extubation (i.e. the number of days from study entry to extubation). The problem that arises is how to handle extubation due to patient death which is clearly different than extubation due to patient recovery. One solution would be to treat successful extubation as a dichotomous variable (either the patient is successfully extubated within some predefined time period or not), and compare the success rates between groups. Unfortunately, comparisons of dichotomous variables require several times as many patients to reach statistical significance as comparisons involving continuous variables, because dichotomous variables discard useful information about the patients. For instance, a patient successfully extubated after 2 days would receive the same consideration as a patient successfully extubated after 29 days in a study assessing extubation at 30 days using the dichotomous approach, and the obvious difference in clinical outcome would be lost. The approach that we favor is using a continous index for ventilator dependence know as ventilator free days. A predefined measurement period, typically 28 days, is specified before the study begins. Patients accrue one point for each day during the measurement period that they are both alive and free of mechanical ventilation. A patient who is extubated on day 2 of the study and remains alive and free of the ventilator for the remainder of the 28–day period would receive a ventilator free days score of 26, whereas the patient who is ventilated until death on day 2 would receive a ventilator free days score of zero. The approach retains the maximum amount of clinical information in a continous variable while controlling for extubation due to death, thereby reducing the number of patients needed to adequately assess the effects of a given treatment on ventilator dependence. We should note that the ventilator free days score, while continuous, is not a normally distributed variable. There are clusters of patients with scores at each end of the scale (zero and 28). Statistical analyses of this variable should employ non-parametric tests.

The failure free days approach can be applied to clinical endpoints other than mechanical ventilation. It can be applied to any organ failure. Treatment regimens can be compared with respect to outcomes such as renal failure free days, shock free days, coma free days, etc., using such tools as the Brussels Organ Failure Table [21, 22].

Assessing Survival Effects of Treatment

The holy grail of endpoints in clinical trials of ARDS patients is survival. Ultimately, we would like to know if any intervention proposed for patients with ARDS is likely to save lives.

Survival is necessarily a dichotomous variable (patients either live or die), and any study whose objective is to determine survival benefit will likely require a very large number of patients (typically a few hundred). In contrast, much smaller studies may be adequate to show differences caused by treatment in continuous physiologic or laboratory variables such as oxygenation, weight change, protein levels, lung compliance, dead space fraction, or even ventilator free days. A rational approach to evaluating new therapies in ARDS may be to first conduct smaller randomized clinical trials to assess these physiologic endpoints, and reserve the larger, more costly, multicenter trials for assessing survival benefits for therapies that have shown promise in the smaller studies. It seems unlikely that a therapy which cannot be shown to impart some physiologic benefit is likely to improve survival in patients with ARDS.

Statistical Power

Any reasonable clinical trial in ARDS should be undertaken with the appropriate statistical power to detect a true difference between treatment groups if such a difference exists. Many of the smaller randomized trials conducted thus far in ARDS, especially those comparing different strategies of mechanical ventilation, have found no survival benefit for any given strategy, but these studies have been severely underpowered to detect such differences. It is relatively easy to obtain results that show no statistically significant differences by including too few patients in the study. The appropriate conclusion from an underpowered negative study is not that the therapy is useless, but rather that the study was not capable of determining whether or not the therapy was useful. Furthermore, continuous outcome variables require far fewer patients to adequately assess than do dichotomous variables. For instance, in a study of diuretic strategy, we estimate that approximately 15 patients per arm would be sufficient to assess a 2.5 kg difference in diuresis or a 50-point difference in PaO_2/FiO_2 ratio, but 150 patients per arm would be needed to demonstrate a 10%-point difference in survival. Other power calculations for our hypothetical study of albumin and diuretics in ARDS are shown in Table 2.

Conclusion

Nearly 30 years have elapsed since ARDS was first described, yet many basic clinical management questions remain to be studied. These questions include the utility (or possible harm) of diuretics and colloid in these patients. We are likely to best utilize our scare clinical research resources if we design small studies with sufficient power to detect physiologic endpoint improvement before embarking on more costly and larger multicenter clinical trials to assess survival benefit. We can enhance our ability to detect meaningful differences caused by treatment if we select patients or outcome variables such that underlying variability is minimized and the information content of the variables is maximized. The factorial design is the most efficient for assessing multiple interventions simultaneously if the target population and available resources permit its use. Clinical studies should include a long enough follow-up period so that meaningful effects of therapy can be assessed, yet short enough that follow-up is not compromised by dropout in one or more treatment arms because of mortality. Finally, the practicalities of highly restrictive trials – low patient recruitment and lack of generalizability – make the decision to conduct the "ideal" clinical trial a complicated and difficult one.

Table 2. Estimates of detectable effect size in outcome variables for the proposed clinical trial of albumin and diuretics in ARDS. The estimates are based on a sample size of 15 patients per arm with the standard deviation derived from a recently completed clinical trial of ibuprofen in sepsis syndrome

Parameter		Mean ± SD	Detectable effect size
Serum protein level (g/dL)	4.0	0.5	0.52
Creatinine change (mg/dL)	0.27	0.40	0.42
Weight change (kg over 5 days)	4.4	2.5	2.6
Minute ventilation (L/min)	15.4	2.5	2.6
PaO_2/FiO_2 ratio	150	50	52
Dynamic compliance (mL/cm H_2O)	23	5.0	5.2
Static compliance (mL/cm H_2O)	36	10	10

References

1. Bernard GR, Artigas A, Brigham KL, et al and the consensus committee (1994) The American-European consensus conference on ARDS. Definitions, mechanisms, relevant outcomes, and clinical trial coordination. Am J Respir Crit Care Med 149:818–824
2. Kaminski MV Jr, Haase TJ (1992) Albumin and colloid osmotic pressure implications for fluid resuscitation. Crit Care Clin 8:311–321
3. Bernard GR, Brigham KL (1995) Increased lung vascular permeability: Mediators and therapies. In: Shoemaker W (ed) Textbook of Critical Care Medicine, 3rd Edn. W. B. Saunders, Philadelphia, PA, pp 674–680
4. Pockaj BA, Yang JC, Lotze MT, et al (1994) A prospective randomized trial evalutating colloid versus crystalloid resuscitation in the treatment of vascular leak syndrome associated with interleukin-2 therapy. J Immunol 15:22–28
5. Virgilio RW, Rice CL, Smith DE, et al (1989) Crystalloid versus colloid resuscitation: Is one better? A randomized clinical study. Surgery 85:129–139
6. Velanovich V (1989) Crystalloid versus colloid fluid resusciation: A meta-analysis of mortality. Surgery 105:65–71
7. Golub R, Sorento JJ Jr, Cantu R Jr, Nierman DM, Moideen A, Stein HD (1994) Efficacy of albumin supplementation in the surgical intensive care unit: A prospective, randomized study. Crit Care Med 22:613–619
8. Greenough A, Emery E, Hird MF, Gamsu HR (1993) Randomised controlled trial of albumin infusion in ill preterm infants. Eur J Ped 152:157–159
9. Brown RO, Bradley JE, Bekemeyer WB, Luther RW (1988) Effect of albumin supplementation during parenteral nutrition on hospital morbidity. Crit Care Med 16:1177–1182
10. Foley EF, Borlase BC, Dzik WH, Bistrian BR, Benotti PN (1990) Albumin supplementation in the critically ill. A prospective randomized trial. Arch Surg 125:739–742
11. Marik PE (1993) The treatment of hypoalbuminemia in the critically ill patient. Heart and Lung 22:166–170
12. Shuster DP (1995) Fluid management in ARDS: "Keep them dry" or does it matter. Intensive Care Med 21:101–103
13. Prewitt RM, McCarthy J, Wood LDH (1981) Treatment of acute low pressure pulmonary edema in dogs. J Clin Invest 67:409–418
14. Huchon GJ, Hopewell PC, Murray JF (1981) Interactions between permeability and hydrostatic pressure in perfused dogs' lungs. J Appl Phys 50:905–911
15. Shoemaker WC, Appel P, Bland R (1983) Use of physiologic monitoring to predict outcome and to assist in clinical decision in critically ill postoperative patients. Am J Surg146:43–50
16. Fowler AA, Hamman RF, Zerbe GO, Benson KN, Hyers TM (1985) Adult respiratory distress syndrome: Prognosis after onset. Am Rev Respir Dis 132:472–478
17. Mitchell JP, Schuller D, Calandrino FS, Schuster DP (1992) Improved outcome based on fluid management in critically ill patients requiring pulmonary artery catheterization. Am Rev Respir Dis 145:990–998
18. Simmons RS, Berdine GG, Seidenfeld JJ, et al (1987) Fluid balance and the adult respiratory distress syndrome. Am Rev Respir Dis 135:924–929
19. Humphrey H, Hall J, Sznajder I, Silverstein M, Wood L (1990) Improved survival in ARDS patients associated with a reduction in pulmonary capillary wedge pressure. Chest 97:1176–1180
20. Wheeler AP, Edens T, Swindell B, et al (1994) Clinical trials of multiple organ failure: The confounding effect of death on measuring organ failure and reversal. Am J Respir Crit Care Med 149:A650 (Abst)
21. Bernard GR, Doig G, Hudson L, et al (1995) Quantification of organ failure for clinical trials and clinical practice. Am J Respir Crit Care Med 151:A323 (Abst)
22. Marshall JC, Cook DJ, Christou NV, Bernard GR, Sprung CL, Sibbald WJ (1995) The multiple organ dysfunction (MOD) score: A reliable descriptor of a complex clinical outcome. Crit Care Med 23:1638–1652

Future Clinical Trials of Mechanical Ventilation in ARDS and ALI

R. Brower

Introduction

Mechanical ventilation (MV) is our primary means for providing respiratory support in patients with severe acute respiratory distress syndrome (ARDS) and acute lung injury (ALI). In many patients, death is likely unless adequate gas exchange can be maintained until specific treatments and supportive therapies can be administered and acute inflammatory and fibroproliferative processes can resolve. However, the goals of MV are frequently difficult to achieve in ARDS/ALI, and there are many limitations and potential adverse effects of traditional MV techniques.

Numerous modifications have been suggested to improve MV techniques in ARDS/ALI [1–11]. In some instances, potentially beneficial short-term effects of new approaches were demonstrated on lung physiology and pathology in animals or humans [4, 12–17]. In other instances, effects on ARDS/ALI mortality were inferred from uncontrolled studies [8, 9]. There are relatively few instances [1, 11] where effects on mortality or other key clinical events were assessed in randomized controlled clinical trials in humans with ARDS/ALI.

The purposes of this chapter are to:
1) review some recent experiences in designing and conducting randomized, controlled trials of new MV strategies in ARDS/ALI;
2) focus on some new ideas for improving MV in ARDS/ALI that may require further clinical testing in the near future; and
3) begin a discussion of key elements of design and conduct of future trials of MV in ARDS/ALI.

Recent and Current Experiences in Clinical Trials

Numerous studies have demonstrated ALI in animals ventilated with large tidal volumes to simulate overdistention in the patent airspaces of the lungs in ARDS patients [7, 16–21]. In uncontrolled studies, mortality rates were surprisingly low when humans with ARDS were ventilated with small tidal volumes (VT) to reduce overdistension injury [8, 9]. Despite the lack of carefully controlled clinical trials demonstrating efficacy, several authors recommended small tidal volume ventilation with permissive hypercapnia (STV/PH) for management of ARDS/

ALI [22–24], and many clinicians adopted this modification of MV in their practices [25]. However, there are numerous potentially adverse effects of STV/PH ventilation, including deterioration of gas exchange [26, 27], circulatory failure from acute acidosis [28–30], and severe dyspnea and agitation requiring increased sedation and neuromuscular blockade. Because the human experience with STV/PH was limited to uncontrolled series, true effects on mortality, time to recovery, and other important clinical events were unknown. Moreover, clinicians had little information regarding goals for VT, airway pressure, acceptable levels of $PaCO_2$, monitoring and adjusting for adverse effects, etc. In the early 1990's, several randomized controlled clinical trials of small VT or "low stretch" ventilation were initiated in Europe and North America to address the concerns and questions raised after the reports of good survival in uncontrolled series.

In Baltimore, a trial was designed to answer some questions regarding adverse effects and establish a framework on which to design a more ambitious trial to assess effects of STV/PH on mortality and other key clinical events. The primary objective of the trial was to determine if STV/PH would cause deterioration in gas exchange. If STV/PH caused worse gas exchange, higher levels of FiO_2 and positive end-expiratory pressure (PEEP) would be necessary to support minimally acceptable levels of arterial oxygenation. This could lead to greater oxygen toxicity, circulatory depression, and barotrauma. Additional objectives of the trial were to assess effects of STV/PH on circulation. If acidosis caused circulatory depression, requirements for vasopressors and intravenous fluids would increase. A third objective was to assess effects on dyspnea and agitation by monitoring requirements for sedatives and neuromuscular blocking agents. Inclusion criteria for this trial were:
1) $PaO_2/FiO_2 < 200$;
2) Bilateral infiltrates on frontal chest radiograph;
3) No suspicion of congestive heart failure or volume overload (if measured, pulmonary artery wedge pressure ≤ 18 mmHg);
4) Intubated and receiving MV. Patients were excluded if > 24 h had elapsed from the time that all inclusion criteria were first met.

Additional criteria were used to exclude patients with conditions where hypercapnia might be contraindicated: pregnancy, age < 18 years, and severe comorbid conditions that would likely affect outcomes of interest.

Rules for controlling ventilator management in the Baltimore trial are summarized in Table 1. These were designed to achieve two main objectives. First, the rules were written to simulate techniques used in the uncontrolled reports of STV/PH in ARDS where mortality rates were lower than expected [8, 9]. This was difficult because many aspects of the previous study techniques were not described explicitly. An upper limit for peak inspiratory alveolar pressure (P_{plat}) of 30 cmH$_2$O was used in the STV/PH group instead of peak airway pressures of ~ 35 cmH$_2$O as in the previous reports because P_{plat} is a more specific indicator of end-inspiratory lung stretch. All patients were ventilated with a volume cycled mode because control of VT and stretch is difficult with pressure-limited modes when patients exert respiratory muscle effort; for ethical and logistical reasons, neuromuscular blockade could not be required for this trial.

Table 1. Baltimore trial of STV/PH: Ventilator management

	Traditional tidal volume	Small tidal volume
Mode	Volume assist/control or SIMV with ≤ 5 cmH$_2$O pressure support	
Tidal Volume	Initial $= 10$–12 mL/kg ideal body weight Decreased to maintain $P_{plat} < 45$–55 cmH$_2$O	Initial $= 8$ mL/kg ideal body weight Decreased to maintain $P_{plat} < 30$ cmH$_2$O
P_{plat}	< 45–55 cmH$_2$O	< 30 cmH$_2$O
Ventilator Set Rate	Adjusted to maintain PaCO$_2 = 30$–45 mmHg if possible	
I/E	$\leq 1/1$ (any flow rate and inspiratory wave form was allowed if Tinsp $<$ Texp)	$\leq 1/1$

Protocol Approved Combinations of FiO$_2$ and PEEP

FiO$_2$	0.50	0.50	0.50	0.60	0.70	0.70	0.70	0.80	0.90	0.90	0.90	1.0
PEEP (cmH$_2$O)	5	7.5	10	10	10	12.5	15	15	15	17.5	20	≥ 20

In both groups, only these combinations of FiO$_2$ and PEEP were allowed.

Oxygenation	$55 \leq$ PaO$_2 \leq 75$ mmHg or $86 \leq$ SpO$_2 \leq 94\%$
	If PaO$_2$ (or SpO$_2$) deviated from the target range, either PEEP or FiO$_2$ was adjusted upward or downward to the next approved FiO$_2$/PEEP combination
Na-bicarbonate administration	pH > 7.30 No bicarbonate allowed $7.2 \leq$ pH ≤ 7.3 Bicarbonate allowed pH ± 7.2 Bicarbonate required

A second objective of the ventilator management rules was to reduce variations within and between groups regarding important ventilator parameters due to differences in clinicians' ventilator management styles. This would have three important benefits:
1) By reducing variance in some measures of interest, it would improve the probability of discerning true treatment effects and reduce the number of patients necessary to enroll to identify these effects;
2) By preventing practice decisions by clinicians who were aware of treatment assignments, potential biases, intentional or inadvertent, were minimized; and
3) Regardless of the outcome of the study, explicit ventilator management rules would provide a firm foundation on which to design subsequent trials or practice guidelines.

Although the main objectives for the ventilator rules were clear and important, it was challenging to write the rules to be acceptable to clinicians whose primary roles were as patient advocates and who frequently maintained strong opinions about optimal ventilator management. Most clinicians will agree that their strong opinions are sometimes based on incomplete knowledge of scientific information (or lack thereof) or on recent or most memorable experiences. Nonetheless, clinicians' primary roles are as patient advocates, and they must do the best they can with the information available to them. To maximize compatibility of clinicians' objectives with those of the trial, extensive discussions were conducted, literature reviews were provided, and recommendations were sought from clinicians from all intensive care units where patients would be recruited. This process resulted in broad support for the objectives and methods of the trial.

In some instances, the rules represented compromises between practice styles. The best example of this is the algorithm for managing PEEP and FiO_2 to maintain adequate arterial oxygenation. Some intensivists preferred to use high FiO_2s before raising PEEP $> 5-10$ cmH_2O. Others preferred to raise PEEP to $15-20$ cmH_2O before raising FiO_2 > 0.50. It was essential to minimize these variations in practice style, independent of treatment group, because a primary objective of the trial was to assess effects of STV/PH on gas exchange by comparing requirements for PEEP and FiO_2. Moreover, it was possible, if not likely, that clinicians would use PEEP and FiO_2 according to different prioritization schemes in patients randomized to the two treatment groups. This would cause additional variance. Adverse or beneficial effects from different levels of FiO_2 and PEEP between groups could further increase variance. Thus, failure to rigorously control use of PEEP and FiO_2 could obscure any effect of STV/PH on gas exchange independent of the effects of clinicians' practice styles.

Although the ventilator management rules for this trial were endorsed by clinicians as well as investigators, they required substantially more attention than was typically given to ventilator management. Therefore, execution of the protocol required substantial additional attention by study personnel to ensure that the procedures were followed. Respiratory therapists and nurses as well as clinicians required frequent educational exercises and re-enforcement. Initiation of ventilator procedures required approximately 2 h per patient by a member of the study team. On subsequent days, approximately 1 h per patient was necessary to remind caregivers of the goals for the dependent parameters (P_{plat}, oxygenation, pH, $PaCO_2$) and the ventilator settings that were allowable to achieve these goals. Computerized decision support tools [31, 32] would have been helpful for improving the clarity of the instructions and the accuracy of caregivers' decisions in executing the protocol, but resources were not available to provide these.

Compliance with the ventilator management rules and achievement of the patient-related objectives were assessed in two ways. First, in 10 patients selected to represent all of the sites where patients were recruited, all ventilator and patient records were reviewed to determine percent of study time that P_{plat} and PaO_2 were out of target ranges. Second, for all 52 patients enrolled in the study, ventilator and patient parameters were reviewed for compliance with the protocol rules and objectives at two randomly selected times. Results of both assessments are shown in Table 2. These data suggest that goals for the patient related objectives (P_{plat} and PaO_2) were met in high percentages of the study time. Moreover, procedures for ventilator management were correct most of the time. Importantly, between-group differences in accuracy of protocol execution were trivial. In most instances when ventilator settings or patient parameters were not accurate relative to protocol requirements, the reasons were slow response times or misunderstandings of protocol procedures by therapists or clinicians. There were very few instances where clinicians purposely deviated from protocol procedures.

Mean values for PEEP and FiO_2 during the first four days after enrollment are shown in Fig. 1. The groups were well matched for requirements for oxygenation support at the time of enrollment (Day 0). The subsequent data suggest that between-group differences in requirements for PEEP and FiO_2 were small or non-existent. Since PaO_2 and SpO_2 goals were the same in both groups, these data do not support the concern that the STV/PH treatment would cause deterioration in gas exchange. Further analysis of these data will be necessary to adjust for differences within and possibly between treatment groups in length of time on MV and also various factors that may affect individual patient's courses.

To address concerns regarding effects of STV/PH on circulation, dyspnea, and agitation, all prescriptions for vasopressors, sedatives, and neuromuscular blocking agents were recorded while study patients received MV. No between-group differences were identified in vasopressor use or sedation. There was also no difference in number of sedatives used per patient day. However, there was a trend towards greater use of neuromuscular blocking agents in the STV/PH group. No attempt was made to control use of these medications, and practices varied sub-

Table 2. Baltimore trial of STV/PH: Assessment of study procedures

% of time P_{plat} and PaO_2 "off-target" until appropriate response (complete review of all values on 10 patients)

	TTV, %	STV/PH, %
P_{plat}	<1	2
PaO_2	11	10

% of randomly selected instances "off-target"

	TTV, %	STV/PH, %
Mode	0	2
PEEP/FiO_2	8	4
Tidal volume	4	0
P_{plat}	0	8
SpO_2	18	14
$PaCO_2$	17	10

TTV = Traditional tidal volume treatment group. STV/PH = Small tidal volume/permissive hypercapnia treatment group

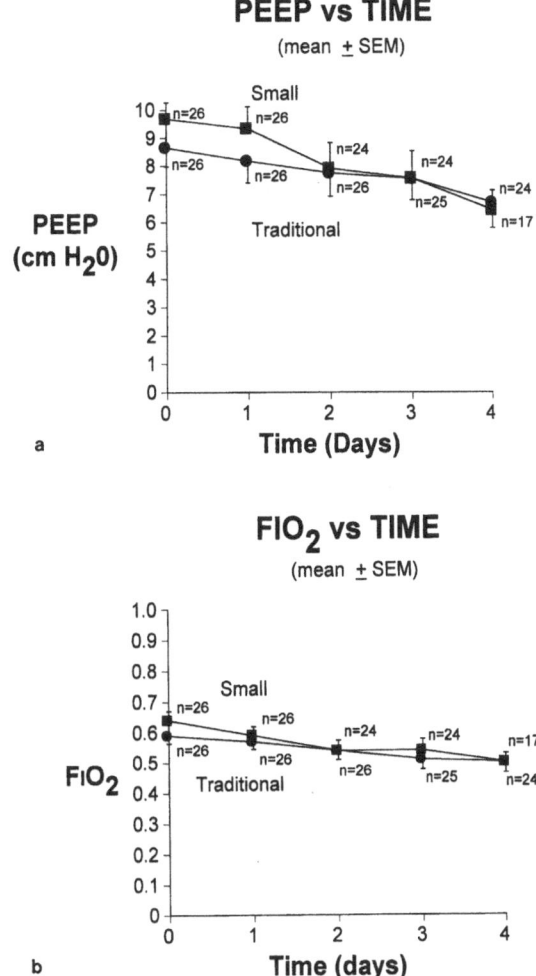

Fig. 1. Baltimore trial of STV/PH. Mean values of PEEP (**a**) and FiO$_2$ (**b**) during the first 4 days after enrollment

stantially among clinicians. Since it was not possible to keep clinical staff blinded to treatment group, it is possible that prescriptions for these medications were affected by clinicians' biases. Therefore, between-group comparisons for these prescriptions must be interpreted conservatively.

Several factors led to the decision by the recently formed National Heart, Lung, and Blood Institute (NHLBI) ARDS Network to conduct a trial of STV/PH. One priority was to address an important question of relevance to a large number of patients. Since positive pressure ventilation is prescribed to most patients with severe ARDS/ALI, and since all intensivists must consider the issues of stretch, tidal volume, and permissive hypercapnia in patients on MV, a trial of STV/PH was an obvious choice. A second reason for the decision to develop a ventilator trial is that clinicians' ventilator management styles vary so greatly, independent of specific patient requirements [33]. If ventilator management were left uncontrolled in clinical trials of pharmacologic agents or other interventions not involving MV, clinicians' ventilator practice variations could reduce chances of discerning true effects of the new agents. Hence, a ventilator trial could provide the foundation for supportive care ventilator management for subsequent trials of other interventions.

Inclusion criteria for the ARDS Network trial include $PaO_2/FiO_2 \leq 300$, allowing entry of patients with ALI as well as ARDS. Numerous exclusion criteria are designed to enhance the probability of discerning any treatment group differences in important outcome variables. Protocol procedures are summarized in Table 3. These procedures were designed using numerous insights from trials of STV/PH in Utah and Baltimore and the collective experiences of network clini-

Table 3. NHLBI, NIH ARDS Network Trial of STV/PH: Ventilator management

	Traditional tidal volume	Small tidal volume
Mode	Volume Assist/Control	
Tidal Volume	Initial = 12 mL/kg ideal body weight Decrease if necessary to achieve P_{plat} goal	Initial = 6 mL/kg ideal body weight Decrease if necessary to 5 or 4 mL/kg to achieve P_{plat} goal
P_{plat}	< 50 cmH$_2$O	< 30 cmH$_2$O
Ventilator Set Rate	Adjusted to maintain pH > 30 if possible. Maximum set rate = 35.	
I/E	1/1–1/3 (any flow rate and inspiratory wave form allowed)	

Protocol Approved Combinations of FiO$_2$ and PEEP
FiO$_2$ 0.30 0.40 0.40 0.50 0.50 0.60 0.70 0.70 0.70 0.80 0.90 0.90 0.90 1.0 1.000
PEEP 5   5   8   8   10   10   10   12   14   14   14   16   18   18 ≥20

In both groups, only these combinations of FiO$_2$ and PEEP are allowed.

Oxygena-tion	$55 \leq PaO_2 \leq 80$ mmHg or $80 \leq SpO_2 \leq 95\%$

If PaO$_2$ (or SpO$_2$) deviates from the target range, either PEEP or FiO$_2$ is adjusted upward or downward to the next approved FiO$_2$/PEEP combination.

Weaning	Weaning procedures attempted each day if FiO$_2$ < 0.40. Weaning proceeds by step-reductions in pressure support beginning at 20 cmH$_2$O and proceeding to 15, 10, and 5 cm H$_2$O at intervals of 1–3 h. Protocol criteria to assess for tolerance to weaning applied at each step. Accelerated weaning allowed for some patients.

cians and investigators. For example, in the Baltimore trial, the difference between treatment groups in mean P_{plat} values during the first several days after enrollment was only ~ 5 cmH$_2$O. One reason for this small separation between treatment groups was that P_{plat} was < 30 cmH$_2$O after the initial decrease in tidal volume (to 8 mL/kg ideal body weight) in ~ 50% of STV/PH patients. This was consistent with the target described in the uncontrolled reports [8, 9], so no further reductions in tidal volume were required in the trial. However, it was apparent that most patients were comfortable on this VT, with little or no additional tachypnea or hypercapnia. More aggressive reductions in VT would have been possible to achieve lower levels of stretch (and P_{plat}) if desired. A second reason for the small separation in P_{plat} between groups in the Baltimore trial was that the protocol VT procedures did not accurately reflect traditional ventilator management. In over half the patients, pre-enrollment VT exceeded the volumes required by the trial procedures for the traditional management group. It was necessary to reduce VT in these patients to levels prescribed in the trial. For the ARDS Network trial, STV/PH tidal volumes will be reduced to 6 mL/kg ideal body weight regardless of P_{plat} and reduced further if necessary to achieve P_{plat} < 30 cmH$_2$O. In the traditional management group, VT will be set initially = 12 mL/kg ideal body weight. These changes in approach will result in greater separation between groups in P_{plat}, providing a better opportunity to discern effects of end-inspiratory stretch on important outcome variables.

The Baltimore trial allowed weaning from MV if FiO$_2$ ≤ 0.50. However, weaning was not always required at this point, and the method of weaning was not controlled. This allowed substantial variations in practice which could affect length of time on MV. Since the trial was not blinded, differences in clinicians' approaches could cause between group differences independent of any effect of treatment. One of the primary outcome variables in the ARDS Network trial is ventilator-free days (number of days of unassisted breathing between enrollment and day 28). Therefore, procedures are explicitly defined in this trial to ensure the same aggressive approach to weaning in both groups of patients.

The first primary outcome variable for the ARDS Network trial is all-cause mortality prior to discharge home off MV. Since mortality in ARDS patients is affected by many factors other than lung injury and the role of stretch in MV, it will be difficult to demonstrate a difference in this endpoint. Therefore, a second primary outcome variable for this trial is "ventilator-free days prior to day 28". If a patient initiates unassisted breathing before day 28 of the study and sustains spontaneous breathing for at least 48 h, then the number of days of unassisted breathing prior to 28 days will be counted. This variable should be more directly related to recovery from respiratory failure from ARDS/ALI and is therefore more likely to show a difference between groups. Additional outcome variables for this trial include organ failure-free days, using the Brussels criteria [34] for defining organ failures.

The first patients were enrolled in the ARDS Network trial in March 1996. The trial is designed with b = 90% and a = 0.05 to demonstrate a 10% reduction in mortality (from 50 to 40%) with the STV/PH treatment. It may continue to a maximum enrollment of 1000 patients. Interim analyses will occur after each 200 patients. An O'Brien-Fleming upper boundary is designed to stop the trial early for superiority of the STV/PH treatment. The trial may also stop early at the interim analyses for futility (very low probability that STV/PH will be superior if more patients are enrolled). However, the trial will not stop early for futility with respect to the mortality endpoint if there are encouraging trends in ventilator-free days in the STV/PH group.

New Ideas for Improving MV in ARDS/ALI

Improving Airspace Recruitment to Prevent Lung Injury

Numerous studies in animals [12, 14–17] strongly suggest that ALI may occur from repeated closing and opening of small unstable airways during tidal ventilation. This ventilation-induced injury may be reduced when some level of PEEP is applied to prevent airway closure during exhalation. Some studies strongly suggest that the levels of PEEP necessary to achieve this objective exceed the levels usually applied to support arterial oxygenation [12, 14, 15]. A recent report suggests more rapid recovery from respiratory failure and reduced mortality in ARDS patients ventilated with a lung protective strategy that included high PEEPs [1].

Some studies suggest that protection against closing-reopening injury may be accomplished by raising PEEP to ~ 2 cmH_2O > the pressure at the end of the lower limb of a quasistatic inflation pressure-volume (P-V) relationship (P_{flex}) [1, 14]. However, there are numerous theoretical and practical limitations to this approach. P-V curves may change quickly in some ARDS/ALI patients in the early phase of illness. Frequent measurements of P_{flex}, each of which requires neuromuscular blockade, may not be acceptable to some patients and clinicians. Moreover, P_{flex} values are frequently not discernible on the P-V curves [35, 36]. Values that can be discerned under quasistatic conditions may not represent the PEEP necessary to maintain airway patency during tidal ventilation.

Another problem with high PEEPs is that they tend to contribute to high airway pressures and overdistention unless VT are simultaneously reduced. Effective ventilation may be sacrificed in favor of imperatives to achieve high levels of recruitment and reduce distention. Many authors and clinicians claim that decreased alveolar ventilation and acute respiratory acidosis are well tolerated, and that salutary effects of reducing ventilation-associated lung injury outweigh adverse effects of acute hypercapnia [22–24]. However, with the exception of one modest study [1], there are no controlled clinical trials in which mortality or other important clinical outcome variables in ARDS/ALI improved despite sacrifice of traditional gas exchange and acid-base objectives. On the other hand, some recently concluded clinical trials of STV/PH did not show trends towards improved survival. Interpretation of mortality results in these trials is limited because of the relatively small numbers of patients enrolled. Moreover, it is possible that the targets for peak lung distention in these studies were inadequate to achieve the intended benefits; or that peak lung distention is not a key determinant of outcome in ARDS/ALI. But it is also possible that adverse effects of PH were more substantial than previously estimated and counteracted the beneficial effects of peak lung distention. Additional studies are necessary to clearly define: 1) the amount of PEEP necessary to achieve lung protective effects of increased lung recruitment; 2) true benefits, if any, from reduced lung distention during inspiration; 3) the magnitudes of salutary effects of these modifications relative to the risks of acute respiratory acidosis.

Recent studies suggest that other factors in addition to PEEP may play important roles in determining airway recruitment. For example, in an oleic acid model of ALI in pigs, shunt decreased, oxygenation improved, respiratory system compliance increased, and wet/dry weight ratios decreased when some animals were ventilated with biologic variability in respiratory rate and VT at the same PEEP and mean airway pressure as control animals [37]. The authors cited previous work that suggested that during each inspiration, there is a variable sequence of airway openings that depends on characteristics of small airways [38]. Opening pressures of each airway segment may change from breath to breath due to alterations in various factors such as thickness and surface tension of airway lining

Table 4. Factors that may affect airway patency

Airway transmural pressure
Intraluminal pressure
- PEEP
- Inspiratory pressure
Surrounding pressure
- Pleural pressure
  transpulmonary pressure
  body position
  respiratory muscle effort
  pleural liquid, air, tubes, ...
- Tethering forces from parenchyma
  transpulmonary pressure
  emphysema, fibrosis, ...

Opening/closing pressures
Lining fluid characteristics
- Surface tension
- Viscosity
- Volume (thickness)
- Distribution
Airway characteristics
- Size (wall thickness, cartilage, smooth muscle, ...)
- Inflammation
- Wall tension
Hysteresis
- Magnitude of opening pressure > closing pressure
Breath-to-breath variability in opening/closing pressures

Time Factors
Durations of inspiration and expiration
Speed of airway opening and closing

fluid and airway wall tension and stress relaxation. Perhaps these breath-to-breath changes in opening pressures are amplified when the lungs are ventilated with variations in VT and respiratory rate. If so, then with hysteresis in airway opening pressures (closing pressures lower than opening pressures), overall airway patency could be enhanced with variable respiratory rate and VT. If the results in pigs with ALI can be replicated and extended to other species, including humans, the implications are potentially great. It may be possible to maintain substantially improved airway patency and prevent ventilation-associated injury without resorting to high PEEPs.

Recent studies in mechanical models and animals have further defined numerous variables that may affect airway patency [39–43]. Airway surface tension is a key determinant of the airway transmural pressure at which a closed airway begins to open. However, once airway transmural pressure exceeds this level, the speed at which a segment of airway opens depends on other factors as well. When the viscosity of airway lining fluid is high, the speed of airway opening may decrease substantially [39]. Although airways typically "pop open" once airway pressure exceeds their opening pressures, high lining fluid viscosity could prevent complete opening during inspiration. Tension in airway walls and tethering forces from surrounding parenchyma may also play important roles in determining airway patency [39–41]. Magnitudes and distributions of pleural pressure and the influence of body position are also important determinants of airway opening, and recent reports suggest that these may be manipulated advantageously in ARDS/ALI patients [44, 45]. An outline of some factors affecting airway opening is given in Table 4. A thorough understanding of these factors and the relationships among them may yield insights that will allow better airway recruitment through improved ventilator management.

Improved Patient-Ventilator Interactions

Severe dyspnea with agitation frequently persist in patients on MV, despite achievement of virtually normal arterial blood gas values. Although ventilators may guarantee normal amounts of ventilation and oxygenation, respiratory muscles frequently continue to contract vigorously [46, 47]. In some patients with acute respiratory failure, substantial amounts of oxygen are consumed with intense respiratory and other muscle activity [48]. In some patients, active efforts to exhale may counteract effects of PEEP; adequate arterial oxygenation may be achievable only with very high FiO_2s and PEEP. In the most severe cases, intensivists may resort to heavy sedation and even neuromuscular blockade to achieve minimal objectives of oxygen delivery to essential organs.

Continued respiratory distress in patients on MV may be related to excessive catecholamines or to effects of pulmonary congestion and inflammation on vagal afferents [49]. However, much respiratory distress and muscular effort may be attributable to dysynchrony between patients' efforts to breathe and the assistance provided by the ventilator [50–52]. In traditional volume-cycled modes, each breath is delivered in a stereotyped manner, with fixed volume, peak inspiratory

Table 5. Potential benefits of improved patient-ventilator synchrony

Decreased oxygen consumption by muscles of respiration and agitation
- decreased FiO$_2$ and PEEP
- increased availability of oxygen to critical organs

Decreased agitation
- decreased requirements for sedatives and neuromuscular blockade
- fewer ventilator days due to over-sedation
- fewer complications from neuromuscular blockade

Increased (biologic) variability in respiratory pattern
- improved airway patency
- decreased shunt
- improved oxygenation
- decreased requirement for PEEP to support oxygenation
- decreased opening-reclosing injury

flow rate and flow waveform, and duration of inspiration. Even when values for these parameters of inspiration are matched to the average values a patient "desires", many breaths are not well matched to the patient's efforts because these efforts vary substantially from breath to breath. Pressure limited modes allow some breath-to-breath variability in flow rate, pattern, and timing, but ventilator response times are frequently inadequate to maintain target levels of support in patients with the greatest respiratory distress. Substantial improvements in ventilator technology and in intensivists' repertoires are necessary to overcome these limitations of MV in patients with ARDS/ALI. Potential benefits of improved MV in ARDS/ALI patients are shown in Table 5.

Conclusion

Several issues should be addressed in deciding future directions for clinical trials of MV in ARDS/ALI:

1) Is it appropriate to utilize scarce resources to study MV? Compelling data from animal and some human studies strongly suggest that traditional MV techniques are associated with adverse effects, and that some modifications of traditional techniques may attenuate these effects. Since most patients with severe ARDS/ALI require MV, there is potential benefit to a large number of patients if substantial improvements in MV can be demonstrated. However, there are obvious risks of some proposed modifications of traditional MV techniques, and it is not apparent that the potential benefits outweigh the potential risks. To demonstrate the true value of these modifications, it will be necessary to conduct randomized, rigorously controlled clinical trials focussed on key clinical outcome variables.

2) Which modifications of MV should be subjected to the rigors and expense of randomized controlled trials, and which if any may be introduced with lesser efforts? Intended beneficial effects of some modifications, such as reduced airway shear force- and stretch-induced ALI, are difficult or impossible to meas-

ure in ARDS/ALI patients. Moreover, some proposed modifications entail risks that are also very difficult to measure and compare meaningfully with the desired beneficial effects. At this time, the true value of these modifications can be demonstrated only in controlled clinical trials with large numbers of patients that focus on key clinical outcome variables that can be measured reliably. Some proposed modifications to traditional MV techniques may not require large-scale randomized controlled trials if the intended benefits, such as reduced work-of-breathing, can be readily measured and if potential adverse effects are not apparent.

3) What outcome variables should be used to design large randomized controlled trials of MV in ARDS/ALI? The "gold-standard" of all-cause mortality at 28–30 days is influenced by many factors in addition to MV technique. Any single new treatment for patients with ARDS/ALI may not reduce mortality by more than a few percent. An effect such as this on mortality would be important, but demonstrating the effect would probably require enrollment of 2000 patients, if not more. It is tempting, therefore, to use other endpoints that relate more directly to the intended effects of the new treatment, such as ventilator-days or time-to-recovery from respiratory failure. A disadvantage of endpoints such as these is that they may hide serious delayed adverse effects of a new treatment. Moreover, they are more likely to be influenced by biases on the parts of clinicians providing clinical care and also study personnel interpreting clinical observations. Therefore, if endpoints such as these are adopted, it will be imperative to develop protocol procedures that rigorously control ventilator management and other supportive care treatments that may affect the endpoints.

4) Is it necessary to control all aspects of ventilator management in a trial designed to test the effects of a change in one parameter, such as tidal volume or P_{plat}? Because of various logistical challenges, it is tempting to design ventilator trials with minimal control of ventilator parameters other than the one that is the focus of the trial. However, because clinicians' ventilator practice styles vary considerably, true treatment effects, if any, may be obscured. If a trial is designed to control most or all ventilator management, patient recruitment may become more difficult because of clinicians' reluctance to relinquish control. However, greater levels of control enhance the value of each experiment and reduce the number of patients necessary to enroll in a trial. Moreover, since it is virtually impossible to keep clinicians and investigators blinded to treatment group, there is the potential for biases in practice styles to affect the outcome of trials. Future trials of MV will benefit from maximal control of ventilator parameters.

5) A fifth issue regarding future trials of MV is how to assure that the experimental procedures are followed as intended. If it is agreed that most or all aspects of ventilator management (not to mention other supportive care) should be rigorously controlled, then each patient becomes a technically challenging experiment. Traditional methods of clinical protocol conduct may not be adequate to achieve satisfactory protocol execution. Recent experiences with moderate levels of control are encouraging, but greater control is probably

necessary, and the complexity of recently developed protocols is daunting. Although computer-based protocols are very challenging to develop, they provide the opportunity to improve performance of complex experimental procedures and maintain more complete records of clinical events of interest. Investigators involved in future trials of MV should give careful consideration to the value of these research tools.

Acknowledgements: Supported by USPHS NIH NHLBI NO1–HR-4603 (ARDS Network).

References

1. Amato MBP, Barbas CSV, Medeiros DM, et al (1995) Beneficial effects of the "open lung approach" with low distending pressures in acute respiratory distress syndrome. Am J Respir Crit Care Med 152:1835–1846
2. Arnold JH, Hanson JH, Toro-Figuero LO, Gutierrez J, Berens RJ, Anglin DL (1994) Prospective, randomized comparison of high-frequency oscillatory ventilation and conventional mechanical ventilation in pediatric respiratory failure. Crit Care Med 22:1530–1539
3. Rasanen J, Cane RD, Downs JB, et al (1991) Airway pressure release ventilation during acute lung injury: A prospective multicenter trial. Crit Care Med 19:1234–1241
4. Tharratt RS, Allen RP, Albertson TE (1988) Pressure controlled inverse ratio ventilation in severe adult respiratory failure. Chest 94:755–762
5. Marcy TW, Marini JJ (1991) Inverse ratio ventilation in ARDS. Chest 100:494–504
6. Patrick W, Webster K, Ludwig L, Roberts D, Wiebe P, Younes M (1996) Non-invasive positive-pressure ventilation in acute respiratory distress without prior chronic respiratory failure. Am J Respir Crit Care Med 153:1005–1111
7. Kolobow T, Moretti MP, Fumagalli R, et al (1987) Severe impairment in lung function induced by high peak airway pressure during mechanical ventilation. Am Rev Respir Dis 135:312–315
8. Hickling KG, Walsh J, Henderson S, Jackson R (1994) Low mortality rate in adult respiratory distress syndrome using low-volume, pressure-limited ventilation with permissive hypercapnia: A prospective study. Crit Care Med 22:1568–1578
9. Hickling KG, Henderson SJ, Jackson R (1990) Low mortality associated with low volume pressure limited ventilation with permissive hypercapnia in severe adult respiratory distress syndrome. Intens Care Med 16:372–377
10. Navalesi P, Hernandez P, Wongsa A, Laporta D, Goldberg P, Gottfried SB (1996) Proportional assist ventilation in acute respiratory failure: Effects on breathing pattern and inspiratory effort. Am J Respir Crit Care Med 154:1330–1338
11. Carlon GC, Howland WS, Ray C, Miodownik S, Griffin JP, Groeger JS (1983) High-frequency jet ventilation. Chest 84:551–559
12. Corbridge TC, Wood LDH, Crawford GP, Chudoba MJ, Yanos J, Sznajder JI (1990) Adverse effects of large tidal volume and low PEEP in canine acid aspiration. Am Rev Respir Dis 142:311–315
13. Witschi HR, Haschek WM, Klein-Szanto AJP, Hakkinen PJ (1981) Potentiation of diffuse lung damage by oxygen: Determining variables. Am Rev Respir Dis 123:98–103
14. Muscedere JG, Mullen JBM, Gan K, Slutsky AS (1994) Tidal ventilation at low airway pressures can augment lung injury. Am J Respir Crit Care Med 149:1327–1334
15. Froese AB, McCulloch PR, Sugiura M, Vaclavik S, Possmayer F, Moller F (1993) Optimizing alveolar expansion prolongs the effectiveness of exogenous surfactant therapy in the adult rabbit. Am Rev Respir Dis 148:569–577
16. Dreyfuss D, Soler P, Basset G, Saumon G (1988) High inflation pressure pulmonary edema. Am Rev Respir Dis 137:1159–1164

17. Webb HH, Tierney DF (1974) Experimental pulmonary edema due to intermittent positive pressure ventilation with high pressures. Am Rev Respir Dis 110:556-560
18. Tsuno K, Miura K, Takeya M, Kolobow T, Morioka T (1991) Histopathologic pulmonary changes from mechanical ventilation at high peak airway pressures. Am Rev Respir Dis 143:1115-1120
19. Parker JC, Hernandez LA, Peevy KJ (1993) Mechanisms of ventilator-induced lung injury. Crit Care Med 21:131-143
20. Parker JC, Hernandez LA, Longenecker GL, Peevy K, Johson W (1990) Lung edema caused by high peak inspiratory pressures in dogs. Am Rev Respir Dis 142:321-328
21. Dreyfuss D, Basset G, Soler P, Saumon G (1985) Intermittent positive-pressure hyperventilation with high inflation pressures produces pulmonary microvascular injury in rats. Am Rev Respir Dis 132:880-884
22. Tuxen DV (1994) Permissive hypercapnic ventilation. Am J Respir Crit Care Med 150:870-874
23. Feihl F, Perret C (1994) Permissive hypercapnia - How permissive should we be? Am J Respir Crit Care Med 150:1722-1737
24. Kacmarek RM, Hickling KG (1993) Permissive hypercapnia. Respir Care 38:373-387
25. Carmichael LC, Dorinsky PM, Higgins SB, et al (1996) Diagnosis and therapy of acute respiratory distress syndrome in adults: An international survey. J Crit Care 11:9-18
26. Hedley-Whyte J, Laver MB, Benedixen HH (1964) Effect of changes in tidal ventilation on physiologic shunting. Am J Physiol 206:891-897
27. Blanch L, Fernandez R, Valles J, Sole J, Roussos C, Artigas A (1994) Effect of two tidal volumes on oxygenation and respiratory system mechanics during the early stage of adult respiratory distress syndrome. J Crit Care 9:151-158
28. Manley ES, Nash CB, Woodbury RA (1964) Cardiovascular responses to severe hypercapnia of short duration. Am J Physiol 207:634-640
29. Tang W, Weil MH, Gazmuri RJ, Bisera J, Rackow EC (1991) Reversible impairment of myocardial contractility due to hypercarbic acidosis in the isolated perfused rat heart. Crit Care Med 19:218-221
30. Wally KR, Lewis TH, Wood LDH (1990) Acute respiratory acidosis decreases left ventricular contractility but increases cardiac output in dogs. Circulation Res 67:628-635
31. East TD, Morris AH, Wallace CJ, et al (1992) A strategy for development of computerized critical care decision support systems. Int J Clin Monitor Comput 8:263-269
32. Henderson S, Crapo RO, Wallace CJ, East TD, Morris AH, Gardner RM (1992) Performance of computerized protocols for the management of arterial oxygenation in an intensive care unit. Int J Clin Monitor Comput 8:271-280
33. Montgomery AB, Luce JM, Murray JF (1989) Retrosternal pain is an early indicator of oxygen toxicity. Am Rev Respir Dis 139:1548-1550
34. Bernard GR, Doig G, Hudson LD, et al (1995) Quantification of organ failure for clinical trials and clinical practice. Am J Respir Crit Care Med 151:A323 (Abst)
35. Ranieri VM, Eissa NT, Corbeil C, et al (1991) Effects of positive end-expiratory pressure on alveolar recruitment and gas exchange in patients with the adult respiratory distress syndrome. Am Rev Respir Dis 144:544-551
36. Ranieri VM, Mascia L, Fiore T, Bruno F, Brienza A, Giuliani R (1995) Cardiorespiratory effects of positive end-expiratory pressure during progressive tidal volume reduction (permissive hypercapnia) in patients with acute respiratory distress syndrome. Anesthesiology 83:710-720
37. Lefevre GR, Kowalski SE, Girling LG, Thiessen DB, Mutch WAC (1996) Improved arterial oxygenation after oleic acid lung injury in the pig using a computer-controlled mechanical ventilator. Am J Respir Crit Care Med 154:1567-1572
38. Suki B, Barabasi A-L, Hantos Z, Petak F, Stanley HE (1994) Avalanches and power-law behaviour in lung inflation. Nature 368:615-618
39. Gaver DP, Samsel RW, Solway J (1990) Effects of surface tension and viscosity on airway reopening. J Appl Physiol 69:74-85
40. Perun ML, Gaver DP (1995) Interaction between airway lining fluid forces and parenchymal tethering during pulmonary airway reopening. J Appl Physiol 79:1717-1728

41. Yap DYK, Liebkemann WD, Solway J, Gaver DP (1994) Influences of parenchymal tethering on the reopening of closed pulmonary airways. J Appl Physiol 76:2095-2105
42. Kamm RD, Schroter RC (1989) Is airway closure caused by a liquid film instability? Respir Physiol 75:141-156
43. Naureckas ET, Dawson CA, Gerber BS, et al (1994) Airway reopening pressure in isolated rat lungs. J Appl Physiol 76:1372-1377
44. Douglas WW, Rehder K, Beynen FM, Sessler AD, Marsh HM (1977) Improved oxygenation in patients with acute respiratory failure: The prone position. Am Rev Respir Dis 115:559-566
45. Fridrich P, Krafft P, Hochleuthner H, Mauritz W (1996) The effects of long-term prone positioning in patients with trauma-induced adult respiratory distress syndrome. Anesth Analg 83:1206-1211
46. Marini JJ, Rodriguez RM, Lamb V (1986) The inspiratory workload of patient-initiated mechanical ventilation. Am Rev Respir Dis 134:902-909
47. Marini JJ, Capps JS, Culver BH (1995) The inspiratory work of breathing during assisted mechanical ventilation. Chest 87:612-618
48. Manthous CA, Hall JB, Kushner R, Schmidt GA, Russo G, Wood LDH (1995) The effect of mechanical ventilation on oxygen consumption in critically ill patients. Am J Respir Crit Care Med 151:210-214
49. Manning HL, Schwartzstein RM (1995) Pathophysiology of dyspnea. N Engl J Med 333:1547-1553
50. Sassoon CSH, Del Rosario N, Fei R, Rheeman CH, Gruer SE, Mahutte CK (1994) Influence of pressure- and flow-triggered synchronous intermittent madatory ventilation on inspiratory muscle work. Crit Care Med 22:1933-1941
51. Gurevitch MJ, Gelmont D (1989) Importance of trigger sensitivity to ventilator response delay in advanced chronic obstructive pulmonary disease with respiratory failure. Crit Care Med 17:354-359
52. Manning HL, Molinary EJ, Leiter JC (1995) Effect of inspiratory flow rate on respiratory sensation and pattern of breathing. Am J Respir Crit Care Med 151:751-757

Future Clinical Trials of Pharmacologic Interventions

E. Abraham

Introduction

Acute respiratory distress syndrome (ARDS) was first described as a clinical entity by Ashbaugh and Petty more than 25 years ago [1]. Since that initial description, there has been growing understanding of the pathophysiologic mechanisms which lead to the development of acute lung injury (ALI) in patient populations at risk. In particular, the roles of proinflammatory cytokines, chemokines, adhesion molecules, and oxygen radicals as mediators of pulmonary inflammation have been characterized. Alterations in neutrophil function, as well as the role of the neutrophil in damaging the lung and contributing to the development of ARDS and ALI have been described. Other chapters in this book have reviewed the mediators and cellular factors which contribute to the development of acute inflammatory lung injury, so that further discussion of the pathophysiology of ARDS is not required in this chapter. Rather, I will try to assess therapeutic approaches to ARDS and ALI which may be beneficial in the next 15 years.

Underlying any discussion of pharmacologic intervention in ALI is the growing realization of the multiplicity of cellular and immunologic mediators which contribute to the development of inflammation in the lungs. Previous clinical trials in sepsis and ARDS have concentrated on blocking a single mediator, with the hope that such intervention could have a meaningful effect on outcome. Such an approach, unless it is directed to a mediator, so central in the inflammatory cascade that inhibiting its actions will affect all downstream events, is unlikely to be of benefit in altering the course of a clinical entity as complicated as ALI. Results from clinical trials have confirmed the problems with blocking single mediators; even antagonizing the actions of a cytokine, such as tumor necrosis factor (TNF-α), which appears to be of major importance in acute inflammatory processes, has, at best, only minimal effects on improving survival in all groups of patients with sepsis-associated ARDS. While such anti-cytokine approaches may provide greater survival benefit in subgroups of septic patients, this need to prospectively stratify patients in order to achieve benefit with such interventions only confirms that a single therapy is unlikely to benefit large groups of patients with ALI.

Most evidence also suggests that ALI is not simply a pulmonary disease, but rather reflects inflammatory processes affecting multiple organ systems. The basis for the view that ALI is a multisystemic disease comes both from outcome data, which demonstrate that few patients with ARDS die from hypoxemia, from epidemiologic studies, which demonstrate that most patients with ARDS do not have "pure" pulmonary injury but rather have multiple organ dysfunction, and from experimental ALI models which show increased expression of cytokines, chemokines, adhesion molecules and other inflammatory mediators in sites distant from the lungs, such as the liver and intestines.

The fact that ALI is usually a component of a multisystemic process strongly suggests that, in order to have a meaningful impact on outcome, pharmacologic interventions will need to have multisystemic effects, and not be simply directed to the lungs. There is already a fairly long history of lung specific therapies failing to alter outcome in patients with ALI or ARDS. For example, in adults, neither surfactant, inhaled nitric oxide, ECMO, nor partial liquid ventilation were able to demonstrate any meaningful impact on survival when used alone in clinical trials.

If one considers the data from completed clinical trials in conjunction with clinical and experimental information which show that multiple mediators are involved in the pathophysiology of ALI, then it becomes apparent that future clinical trials investigating pharmacologic interventions for ALI should use agents or combinations of agents that have systemic effects and that affect more than one point in the inflammatory cascade. There are several pharmacologic approaches that are presently being utilized in early clinical trials or that will become available over the next several years that meet this requirement for multisystemic effects on multiple points in the inflammatory cascade. I will review that future potential of these therapies with the understanding that divination is fraught with danger, as even the oracles at Delphi frequently found.

Anti-Cytokine Interventions

Both interleukin-1 (IL-1) and TNF-α have been targets of anti-cytokine therapies in clinical trials of patients with sepsis with or without septic shock. Most of the patients included in these studies had ALI as a result of their septic process. The studies can therefore be used to assess the utility of these anti-cytokine therapies in sepsis-induced ALI.

The agent used to block the effects of IL-1 in these trials was the IL-1 receptor antagonist (IL-1ra), a naturally occurring molecule which binds to the IL-1 receptor in a non-activating manner, thereby serving as a competitive inhibitor of the effects of IL-1. Several different approaches have been taken to blocking the effects of TNF-α, including the use of murine monoclonal antibodies and antibody F(ab')2 fragments, as well as fusion protein constructs consisting of the extramembrane parts of either the Type I (p55) or Type II (p75) TNF receptor joined to the constant portion (Fc) of a human IgG1 antibody molecule.

Three studies were undertaken examining the utility of the IL-1ra in patients with sepsis. In the initial open-label clinical trial in 99 septic patients, a dose-dependent, 28 day survival benefit was found with IL-1ra treatment [2]. However, when IL-1ra was examined in a double-blinded study of 893 patients, no significant overall benefit was associated with treatment with this agent [3]. In a retrospective analysis using an APACHE III modified sepsis scoring system, patients with a predicted mortality > 24% appeared to show improved survival when treated with IL-1ra. Unfortunately, a third study in 696 patients failed to demonstrate a statistically significant reduction in mortality in this group of patients with high predicted mortality when given IL-1ra compared to those receiving standard therapy [4].

In contrast to the situation with blocking IL-1, where little benefit could be demonstrated, therapies with anti-TNF agents appear capable of improving survival in prospectively identifiable patient groups. Additionally, the study with the p55 TNF receptor fusion protein complex provides data which demonstrate that such therapy, at least in patients with severe sepsis, with or without early septic shock, decreases time on the ventilator and days in the intensive care unit for intubated patients with ALI [5].

The initial study to demonstrate potential benefit of anti-TNF-α therapy was the NORASEPT I trial, which examined a murine IgG1 monoclonal antibody in the therapy of severe sepsis and septic shock [6]. Entry criteria for this study included the presence of at least one organ system dysfunction (i.e. decreased urine output, hypoxemia, lactic/metabolic acidosis, altered mental status, or disseminated intravascular coagulation, DIC) for less than 12 h prior to enrollment in patients with the clinical diagnosis of infection. Of note, at the time of randomization, over 50% of patients had respiratory failure, and almost all of these patients met criteria for ALI. Separate randomization lists were used for patients with or without shock at the time of study entry. A total of 994 patients were entered in NORASEPT I, of which approximately half were in shock at the time of randomization. Overall, there was no statistically significant benefit associated with anti-TNF therapy. However, quite different results were seen when the two prospectively defined subgroups were examined. In patients with septic shock, a statistically significant reduction in mortality was present during the first 2 weeks following therapy with either 7.5 or 15 mg/kg monoclonal anti-TNF-α antibody compared to placebo. In contrast, no benefit was found with anti-TNF-α therapy in patients who were not in shock at study entry.

A second study (INTERSEPT) with the murine monoclonal anti-TNF-α antibody was undertaken in 14 countries, primarily in Europe [7]. Although the INTERSEPT study initially enrolled septic patients with and without shock, after the results of NORASEPT I were available, only shock patients were entered into INTERSEPT. A total of 564 patients, of which 420 in septic shock, were enrolled in the INTERSEPT study. Day 28 mortality was reduced by 14.3% in patients who received 3 mg/kg monoclonal anti-TNF-α antibody, with no reduction in mortality found in the patients given 15 mg/kg.

The utility of the F(ab')2 fragments of a murine IgG3 monoclonal antibody to TNF-α has been examined in patients with severe sepsis or septic shock [7]. There were 122 patients entered in the clinical trial, and no increase in survival from sepsis for the patients receiving anti-TNF treatment was present in the overall study population. However, a retrospective stratification of patients by IL-6 concentration suggested beneficial effects for the drug in patients (n = 37) with baseline circulating IL-6 concentrations greater than 1000 pg/mL, with mortality decreasing from 80% in the placebo group to 35% in patients who received the highest dose (1 mg/kg) of the anti-TNF-α therapy.

Two studies have used soluble TNF receptor constructs as anti-TNF agents. In the first of these studies, the molecule used consisted of the extramembrane components of the human type II (p75) receptor joined to the Fc portion of a human IgG1 antibody molecule [8]. Patients (n = 141) with septic shock, with or without associated organ system dysfunction, were entered into the study. A statistically significant (p = 0.014) dose-dependent increase in mortality was found in patients treated with this p75 soluble TNF receptor construct, with mortality rising from 30% in the placebo group to 53% in the patients treated with the highest dose (1.5 mg/kg) of the anti-TNF compound.

A recently completed study examined the role of a p55 TNF receptor fusion protein construct in which separate randomization lists were used for patients with severe sepsis with or without early shock and also for those with refractory septic shock [5]. The doses of the p55 TNF receptor complex used in this study (0.008, 0.042, and 0.08 mg/kg) were substantially lower than those administered in the p75 TNF receptor complex clinical trial. In this study, refractory septic shock was defined as hypotension that was unresponsive to fluid for at least 2 h prior to enrollment associated with at least one organ dysfunction (i.e. hypoxemia, metabolic acidosis, decreased urine output, or DIC). The severe sepsis group consisted of patients having at least two organ dysfunctions, with or without fluid unresponsive hypotension for less than 2 h prior to enrollment.

Therapy with 0.08 mg/kg of the p55 TNF receptor fusion protein complex, but not other doses, was associated with a 36% reduction (p = 0.07) in day 28 mortality in the prospectively defined patient group with severe sepsis with or without early septic shock. In contrast, no apparent beneficial effects were seen with any dose of the p55 receptor complex in patients with refractory septic shock.

There are several possible explanations for the marked differences in the outcomes of septic patients treated with the p55 or p75 TNF receptor fusion protein constructs. The enhanced mortality associated with treatment with the p75 TNF receptor molecule may be related to the extremely high doses used in the study. Although potency estimates are difficult to quantitate, the soluble TNF receptor complex appeared to inactivate TNF-α approximately 100 times as well as the monoclonal antibodies, so that therapy with a dose of 1.5 mg/kg of this human protein with a long half life would be expected to completely neutralize TNF-α for a prolonged period. TNF-α is an essential component of normal inflammatory responses, and prolonged neutralization of its activity may have potent immunosuppressive effects leading to increased mortality. An additional potentially important reason for the seemingly opposite effects of the p75 and the p55 TNF receptor fusion proteins in septic patients relates to the differing kinetic affinities of the two molecules. Although both molecules rapidly bind TNF-α, TNF-α is released much more quickly from the p75 receptor complex than from the p55 fusion protein [10]. These differences in kinetic affinity may have *in vivo* significance. In a series of experiments in mice given intravenous infusions of E. coli, therapy with the p75 TNF receptor complex decreased the magnitude of the initial rise in circulating TNF-α which occurred in untreated mice after the administration of E. coli [9]. However, whereas TNF-α rapidly disappeared from the circulation in untreated mice, administration of the p75 TNF receptor complex was associated with prolonged increases in circulating levels of TNF-α. In contrast, in bacteremic mice treated with the p55 TNF receptor complex molecule, no TNF-α was present in the circulation at any time after the E. coli infusion.

Approximately 2300 patients were included in the 5 studies investigating anti-TNF therapies. Four of the studies, compromising over 2000 patients, showed survival benefits in patients treated with the anti-TNF agent. As noted above, there are strong reasons to believe that it was the dose and/or possibly the nature of the agent itself that explained the contradictory results in the 141 patient p75 TNF receptor trial, rather than the anti-TNF approach. In the three largest studies, benefit with anti-TNF therapies was apparent in prospectively defined patient populations. Although none of the studies showed statistically significant reduction in mortality at day 28 after anti-TNF therapy, none of the studies was powered to achieve statistical significance at this time point. Taken together, the results from the anti-TNF clinical trials give strong reasons for optimism relating to this therapeutic approach in clinically definable patient populations. In particular, these studies suggest that the patients who benefit from anti-TNF therapies are those with severe sepsis causing the failure of at least two organ systems, if not associated with shock, as well as patients with shock of less than 6 h duration, if associated with at least one organ system dysfunction. It appears unlikely that patients with prolonged refractory septic shock benefit from TNF blockade and, in fact, the inclusion of such patients in the NORASEPT I and INTERSEPT studies may have diminished the apparent effect of treatment with the monoclonal anti-TNF-α antibody. The anti-TNF clinical trials also indicate that such therapies are not of use in the less ill septic patients with only a single organ failure. Finally, the studies strongly suggest that the dose of the anti-TNF agent is also crucial; use of a dose that results in prolonged TNF blockade after initial resolution of the sepsis-induced organ failure may provide no further benefit, and may even be harmful.

Three large Phase III studies are presently underway to confirm the benefit that was suggested by the initial clinical trial with the anti-TNF agent. These ongoing clinical studies are examining the monoclonal anti-TNF-α antibody used in NORASEPT I and INTERSEPT, the p55 TNF receptor fusion protein construct, and murine monoclonal antibody F(ab')2 fragments. The initial results from these studies should be available in the latter part of 1997 and will be crucial in determining the role of anti-TNF therapies in critically ill septic patients.

The available data, while they do suggest that anti-TNF therapies may be of use in certain septic populations with ALI, also can be interpreted as showing that the role for anti-TNF therapy will be relatively limited in the overall patient population with ALI. Even in patient groups with sepsis-induced ALI associated with other organ dysfunction, the improvement in survival with anti-TNF therapy is likely to be modest, suggesting that additional benefit may be achieved if such therapy be combined with additional agents which affect other proinflammatory mediators.

Administration of IL-10, an anti-inflammatory cytokine produced by Th2 cells, represents a potential therapy for ALI. IL-10, because it has systemic effects and down-regulates the production of multiple pro-inflammatory cytokines produced by macrophages and Th1 cells, including TNF-α and interferon gamma (IFN-γ), meets the proposed requirements for an effective future therapy in ALI [11]. In sepsis models such as those associated with endotoxin injection, and in models of ALI such as that produced by intratracheal instillation of TNF-α, the administration of IL-10 improves survival [12].

Because circulating levels of IL-10 are already markedly elevated in patients at risk for or with ALI and in septic patients, it is unclear if therapy with additional IL-10 can have a meaningful impact on outcome in these patient groups. A therapeutic concern relating to IL-10 is the fact that therapy with this cytokine increases mortality in animals with a localized pulmonary infection, such as Klebsiella pneumonia [13]. Because many patients with ALI may have either pre-existent localized infections, such as a nosocomial pneumonia, or may develop such infections while intubated in the ICU, there may be significant safety concerns with the use of IL-10 in this patient population.

Therapies Able to Affect Intracellular Signalling

Interaction of lipopolysaccharide (LPS, endotoxin), Gram-positive exotoxins, and cytokines, such as TNF-α, with their cellular receptors leads to increased transcription of immunoregulatory genes. In part, this enhanced expression of immunoregulatory genes appears to result from phosphorylation and activation of transcriptional regulatory factors as well as cytoplasmic proteins affecting the activation of these regulatory molecules. Cytoplasmic and nuclear kinases, including members of the mitogen activated protein (MAP) kinase family as well as JAK-STAT kinases, appear to have an important role in phosphorylating and activating regulatory proteins responsible for transducing extracellular signals to the nucleus.

Binding sites for the nuclear transcriptional regulatory factor NF-κB are present in the promoter regions of many of the pro-inflammatory mediators important in producing organ system dysfunction, including ALI, after sepsis or shock [14]. For example, the TNF-α promoter contains 4 NF-κB sites, and binding regions for NF-κB are also found in the promoters for other cytokine genes, such as IL-8, as well as in those for adhesion molecules, such as ICAM-1, and complement proteins, such as C4.

NF-κB is normally sequestered in the cytoplasm through association of the p50/p65 heterodimer with an inhibitory IkB protein [15]. However, activation stimuli lead to the ubiquination and then proteolysis of IkB, allowing the p50/p65 heterodimer to translocate to the nucleus, bind to specific sequences in gene promoters, and then, in conjunction with other transcriptional factors, induce transcription of those genes to whose promoters it has bound.

Both *in vitro* and *in vivo* experiments have demonstrated that reactive oxygen intermediates, including both H_2O_2 and O_2^-, can lead to activation of NF-κB [16–18]. Similarly, endotoxin, presumably through p38 kinase-associated pathways, also has been shown to lead to NF-κB activation [19]. In experimental models of ALI, such as that induced by blood loss and resuscitation, NF-κB is activated in pulmonary cell populations, and such activation is correlated with increased levels of mRNA for proinflammatory and immunoregulatory cytokines which have NF-κB binding sites in their promoters [17]. Endotoxin-induced models of lung injury are also associated with increased NF-κB activation in the lungs [19]. Of critical importance is the fact that NF-κB is activated in alveolar macrophages obtained from patients with ARDS, suggesting that ongoing activation of NF-κB may contribute to the proinflammatory state which is present in the lungs of these patients [20].

Because of the presence of NF-κB binding sites in the promoters of multiple genes important in modulating the inflammatory response, NF-κB is an attractive target for future therapies aimed at preventing or treating organ system dysfunction associated with shock states. While there is presently highly suggestive data indicating that NF-κB does occupy a central role in initiating and augmenting the inflammatory response in endotoxemia and other conditions associated with increased generation of reactive oxygen intermediates, direct demonstration of such actions will require the development of agents which specifically block activation of NF-κB.

There is tremendous enthusiasm for the development of therapies able to prevent activation of NF-κB. Several groups of agents which are capable of blocking NF-κB activation have been described. However, to date all of these agents have additional actions beyond blocking NF-κB activation and most of these agents also have significant toxicities which would limit their use in the clinical setting. Given the intense interest in affecting NF-κB activation, it is likely that more specific pharmacologic agents with acceptable toxicity profiles will be available in the future for testing in pro-inflammatory conditions such as ALI. Because of the central role that NF-κB appears to occupy in terms of modulating inflammatory and immunoregulatory responses, it will be important to remember that agents able to affect NF-κB activation will have widespread effects on immune function, with the important risk of potently inhibiting inflammatory response and producing an immunosuppressed condition. The challenge will be to define the appropriate settings for the utilization of such therapies.

Because of the difficulties in modifying the actions of a commonly used intracellular signalling pathway, such as that involving NF-κB, it may be more useful clinically to develop compounds which can affect intracellular signalling through inhibiting pathways activated by mediators commonly increased in the setting of organ dysfunction, such as ALI, associated with critical illness. An example of such an approach would be through blockade of the activation and phosphorylation of the p38 MAP kinase [21]. The p38 MAP kinase is activated by cytokines, such as IL-1 and TNF-α, as well as LPS, osmotic stress, and activated platelets [22]. Functionally, activation of p38 MAP kinase results in actin assembly and adherence, but not other aspects of neutrophil activation, such as migration, superoxide production, or granule enzyme release [21]. Therefore, one could theoretically achieve modification of neutrophil function with a p38 inhibitor, without totally inactivating all neutrophil activities. Pharmacologic inhibitors of p38 are becoming available, show activity in improving outcome in endotoxin models, and may have future utility in modifying and improving outcome from inflammatory conditions, such as ALI, without producing inappropriate immunosuppression, such as might be expected with NF-κB inhibitors.

Interaction of TNF-α, IL-1β, and IL-1α initiate their intracellular signalling pathways through increasing acidic sphingomyelinase and affecting ceramide concentrations [23]. Interruption of inflammatory mechanisms initiated by these cytokines can be achieved through inhibiting these sphingomyelinase-induced mechanisms. Pharmacologic agents able to block cytokine-induced sphingomyelinase activation are being developed and may have therapeutic utility in cytokine-driven pro-inflammatory states, such as ALI.

Therapies Able to Modify Neutrophil Function

Neutrophils have an important role in inflammatory reactions such as that present in ALI. Experimental data suggests that inhibition of neutrophil activation can improve outcome in models of ALI. Clinically, a similar situation has been noted in neutropenic patients, where the severity of lung injury worsens as the neutropenia resolves, and the patient is now able to develop a neutrophil replete inflammatory response in the lungs.

Several therapies which modify neutrophil function have shown promising results in experimental models of lung injury and may demonstrate utility in clinical trials. As mentioned above, inhibition of p38 MAP kinase modifies some, but not all, neutrophil functions [21] and shows the ability to improve survival in endotoxemia models. Both oral and intravenous formulations of p38 inhibitors will soon be available for clinical trials and may show benefit in improving outcome from ALI. Other therapies that affect neutrophil function and which may be useful in treating the multiorgan inflammatory response of which ALI is often a part include liposomal prostaglandin E1 as well as monoclonal antibodies and other compounds blocking neutrophil-adhesion molecule interactions.

The effects of liposomal prostaglandin E1 on neutrophil function appear to be due to both the liposome and PGE1 moieties. Liposomes are endogenously opsonized with C3bi and thus bind to the neutrophil CRE (CD11b/CD18) receptor. Opsonized liposome engagement of CR3 results in an increase in cyclic adenosine monophosphate (cAMP) and a down-regulation of CD18 expression on the neutrophil surface. PGE1 engagement of its EP2 counterreceptor also increases intracellular cAMP. Concomitant administration of liposomes and PGE1, as with liposomal PGE1, results in an additive increase in intracellular cAMP and a down-regulation of CD18 that exceed those effects of either component administered alone [24]. In animal models, administration of liposomal PGE1 improved outcome in neutrophil-mediated models of inflammation. In particular, liposomal PGE1 diminished the severity of capillary leak and neutrophil infiltration in IL-1-induced ALI in rats.

A small Phase II study evaluated the safety and efficacy of liposomal PGE1 in the treatment of patients with ARDS [25]. In that study, treatment with liposomal PGE1 was associated with improved oxygenation, increased lung compliance, and decreased ventilatory dependency compared to placebo. Two large Phase III studies are in progress to examine more completely the role of liposomal PGE1 in the therapy of patients with ARDS. The results of those studies should be available in 1997.

Increased pulmonary expression of adhesion molecules, including p-selectin and ICAM-1, important in inducing neutrophil influx into the lung, occurs in experimental models of ALI. Patients at risk for ARDS also show increased circulating levels of soluble ICAM and p-selectin, consistent with increased endothelial expression of these molecules, with subsequent shedding into the circulation [26, 27].

The administration of monoclonal antibodies to p-selectin prevents pulmonary accumulation of neutrophils and subsequent pulmonary vascular injury in experimental models of ALI [28]. Oligosaccharides which are ligands for p-selectin can also decrease p-selectin-dependent lung injury in experimental models [29]. A similar improvement in neutrophil infiltration, edema, and bronchoalveolar fluid protein concentration is seen after therapy with monoclonal anti-ICAM-1 antibodies in some models of ALI [30].

Both anti-p-selectin and anti-ICAM-1 therapies thus represent potential pharmacologic interventions which will have multisystemic effects and interrupt the important common pathway in the inflammatory cascade which the neutrophil occupies. The risk with these therapies rests in their potential immunosuppressive actions. Blocking neutrophil adhesion may render a patient overly susceptible to nosocomial infection, so that even though the outcome from ALI is improved, the patient then suffers from the effects of a secondary infection. This issue of immunosuppression in various experimental models appears to be less severe with anti-p-selectin therapies than with anti-ICAM-1 interventions, but these results may reflect the experimental models chosen and may not predict the potential immunosuppressive effects of these therapies in critically ill patients.

Anti-Oxidants

Benefits from anti-oxidant therapies may accrue at several stages in the inflammatory process. Amelioration of oxidant damage produced by neutrophil degranulation and oxidative burst might result from such therapy. Additionally, increased intracellular oxidant generation appears to be important in activating nuclear transcriptional regulatory factors, including NF-κB and the cAMP responsive element binding protein (CREB), which are important in increasing the transcription of immunoregulatory cytokine, adhesion molecule, and other pro-inflammatory mediator genes [17, 19]. Antioxidant therapies, such as inhibition of xanthine oxidase or N-acetylcysteine (NAC), in experimental models of ALI and systemic inflammation are able to prevent NF-κB activation and pro-inflammatory cytokine expression among pulmonary cell populations [17, 19].

The results of clinical trials with antioxidant therapies in patients with ARDS do not show any clear benefit, but these findings may reflect the pharmacologic agents used or the patient population studied rather than the inadequacy of this approach in ALI. Several small studies suggested a more rapid reversal of ALI and ARDS. In particular, a recent study examined the utility of NAC and procysteine in 46 patients with ARDS [31]. Both NAC and procysteine-repleted red blood cell glutathione, but neither antioxidant resulted in any effect on survival compared to placebo. Time on the ventilator was not significantly reduced by either procysteine or NAC compared to placebo. There was, however, trends towards improvement in organ failure free days in patients treated with either NAC or procysteine compared to placebo.

Future trials with anti-oxidant agents will probably require early initiation of therapy in patients at risk for ALI, given the extremely rapid activation of NF-κB in experimental models of ARDS. However, the continued activation of NF-κB found in the alveolar macrophages of patients with ARDS [20] suggests that appropriate anti-oxidant therapy may have some benefit in this setting as well, if such activation of NF-κB is driven by oxidants and not through other mechanisms, such as cytokine-induced signalling pathways. At present, the relative importance of the intracellular signalling pathways which are activated in patients with ARDS and which lead to activation of NF-κB in this setting are unknown, and understanding of this issue will be important in designing future studies with antioxidants. Additionally, the relative importance of NF-κB as compared to other transcriptional factors, such as CREB or AP-1, in producing a continued pulmonary inflammatory response in patients with ALI remains to be determined. Finally, the appropriate anti-oxidant agent to be used in these patients remains to be determined. It is unclear from the various *in vitro* and *in vivo* experimental models if H_2O_2 or O_2 is more important in activating NF-κB. The selection of anti-oxidant therapy may be dependent on which of these reactive oxygen intermediates plays the more important role in activating NF-κB, as well as such practical considerations as achieving adequate intracellular levels of such therapeutic agents.

Combination Therapies

At the beginning of this chapter, reference was made to the need for ALI therapies to have multisystemic effects and to affect several steps in the inflammatory cascade. An important method for achieving such aims will be to combine treatments. Experimental work has demonstrated the utility of such an approach in pro-inflammatory conditions such as sepsis where blockade of IL-1 and TNF-α resulted in much greater improvement in survival than inhibiting only one of these cytokines.

Improvement in the pulmonary inflammatory response coupled with therapy which affects ongoing systemic inflammation may be of benefit in improving outcome in ALI. For example, anticytokine therapies or liposomal prostaglandin E1 may have enhanced benefit if they are used in conjunction with lung specific interventions such as partial liquid ventilation with perfluorocarbons, inhaled nitric oxide, or low stretch ventilatory modalities.

Practical issues relating to proprietary interests surrounding novel agents for ALI and other indications often preclude studying combination therapies. Additionally, study design issues often prevent investigating combination therapy. Any study with two experimental agents will necessitate at least 4 arms, comprising placebo, each agent alone, and the combination of agents. If the optimal dose of each agent is unknown, as is frequently the case, then additional study arms will be required. Even with 4 treatment arms, the size of the study to achieve adequate power in determining a meaningful effect on outcome may be too great to be practical.

Of note, the National Institutes of Health (NIH) ARDS Network (a consortium of 10 US medical centers with expertise in ALI/ARDS clinical research) is investigating the combination use of ketoconazole and low tidal volume ventilation in its first study. This clinical trial, which will enroll up to 1000 patients, will be able to show if any meaningful interaction can be achieved with the combination of these two approaches to the therapy of ALI. Because of the structure of the NIH ARDS Network, it can be anticipated that future clinical trials developed by this group of medical centers will also investigate various potentially beneficial combinations of therapies.

Conclusion

The next 15 years hold tremendous promise for the development of pharmacologic therapies able to improve the survival of patients with ALI. Our increased understanding of the multiple pathways leading to the clinical pattern of ALI will allow development of a spectrum of therapeutic agents which can be combined to effectively modulate inflammatory reactions producing lung injury in critically ill patients. The challenge will be in defining for the individual patient the appropriate combination and the timing for the delivery of that combination which will result in the greatest impact on outcome.

References

1. Ashbaugh DG, Bigelow DB, Petty TL, Levine BE (1967) Acute respiratory distress in adults. Lancet 2:319–323
2. Fisher CJ, Slotman GJ, Opal SM, et al (1994) Initial evaluation of human recombinant interleukin-1 receptor antagonist in the treatment of sepsis syndrome: A randomized, open-label, placebo-controlled multicenter trial. Crit Care Med 22:12–21
3. Fisher CJ, Dhainaut JF, Opal SM, et al (1994) Recombinant human interleukin-1 receptor antagonist in the treatment of patients with sepsis syndrome. JAMA 271:1836–1843
4. Opal SM, Fisher CJ, Pribble JP, et al (1997) The confirmatory interleukin-1 receptor antagonist trial in severe sepsis: A phase III randomized, double-blind, placebo-controlled, multicenter trial. Crit Care Med (In press)
5. Abraham E (1996) Status report of soluble receptors in the treatment of septic shock. Presented at IBC Sixth Annual International Symposium on Sepsis, Boston, USA (Abst)
6. Abraham E, Wunderink R, Silverman H, et al (1995) Monoclonal antibody to human tumor necrosis factor alpha (TNFa MAb): Efficacy and safety in patients with the sepsis syndrome. JAMA 273:934–941
7. Cohen J, Carlet J, for the INTERSEPT Study Group (1996) INTERSEPT: An international, multicenter, placebo-controlled trial of monoclonal antibody to human tumor necrosis factor-α in patients with sepsis. Crit Care Med 24:1431–1440

8. Reinhart K, Wiegand-Lohnert C, Grimminger F, et al (1996) Assessment of the safety and efficacy of the monoclonal anti-tumor necrosis factor antibody-fragment, MAK 195F, in patients with sepsis and septic shock: A multicenter, randomized, placebo-controlled, dose-ranging study. Crit Care Med 24:733–742

9. Fisher CJ, Agosti JM, Opal SM, et al (1996) Treatment of patients with septic shock with tumor necrosis factor receptor Fc fusion protein. N Engl J Med 334:1697–1702

10. Evans TJ, Moyes D, Carpenter A, et al (1994) Protective effect of 55– but not 75–kD soluble tumor necrosis factor receptor-immunoglobulin G fusion proteins in an animal model of Gram-negative sepsis. J Exp Med 180:2173–2179

11. Moore KW, O'Garra A, de Waal Malefyt R, Vieira P, Mosmann TR (1993) Interleukin 10. Ann Rev Immunol 11:165–190

12. Howard M, Muchamuel T, Andrade S, Menon S (1993) Interleukin-10 protects mice from lethal endotoxemia. J Exp Med 177:1205–1208

13. Greenberger MJ, Strieter RM, Kunkel SL, Danforth JM, Goodman RE, Standiford TJ (1995) Neutralization of IL-10 increases survival in a murine model of Klebsiella pneumonia. J Immunol 155:722–729

14. Abraham E (1996) Alterations in transcriptional regulation of proinflammatory and immunoregulatory cytokine expression by hemorrhage, injury, and critical illness. New Horizons 4:184–193

15. Baeuerle PA, Baltimore D (1996) NF-κB: Ten years after. Cell 87:13–20

16. Schreck R, Rieber P, Baeuerle PA (1991) Reactive oxygen intermediates as apparently widely used messengers in the activation of the NF-kappa B transcription factor and HIV 1. EMBO J 10:2247–2258

17. Shenkar R, Schwartz MD, Terada L, Repine J, McCord J, Abraham E (1996) Hemorrhage activates NF-κB in murine lung mononuclear cells *in vivo*: Role of xanthine oxidase-derived superoxide anion. Am J Physiol (Lung Cell Mol Physiol) 270:L729–L735

18. Satriano J, Schlondorff D (1994) Activation and attenuation of transcription factor NF-κB in mouse glomerular mesangial cells in response to tumor necrosis factor-α, immunoglobulin G, and adenosine 3′:5′-cyclic monophosphate. J Clin Invest 94:1629–1636

19. Blackwell TS, Blackwell TR, Holden EP, Christman BW, Christman JW (1996) *In vivo* antioxidant treatment suppresses nuclear factor-kB activation and neutrophilic lung inflammation. J Immunol 157:1630–1637

20. Schwartz MD, Moore EE, Moore FA, et al (1996) NF-κB is activated in alveolar macrophages from patients with acute respiratory distress syndrome. Crit Care Med 24:1285–1292

21. Nick JA, Avdi NJ, Gerwins P, Johnson GL, Worthen GS (1996) Activation of a p38 mitogen-activated protein kinase in human neutrophils by lipopolysaccharide. J Immunol 156:4867–4875

22. Raingeaud J, Gupta S, Rogers JS, et al (1995) Proinflammatory cytokines and environmental stress cause p38 mitogen-activated protein kinase activation by dual phosphorylation on tyrosine and threonine. J Biol Chem 270:7420–7426

23. Kolesnick R, Golde DW (1994) The sphingomyelin pathway in tumor necrosis factor and interleukin-1 signaling. Cell 77:325–328

24. Eierman DF, Yagami M, Erme SM, et al (1995) Endogenously opsonized particles divert prostanoid action from lethal to protective in models of experimental endotoxemia. Proc Natl Acad Sci USA 92:2815–2819

25. Abraham E, Park Y, Covington P, Conrad SA, Schwartz M (1996) Liposomal prostaglandin E1 (TLC C-53) in acute respiratory distress syndrome (ARDS): A placebo-controlled, randomized, double-blind, multicenter clinical trial. Crit Care Med 24:10–15

26. Law MM, Cryer HG, Abraham E (1994) Elevated levels of soluble ICAM-1 correlate with the development of multiple organ failure in severely injured trauma patients. J Trauma 37:100–109

27. Sakamaki F, Ishizaka A, Handa M, et al (1995) Soluble form of p-selectin in plasma is elevated in ALI. Am J Respir Crit Care Med 151:1821–1826

28. Kushimoto S, Okajima K, Uchiba M, Murakami K, Okabe H, Takatsuki K (1996) Pulmonary vascular injury induced by hemorrhagic shock is mediated by p-selectin in rats. Thrombosis Res 82:97–106

29. Mulligan MS, Paulson JC, De Frees S, Zheng ZL, Lowe JB, Ward PA (1993) Protective effects of oligosaccharides in P-selectin-dependent lung injury. Nature 364:149–151
30. Nagase T, Ohga E, Sudo E, et al (1996) Intercellular adhesion molecule-1 mediates acid aspiration-induced lung injury. Am J Respir Crit Care Med 154:504–510
31. Bernard GR, Dupont W, Edens T, et al (1994) Antioxidants in the acute respiratory distress syndrome (ARDS) Am J Respir Crit Care Med 149:A241 (Abst)

Subject Index

Springer-Verlag
and the Environment

We at Springer-Verlag firmly believe that an international science publisher has a special obligation to the environment, and our corporate policies consistently reflect this conviction.

We also expect our business partners – paper mills, printers, packaging manufacturers, etc. – to commit themselves to using environmentally friendly materials and production processes.

The paper in this book is made from low- or no-chlorine pulp and is acid free, in conformance with international standards for paper permanency.